A Clinical Guide to Tissue Diseases

A Clinical Guide to Tissue Diseases

Editor: Omar Hebert

hayle medical

New York

Hayle Medical,
750 Third Avenue, 9th Floor,
New York, NY 10017, USA

Visit us on the World Wide Web at:
www.haylemedical.com

ISBN 978-1-64647-594-0 (Hardback)

Cataloging-in-Publication Data

A clinical guide to tissue diseases / edited by Omar Hebert.
p. cm.
Includes bibliographical references and index.
ISBN 978-1-64647-594-0
1. Connective tissues--Diseases. 2. Connective tissues--Diseases--Treatment.
3. Connective tissues--Diseases--Diagnosis. 4. Tissues--Diseases. I. Hebert, Omar.
RC924 .C55 2023
616.77--dc23

Contents

Preface

Every book is a source of knowledge and this one is no exception. The idea that led to the conceptualization of this book was the fact that the world is advancing rapidly; which makes it crucial to document the progress in every field. I am aware that a lot of data is already available, yet, there is a lot more to learn. Hence, I accepted the responsibility of editing this book and contributing my knowledge to the community.

A tissue refers to a distinct material comprising of special cells, which work together in coordination to carry out a particular function. There are four types of tissues, namely, connective tissue, epithelial tissue, muscle tissue and nervous tissue. Connective tissue diseases are a set of medical conditions in which the connective tissues of the body are the primary target of pathology. There are several types of connective tissue diseases, such as systemic lupus erythematosus, marfan syndrome, granulomatosis with polyangiitis (GPA), and microscopic polyangiitis. The signs and symptoms of these diseases include weakness, fatigue and fever. Some of the major epithelial tissue diseases and conditions include celiac disease, asthma, human papilloma virus (HPV), vertigo, and certain types of cancer. Medications, vitamin supplements and physical therapy can be used to treat these diseases. This book aims to understand the clinical perspectives of tissue diseases. It presents researches and studies performed by experts across the globe. This book is a vital tool for all researching and studying these diseases.

While editing this book, I had multiple visions for it. Then I finally narrowed down to make every chapter a sole standing text explaining a particular topic, so that they can be used independently. However, the umbrella subject sinews them into a common theme. This makes the book a unique platform of knowledge.

I would like to give the major credit of this book to the experts from every corner of the world, who took the time to share their expertise with us. Also, I owe the completion of this book to the never-ending support of my family, who supported me throughout the project.

Editor

1

Interferons (*IFN-A/-B/-G*) Genetic Variants in Patients with Mixed Connective Tissue Disease (MCTD)

Agnieszka Paradowska-Gorycka [1,*], Anna Wajda [1], Barbara Stypinska [1], Ewa Walczuk [1], Marcela Walczyk [2], Anna Felis-Giemza [2], Aleksandra Poluch-Lewandowska [2] and Marzena Olesińska [2]

1 Department of Molecular Biology, National Institute of Geriatrics, Rheumatology and Rehabilitation, Warsaw 02-637, Poland; annawajda2046@gmail.com (A.W.); barbara.stypinska@wp.pl (B.S.); ewa.walczuk@spartanska.pl (E.W.)

2 Department of Connective Tissue Diseases, National Institute of Geriatrics, Rheumatology and Rehabilitation, Warsaw 02-637, Poland; marcela.walczyk@gmail.com (M.W.); annafelis@wp.pl (A.F.-G.); poluchola@gmail.com (A.P.-L.); marzena.olesinska@vp.pl (M.O.)

* Correspondence: paradowska_aga@interia.pl

Abstract: Mixed connective tissue disease (MCTD) is a rare complex autoimmune disease in which autoantigens are recognized by endosomal TLRs. Their activation induces a higher secretion of the type I interferons, IFN-γ and the up-regulation of the INF-inducible genes. The present study aimed to investigate whether SNPs that are located in the IFN-A, IFN-B, and IFN-G genes are associated with MCTD. 145 MCTD patients and 281 healthy subjects were examined for IFN-A, IFN-B, and IFN-G genetic variants by TaqMan SNP genotyping assay. ELISA determined IFN-α/-β/-γ serum levels. Among the seven tested SNPs, four polymorphisms: IFN-A rs10757212, IFN-A rs3758236, IFN-G rs2069705, IFN-G rs2069718, as well as INF-G rs1861493A/rs2069705A/rs2069718G haplotype were significantly associated with a predisposition for MCTD. Raynaud's phenomenon, erosive arthritis, swollen hands and fingers, and sclerodactyly were significantly more frequently observed in MCTD patients with IFN-G rs2069718 G allele than in patients with IFN-G rs2069718 A allele. We also found that anti-U1-A autoantibodies most frequently occurred in MCTD patients with rs2069718 GA genotype, while the IFN-G rs2069705 AG and rs2069718 GA genotypes might be a marker of anti-Ro60 presence in MCTD patients. Our results indicate that IFN-G genetic variants may be potential genetic biomarkers for MCTD susceptibility and severity.

Keywords: MCTD; genetics; IFN; pathogenesis

---

1. Introduction

Autoimmune, systemic connective tissue diseases affect a small percentage of the general population. However, those diseases are chronic, they begin at a relatively young age and lead to progressive disability, which is an important social and medical problem. Mixed connective tissue disease (MCTD) is one of the least frequent among these disorders. The prevalence of MCTD is still uncertain, but it has been estimated at 10/100,000 in the Caucasian population. Sharp et al. first described MCTD in 1972 [1] as a new entity distinct from other connective tissue diseases (CTDs) [2]. In MCTD, like other systemic CTDs, complex interactions between disease-related phenomena, including chronic inflammation, dyslipidemia, thrombotic events, proliferative vascular arteriopathy, production of autoreactive autoantibodies, and humoral autoimmune processes, can be observed [3]. The presence of high-titer of anti-U1-snRNP antibodies (autoantibodies against the U1-small nuclear ribonucleoprotein antigen) in serum is an important hallmark of MCTD, which is a part of the diagnostic criteria for

MCTD [3–6]. Moreover, U1-RNP, which is a complex of U1-snRNA (small nuclear RNA) and small nuclear RNP, are the putative target of autoimmunity in the pathogenesis of MCTD. The U1-RNA molecule and the specific protein, U1 small nuclear ribonucleoprotein 70 kDa (snRNP70 or U1-70K), are both involved in the formation of network interactions between immune cells and their receptors, leading to autoimmunity, inflammation, and consequently to tissue damage [7–12]. The U1-snRNP immune complex, which contains its own RNA molecule, might induce an immune response through the involvement of specific autoreactive endosomal Toll-like receptors (TLRs) [7]. MCTD-associated autoantigens are recognized by endosomal TLRs, where activation induces a higher secretion of the type I interferons (IFN I), IFN-γ, up-regulation of the IFN-inducible genes (called IFN signature), as well as higher production of the specific autoantibodies [7,10,13,14]. The type I interferons, such as IFN-α and IFN-β, as well as IFN-γ (which is the only one type II class of interferons), are a family of pleiotropic cytokines with a wide spectrum of effects on adaptive and innate immune processes [15–17]. They have a key role in the initiation and progression of autoimmune disease by the promotion of the prolonged survival of activated T lymphocytes, differentiation of the T helper 17 cells (Th17), higher expression of the proinflammatory cytokines and chemokines, as well as by the increase the production of B lymphocyte stimulator and stimulation of B cells proliferation [15,18,19]. Although the detailed etiopathogenesis of systemic CTDs is not established, the growing volume of published studies has confirmed that excessive immunological activation with TLRs and IFNs is very important/one of the crucial pathogenic mechanisms of these diseases [20–23]. Moreover, the studies also highlighted that the overexpression of IFN-inducible genes (IFN signature) is a marker for patients with active and severe CTD [24].

Given the causative role of the type I and II interferons in human autoimmune diseases, including their role in the initiation of the disease processes and in the molecular pathogenesis of connective tissue diseases [14,25,26], we decided to explore whether single nucleotide polymorphisms (SNPs) that are located in the *IFN-A* (encodes IFN-α), *IFN-B* (encodes IFN-β), and *IFN-G* (encodes IFN-γ) genes may also be associated with MCTD while using a case-control study.

2. Materials and Methods

2.1. Subjects

A total of 145 MCTD patients and 281 healthy participants were included in the present study. Healthy participants were recruited from the Regional Center for Blood Donation and Blood Treatment in Warsaw, and they did not have a history of autoimmune and/or inflammatory disease at the time of sampling. All of the MCTD patients were recruited at the Department of Connective Tissue Diseases of the National Institute of Geriatrics, Rheumatology, and Rehabilitation. MCTD patients, as well as healthy subjects, were of Caucasian origin. The MCTD patients met Alarcon-Segovia and Villarreal classification criteria, which were chosen due to their very high specificity for MCTD. Patients with MCTD, who met the classification criteria for two connective tissue diseases at the same time, were excluded from the study. A set of objective and subjective methods to assess the damage in MCTD, as well as disease activity, were developed specifically for the purpose of this study since guidelines to evaluate the disease status of MCTD patients have not been yet established. The activity index, developed at our Institute and based on the Systemic Lupus Erythematosus Disease Activity Index (SLEDAI) for SLE activity assessment, was used to evaluate the clinical activity of MCTD. Applied MCTD activity scale includes the assessment of clinical and laboratory symptoms that indicate active disease. The assigned number of points was calculated for each symptom indicating the activity of the disease, which was found in the last 28 days. The activity index (AI) for a given patient was the sum of all points, with a maximum of 52. In the Mixed Connective Tissue Disease–Activity Index (MCTD-AI), the most important organ symptoms (such as lung involvement, pulmonary hypertension, and vasculitis) that are not present in lupus are taken into account (Table S1 in Supplementary Files). The use of the MCTD-AI scale enables the estimated stratification of patients. Similarly, based on the

Systemic Lupus International Collaborating Clinics/American College of Rheumatology (SLICC/ACR) damage index (DI), which assesses damage in SLE, we have developed an MCTD damage scale consisting of clinical symptoms caused by a permanent result of the disease, its treatment or related diseases—Mixed Connective Tissue Disease—Damage Index (MCTD-DI) (Table S2 in Supplementary Files). For every symptom of damage that has occurred during MCTD and has lasted for at least six months, one point was scored, if the episode recurred—two points. The damage index for a given MCTD patient was the sum of all points. SLICC/ACR scale. The identification of antinuclear antibodies (ANA) was performed by indirect immunofluorescence (IF) on the Hep2 cell lines (Euroimmun Polska, Wroclaw, Poland). Autoantibodies to Sm, Ro, La, RibP, PCNA, CENPB, Scl-70, Jo-1, His, dsDNA were measured in sera while using DOT-blot tests (recomLine ANA/ENA, Mikrogen Diagnostik, Neuried, Germany). The presence of anti-U1-RNP was determined by electrochemiluminescence (ECLIA) using streptavidin-coated paramagnetic beads (UNICAP100, Phadia, Sweden). The Research Ethics Committee of the National Institute of Geriatrics, Rheumatology, and Rehabilitation in Warsaw approved the presented clinical investigation (of 14 January 2016). All participants, patients, and healthy donors gave informed written consent and research was conducted in accordance with the Declaration of Helsinki.

2.2. Genomic DNA Extraction

Genomic DNA was extracted from 200 μL of whole blood samples from MCTD patients and healthy subjects while using the QIAamp DNA Blood Mini Kit (Qiagen, Hilden, Germany) in accordance with the manufacturer's instructions. All of the extracted DNA samples were standardized to give a final concentration of 1.8 ng/uL and stored at −80 °C until the next analyses.

2.3. SNP Selection and Genotyping

The IFNs polymorphisms were selected based on SNPs position in the gene, possible functional effect, or association with other autoimmune diseases. The SNPs with a minor allele frequency (MAF) <0.05 (<5%) were excluded. The DNA samples were genotyped for SNPs of *IFN-A* rs10757212 and rs3758236, *IFN-B* rs7873167, and rs10964831, and *IFN-G* rs1861493, rs2069705, and rs2069718 using TaqMan allelic discrimination assay (used assay ID: C__11843895_10, C__27475238_10, C__29146577_10, C__31290012_10, C___2683476_10, C__15944115_20, C__15799728_10, respectively, Applied Biosystems, Foster City, CA, USA). The TaqMan SNP genotyping assays were performed by a QuantStudio 5 detection system (Life Technologies, Carlsbad, CA, USA), which were carried out in 384-well plates in a 7.5 μL reaction volume containing 1.8 ng genomic DNA, 0.35 μL assay mix (20×) and 3.75 μL Taqman universal PCR master mix (2×). The reaction was performed with the following amplification protocol: denaturation at 95 °C for 10 min., followed by 40 cycles of denaturation at 92 °C for 15 s, and annealing and extension at 60 °C for 1 min.

2.4. Quantitative Analysis of IFNs

The concentrations of IFN-α/-β/-γ in serum of MCTD and healthy subjects were measured by colorimetric sandwich enzyme-linked immunosorbent assay (ELISA) (SunRed Biological Technology, Shanghai, China). The ELISA test was performed in accordance with the manufacturers' instructions. For analysis we used 40 μL of serum. The ELISA standard ranges were 6–2000 pg/mL for IFN-α, 8–2000 ng/L for IFN-β, and 2–600 ng/L for IFN-γ.

2.5. Statistical Analysis

All data were presented as a median (interquartile range, IQR) for non-normally distributed continuous variables or as mean ± SD for normally distributed continuous variables. The accordance of genotype distribution with Hardy–Weinberg Equilibrium (HWE) was performed while using the HWE exact test with "genetics" R package (Gregory Warnes, with contributions from Gregor Gorjanc, Friedrich Leisch and Michael Man. (2019); genetics: Population Genetics. R package version

1.3.8.1.1. https://CRAN.R-project.org/package). Logistic regression was used to evaluate genotype and allele distribution between groups (OR, 95% confidence intervals, p-value); the results were adjusted by age and gender accordingly. The analysis was calculated under dominant, codominant, overdominant and recessive, and allelic models. The presence of linkage disequilibrium (LD), as well as a coefficient (D′ and r2) for haplotypes, was carried out while using the SHEsis software, available at http://analysis.bio-x.cn. Differences between tested SNPs, disease activity parameters and cytokines serum concentrations were analyzed while using the Kruskal–Wallis Test, Mann–Whitney test, or analysis of variance for continuous variables and χ^2 or Fisher exact test for categorical variables. A p-value < 0.05 indicated a statistically significant result.

3. Results

3.1. MCTD Patients Clinical Characteristics and Autoantibodies Profile

A set of objective and subjective methods to assess the damage in MCTD as well as disease activity were developed specifically for the purpose of this study since guidelines to evaluate the disease status of MCTD patients have not been yet established.

The median value of MCTD-AI was 9.4 points (lowest—0, highest—32 points). In 40% of our MCTD patients, MCTD-DI was at or below six points and these patients had symptoms of organ involvement.

Median value of MCTD -DI was 5 (lowest value—0, highest—12). Damage most commonly affected skin, musculoskeletal and cardiovascular systems, and lungs. Table 1 summarizes the clinical characteristics of MCTD patients. The clinical picture of MCTD was variable. Some symptoms, such as skin lesions typical for SLE, swelling of the hands, arthropathy, inflammation, and involvement of the muscle, were mostly occurring early in the course of the disease. The major clinical features of MCTD patients were Raynaud's phenomenon (96.7%), hands edema (91.9%), polyarthritis (93.94%), leuco/thrombocytopenia (64.65%), and myopathy (66.67%). 97% of our MCTD patients presented with Raynaud's phenomenon right at the onset of the disease. ANA in titer >1:320 was detected in 88% of MCTD patients. All of the MCTD patients had anti-U1-RNP antibodies: anti-70K was detected in 76% of patients, anti-A in 84% of patients, and anti-C in 79% of patients (Table 2).

Table 1. Clinical and biochemical characteristics of the study group.

Parameter		MCTD Patients	
		N	*n* (%)
sex	men	99	15 (15.15%)
	women		84 (84.85%)
Damage index (median range (min–max)) MCTD-DI		83	5 (0–12)
Activity index (median range (min–max)) MCTD-AI		83	9.4 (0–32)
Disease duration (months; median range (min–max))		99	96.0 (10-420)
course of disease: single-phase		99	12 (12.12%)
course of disease: multiphase			28 (28.28%)
course of disease: chronic progressive			59 (59.6%)
Raynaud's phenomenon		99	96 (96.97%)
Sjogren's syndrome		99	22 (22.2%)
Hands edema		99	91 (91.92%)
deformative and/or erosive arthritis		99	13 (13.13%)
Poikiloderma		99	30 (30.3%)
Polyarthritis		99	93 (93.94%)
swollen hand and fingers		99	89 (89.8%)
Lymphadenopathy		99	26 (26.26%)
facial erythema		99	42 (42.42%)
pericarditis/pleuritis		99	16 (16.16%)
Leuco/thrombocytopenia		99	64 (64.65%)
Sclerodactyly		99	34 (34.34%)

Table 1. *Cont.*

Parameter	MCTD Patients	
	N	*n* (%)
pulmonary fibrosis	99	30 (30.3%)
Pulmonary arterial hypertension (PAH)	99	12 (12.12)
esophageal involvement/dysphagia	99	22 (22.22%)/21 (21.21%)
Myopathy	99	66 (66.67%)
Cardiomyopathy or ventricular dysfunction documented by echocardiography (chamber?)	99	4 (4.04%)
Therapeutic profiles:		
Azathioprine		6 (6%)
Methotrexate		23 (23%)
Prednisone		76 (77%)
Chloroquine		58 (59%)

N—number of patients with clinical information; *n*—number of patients with positive clinical manifestation.

Table 2. Autoantibody profile in the mixed connective tissue disease (MCTD) group.

Autoantibody Target	MCTD Patients	
	N	*n* (%)
RF	97	36 (37%)
anti-CCP	70	3 (4%)
anti-U1-RNP	99	99 (100%)
anti-70K	99	75 (76%)
anti-A	99	83 (84%)
anti-C	98	78 (79%)
anti-SmB	97	29 (30%)
anti-SmD	99	6 (6%)
anti-Ro60	99	10 (10%)
anti-Ro52	99	24 (24%)
anti-La	99	2 (2%)
anti-RibP	99	3 (3%)
anti-PCNA	99	1 (1%)
anti-CENP B	99	0
anti-Scl-70	99	2 (2%)
anti-Jo-1	99	1 (1%)
anti-His	98	13 (13%)
anti-dsDNA	99	13 (13%)

N—number of patients with clinical information; *n*—number of patients with positive clinical manifestation;.RF—rheumatoid factor; anti-CCP—anti-cyclic citrullinated peptide autoantibodies, aCCP; anti-RibP—anti-protein ribosomal P; anti-PCNA—antibodies directed against proliferating cell nuclear antigen; anti-CENP B—anti-Centromere Protein B; anti-Scl-70 - anti-topoisomerase I; anti-Jo-1—antihistidyl transfer RNA [t-RNA] synthetase; anti-dsDNA—anti-double stranded DNA.

3.2. Association of IFN-A, IFN-B and IFN-G Genetic Variants with Risk of MCTD

In the first step, we determined whether *IFN-A*, *IFN-B*, and *IFN-G* gene variants were associated with MCTD severity.

Among seven examined SNPs, the distributions of six SNPs genotypes (rs10757212, rs3758236, rs7873167, rs10964831, rs1861493, and rs2069705) were consistent with the Hardy–Weinberg equilibrium (HWE) in both MCTD patients and healthy subjects (Table S3 in Supplementary Files). The *IFN-G* rs2069718 genotype distribution was in HWE in controls, but it showed deviation from HWE in MCTD patients ($p = 0.02$, Table S3 in Supplementary Files). However, the genotyping was randomly repeated on 20% selected samples (10% for MCTD group and 10% for control groups), giving complete conformity of the result.

Next, we compared the minor allele frequencies (MAF) between our study groups and another European ancestry (EUR) while using 1000 genome bases. The MAF was found to be the lowest for *IFNA* rs3758236 A allele in MCTD patients (A: 0.11) and for *IFN-B* rs7873167 G allele in MCTD patients and controls (G: 0.11); while the highest was for *IFN-G* rs2069705 G allele in the controls (G: 0.52) (Table S3 in Supplementary Files). Generally, the MAF of all examined genetic variants in our cohorts were similar to those in the European ancestry.

In Table 3 we have shown genotype distribution and allele frequencies for seven genotyped SNPs in MCTD patients and healthy subjects. Four different genetic models: codominant, dominant, recessive, and overdominant, were tested to explore the relation of INFs genetic variants with MCTD risk. Among the seven tested SNPs, four polymorphisms (*IFN-A* rs10757212, *IFN-A* rs3758236, *IFN-G* rs2069705, *IFN-G* rs2069718) were significantly associated with a predisposition for MCTD. For *IFN-A* rs10757212 and *IFN-G* rs2069705, the recessive model revealed significant differences between the MCTD patients and healthy subjects. We observed that the *IFN-A* rs10757212 GG + GA genotype and *IFN-G* rs2069705 AA + AG genotype was significantly higher in MCTD patients when compared to controls ($p = 0.01$ and $p = 0.03$, respectively). For *IFN-A* rs3758236 the codominant, dominant, and recessive models yielded significant differences between MCTD patients and controls. The *IFN-A* rs3758236 TT genotype under the codominant and dominant models and *IFN-A* rs3758236 TT + TA genotype under the recessive model were more frequently observed in MCTD patients than in the controls ($p = 0.03$, $p = 0.04$ and $p = 0.02$, respectively). The *IFN-A* rs3758236 A allele were also more frequently observed in MCTD patients than in healthy subjects (89% vs 82%, $p = 0.04$). For *IFN-G* rs2069718 GG genotype under the codominant model and rs2069718 GG + GA genotype under the recessive models have shown an association with MCTD risk ($p = 0.02$ and $p = 0.008$, respectively). The frequencies of the G allele of the *IFN-G* rs2069718 also significantly differed between MCTD patients and healthy subjects (60% vs 48%, $p = 0.008$). With respect to *IFN-B* rs7873167, IFN-B rs10964831, and *IFN-G* rs1861493, there were no differences in the genotype distribution and allele frequencies between MCTD patients and healthy subjects ($p > 0.05$, Table 3).

Table 3. Genotype distribution and allele frequencies of the interferons (IFNs) polymorphisms in MCTD patients and healthy subjects (adjusted by sex and age).

Genetic Model	Genotype	MCTD *n* (%)	Control *n* (%)	OR	*p*-Value
		***IFN-A* rs10757212**			
Codominant	GG	65 (67%)	173 (64%)	1	**0.05**
	GA	31 (32%)	79 (29%)	1.02 (0.6–1.75)	
	AA	1 (1%)	19 (7%)	0.15 (0.02–1.15)	
Dominant	GG	65 (67%)	173 (63.8%)	1	0.5
	GA + AA	32 (33%)	98 (36.2%)	0.86 (0.51–1.45)	
Recessive	GG + GA	96 (99%)	252 (93%)	1	**0.01**
	AA	1 (1%)	19 (7%)	0.14 (0.02–1.13)	
Overdominant	GG + AA	66 (68%)	192 (71%)	1	0.6
	GA	31 (32%)	79 (29%)	1.11 (0.66–1.9)	
Allele	G	161 (83%)	425 (78%)	1	
	A	33 (17%)	117 (22%)	0.74 (0.46–1.14)	0.2
		***IFN-A* rs3758236**			
Codominant	TT	74 (79%)	192 (68%)	1	**0.03**
	TA	19 (20%)	78 (28%)	0.66 (0.36–1.2)	
	AA	1 (1%)	11(4%)	0.14 (0.02–1.12)	
Dominant	TT	74 (79%)	192 (68%)	1	**0.04**
	TA + AA	20 (21%)	89 (32%)	0.56 (0.31–1.01)	
Recessive	TT + TA	93 (99%)	270 (96%)	1	**0.02**
	AA	1(1%)	11 (4%)	0.15 (0.02–1.24)	
Overdominant	TT + AA	75 (80%)	203 (72%)	1	0.2
	TA	19 (20%)	78 (28%)	0.71 (0.39–1.29)	
Allele	T	167 (89%)	462 (82%)	1	
	A	21 (11%)	100 (18%)	0.58 (0.35–0.96)	**0.04**

Table 3. *Cont.*

Genetic Model	Genotype	MCTD *n* (%)	Control *n* (%)	OR	*p*-Value
		***IFN-B* rs7873167**			
Codominant	TT	77 (79%)	221 (80%)	1	0.7
	TG	18 (19%)	53 (19%)	1.06 (0.57–1.98)	
	GG	2 (2%)	3 (1%)	2.18 (0.32–14.86)	
Dominant	TT	77 (79%)	221 (80%)	1	0.7
	TG + GG	20 (21%)	56 (20%)	1.12 (0.61–2.05)	
Recessive	TT + TG	95 (98)	274 (99%)	1	0.4
	GG	2 (2%)	3 (1%)	2.16 (0.32–14.63)	
Overdominant	TT + GG	79 (81%)	224 (81%)	1	0.8
	TG	18 (19%)	53 (19%)	1.05 (0.56–1.95)	
Allele	T	172 (89%)	495 (89%)	1	
	G	22 (11%)	59 (11%)	1.07 (0.64–1.80)	0.7
		***IFN-B* rs10964831**			
Codominant	AA	66 (70%)	163 (73%)	1	0.6
	AT	26 (28%)	59 (26%)	1.15 (0.64–2.05)	
	TT	2 (2%)	3 (1%)	2.45 (0.35–17.21)	
Dominant	AA	66 (70%)	163 (73%)	1	0.5
	AT + TT	28 (30%)	62 (27%)	1.2 (0.68–2.12)	
Recessive	AA + AT	92 (98%)	222 (99%)	1	0.3
	TT	2 (2%)	3 (1%)	2.39 (0.34–16.66)	
Overdominant	AA + TT	68 (72%)	166 (74%)	1	0.6
	AT	26 (28%)	59 (26%)	1.13 (0.63–2.02)	
Allele	A	158 (84%)	385 (85%)	1	
	T	30 (16%)	65 (15%)	1.12 (0.70–1.80)	0.6
		***IFN-G* rs1861493**			
Codominant	AA	38 (48%)	33 (55%)	1	0.5
	AG	34 (42%)	21 (35%)	1.56 (0.69–3.53)	
	GG	8 (10%)	6 (10%)	1.03 (0.27–3.98)	
Dominant	AA	38 (48%)	33 (55%)	1	0.3
	AG + GG	42 (52%)	27 (45%)	1.44 (0.66–3.11)	
Recessive	AA + AG	72 (90%)	54 (90%)	1	0.8
	GG	8 (10%)	6 (10%)	0.84 (0.23–3.11)	
Overdominant	AA + GG	46 (58%)	39 (65%)	1	0.2
	AG	34 (42%)	21 (35%)	1.55 (0.7–3.41)	
Allele	A	110 (69%)	87 (73%)	1	
	G	50 (31%)	33 (27%)	1.20 (0.71–2.02)	0.5
		***IFN-G* rs2069705**			
Codominant	AA	36 (38%)	68 (32%)	1	0.09
	AG	49 (52%)	99 (47%)	0.86 (0.49–1.51)	
	GG	10 (10%)	45 (21%)	0.41 (0.18–0.95)	
Dominant	AA	36 (38%)	68 (32%)	1	0.2
	AG + GG	59 (62%)	144 (68%)	0.73 (0.42–1.25)	
Recessive	AA + AG	85 (90%)	167 (79%)	1	**0.03**
	GG	10 (10%)	45 (21%)	0.45 (0.21–0.98)	
Overdominant	AA + GG	46 (48%)	113 (53%)	1	0.6
	AG	49 (52%)	99 (47%)	1.12 (0.67–1.88)	
Allele	A	121 (64%)	235 (55%)	1	
	G	69 (36%)	189 (45%)	0.71 (0.50–1.01)	0.06
		***IFN-G* rs2069718**			
Codominant	GG	31 (32%)	35 (23%)	1	**0.02**
	GA	55 (57%)	77 (50%)	0.83 (0.43–1.59)	
	AA	11 (11%)	41 (27%)	0.32 (0.13–0.79)	
Dominant	GG	31 (32%)	35 (23%)	1	0.1
	GA + AA	66 (68%)	118 (77%)	0.66 (0.35–1.23)	
Recessive	GG + GA	86 (89%)	112 (73%)	1	**0.008**
	AA	11 (11%)	41 (27%)	0.36 (0.16–0.8)	

Table 3. *Cont.*

Genetic Model	Genotype	MCTD *n* (%)	Control *n* (%)	OR	*p*-Value
Overdominant	GG + AA	42 (43%)	76 (50%)	1	0.3
	GA	55 (57%)	77 (50%)	1.28 (0.73–2.25)	
Allele	G	117 (60%)	147 (48%)	1	
	A	77 (40%)	159 (52%)	0.61 (0.42–0.88)	**0.008**

$p \leq 0.05$ was considered as significant, all significant *p*-value was bolded.

3.3. Genetic Association of IFNs Haplotypes with MCTD

The SHEsis program has been used. The analysis revealed a quite strong LD between *IFN-G* rs2069705 and rs2067918 with D′ = 0.77 and $r^2 = 0.5$. In other examined genetic variants, we observed a weak LD, as the r^2 value between all of them is considerably low ($r^2 < 0.3$).

The following sequence: *IFN-A* rs10757212 G/A, *IFN-A* rs3758236 T/A, *IFN-B* rs7873167 T/G, IFN-B rs10964831 A/T were used to create the haplotypes because the *INF-A* and *INF-B* genes are located on the same chromosome 9. Sixteen potential haplotypes were formed in both MCTD patients and healthy subjects; however, the haplotypes with frequency of <0.03 are ignored (Table 4). The most frequent haplotype observed in both studied groups was GTTA (59% of MCTD patients and 50% of HC, $p = 0.07$). Other haplotypes occur with moderate frequency. The frequency of ATTA and GATA haplotypes was significantly higher in healthy subjects than in MCTD patients ($p = 0.03$ and $p = 0.01$, respectively), thus conferring disease protection nature to these haplotypes.

Table 4. Haplotype analysis results among two single nucleotide polymorphisms (SNPs) in IFN-A locus, two SNPs in IFN-B locus and three SNPs in INF-G locus.

Haplotype IFN-A rs10757212 G/A, IFN-A rs3758236 T/A, IFN-B rs7873167 T/G, IFN-B rs10964831 A/T	**Frequency**	**MCTD Patients**	**Controls**	***p*-Value**
GTTA	0.53	0.59	0.50	0.07
GTTT	0.11	0.13	0.10	0.2
AATA	0.06	0.08	0.05	0.5
GTGA	0.06	0.06	0.06	0.7
ATTA	0.10	0.05	0.12	**0.03**
GATA	0.07	0.02	0.08	**0.01**
Haplotype IFN-G rs1861493 A/G, rs2069705 A/G, rs2069718 G/A	**Frequency**	**MCTD Patients**	**Controls**	***p*-Value**
AAG	0.46	0.58	0.36	**<0.0001**
GAG	0.04	0.05	0.03	0.1
AGA	0.1	0.1	0.09	0.4
GGA	0.25	0.23	0.25	0.3
AAA	0.08	0.03	0.14	**0.0003**
AGG	0.05	0.004	0.1	**<0.0001**

p values in bold face are considered as significant.

For *INF-G*, gene haplotypes were separately created because this gene is located on chromosome 12. To create the haplotypes, *INF-G* polymorphisms were tested in the following sequence: rs1861493 A/G, rs2069705 A/G, and rs2069718 G/A. We observed that eight potential haplotypes were created; however, the haplotypes with frequency of <0.03 were ignored (Table 4). The most common haplotype was AAG, which was observed in 58% of MCTD patients and in 36% of healthy subjects. This AAG haplotype was also significantly associated with the risk for MCTD ($p < 0.0001$). In contrast, the AAA and AGG haplotypes, which were the minor haplotypes in MCTD patients, were significantly associated with a lower risk of MCTD (AAA: 3% in MCTD vs 13% in HC, $p = 0.0003$; AGG: 0.4% in MCTD vs 10% in HC, $p < 0.0001$; Table 4).

3.4. Correlation of the IFNs Genetic Variants with Clinical Variables in Patients with MCTD

Hence, it could conceivably be hypothesized that all three interferons, *IFN-A*, *IFN-B*, and *IFN-G*, may be good candidate genes to play a part in MCTD autoimmune process, we analyzed whether examined IFNs genetic variants may have an impact on MCTD phenotype. We tested the genotype frequencies of IFNs polymorphisms, in different genetic models (codominant (Table 5), dominant (Table 6) and recessive (Table 7)). Tables 5–7 only present significant association or association with tendency. Pulmonary fibrosis and poikiloderma were more frequently observed in MCTD patients with *IFN-A* rs3758236 TT genotype than in MCTD patients with *IFN-A* rs3758236 TA or AA genotype (Table 5, $p = 0.03$ and $p = 0.04$, respectively). Rheumatoid factor was more frequent in MCTD patients with *IFN-B* rs7873167 TT genotype when comparing to MCTC patients with other genotypes ($p = 0.01$). The MCTD patients with *IFN-B* rs10964831 TT genotype were characterized by significantly higher damage index than other MCTD patients (TT: 33.5 ± 31.5, AT: 12.577 ± 3.145, AA: 7.879 ± 1.364, $p = 0.01$). In MCTD patients with *IFN-G* rs1861493 AG genotype, we observed more frequent occurrence of rheumatoid factors (Table 5, $p = 0.03$) as well as a tendency towards the more frequent occurrence of lymphadenopathy (Table 5, $p = 0.06$) and enlargement of lymph nodes (Table 5, $p = 0.06$) when compared to MCTD patients with *IFN-G* rs1861493 AA or GG genotypes (Table 5). Moreover, in the carriers of the polymorphic *IFN-G* rs1861493 G allele Sjogren's syndrome and poikiloderma were present considerably more frequently than in patients with two wild-type alleles (Table 6, $p = 0.02$ and $p = 0.03$, respectively). The swollen hands and fingers were more frequently observed in MCTD patients with *IFN-G* rs2069705 A allele than in the carriers of *IFN-G* rs2069705 GG genotype (Table 7, $p = 0.03$). In the carriers of *IFN-G* rs2069705 A allele, we also observed a tendency to the more frequent presence of sclerodactyly (Table 7, $p = 0.07$). In contrast, in the carriers of *IFN-G* rs2069705 G allele, we observed a tendency for the presence of pericarditis and poikiloderma to appear more frequently (Table 6, $p = 0.07$ and $p = 0.06$, respectively). Additionally, Raynaud's Phenomenon and erosive arthritis were more often present in the MCTD patients with *IFN-G* rs2069718 GA genotype than in the MCTD patients with other genotypes. Moreover, the erosive arthritis was not present in MCTD patients with *IFN-G* rs2069718 AA genotype (Table 5). Furthermore, swollen hands and fingers, as well as sclerodactyly, were more frequently observed in MCTD patients with *IFN-G* rs2069718 G allele than in MCTD patients with IFN-G rs2069718 A allele (Table 7, both $p = 0.04$).

Table 5. Correlation between *IFN-A, IFN-B, IFN-G* genotypes (codominant model), and clinical pathology parameters in MCTD.

Parameter/Genotype	MCTD *n* (%)	OR, 95%CI	*p*-Value
	IFN-A rs3758236		
pulmonary fibrosis			
TT	24 (88.9%)	1	**0.03**
TA	2 (7.4%)	0.25 (0.05–1.15)	
AA	1 (3.7%)		
poikilodermy			
TT	19 (65.5%)	1	**0.04**
TA	10 (34.5%)	3.22 (1.14–9.11)	
AA	0 (0%)	0	
	IFN-B rs7873167		
RF presence			
TT	24 (68.6%)	1	**0.01**
TG	11 (31.4%)	3.97 (1.31–12.01)	
GG	0 (0%)	0	
lymphadenopathy			
TT	18 (69.2%)	1	0.06
TG	6 (23.1%)	1.64(0.54–4.99)	
GG	2 (7.7%)		

Table 5. *Cont.*

Parameter/Genotype	MCTD *n* (%)	OR, 95%CI	*p*-Value
	IFN-G rs1861493		
RF presence			
AA	9 (31%)	1	**0.03**
AG	18 (62.1%)	3.62 (1.33–9.92)	
GG	2 (6.9%)	1.29(0.21–7.82)	
Sjogren's Syndrome			
AA	3 (20%)	1	0.06
AG	9 (60%)	4.29(0.98–18.72)	
GG	3 (20%)	6.67(0.89–49.67)	
lymphadenopathy			
AA	6 (30%)	1	0.06
AG	13 (65%)	3.3(108–10.05)	
GG	1 (5%)	0.76 (0.08–7.37)	
poikilodermy			
AA	7 (29.2%)	1	0.09
AG	14 (58.3%)	3.1(1.07–9.01)	
GG	3 (12.5%)	2.66(0.51–13.83)	
lymphadenopathy			
AA	6 (30%)	1	0.06
AG	13 (65%)	3.3 (1.08–10.05)	
GG	1 (5%)	0.76 (0.08–7.37)	
	IFN-G rs2069705		
swollen hands and finger			
AA	34 (39.1%)	1	0.09
AG	46 (52.9%)	0.9 (0.14–5.7)	
GG	7 (8%)	0.14 (0.02–0.98)	
sclerodactyly			
AA	10 (32.3%)	1	0.09
AG	20 (64.5%)	1.79 (0.71–4.52)	
GG	1 (3.2%)	0.29 (0.03–2.58)	
	IFN-G rs2069718		
Raynaud phenomenon			
GG	31 (33%)	1	**0.03**
GA	54 (57.4%)	0	
AA	9 (9.6%)	0	
erosive arthritis			
GG	1 (7.7%)	1	**0.02**
GA	12 (92.3%)	8.37 (1.03–67.86)	
AA	0 (0%)	0	

p values in bold face are considered as significant.

Table 6. Correlation between *IFN-A, IFN-B, IFN-G* genotypes (dominant model), and clinical pathology parameters in MCTD.

	IFN-A rs3758236		
poikilodermy			
TT	19 (65.6%)	1	**0.04**
TA + AA	10 (34.5%)	2.89 (1.04–8.03)	
	IFN-G rs1861493		
Sjogren's syndrome			

Table 6. *Cont.*

AA	3 (20%)	1	**0.02**
AG + GG	12 (80%)	4.71 (1.14–19.48)	
poikilodermy			
AA	7 (29.2%)	1	**0.03**
AG + GG	17 (70.8%)	3.01 (1.08–8.4)	
	IFN-G rs2069705		
pericarditis			
AA	3 (18.8%)	1	0.07
AG + GG	13 (81.2%)	3.11 (0.82+11.79)	
poikilodermy			
AA	7 (24.1%)	1	0.06
AG + GG	22 (75.9%)	2.46 (0.92–6.56)	

p values in bold face are considered as significant.

Table 7. Correlation between *IFN-A, IFN-B, IFN-G* genotypes (recessive model) and clinical pathology parameters in MCTD.

	IFN-G rs2069705		
swollen hands and fingers			
AA + AG	89 (92%)	1	**0.03**
GG	7 (8%)	0.15 (0.03 + 0.74)	
Sclerodactyly			
AA + AG	30 (96.8%)	1	0.08
GG	1 (3.2%)	0.2 (0.02+1.69)	
	IFN-G rs2069718		
swollen hands and fingers			
GG + GA	81 (91%)	1	**0.04**
AA	8 (9%)	0.16 (0.03+0.82)	
Sclerodactyly			
GG + GA	31 (96.9%)	1	**0.04**
AA	1 (3.1%)	0.18 90.02+1.45)	

p values in bold face are considered as significant.

3.5. INFs Gene Polymorphisms Association with Serologic Profile of MCTD Patients

Analysis of the association between the *IFN-G* genetic variants and autoantibody profiles in patients with MCTD was the next stage of present research. The *IFN-A* and *IFN-B* gene polymorphisms, which were examined in this study, were excluded for this analysis because we have only 1 or 2 patients with polymorphic genotype. The frequencies of all examined *IFN-G* polymorphisms were compared between the MCTD patients with the presence of autoantibodies and MCTD patients without autoantibodies (Table 8a,b). The results showed an significant association between *IFN-G* rs1861493 A/G and RF ($p = 0.03$) and anti-DNA ($p = 0.01$) presence; between *IFN-G* rs2069705 A/G genetic variant and anti-U1-A ($p = 0.03$), anti-Ro60 ($p = 0.009$), and anti-DNA ($p = 0.02$) presence; as well as between IFN-G rs2069718 G/A and RF ($p = 0.08$), anti-U1-RNP (0.056), anti-Ro60 ($p = 0.02$), and anti-DNA ($p = 0.04$) presence. Anti-U1-A most frequently occurred in MCTD patients with rs2069705AG and rs2069718 GA genotype. In MCTD patients with the *IFN-G* rs1861493 AG genotype, the rheumatoid factor was present more often than in other genotypes ($p = 0.03$). In contrast, in MCTD patients with the *IFN-G* rs1861493 GG genotype, we did not observe anti-Ro60 antibodies. Similarly, in MCTD patients with the *IFN-G* rs2069705AA and *IFN-G* rs2069718 GG genotypes, we did not observe anti-CCP antibodies.

Table 8. IFNs genotypes in relation to antibody profiles in MCTD patients.

(a)

Genotype	Anti-U1-70K		Anti-U1-A		Anti-U1-C		Anti-SmB		Anti-SmD	
	(−)	(+)	(−)	(+)	(−)	(+)	(−)	(+)	(−)	(+)
INF-G rs1861493 A/G										
AA	12 (32%)	26 (68%)	7 (18%)	31 (82%)	8 (21%)	30 (79%)	27 (71%)	11 (29%)	36 (95%)	2 (5%)
AG	6 (18%)	28 (82%)	5 (15%)	29 (85%)	5 (15%)	29 (85%)	21 (62%)	13 (38%)	31 (91%)	3 (9%)
GG	1 (13%)	7 (87%)	3 (38%)	5 (62%)	2 (25%)	6 (75%)	6 (75%)	2 (25%)	7 (87%)	1 (13%)
***p*-value**	0.3		0.3		0.7		0.6		0.7	
INF-G rs2069705 A/G										
AA	9 (25%)	27 (75%)	8 (22%)	28 (78%)	5 (14%)	31 (86%)	23 (64%)	13 (36%)	34 (94%)	2 (6%)
AG	13 (27%)	36 (73%)	4 (8%)	45 (92%)	9 (18%)	40 (82%)	33 (67%)	15 (31%)	34 (94%)	2 (6%)
GG	3 (30%)	7 (70%)	4 (40%)	6 (60%)	4 (40%)	6 (60%)	8 (80%)	2 (20%)	9 (90%)	1 (10%)
***p*-value**	0.9		**0.03**		0.1		0.6		0.9	
IFN-G rs2069718 G/A										
GG	8 (26%)	23 (74%)	6 (19%)	25 (81%)	6 (19%)	25 (81%)	21 (68%)	10 (32%)	30 (97%)	1 (3%)
GA	12 (22%)	43 (78%)	5 (9%)	50 (91%)	10 (18%)	45 (82%)	37 (67%)	17 (31%)	52 (95%)	3 (5%)
AA	4 (36%)	7 (64%)	4 (36%)	7 (64%)	4 (36%)	7 (64%)	9 (82%)	2 (18%)	10 (91%)	1 (9%)
***p*-value**	0.6		**0.05**		0.4		0.6		0.7	

(b)

Genotype	RF		Anti-CCP		Anti-Ro60		Anti-Ro52		Anti-His		Anti-dsDNA	
	(−)	(+)	(−)	(+)	(−)	(+)	(−)	(+)	(−)	(+)	(−)	(+)
INF-G rs1861493 A/G												
AA	29 (76%)	9 (24%)	29 (100%)	0	36 (95%)	2 (5%)	31 (82%)	7 (18%)	34 (89%)	4 (11%)	34 (89%)	4 (11%)
AG	16 (47%)	18 (53%)	25 (89%)	3 (11%)	29 (85%)	5 (15%)	22 (65%)	12 (35%)	27 (79%)	7 (21%)	30 (88%)	4 (12%)
GG	5 (71%)	2 (29%)	3 (100%)	0	8 (100%)	0	6 (75%)	2 (25%)	7 (87%)	1 (13%)	4 (50%)	4 (50%)
***p*-value**	**0.03**		0.2		0.2		0.3		0.5		**0.01**	
INF-G rs2069705 A/G												
AA	25 (71%)	10 (29%)	26 (100%)	0	36 (100%)	0	31 (86%)	5 (14%)	32 (89%)	4 (11%)	33 (92%)	3 (8%)
AG	27 (55%)	22 (45%)	35 (95%)	2 (5%)	40 (82%)	9 (18%)	33 (67%)	16 (33%)	41 (84%)	8 (16%)	43 (88%)	6 (12%)
GG	6 (67%)	3 (33%)	9 (90%)	1 (10%)	10 (100%)	0	8 (80%)	2 (20%)	8 (80%)	2 (20%)	6 (60%)	4 (40%)
***p*-value**	0.3		0.1		**0.009**		0.1		0.7		**0.02**	

Table 8. *Cont.*

Genotype	RF		Anti-CCP		Anti-Ro60		Anti-Ro52		Anti-His		Anti-dsDNA	
	(−)	(+)	(−)	(+)	(−)	(+)	(−)	(+)	(−)	(+)	(−)	(+)
IFN-G rs2069718 G/A												
GG	20 (67%)	10 (33%)	21 (100%)	0	31 (100%)	0	26 (84%)	5 (16%)	27 (87%)	4 (13%)	28 (90%)	3 (10%)
GA	33 (60%)	22 (40%)	39 (95%)	2 (5%)	46 (84%)	9 (16%)	39 (71%)	16 (29%)	47 (85%)	8 (15%)	50 (91%)	5 (9%)
AA	7 (70%)	3 (30%)	5 (83%)	1(17%)	11 (100%)	0	9 (82%)	2 (18%)	9 (82%)	2 (18%)	7 (64%)	4 (36%)
p-value	**0.08**		0.2		**0.02**		0.4		0.9		**0.04**	

(−) negative, n (%) of MCTD patients without autoantibody presence. (+) positive, n (%) of MCTD patients with autoantibody presence.

We also observed that *IFN-G* rs1891493 AG might be a marker of anti-CCP presence in MCTD patients; furthermore, the *IFN-G* rs2069705 AG and *IFN-G* rs2069718 GA genotypes might be a marker of anti-Ro60 presence in MCTD patients (Table 8b).

3.6. Variation in IFN-α/-β/-γ Serum Levels in Relation to IFN-A/-B/-G Gene Polymorphisms

The last part of our analysis was to determine the impact of IFNs genetic variants on interferons serum levels in patients with MCTD and controls. In our study, we observed that IFN-α showed the highest level in serum in MCTD patients (median: 650.7 pg/mL), while IFN-γ was at the lowest level in serum (median: 31.9 ng/L). Analysis of IFN-α/-β/-γ levels in serum in MCTD patients and healthy subjects in relation to all examined IFN-A/-B/-G genetic variants revealed no association between IFN-A/-B/-G different genotypes and IFN-α/-β/-γ levels in serum among MCTD patients and as well as in the control groups.

4. Discussion

The current investigation is the first, which showed the association between type I and II interferons genetic variants and MCTD. The fact that MCTD is a rare complex disease makes the recruitment of large sample size challenging. Therefore, we believe that our group of 145 MCTD patients with a very detailed characteristic is the added value of this work and the findings of this study may also be significant for clinical practice. The interferons play a very important role in the pathogenesis of the autoimmune diseases and they are produced in response to inflammatory stimuli. The interaction between type I (IFN-α and IFN-β) as well as type II (IFN-γ) interferons and immune cells leads to the induction of many aspects of the immune response. Type I and II interferons have both pleiotropic cellular effects, such as cell cycle, proliferation, and differentiation regulation, and antiproliferative effects, such as the regulation of DNA replication and modulation of gene expression [27]. The role of interferons in the braking of the immune system homeostasis and leading to the initiation and progression of the immune processes makes IFNs genes a potential candidate for MCTD susceptibility/severity.

The present study demonstrates, for the first time, the association between *IFN-A, IFN-B,* and *IFN-G* genetic variants and MCTD risk, phenotype, and serological profile. Several studies have reported that the dysregulation of the IFN system occurs in connective tissue diseases, such as systemic lupus erythematosus (SLE), systemic sclerosis (SSc), or rheumatoid arthritis (RA) [24]. Genome wide-association studies (GWAS) identified IFN and IFN-inducible genes as loci that contribute to CTDs susceptibility and/or severity [26,28–32]. To date, there is no GWAS published for MCTD. Our results showed a significant association of the *IFN-A* rs10757212, *IFN-A* rs3758236, *IFN-G* rs2069705, and *IFN-G* rs2069718 gene polymorphisms with the occurrence of MCTD. The present study also demonstrated that *INF-G* rs1861493A/rs2069705A/rs2069718G haplotype, which was observed in 58% of MCTD patients, was significantly associated with MCTD risk. Our results indicated that *IFN-A*, as well as *IFN-G* genetic variants, might be potential genetic biomarkers for MCTD susceptibility. Although we found that the IFN-α/-β/-γ levels in serum in MCTD patients were higher than in healthy subjects in the present study, we did not detect the association between interferons genetic variants and IFN serum levels. This may be due to a small sample size of our study group or that the SNPs located in the IFNs genes may have an impact on the changing structure of their protein rather than the regulation of serum protein levels. Moreover, changes in the protein structure can lead to a modification of the IFN affinity for its receptors that are involved in the immune pathways. On the other hand, epigenome-wide association studies (EWAS) in MCTD patients [33] and Genome-wide transcriptional profiling in SLE or SSc patients [24,34,35] confirmed the overexpression of IFN-inducible genes, known as the "interferon (IFN) signature" in these patients. The overexpression of interferon signature occurs early in the hematopoietic process and correlates with disease activity. Our results also demonstrated that the *IFN-G* genetic variant at position rs2069718 G/A might be associated with some clinical symptoms of MCTD, such as Raynaud's Phenomenon, erosive arthritis, swollen hands and fingers, and sclerodactyly. The clinical picture of MCTD develops over time. Usually, the first symptom is Raynaud's Phenomenon, which is accompanied by swollen hands and fingers, erosive arthritis, and skin involvement. Raynaud's Phenomenon and erosive arthritis, as two of the most devastating complications of MCTD, at the time blood sampling were observed in 97% and 94% of MCTD patients, respectively. In our study, we observed that both Raynaud's Phenomenon and erosive arthritis were more often present in MCTD patients with the *IFN-G* rs2069718 GA genotype than in MCTD patients with other genotypes. Moreover, the erosive arthritis was not present in MCTD patients with the *IFN-G* rs2069718 AA genotype. Further, swollen hands and fingers, as well as sclerodactyly, were considerably more frequently observed in MCTD patients with *IFN-G* rs2069718 G allele than in MCTD patients with IFN-G rs2069718 A allele. The characteristics of autoimmune CTDs include the presence of autoantibodies, which are involved in the disease pathogenesis, in combination with particular clinical parameters. In MCTD patients, different autoantibodies are described and they may be a partial explanation of diverse clinical phenotype. Autoantibodies against RNA-associated proteins, such as anti-U1-RNP, Anti-Sjögren's-syndrome-related antigen A (anti-SSA; anti-Ro60; and, anti-Ro52), and anti-Sjögren's syndrome type B (anti-SSBalso known asanti-La) can enhance the immune response. The most common antibodies that are observed in MCTD patients are anti-U1-RNP (present in all our patients), anti-U1-70K (present in 76% of our patients), anti-U1-A (present in 84% of our patients), and anti-U1-C (present in 79% of our patients). In the anti-RNP response, autoantibodies against U1-70K and Sm-B/B proteins appear first, and then autoantibodies directed against U1-A and -C and at the end autoantibodies directed against Sm-D [9]. In the present study, we observed that the anti-U1-A autoantibodies were the most frequently occurring in MCTD patients with rs2069718 GA genotype. Anti-U1-RNP antibodies through the upregulation of the intracellular adhesion molecule-1, endothelial leukocyte adhesion molecule-1, and major histocompatibility complex (MHC) class II molecules expression may lead to the hyperplasia, obliterated vasculopathy, and pulmonary arterial hypertension (PAH). Moreover, in MCTD patients, autoantibody titers against the U1-RNP may correlate with disease activity [36]. Autoantibodies against RNA binding protein Ro60, which regulate IFN stimulated gene expression [16], were present in 10% of our MCTD patients. Our results indicate that IFN-G rs2069705 AG and rs2069718 GA genotypes may be markers of anti-Ro60 presence in MCTD patients (anti-Ro60 were not present in MCTD patients with other IFN-G rs2069705 and rs2069718 genotypes).

However, our study has severallimitations. First, our sample size is relatively small and might lead to a limited statistical impact on the accuracy and precision of the results. However, MCTD is a very rare disease and the recruitment of a large sample size is challenged. We determined the alpha coefficient = 0.05 to avoid the type 1 error. This is a value that allows for 95% to avoid the first type of error. Although in some analyses (e.g., autoantibodies profiles) we found statistical significance results, the small number of selected subgroups of MCTD patients does not allow for high test power. The second limitation of this study is the absence of precise measures of clinical activity of MCTD—for the purpose of this study we constructed a set of objective and subjective methods to assess the damage in MCTD as well as disease activity. These methods were developed based on the tools that were employed in SLE. Third, our study was performed in Polish Caucasians subjects only. Future prospective studies involving other populations with different ethnicities are needed and would be interesting.

5. Conclusions

In conclusion, our results add novel evidence in elucidating the genetic predisposition among MCTD patients. This was the first study to show that IFN-A and IFN-G play unique roles in the development of MCTD. What is more, we first demonstrated that IFN-B, as well as IFN-G, play a special/exceptional role in the MCTD phenotype. Our study indicates that IFN-G genetic variants could be potential biomarkers for MCTD susceptibility and severity.

Author Contributions: A.P.-G. conceived, designed and performed experiments, analyzed and interpreted of data and wrote the manuscript. A.W. and E.W. performed experiments. M.W., A.F.-G. and M.O. were involved in the classification of patients with rheumatoid arthritis, clinical check of patients and treatment control. B.S. performed statistical analysis. All authors read and approved the final version.

Acknowledgments: The technical assistance of Wieslawa Frankowska is gratefully acknowledged. We are also grateful to all of the MCTD patients and healthy subjects whose cooperation made this study possible.

References

1. Sharp, G.C.; Irvin, W.S.; Tan, E.M.; Gould, R.G.; Holman, H.R. Mixed connective tissue disease—An apparently distinct rheumatic disease syndrome associated with a specific antibody to an extractable nuclear antigen (ENA). *Am. J. Med.* **1972**, *52*, 148–159. [CrossRef]
2. Minkin, W.; Rabhan, N. Mixed connective tissue disease. *Arch. Dermatol.* **1976**, *112*, 1535–1538. [CrossRef]
3. Ortega-Hernandez, O.D.; Shoenfeld, Y. Mixed connective tissue disease: An overview of clinical manifestations, diagnosis and treatment. *Best Pract. Res. Clin. Rheumatol.* **2012**, *26*, 61–72. [CrossRef] [PubMed]
4. Aringer, M.; Steiner, G.; Smolen, J.S. Does mixed connective tissue disease exist? Yes. *Rheum. Dis. Clin. N. Am.* **2005**, *31*, 411–420. [CrossRef]
5. Greidinger, E.L.; Hoffman, R.W. Autoantibodies in the pathogenesis of mixed connective tissue disease. *Rheum. Dis. Clin. N. Am.* **2005**, *31*, 437–450. [CrossRef]
6. Tani, C.; Carli, L.; Vagnani, S.; Talarico, R.; Baldini, C.; Mosca, M.; Bombardieri, S. The diagnosis and classification of mixed connective tissue disease. *J. Autoimmun.* **2014**, 46–49. [CrossRef]
7. Kattah, N.H.; Kattah, M.G.; Utz, P.J. The U1-snRNP complex: Structural properties relating to autoimmune pathogenesis in rheumatic diseases. *Immunol. Rev.* **2010**, *233*, 126–145. [CrossRef]
8. Casciola-Rosen, L.A.; Miller, D.K.; Anhalt, G.J.; Rosen, A. Specific cleavage of the 70-kDa protein component of the U1 small nuclear ribonucleoprotein is a characteristic biochemical feature of apoptotic cell death. *J. Biol. Chem.* **1994**, *269*, 30757–30760.
9. Paradowska-Gorycka, A. U1-RNP and TLR receptors in the pathogenesis of mixed connective tissue disease. Part I. The U1-RNP complex and its biological significance in the pathogenesis of mixed connective tissue disease. *Reumatologia* **2015**, *53*, 94–100. [CrossRef]
10. Keith, M.P.; Moratz, C.; Tsokos, G.C. Anti-RNP immunity: Implications for tissue injury and the pathogenesis of connective tissue disease. *Autoimmun. Rev.* **2007**, *6*, 232–236. [CrossRef]
11. Hof, D.; Raats, J.M.; Pruijn, G.J. Apoptotic modifications affect the autoreactivity of the U1 snRNP autoantigen. *Autoimmun. Rev.* **2005**, *4*, 380–388. [CrossRef]
12. Hoffman, R.W.; Maldonado, M.E. Immune pathogenesis of Mixed Connective Tissue Disease: A short analytical review. *Clin. Immunol.* **2008**, *128*, 8–17. [CrossRef] [PubMed]
13. Li, J.; Wang, X.; Zhang, F.; Yin, H. Toll-like receptors as therapeutic targets for autoimmune connective tissue diseases. *Pharmacol. Ther.* **2013**, *138*, 441–451. [CrossRef] [PubMed]
14. Ronnblom, L. The importance of the type I interferon system in autoimmunity. *Clin. Exp. Rheumatol.* **2016**, *34*, S21–S24.
15. Bengtsson, A.A.; Rönnblom, L. Role of interferons in SLE. *Best Pract. Res. Clin. Rheumatol.* **2017**, *31*, 415–428. [CrossRef]
16. Psarras, A.; Emery, P.; Vital, E.M. Type I interferon-mediated autoimmune diseases: Pathogenesis, diagnosis and targeted therapy. *Rheumatology (Oxford)* **2017**, *56*, 1662–1675. [CrossRef]
17. Chen, J.Y.; Wang, C.M.; Chen, T.D.; Jan Wu, Y.J.; Lin, J.C.; Lu, L.Y.; Wu, J. Interferon-λ3/4 genetic variants and interferon-λ3 serum levels are biomarkers of lupus nephritis and disease activity in Taiwanese. *Arthritis Res. Ther.* **2018**, *20*, 193. [CrossRef]
18. McNab, F.; Mayer-Barber, K.; Sher, A.; Wack, A.; O'Garra, A. Type I interferons in infectious disease. *Nat. Rev. Immunol.* **2015**, *15*, 87–103. [CrossRef]
19. Eloranta, M.L.; Alm, G.V.; Ronnblom, L. Disease mechanisms in rheumatology–tools and pathways: Plasmacytoid dendritic cells and their role in autoimmune rheumatic diseases. *Arthritis Rheum.* **2013**, *65*, 853–863. [CrossRef]

20. Yu, S.L.; Chan, P.K.; Wong, C.K.; Szeto, C.C.; Ho, S.C.; So, K.; Yu, M.M.; Yim, S.F.; Cheung, T.H.; Wong, M.C.; et al. Antagonist-mediated down-regulation of Toll-like receptors increases the prevalence of human papillomavirus infection in systemic lupus erythematosus. *Arthritis Res. Ther.* **2012**, *14*, R80. [CrossRef]
21. Chauhan, S.K.; Singh, V.V.; Rai, R.; Rai, M.; Rai, G. Distinct autoantibody profiles in systemic lupus erythematosus patients are selectively associated with TLR7 and TLR9 upregulation. *J. Clin. Immunol.* **2013**, *33*, 954–964. [CrossRef] [PubMed]
22. Midgley, A.; Thorbinson, C.; Beresford, M.W. Expression of Toll-like receptors and their detection of nuclear self-antigen leading to immune activation in JSLE. *Rheumatology (Oxford)* **2012**, *51*, 824–832. [CrossRef] [PubMed]
23. El-Sherbiny, Y.M.; Psarras, A.; Md Yusof, M.Y.; Hensor, E.M.A.; Tooze, R.; Doody, G.; Mohamed, A.A.A.; McGonagle, D.; Wittmann, M.; Emery, P.; et al. A novel two-score system for interferon status segregates autoimmune diseases and correlates with clinical features. *Sci. Rep.* **2018**, *8*, 5793. [CrossRef]
24. Ramos, P.S.; Williams, A.H.; Ziegler, J.T.; Comeau, M.E.; Guy, R.T.; Lessard, C.J.; Li, H.; Edberg, J.C.; Zidovetzki, R.; Criswell, L.A.; et al. Genetic analyses of interferon pathway-related genes reveal multiple new loci associated with systemic lupus erythematosus. *Arthritis Rheum.* **2011**, *63*, 2049–2057. [CrossRef] [PubMed]
25. Kariuki, S.N.; Ghodke-Puranik, Y.; Dorschner, J.M.; Chrabot, B.S.; Kelly, J.A.; Tsao, B.P.; Kimberly, R.P.; Alarcón-Riquelme, M.E.; Jacob, C.O.; Criswell, L.A.; et al. Genetic analysis of the pathogenic molecular sub-phenotype interferon-alpha identifies multiple novel loci involved in systemic lupus erythematosus. *Genes Immun.* **2015**, *16*, 15–23. [CrossRef] [PubMed]
26. Niewold, T.B. Interferon alpha as a primary pathogenic factor in human lupus. *J. Interferon Cytokine Res.* **2011**, *31*, 887–892. [CrossRef] [PubMed]
27. Ghodke-Puranik, Y.; Dorschner, J.M.; Vsetecka, D.M.; Amin, S.; Makol, A.; Ernste, F.; Osborn, T.; Moder, K.; Chowdhary, V.; Eliopoulos, E.; et al. Lupus-Associated Functional Polymorphism in PNP Causes Cell Cycle Abnormalities and Interferon Pathway Activation in Human Immune Cells. *Arthritis Rheumatol.* **2017**, *69*, 2328–2337. [CrossRef] [PubMed]
28. Ghodke-Puranik, Y.; Imgruet, M.; Dorschner, J.M.; Shrestha, P.; McCoy, K.; Kelly, J.A.; Marion, M.; Guthridge, J.M.; Langefeld, C.D.; Harley, J.B.; et al. Novel genetic associations with interferon in systemic lupus erythematosus identified by replication and fine-mapping of trait-stratified genome-wide screen. *Cytokine* **2019**. [CrossRef]
29. Morris, D.L.; Sheng, Y.; Zhang, Y.; Wang, Y.F.; Zhu, Z.; Tombleson, P.; Chen, L.; Cunninghame Graham, D.S.; Bentham, J.; Roberts, A.L.; et al. Genome-wide association meta-analysis in Chinese and European individuals identifies ten new loci associated with systemic lupus erythematosus. *Nat. Genet.* **2016**, *48*, 940–946. [CrossRef]
30. Teruel, M.; Alarcon-Riquelme, M.E. The genetic basis of systemic lupus erythematosus: What are the risk factors and what have we learned. *J. Autoimmun.* **2016**, *74*, 161–175. [CrossRef]
31. Järvinen, T.M.; Hellquist, A.; Zucchelli, M.; Koskenmies, S.; Panelius, J.; Hasan, T.; Julkunen, H.; D'Amato, M.; Kere, J. Replication of GWAS-identified systemic lupus erythematosus susceptibility genes affirms B-cell receptor pathway signaling and strengthens the role of IRF5 in disease susceptibility in a Northern European population. *Rheumatology (Oxford)* **2012**, *51*, 87–92. [CrossRef] [PubMed]
32. Skaug, B.; Assassi, S. Type I interferon dysregulation in Systemic Sclerosis. *Cytokine* **2019**. [CrossRef] [PubMed]
33. Carnero-Montoro, E.; Barturen, G.; Povedano, E.; Kerick, M.; Martinez-Bueno, M.; Precisesads Clinical Consortium; Ballestar, E.; Martin, J.; Teruel, M.; Alarcón-Riquelme, M.E. Epigenome-Wide Comparative Study Reveals Key Differences Between Mixed Connective Tissue Disease and Related Systemic Autoimmune Diseases. *Front. Immunol.* **2019**, *10*, 1880. [CrossRef] [PubMed]
34. Carnero-Montoro, E.; Alarcón-Riquelme, M.E. Epigenome-wide association studies for systemic autoimmune diseases: The road behind and the road ahead. *Clin. Immunol.* **2018**, *196*, 21–33. [CrossRef] [PubMed]
35. Teruel, M.; Sawalha, A.H. Epigenetic variability in systemic lupus erythematosus: What we learned from genome-wide DNA methylation studies. *Curr. Rheumatol. Rep.* **2017**, *19*, 32. [CrossRef] [PubMed]
36. Hof, D.; Cheung, K.; de Rooij, D.J.; van den Hoogen, F.H.; Pruijn, G.J.; van Venrooij, W.J.; Raats, J.M. Autoantibodies specific for apoptotic U1-70K are superior serological markers for mixed connective tissue disease. *Arthritis Res. Ther.* **2005**, *7*, R302–R309. [CrossRef] [PubMed]

2

N-Glycosylation Regulates Pannexin 2 Localization but is Not Required for Interacting with Pannexin 1

Rafael E. Sanchez-Pupo, Danielle Johnston and Silvia Penuela *

Department of Anatomy and Cell Biology, Schulich School of Medicine & Dentistry, University of Western Ontario, London, ON N6A5C1, Canada; rsnchezp@uwo.ca (R.E.S.-P.); Danielle.Johnston@schulich.uwo.ca (D.J.)

* Correspondence: spenuela@uwo.ca

Abstract: Pannexins (Panx1, 2, 3) are channel-forming glycoproteins expressed in mammalian tissues. We previously reported that N-glycosylation acts as a regulator of the localization and intermixing of Panx1 and Panx3, but its effects on Panx2 are currently unknown. Panx1 and Panx2 intermixing can regulate channel properties, and both pannexins have been implicated in neuronal cell death after ischemia. Our objectives were to validate the predicted N-glycosylation site of Panx2 and to study the effects of Panx2 glycosylation on localization and its capacity to interact with Panx1. We used site-directed mutagenesis, enzymatic de-glycosylation, cell-surface biotinylation, co-immunoprecipitation, and confocal microscopy. Our results showed that N86 is the only N-glycosylation site of Panx2. Panx2 and the N86Q mutant are predominantly localized to the endoplasmic reticulum (ER) and cis-Golgi matrix with limited cell surface localization was seen only in the presence of Panx1. The Panx2 N86Q mutant is glycosylation-deficient and tends to aggregate in the ER reducing its cell surface trafficking but it can still interact with Panx1. Our study indicates that N-glycosylation may be important for folding and trafficking of Panx2. We found that the un-glycosylated forms of Panx1 and 2 can readily interact, regulating their localization and potentially their channel function in cells where they are co-expressed.

Keywords: pannexin; Panx1; Panx2; post-translational modification; traffic; N-glycosylation; channels; subcellular localization

---

1. Introduction

Pannexins (Panx1, Panx2, and Panx3) are membrane-spanning glycoproteins capable of forming large pore channels that allow the passage of ions and macromolecules involved in paracrine and autocrine signaling [1,2]. Panx1 is the most widely expressed pannexin and the most studied, with evidence supporting that its channels act as ATP and Ca^{2+} conduits [3–6] and are implicated in critical cellular processes such as cell death after brain ischemia [7] and inflammation [8]. On the other hand, Panx2 is the largest member of the family and its expression was thought to be restricted to the central nervous system (CNS). Recently, it has been reported that Panx2 can also be expressed in other tissues such as skin, kidney and liver [9,10], while Panx3 is predominantly expressed in skin, cartilage and bone [4,5,11–13]. In contrast to the hexameric type of channels formed by Panx1, it has been suggested that Panx2 can form octameric or heptameric channels [14] and it is still unclear whether its channel function would be similar to the other family members. Interestingly, Panx1 and Panx2 expression have been found to overlap in adult rodent brains although they are inversely regulated throughout development, with Panx1 being more abundant in neonatal and young tissues, whereas Panx2 is more abundant in the adult [15–18]. Under ischemic conditions, both Panx1 and Panx2 are expressed in the brain and their overlapping channel functions contribute to neurodegeneration. In fact, the deletion of Panx1 and Panx2 in a double knockout mouse model was necessary to observe a reduction in cell death after ischemia, perhaps due to their redundant and/or complementary functions [19].

N-glycosylation is a posttranslational modification that occurs in the endoplasmic reticulum (ER) and is recognized to have profound effects on protein folding and trafficking of membrane-bound proteins [20]. The prediction of putative N-linked glycosylation sites for pannexins has been done in the past, and it has been demonstrated that Panx1 and Panx3 have sites for N-linked glycosylation at Asn (N) 254 and N71, respectively. These studies comprised further characterization using enzymatic digestion with endoglycosidases that confirmed that all three members of the pannexin family are differentially N-glycosylated but not O-glycosylated [11,21]. However, for Panx2 the predicted site of N-glycosylation at residue N86 remains to be validated [22].

Unlike other pannexins, Panx2 is only modified to a high-mannose glycosylation species (termed as Gly-1) and presents a predominantly intracellular localization that has been associated with this lower level of N-glycosylation [22–26]. Previous evidence supports the concept that complex glycoprotein species (Gly-2) (further processed at Golgi) present in Panx1 and Panx3 traffic readily to the cell surface [22]. However, our group and others have stated that under certain circumstances Panx2 can also translocate to the plasma membrane [14,17,22], but it is still unclear whether glycosylation plays a role in regulating Panx2 trafficking.

Panx2 has been shown to interact with Panx1, and when co-expressed together they can form heteromeric channels with reduced channel properties compared to homomeric ones [22,27]. Although this has only been tested in ectopic expression systems it has been suggested that it might function as a mode of regulation in cells that endogenously express both proteins. Interestingly, the Panx1/Panx2 interaction only occurs with the Gly-0 and Gly-1 species of Panx1 [22] and it is unknown whether Panx2 glycosylation has any impact on the formation of these intermixed channels. Since previous studies have shown that Panx1 and Panx2 are often co-expressed in the same cells under normal conditions [15,18,27–30], and that their co-expression modulates important processes such as ischemia-induced neurodegeneration and brain damage in vivo [31], it is important to understand how these channels may be regulated by post-translational modifications (PTMs) such as N-glycosylation, and how this PTM may regulate their interaction.

The present study aimed to validate the predicted N-linked-glycosylation site of Panx2 and determine its role in the regulation of the subcellular localization and intermixing of Panx2 with Panx1. We generated a Panx2 mutant protein completely devoid of N-glycosylation that, when overexpressed, exhibits a high level of intracellular aggregation with decreased traffic to the plasma membrane compared with wild-type Panx2. We found that N-glycosylation of Panx2 is not required for Panx1/Panx2 intermixing but facilitates Panx2 trafficking and localization at the plasma membrane when co-expressed with Panx1. The intracellular localization of un-glycosylated Panx2 reduces its co-localization with Panx1 at the cell surface and may impact their channel function in cells that co-express both glycoproteins, such as neurons. Collectively, we propose that N-glycosylation may be necessary for proper processing of Panx2 at the endoplasmic reticulum, regulating its intracellular distribution, but it is not required for interacting with Panx1.

2. Results

2.1. Characterization of the Panx2 N-Glycosylation Site at Asparagine 86

Previous research has shown that ectopic expression of full-length mouse Panx2 presented N-glycosylated species with high-mannose modification [22]. Based on the analysis of the canonical sequence of Panx2 (UniProt ID: Q6IMP4-1), this modification might occur at asparagine 86 (Asn86 or N86) that is located in the first extracellular loop of Panx2 [20] (Figure 1A). To validate this prediction, we generated a full-length Panx2 mutant (Panx2^{N86Q}, referred here as N86Q) with the substitution of the N86 with a glutamine (Gln, Q) that prevents the attachment of N-linked glycans to this specific site. As shown in Figure 1B, Western blotting (WB) of overexpressed constructs of N86Q and wild-type

Panx2 (as glycosylated control) indicated that the electrophoretic band corresponding to N86Q mutant migrated faster than its wildtype counterpart, characteristic of a reduction in molecular weight.

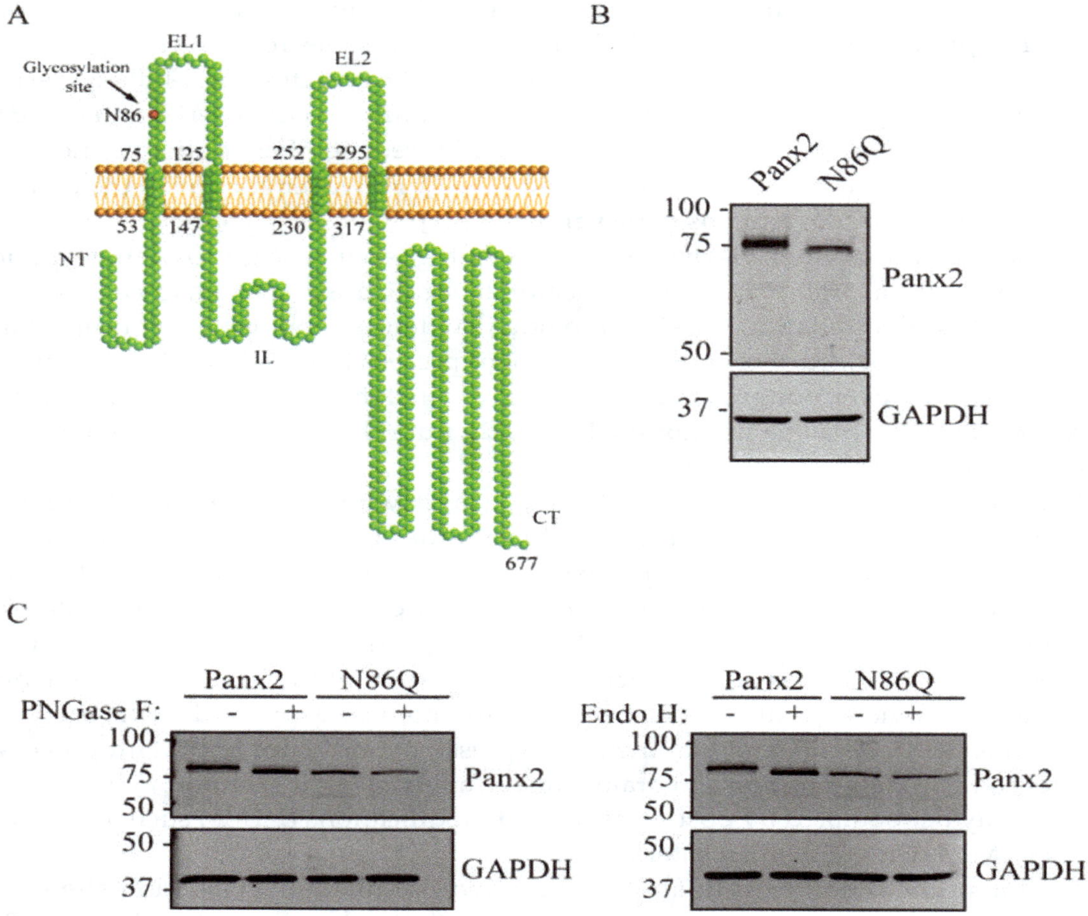

Figure 1. Asn86 is the N-glycosylation site of Panx2. (**A**) Based on sequence analysis, Panx2 (Uniprot ID: Q6IMP4-1) is predicted to contain four transmembrane domains, one intracellular (IL) and two extracellular loops (EL). The predicted N-glycosylation site is located at Asn86 in the first extracellular loop (EL1) (red residue). (**B**) Western blot (WB) comparing wildtype Panx2 and mutant N86Q, the latter shows a faster migrating band than the wildtype counterpart, indicative of decreased molecular weight. (**C**) Cell lysates of HEK293T transiently expressing Panx2 and N86Q mutant were subjected to enzymatic digestions with PNGase F and EndoH N-glycosidases. WB analysis confirmed that N86 is the only glycosylation site for Panx2 since only the wildtype protein exhibited a band shift after treatment with both glycosidases, and the de-glycosylated Panx2 band ran to the same position as the N86Q mutant. GAPDH was used as loading control. Molecular weights are noted in kDa.

To analyze whether N-glycosylation was prevented in the N86Q mutant, enzymatic de-glycosylation with endoglycosidase H (Endo H) and Peptide-N-Glycosidase F (PNGase F) were applied to the protein lysates and analyzed by WB (Figure 1C). Both de-glycosylation treatments did not cause any shift in migration of the N86Q band. Yet, wild-type Panx2 exhibited a small shift after treatment which relocated the migration of this band to the same position as that of the faster migrating N86Q mutant. Thus, the differences in the electrophoretic migration of the N86Q compared with the wild-type (WT) Panx2 can be explained by differences in molecular weight due to the absence of N-glycosylation. These findings validate N86 as the only N-glycosylation site present in Panx2 as was predicted by Penuela and others [22].

2.2. *N86Q Forms Intracellular Aggregates*

To determine whether glycosylation of Panx2 has any effect on its subcellular localization, we ectopically expressed Panx2 WT and N86Q in different reference cell lines and evaluated whether the intracellular distribution observed was dependent on the cell type as has been reported for Panx1 and Panx3 [32]. Because our group has demonstrated before [21] that Panx1 influences Panx2 trafficking, we selected Normal Rat Kidney cells (NRK), that in our experience have very low expression of endogenous Panx1 (Figure 2D), and "adherent" human embryonic kidney cells (AD293) that endogenously express the human ortholog PANX1 (Figure 3D). Likewise, these cell lines were selected as they are suitable transfection hosts with a relatively large cytoplasm which facilitates the visualization of the subcellular localization of proteins.

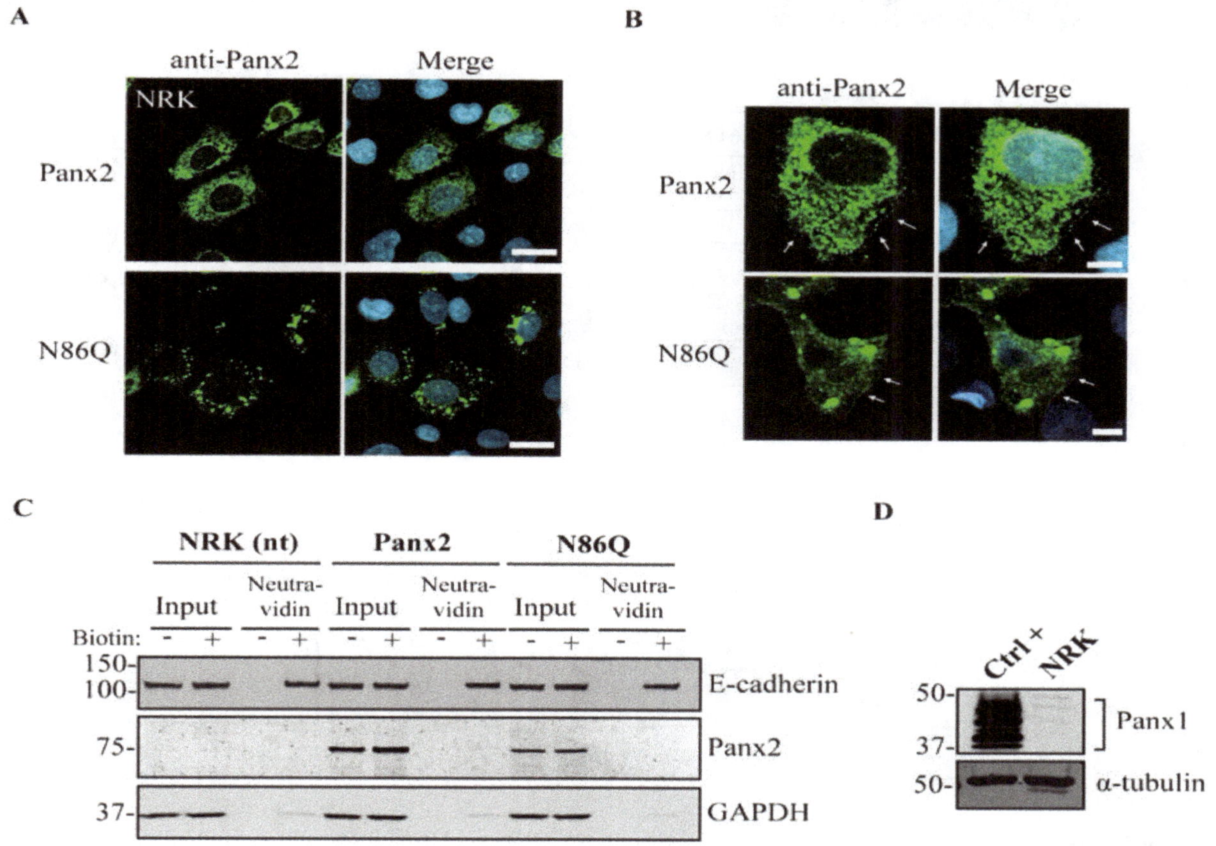

Figure 2. Panx2 has a predominantly intracellular localization, and its N-glycosylation-deficient mutant (N86Q) forms aggregates in NRK cells with low endogenous Panx1 protein expression. (**A**) Confocal micrographs of Panx2 and N86Q ectopically expressed in NRK cells, immunolabeled with anti-Panx2 antibody (green), revealed that Panx2 is predominantly localized intracellularly. The mutant N86Q is also localized intracellularly but appeared mostly as punctate aggregates. Nuclei (blue) were counterstained with Hoechst 33342. Scale bars = 20 μm. (**B**) Representative images of a small subpopulation of NRK cells expressing Panx2 or N86Q that showed minimal apparent localization at the cell surface (indicated with white arrows). Scale bars = 5 μm. (**C**) Western blot analysis of cell-surface-biotinylated proteins with EZ-Link™ Sulfo-NHS-SS-Biotin pulled down with NeutrAvidin® beads showed very low detection of Panx2 but not the N86Q mutant at the cell surface of NRK cells. E-cadherin was used as a positive control of cell surface protein labeling and GAPDH was used as a negative control of intracellular proteins (no biotin internalization). Non-transfected NRKs (nt) were used as a negative control. (**D**) Western blot of protein lysate from NRK cells indicated that these cells have very low detectable levels of endogenous Panx1. Overexpressed Panx1 was used as positive control (Ctrl +) and endogenous α-tubulin was used as protein loading control. Molecular weights noted in kDa.

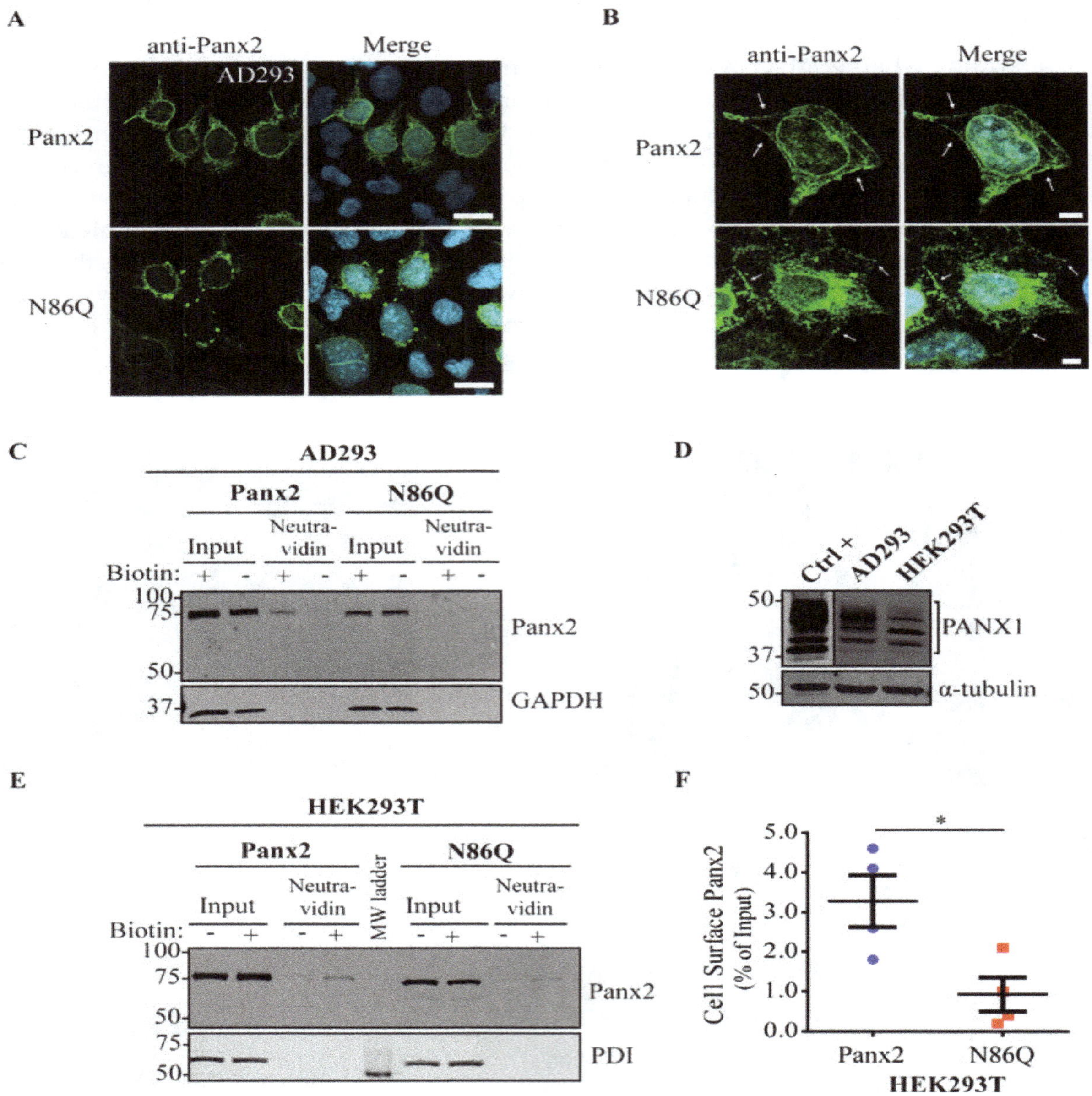

Figure 3. Analysis of Panx2 and N86Q localization in AD293 and HEK293T cells expressing endogenous PANX1. (**A**) Immunolabeling of Panx2 and N86Q mutant (green) showed that both localized mostly intracellularly, but the N86Q mutant aggregated intracellularly in AD293 cells. Scale bars = 20 μm. (**B**) A subpopulation of AD293 cells displayed Panx2 localization at the cell surface, less evident with the N86Q mutant (indicated with white arrows) Scale bars = 5 μm. Nuclei (blue). (**C**) Cell Surface Biotinylation Assays on AD293 cells showed a weak detection of the Panx2 wildtype but not N86Q mutant in surface-labeled fractions. GAPDH was used as a control for biotin internalization. (**D**) Immunoblots of AD293 and HEK293T cells confirmed that both cell lines express endogenous PANX1. Overexpressed human PANX1 served as positive control (Ctrl +) and endogenous α-tubulin was used as loading control. Line dividing upper panel of PANX1 WB indicates differences in exposure of the same blot to show a better detection of endogenous PANX1 compared to the overexpressed positive control. (**E**) Cell surface biotinylation experiments performed on HEK293T cells showed that overexpressed Panx2 and the mutant N86Q are detectable at the cell surface. Protein disulfide-isomerase (PDI) was used as a control for biotin internalization. (**F**) Densitometric analysis and quantification of cell surface biotinylation experiments performed in HEK293T cells revealed a significant reduction of N86Q cell surface detection compared to Panx2. Cell surface detection was calculated relative to the total protein in input lanes. Statistical significance was considered when $p < 0.05$ (* $p = 0.0286$, $N = 4$ independent experiments), Mann Whitney U test. Error bars denote mean ± S.E.M. Molecular weights

Confocal immunofluorescence imaging revealed an intracellular localization of ectopic Panx2 (Figures 2A and 3A, top panel), with perinuclear distribution and spread in intracellular compartments. Interestingly, in both cell types assayed, the mutant N86Q localized intracellularly with large subpopulations forming punctate aggregates (Figures 2A and 3A, bottom panel).

2.3. Limited Panx2 Localization at the Cell Surface Is Reliant on N-Glycosylation Status and the Level of Panx1

Despite the predominant intracellular localization, in a subpopulation of cells, Panx2 and the N86Q mutant (to a lesser extent) were apparent in limited regions of the cell surface (Figures 2B and 3B, arrows). To corroborate these results, cell surface biotinylation assays followed by immunoblotting were conducted using a cell-impermeable biotinylation reagent (Sulfo-NHS-SS-Biotin). Cell-surface biotinylation experiments in NRKs (low endogenous Panx1, Figure 2D) showed a faint band of Panx2 and no detection of N86Q at the cell surface in the neutravidin pull-downs (Figure 2C). Also, AD293 cells (with a higher level of endogenous PANX1, Figure 3D) exhibited low Panx2 and no detectable N86Q mutant protein at the cell surface (Figure 3C). However, in subsequent experiments we also used human embryonic kidney (HEK293T) cells (Figure 3D) that have been used in previous studies [11,22], because of their increased transfection efficiency and enhanced protein expression due to the SV40 T-antigen [33]. After ectopic expression in HEK293T cells, we performed the same cell-surface biotinylation assays and noticed that Panx2 WT protein was detected (approximately 4% of the total Panx2 expression) at the cell surface (Figure 3E). Under these overexpression conditions, the N86Q mutant was also detected in the biotinylated-protein fractions (Figure 3E) but there was a significant ($p = 0.0286$, $N = 4$) reduction (to ~1% of its total amount) in the cell surface protein pool of the mutant (Figure 3F). Therefore, although the Panx2 cell membrane trafficking is reduced when Panx2 is not N-glycosylated at N86, its cell surface localization is not completely abrogated when overexpressed in HEK293T cells.

2.4. Panx2 and N86Q Aggregates Localize to the Endoplasmic Reticulum and Golgi Apparatus

Because of the prominent intracellular localization of both Panx2 and the mutant N86Q, we were interested in determining the subcellular compartments to which these proteins could be trafficking. We transiently expressed these proteins in AD293 cells and used immunolabeling with different organelle markers to assess their intracellular location by confocal microscopy (Figures 4 and 5).

As shown in Figure 4A, Panx2 immunolabeling exhibits a broad cytoplasmic distribution highly overlapping (Pearson's Colocalization Coefficient $(PCC)_{Panx2\text{-}PDI} = 0.49 \pm 0.02$; $n = 41$, $N = 3$) with the chaperone protein disulfide-isomerase (PDI), a known marker of the endoplasmic reticulum (ER). The mutant N86Q had significantly ($p < 0.0001$) less overlap ($PCC_{N86Q\text{-}PDI} = 0.34 \pm 0.03$, $n = 57$, $N = 3$) with PDI although there was also a more punctate distribution of PDI that co-localized with N86Q. These observations suggest that N86Q is being confined to some punctate regions enriched in PDI, along with other subcellular organelles. We also observed an apparent alteration of the ER morphology when N86Q was expressed.

Quantitation of colocalization with cis-Golgi marker (GM130) (Figure 4B) showed a significantly ($p = 0.0001$) higher colocalization with the N86Q mutant ($PCC_{N86Q\text{-}GM130} = 0.43 \pm 0.04$; $n = 41$, $N = 3$) than with Panx2 WT ($PCC_{Panx2\text{-}GM130} = 0.23 \pm 0.03$; $n = 30$, $N = 3$). In this case, cells that overexpressed Panx2 WT exhibited changes in the distribution of GM130 compared to un-transfected ones (in the same field of view, Figure 4B). These changes were more pronounced in AD293 cells overexpressing the mutant N86Q, in which not only the cis-Golgi morphology changed, but GM130 also appeared to accumulate within N86Q aggregates.

On the other hand, lysosome-associated membrane protein 2 (Lamp-2) and the fixable and cell permeant Mitotracker™ Red CMXRos were assayed to label lysosomes/late endosomes, and active mitochondria, respectively. We did not observe colocalization with Lamp-2 ($PCC_{Panx2\text{-}Lamp\text{-}2} = -0.08 \pm 0.01$; $n = 59$, $N = 3$; $PCC_{N86Q\text{-}Lamp\text{-}2} = -0.05 \pm 0.02$; $n = 49$, $N = 3$) or Mitotracker ($PCC_{Panx2\text{-}Mitotracker} = -0.08 \pm 0.03$; $n = 25$, $N = 3$; $PCC_{N86Q\text{-}Mitotracker} = -0.13 \pm 0.06$; $n = 31$, $N = 3$), and there was no difference in the distribution of both markers upon overexpression of Panx2 WT or N86Q.

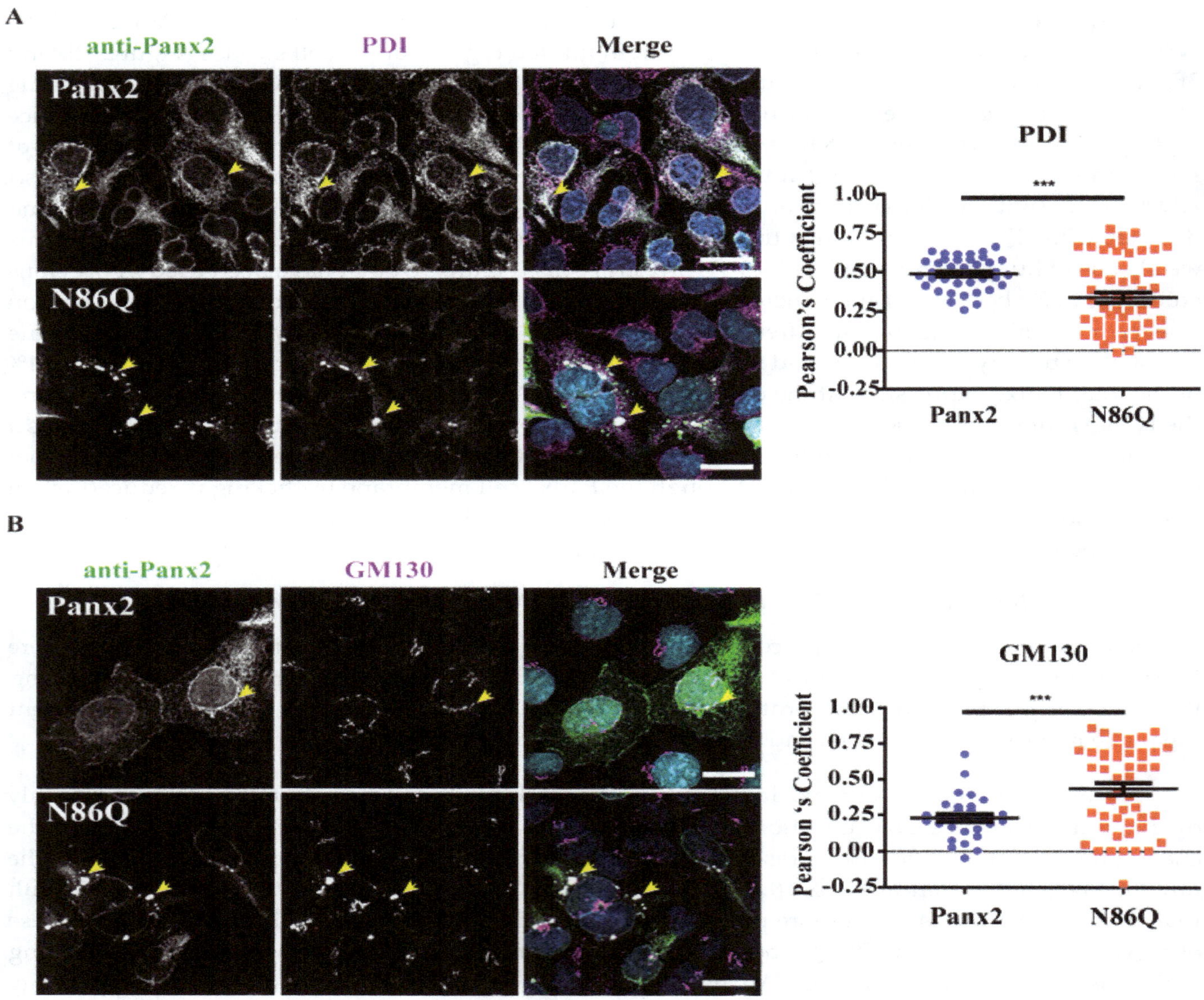

Figure 4. Panx2 and N86Q colocalize with markers of the endoplasmic reticulum and Golgi. Representative confocal micrographs of Panx2 and N86Q ectopically expressed in AD293 cells. Co-immunolabeling with anti-Panx2 antibody (green) and organelle markers (magenta): (**A**) PDI, endoplasmic reticulum (ER); (**B**) GM-130, cis-Golgi matrix. Panx2 has a perinuclear localization and is spread intracellularly in the cytoplasm partially colocalizing with markers of the endoplasmic reticulum and Golgi. N86Q aggregates also overlap with ER and Golgi markers and disrupt their distribution. Yellow arrowheads indicate representative regions of colocalization. Nuclei (blue) were counterstained with Hoechst 33342. Scale bars = 20 μm. Pearson Correlation Coefficients (right) were calculated for multiple regions of interest (ROI)s corresponding to double-labeled cells. Statistical significance was considered when $p < 0.05$ (*** $p \leq 0.0001$, $N = 3$ independent experiments), using unpaired two-tailed t test with Welch's correction. Error bars denote mean ± S.E.M.

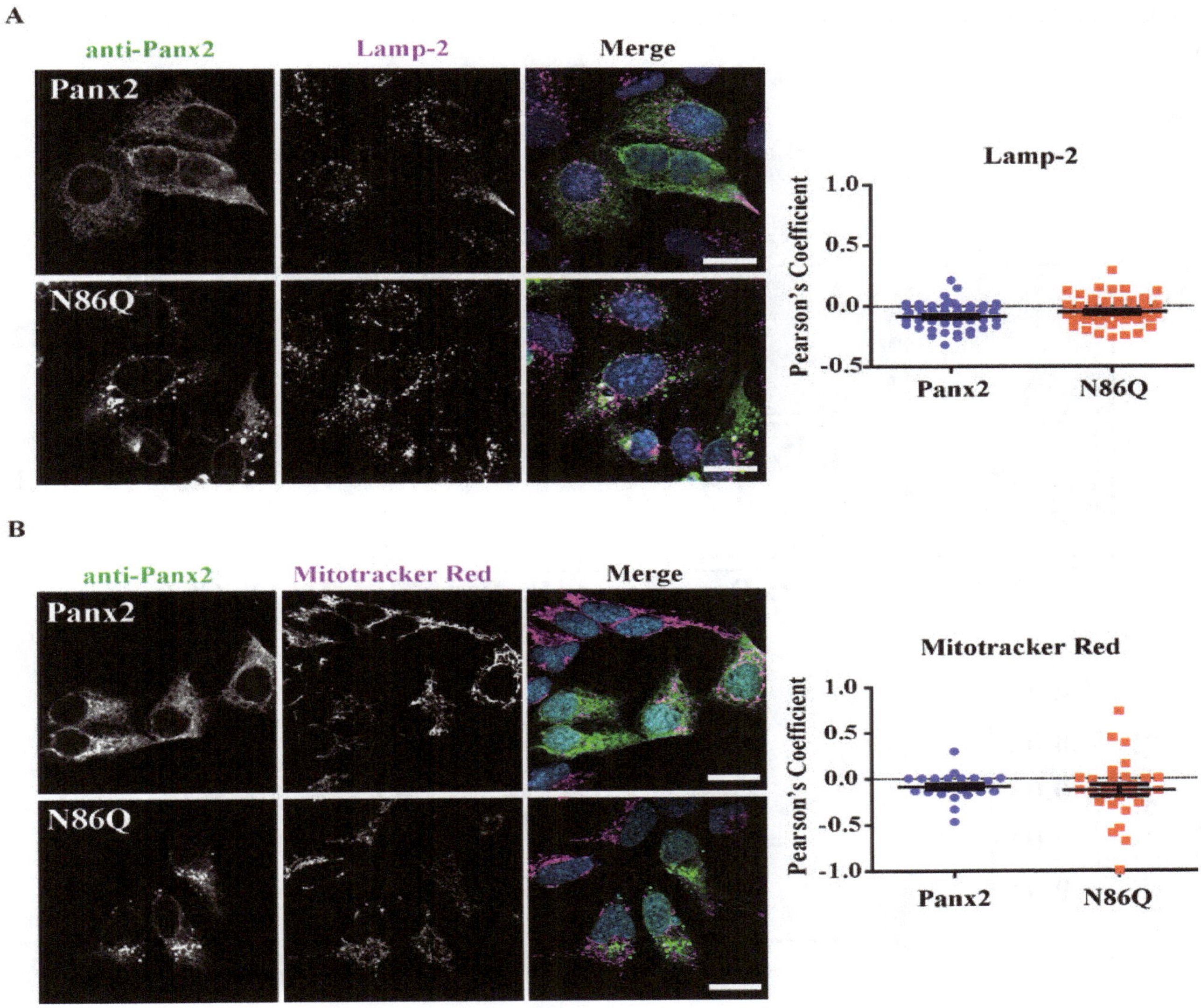

Figure 5. Panx2 and N86Q do not localize to late endosomes/lysosomes or mitochondria. Confocal micrographs of Panx2 and N86Q ectopically expressed in AD293 cells. Co-immunolabeling with anti-Panx2 antibody (green) and organelle markers (magenta): (**A**) Lamp-2, lysosomes and late endosomes, and (**B**) Mitotracker® Red, mitochondria showed that neither Panx2 or N86Q mutant exhibited significant overlap with the markers. Nuclei (blue) were counterstained with Hoechst 33342. Nuclei (blue) were counterstained with Hoechst 33342. Scale bars = 20 μm. Pearson Correlation Coefficients (right) were calculated for multiples ROIs corresponding to double-labeled cells. There was no statistical significance ($p > 0.05$, $N = 3$, unpaired two-tailed t test with Welch's correction) in the degree of colocalization between Panx2 and N86Q with the markers. Error bars denote mean ± S.E.M.

2.5. Panx2 N-Glycosylation Is Not Required for the Interaction with Panx1

Due to our previous report [22] in which we showed that glycosylation regulates intermixing of pannexins and that Panx2 interacts only with the core (non-glycosylated, Gly-0) and high-mannose species (Gly-1) of Panx1, we were interested in determining what would be the outcome with the un-glycosylated species of Panx2. For these experiments, Panx1 was ectopically co-expressed with either Panx2 or non-glycosylated N86Q mutant in HEK293T cells. Using co-immunoprecipitation assays (co-IP, Figure 6A), we observed that both Panx2 and N86Q can co-IP in a complex with Panx1 and occasionally, although not statistically significant ($p > 0.05$, $N = 4$) (Figure 6B,C), N86Q pulled down more Panx1 than the WT Panx2. In addition, consistently with what was reported before by

Penuela et al. (2009), we noticed that only Gly-0 and Gly-1 Panx1 species interacted with both variants of Panx2.

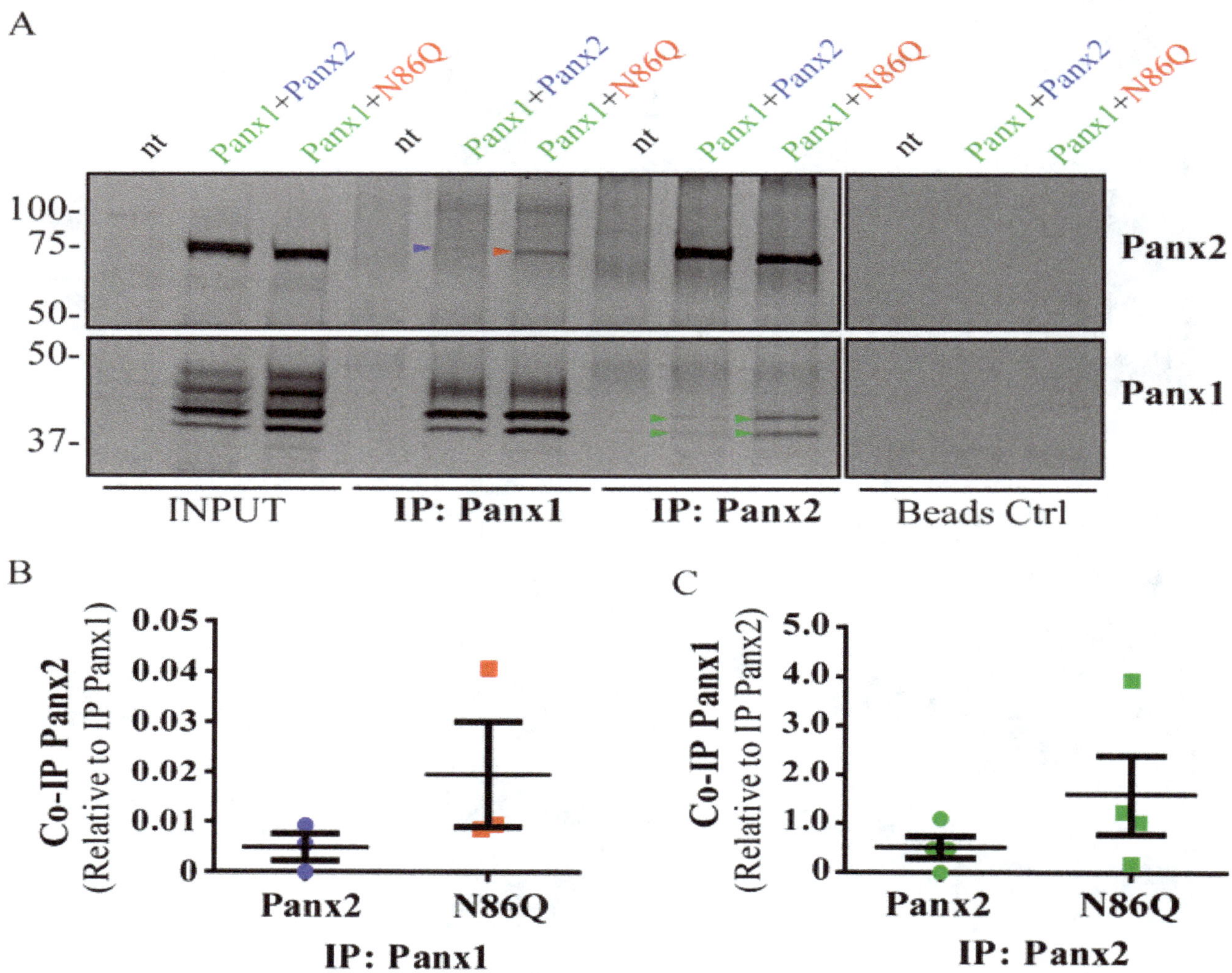

Figure 6. Panx2 glycosylation is not required for the interaction with Panx1 by immunoprecipitation. (**A**) Reciprocal co-immunoprecipitation (co-IP) experiments showed that both Panx2 and N86Q co-IP in a complex with overexpressed Panx1 in HEK293T cells. Colored arrowheads denote bands of co-IP proteins detected in WB. (**B**,**C**) Quantitative analysis (see Materials and Methods Section 4.8) of co-IP shows that the interaction of N86Q with Panx1 is not significantly different ($p > 0.05$, $N = 4$) than with Panx2, and in both cases the complexes only involved the lower glycosylated species of Panx1 (Gly-0 and Gly-1). Beads Ctrl denote control IPs done in parallel without antibodies. Protein sizes in kDa.

Due to the lack of available antibodies from different species to perform double immunolabeling of both pannexins, we used C-terminal FLAG-tagged Panx2 and N86Q that were co-expressed with Panx1 in HEK293T cells. Confocal imaging of Panx2-FLAG or N86Q-FLAG co-expressed with Panx1 (Figure 7A) showed that Panx2-FLAG exhibits both an intracellular and cell surface localization overlap with Panx1 (see Linescan analysis, Figure 7A). N86Q-FLAG formed mostly intracellular aggregates like its untagged counterpart (Figure 3A). A small subpopulation of N86Q-FLAG could still be seen at the cell surface colocalizing with Panx1 (see Linescan analysis, Figure 7B), but to a lesser degree than Panx2-FLAG. Taken together, these findings suggest that the glycosylation of Panx2 is not required for the interaction of Panx1/Panx2 but can determine the differential localization of glycosylated and un-glycosylated species.

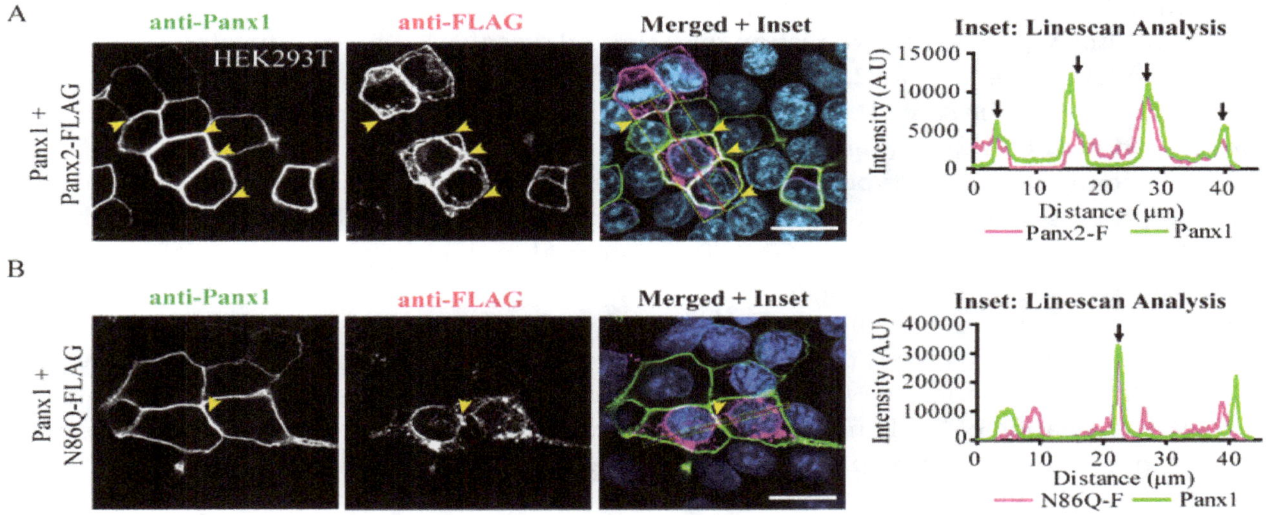

Figure 7. N-glycosylation may enhance plasma membrane localization of Panx2 when co-expressed with Panx1. Confocal micrographs of (**A**) Panx2-FLAG or (**B**) N86Q-FLAG (magenta) ectopically co-expressed with mouse Panx1 (green) in HEK293T cells. 72 h post-transfection Panx2-FLAG partially colocalized with Panx1 at the cell membrane (see black arrows in Linescan, **panel A**) with a subpopulation still in intracellular compartments. N86Q-FLAG formed intracellular aggregates and showed limited colocalization with Panx1 at the plasma membrane (see black arrows in Linescan, **panel B**). Yellow arrowheads denote regions of colocalization of Panx1 and FLAG labeling also depicted with black arrows in the corresponding linescans. Insets: Linescans showing the overlapping (black arrows) between fluorescence peaks to denote colocalization. Nuclei (blue, Hoechst 33342). Scale bars = 20 μm.

3. Discussion

Pannexins are a family of channel proteins implicated in important physiological and pathological functions and most of the current research has been conducted to analyze their level of expression and distribution within mammalian tissues and their role in diverse diseases [34]. However, there is still a need to understand the biophysical properties of these channels and the different ways of regulation that prevent the detrimental effects of their exacerbated channel activity. Pannexins are N-glycosylated and as integral membrane proteins, this modification seems to be essential in regulating their trafficking, as was demonstrated formerly for Panx1 and Panx3 [11,22]. Unlike the other pannexins, Panx2 is modified only to a high-mannose glycosylation (Gly-1) which is known to be an early post-translational modification occurring in the ER lumen. For many other glycoproteins, this step is generally followed by further oligosaccharide editing in the Golgi (complex glycosylation). To date, there is no evidence showing further processing of Panx2 in Golgi and only studies in Panx1 and Panx3 showed that trafficking of these two pannexins to the plasma membrane is mediated by Sar1-dependent COPII vesicles [35] with N-glycosylation affecting their final delivery [11,36,37]. This suggests that N-glycosylation regulates the route of pannexin trafficking and modifies their localization and channel formation in immortalized culture cells. A previous report of Panx2 localization pointed to a predominantly intracellular distribution that can also be modified by other PTMs like palmytoilation, which can determine its subcellular localization in neurons [17].

Panx2 seems to be mostly intracellularly localized, but in some instances, it can also translocate to the plasma membrane [14,17]. However, the exact site of N-glycosylation and whether this modification affects Panx2 trafficking was unknown. In this study, we sought to determine the N-glycosylation site by generating a glycosylation-deficient mutant (N86Q) based on the predicted N-linked glycosylation site reported by Penuela et al. [22]. For our experiments we transfected constructs encoding mouse Panx2 and an N86Q mutant into HEK293T cells. Our results showed that N86Q substitution generated a Panx2 mutant with a faster-migrating electrophoretic band compared to Panx2 WT, that does not shift after specific N-glycosidase digestion with endoglycosidases, thus confirming that N86 is the only N-glycosylation site for Panx2. In the other cell lines assayed (NRK and AD293) we also observed that overexpression of the same Panx2 WT and N86Q constructs exhibited the same electrophoretic properties seen with HEK293T (Figures 2C and 3C).

Independently of the cell-type used for ectopic expression, the N86Q mutant appeared to form punctate aggregates that were localized to intracellular compartments along with the ER-chaperone PDI, and the cis-Golgi matrix marker GM130. Compared to the N-glycosylation-deficient mutants of Panx1 and Panx3 [11], un-glycosylated Panx2 exhibited an exacerbated abnormal intracellular aggregation. This raises the possibility that the lack of N-glycosylation may have affected proper protein folding of Panx2, which is the largest member of the pannexin family. We cannot rule out that the intracellular accumulation of N86Q could be an artifact of overexpression, that concomitant with the lack of glycosylation of the Panx2 mutant, might have induced misfolding and ER-stress [38].

A previous study in murine postnatal hippocampal neural progenitor cells (NPC)s [17] showed that treatment with glycosidases had no effect on endogenous Panx2 electrophoretic mobility, suggesting that they were un-glycosylated. That study relied on antibody detection of endogenous Panx2, and the protein bands identified were of lower molecular weight than the predicted full-length Panx2 used in this study (677 aa, [39]). Further studies are needed to determine first, if the expression of certain un-glycosylated endogenous isoforms of Panx2 is cell-type specific, and second, whether glycosylation has measurable effects on the Panx2 cellular function. To date, there are no reports of mutations in the *Panx2* gene, but our results would predict significant changes in Panx2 behavior if its glycosylation is affected. It is also possible that the un-glycosylated form of Panx2 may be preferentially expressed in some cells and tissues determining the primary function of the Panx2 channel and its subcellular localization.

In our study, we detected large intracellular subpopulations of Panx2 likely localized in the ER, and partially colocalized with cis-Golgi marker. Interestingly, we found that overexpression of the N86Q mutant changed the distribution of PDI and GM130 compared to Panx2 WT, suggesting that the formation of aggregates may disrupt the morphology of ER and cis-Golgi. GM-130 is a peripheral membrane protein in *cis*-Golgi matrix that is important for maintenance of Golgi structure [40], and the regulation of ER-to-Golgi transport of proteins and glycosylation [41]. It is possible that the aggregation of N86Q may interfere with the mutant protein transport from the ER causing accumulation of GM130.

As reviewed by Boyce et al. [42], pannexins contain putative recognition sequences for endocytic and endo-lysosomal targeting which could account for the control of pannexin trafficking. Interestingly, recently published work by Boassa et al., described the localization of a recombinant Panx2 fused to mini-SOG tag that was transiently expressed in HeLa cells [26]. These authors used correlated light and electron microscopy imaging to detect Panx2 localization at cytoplasmic protrusions. Also, immuno-colocalization in HEK293T cells using assorted vesicular markers displayed Panx2 WT (untagged) localized to early or recycling endosomes rather than ER. Although, they mentioned in the manuscript that when the ER marker calnexin was used they detected colocalization with overexpressed Panx2 in HEK293T cells. Our findings are consistent with these reports [24], since we found Panx2 primarily in the ER (Figure 4A). However, we did not find conclusive evidence of Panx2 in endo-lysosome compartments (Figure 5A) as others have reported [25,26]. Based on our results, it is possible that Panx2 may have an intracellular channel function in the ER, similar to the proposed calcium-leak channels formed by Panx1 and Panx3 [6].

In some instances, Panx2 distribution exhibited limited cell surface localization that was more apparent when higher endogenous or ectopic Panx1 protein was expressed in the studied cell lines. This is consistent with our previous observation of increased Panx2 at the cell surface when co-expressed with Panx1 under overexpression conditions [22]. Here, we used three different cells lines with varying levels of endogenous Panx1 and a different capacity of protein production. We noticed that in cells with low endogenous Panx1 (e.g., NRKs), there was barely any Panx2 at the cell surface based on immunolabeling and cell surface biotinylation pull-downs. In the case of AD293 and HEK293T cells, it was possible to detect low levels of overexpressed Panx2 at the cell surface, while the mutant Panx2 (N86Q) had a detectable but significantly decreased presence only at the cell membrane of HEK293T cells. This result could be attributed to the increased protein expression in HEK293T cells that contains the SV40 T-antigen and have high transfection efficiency. This feature might have allowed the overexpressed Panx2 to bypass mechanisms of protein quality control resulting in more Panx2 trafficking to the plasma membrane [43].

Further research is needed to evaluate endogenous Panx2 in terms of N-glycosylation and subcellular localization of its isoforms, and to examine if Panx2 can form channels at the plasma membrane under physiological conditions. To date, limited studies have attempted to evaluate the Panx2 channel function [14,15] and several factors make it difficult to test Panx2 channel activity, such as its intracellular localization, the lack of evidence of in vivo functional channel formation [27] and the unknown mechanisms of activation [14].

Work done by Bruzzone et al. [15], showed that Panx1 and Panx2 were abundantly expressed in the CNS, and co-injection of both pannexin RNAs in paired *Xenopus* oocytes resulted in the formation of heteromeric channels with functional characteristics different from those formed by Panx1 monomers but with similar pharmacological sensitivity [27]. Ambrosi et al. [14] suggested that Panx1/Panx2 heteromeric channels tend to be unstable and they attributed that to differences in monomers size and oligomeric symmetry between these two pannexins. We have previously shown that Panx1 and Panx2 do form a complex as determined by co-IP experiments. Interestingly, when both pannexins are co-expressed, the level of interaction between Panx2 and glycosylated-species of Panx1 is dependent of the glycosylation of the latter [22]. Here, we showed in vitro, that the Panx2 glycosylation-deficient mutant can readily form complexes with Panx1, thus Panx2 glycosylation is not required for intermixing of the two pannexins. In fact, although it was not statistically significant, N86Q seemed to pull-down Panx1 more efficiently than the WT Panx2. However, in confocal images the N86Q aggregates did not show higher overlap with Panx1-immunolabeling than Panx2 WT. Consistent with our previous report [22], complex N-glycosylation of Panx1 hinders their interaction, since both Panx2 and N86Q interacted only with the Gly-0 and Gly-1 forms of Panx1. Taken together, these results suggest that in an ectopic expression system, glycosylation of Panx2 is not required for Panx1/Panx2 intermixing, but it does help with the transport of Panx2 to the cell surface, which is also increased by the presence of Panx1.

Finally, we propose that N-glycosylation of pannexins is an important post-translational modification that partially regulates their subcellular localization. Whether N-glycosylation represents a post-translational mechanism that regulates trafficking and Panx1/Panx2 interactions in vivo would be important questions to address in future studies. In cells where both pannexins are co-expressed, glycosylation may act as a form of regulation defining whether these channels will serve as intracellular or plasma membrane channels with different physiological and pathological functions.

4. Materials and Methods

4.1. Cell Lines, Constructs and Transient Transfections

Media, supplements and reagents were obtained from GIBCO® and Invitrogen™ (Carlsbad, CA, USA). Normal rat kidney (NRK) (ATCC® CRL-6509™) and human embryonic kidney cells (HEK293T) (ATCC® CRL-3216™) were obtained from ATCC (Manassas, VA, USA). Adherent HEK293 cells (AD293, Cat# 240085) were obtained from Agilent Technologies, Inc. (Santa Clara, CA, USA). Cell cultures were grown in high-glucose DMEM supplemented with 10% fetal bovine serum (FBS), 100 U/mL penicillin, 100 μg/mL streptomycin and 2mM L-Glutamine. At ~50% of confluency, cells were transfected adding Lipofectamine 3000 (Invitrogen™) following manufacturer directions. 2 μg of pcDNA3.1 (Invitrogen™) plasmids encoding mouse Panx2 [22] or Panx2^{N86Q} or their respective FLAG-tagged versions were used for transfections in 35 mm culture plates. After 48 h for single transfections and 72 h for co-transfections, proteins were extracted, and expression levels were determined by Western blot. For co-transfections experiments with mPanx1 plasmid [11], levels were reduced to 0.5 μg of DNA.

4.2. Mutagenesis and Cloning of New FLAG-Tagged Panx2 Constructs

As described previously [11], Panx2 has a predicted N-glycosylation consensus site located at asparagine (N) 86 on the first extracellular loop. Site-directed mutagenesis service (NorClone Biotech Labs, London, ON, Canada) was used to generate a new expression Panx2 construct encoding a replacement of asparagine by glutamine at position 86, referred to as Panx2 N86Q. FLAG-tagged Panx2 was obtained by inserting a single FLAG sequence with In-Fusion HD Cloning Kit (Clontech Laboratories, Inc., Takara Bio, Inc., Mountain View, CA, USA) at the end of the coding region of the Panx2 C-termini. Primers used for FLAG insertion were Forward: 5′-GTTTAAACTTAAGCTTCATGCACCACCTCCTGGAG-3′ and Reverse: 5′-GCCCTCTAGACTCGAGCTCACTTGTCATCGTCGTCCTTGTAATCAAACTCCACAGTACT-3′. All the constructs were verified by sequencing.

4.3. Protein Extractions and Western Blots

For co-immunoprecipitation (Co-IP) assays, cell lysates were obtained using a Triton-based extraction buffer (IP buffer) (1% Triton X-100, 150 mM NaCl, 10 mM Tris, 1 mM EDTA, 1 mM EGTA, 0.5% NP-40). The rest of the protein extractions were performed with SDS-based buffer (RIPA buffer) (0.1% SDS, 50 mM Tris-HCl, pH 8.0, 150 mM NaCl, 1% NP-40 and 0.5% Sodium Deoxycholate). In each case, lysis buffers were complemented with a final concentration of 1 mM NaF, 1 mM Na_3VO_4, and one tablet of cOmplete™-mini, EDTA-free Protease Inhibitor Cocktail (Roche, Mannheim, Germany). Total protein concentrations were quantitated with Pierce™ BCA Protein Assay Kit (Thermo Scientific, Rockford, IL, USA). For Western Blots, 50 μg of total protein were resolved in 8% SDS-PAGE and transferred onto nitrocellulose membranes using an iBlot™ Blotting System (Invitrogen, Carlsbad, CA, USA). Membranes were blocked with 3% bovine serum albumin (BSA, Burlington, ON, Canada) and 0.05% Tween 20-Phosphate Buffer Saline (T-PBS) for 45 min at room temperature and probed overnight with a 1:1000 dilution of the rabbit affinity-purified antibodies anti-Panx2-CT-523 [22]. Mouse monoclonal anti-FLAG® M2 (Sigma, St. Louis, MO, USA, Cat# F3165), monoclonal mouse anti-GAPDH (Millipore, Burlington, MA, USA, Cat# MAB374, RRID: AB_2107445), and anti-α-Tubulin (Millipore-Sigma Cat# 05-829, clone DM1A) antibodies were used at 1:2000, 1:1000 and 1:5000 dilutions, respectively. For detection, IRDye-800 and -680RD (Life Technologies™, Carlsbad, CA, USA) were used as secondary antibodies at 1:10,000 dilution and the membranes were scanned on a Li-Cor Odyssey infrared system (Li-Cor, Lincoln, NL, USA). In most cases, GAPDH was used as a loading control.

4.4. Immunofluorescence, Confocal Imaging, Linescans and Colocalization Analysis

Cells were grown on coverslips at ~70% of confluency and were transfected as described previously in Section 4.1. After 48 h of transfection, coverslips were washed with D-PBS (Gibco®) and fixed with ice-cold 80% methanol and 20% acetone for 15 min at 4 °C. Coverslips were blocked with 2% BSA-PBS for 1h and primary antibodies were used diluted in blocking buffer as follows: polyclonal anti-Panx2-CT (2 mg/mL, 1:100 dilution), polyclonal anti-Panx1-CT (1 mg/mL, 1:100 dilution), anti-PDI monoclonal antibody (1 mg/mL, 1:400 dilution) (1D3, Enzo® Life Sciences, Burlington, ON, Canada, ADI-SPA-891-D), cis-Golgi marker anti-GM130 (1 mg/mL, 1:300) (Abcam, Toronto, ON, Canada, Prod#: ab169276), anti-FLAG® M2 (1 mg/mL, 1:500) (F3165, Sigma, St. Louis, MO, USA), mouse monoclonal anti-Lamp-2 (1 mg/mL, 1:300) (DHSB, clone H4B4). Coverslips were incubated with primary antibodies for 1 h at room temperature, then washed with PBS and incubated with the secondary antibodies: Alexa Fluor 488 goat anti-rabbit IgG (2 mg/mL, 1:700) or goat anti-mouse antibody Alexa Fluor 647 (2 mg/mL, 1:400) (Life Technologies), that were selected to avoid bleed-through between dyes. Mitochondrial labeling was performed by using MitoTracker™ Red CMXRos (M7512, Thermofisher, Life Technologies, Eugene, OR, USA) as per manufacturer directions, and cells were fixed with freshly prepared paraformaldehyde (4%) and then permeabilized with 0.1% Triton X-100 before the blocking step. Coverslips were rinsed with PBS followed by water once and counterstained with Hoechst 33342 (H3570, Life Technologies™, Eugene, OR, USA) (1:1000, in water) for 5 min to stain nuclei and then were mounted with the custom-made Airvol mounting medium. Imaging was performed with an LSM 800 Confocal Microscope (Carl Zeiss, Oberkochen, Germany) using a Plan-Apochromat 63x/1.40 Oil DIC objective (Carl Zeiss, Oberkochen, Germany). Image acquisition for colocalization was performed with sequential laser scanning and with the multitracking feature of the Zeiss software with settings to avoid wrong excitation-crosstalk and bleed-through of the channels. Colocalization was quantitated with the colocalization plug-in of the Zeiss software (ZEN, version 2.3, blue edition). Regions of interest (ROI) were drawn in dual-labeled cells selecting individual cells expressing Panx2 or the mutant and co-stained with organelle markers. Controls of single-labeled cells were used to determine thresholds of intensities for each single channel and a manual thresholding was used to determine the region of pixels colocalized in the intensities scatterplots. Pearson correlation coefficient was determined for each cell as a measure of colocalization and was expressed as means $\pm$ S.E.M., representative of at least three independent transfections. Linescans using Zeiss software tool were used to detect overlaps of fluorescence peaks in cells co-transfected with Panx1.

4.5. Cell Surface Biotinylation Assays

Cell surface biotinylation assays were performed as described in Reference [22]. Briefly, cells were grown in 60 mm plates and used for biotinylation 72 h following transfection with Panx2 or N86Q constructs. After, culture media was aspirated, the cell monolayer was rinsed twice with ice-cold D-PBS supplemented with Ca^{2+} and Mg^{2+} (Gibco®). Then, cells were incubated only with D-PBS (non-labeling as a negative control) or with a solution of 1.5 mg/mL EZ-Link™ Sulfo-NHS-SS-Biotin (Thermo Scientific, Rockford, IL, USA) in D-PBS for 30 min on ice and covered from light. Plates were washed once again with D-PBS and then incubated with 100 mM glycine dissolved in D-PBS for 30 min to quench the remaining labeling biotin washed once more with D-PBS. Lysates were prepared using RIPA buffer as described before. For pull-down of cell surface biotinylated proteins, 250 µg of total protein was incubated overnight with 50% slurry of 50 µL NeutrAvidin agarose beads (Thermo Scientific, Rockford, IL, USA). Samples from lysates and initial flow-through wash were collected, the beads were spun down (at 500× *g*, 4 °C) and then washed three times with RIPA buffer. The samples and the beads were then mixed with 2X Laemmli buffer and 10% β-mercaptoethanol and placed at 95 °C in heat block for 5 min. 50 µg of total protein from lysates and the beads supernatant were resolved in parallel with 8% SDS-PAGE gel and then transferred to nitrocellulose membranes as previously described. PDI or GAPDH were used as controls of non-specific biotinylation of intracellular/cytoplasmic proteins and E-cadherin was used as positive control of cell surface protein.

4.6. Co-Immunoprecipitation (Co-IP) Assays

Co-immunoprecipitation (Co-IP) of protein complexes was performed at 4 °C by incubating overnight 1 mg of total protein from pre-cleared (with Protein A/G beads alone) lysates with 5 µg/mL of rabbit polyclonal anti-Panx2-CT or anti-Panx1-CT affinity-purified antibody crosslinked to Pierce Protein A/G-Agarose beads (Thermo Scientific); the same amount of beads (~30 µL) were used for IP in each case. Control experiments to evaluate unspecific binding to the beads were performed in parallel using beads with no antibody. To remove un-bound proteins, four washes with 500 µL of ice-cold IP buffer were performed. Then, beads were dried by aspiration and re-suspended in 2X Laemmli buffer (10% (*v:v*) β-mercaptoethanol), boiled for 5 min, spun down and the supernatants (IP samples) were used for WB. For WB analysis, 50 µg of protein of each lysate was loaded into the INPUT lanes and ran along with the IP samples. The intensities of the bands in each lane were obtained by densitometry and were used for quantitation.

4.7. De-Glycosylation Assays

Lysates from HEK293T cells ectopically expressing mouse Panx2 and the N86Q were used for validation of N-glycosylation site of the mouse Panx2 construct. Enzymatic de-glycosylation with Peptide-N-glycosidase F (PNGase F) and Endoglycosidase H (EndoH) were used to detect the presence of all complex forms of N-glycosylation and high-mannose modification, respectively. PNGase F (Roche, Indianapolis, IN, USA) and EndoH (New England Biolabs Ipswich, MA, USA) digestions were performed according to their manufacturer's instructions. Briefly, at least 35 µg of total protein was denatured at 100 °C for 5 min in denaturing buffer (0.1% (*v*/*v*) SDS, 0.05 M 2-mercaptoethanol, 50 mM phosphate buffer, pH 7.5) and subsequently incubated for 1h at 37 °C with 10 units of the PNGase F, 0.7% (*v*/*v*) of Triton X-100 or 2500 U of Endo H in supplier's digestion buffer. In the parallel control, samples were assayed without endoglycosidases. Protein samples were separated on an 8% SDS-polyacrylamide gel electrophoresis gel (PAGE) and transferred to nitrocellulose membranes for WB.

4.8. Densitometric Analysis of Western Blots

Densitometry analysis was performed in the Odyssey Application Software Version 3.0.16 (LI-COR Biosciences, Lincoln, NL, USA) as follows: For cell surface biotinylation experiments, the fraction of biotinylated-protein detected at the cell surface was calculated using the integrated intensity (I.I.) of protein bands detected in the Neutravidin lanes divided by the I.I. of protein bands detected in their corresponding input-lysate lanes. For Co-IP experiments, quantitative analysis was performed by calculating the ratio of the I.I detected for Co-IP protein divided by the I.I of the IP-target protein. Quantitation results were expressed as means ± S.E.M. representative of at least three independent experiments.

4.9. Statistics

Statistical analysis was performed using the statistical package of GraphPad Prism® Ver. 5.03 (GraphPad Software, Inc., San Diego, CA, USA). Cell surface biotinylation data were analyzed with non-parametric Mann-Whitney U test for unpaired data. Data derived from quantitation of Co-IP assays and colocalization were analyzed with a two-tailed unpaired t test with Welch's correction. A probability of $p < 0.05$ was considered as statistically significant.

Author Contributions: R.E.S.-P. devised and performed the experiments, analysis of data. R.E.S.-P. and S.P. wrote the manuscript. D.J., assisted on the design of mutagenesis, and provided technical help in immunostaining and imaging and revised the manuscript. S.P. designed the original project, devised experiments, served as scientific advisor and provided critical revision of results and manuscript.

Abbreviations

AD293	Adherent human embryonic kidney cells
ATP	Adenosine triphosphate nucleotide
CNS	Central nervous system
Co-IP	Co-immunoprecipitation
Endo H	Endoglycosidase H
ER	Endoplasmic reticulum
GAPDH	Glyceraldehyde 3-phosphate dehydrogenase
GM130	Golgi matrix protein 130 kDa
HEK293T	Human embryonic kidney cells with SV40 T-antigen
IP	Immunoprecipitation

LAMP2	Lysosome-associated membrane glycoprotein 2
NPC	Neural progenitor cells
NRK	Normal rat kidney cells
PDI	Protein disulfide isomerase
PNGase F	Peptide-N-glycosidase F
PTM	Posttranslational modification
SV40	Simian vacuolating virus 40

References

1. Sosinsky, G.E.; Boassa, D.; Dermietzel, R.; Duffy, H.S.; Laird, D.W.; MacVicar, B.; Naus, C.C.; Penuela, S.; Scemes, E.; Spray, D.C.; et al. Pannexin channels are not gap junction hemichannels. *Channels* **2011**, *5*, 193–197. [CrossRef] [PubMed]
2. Panchin, Y.; Kelmanson, I.; Matz, M.; Lukyanov, K.; Usman, N.; Lukyanov, S. A ubiquitous family of putative gap junction molecules. *Curr. Biol.* **2000**, *10*, R473–R474. [CrossRef]
3. Bao, L.; Locovei, S.; Dahl, G. Pannexin membrane channels are mechanosensitive conduits for atp. *FEBS Lett.* **2004**, *572*, 65–68. [CrossRef] [PubMed]
4. Iwamoto, T.; Nakamura, T.; Doyle, A.; Ishikawa, M.; de Vega, S.; Fukumoto, S.; Yamada, Y. Pannexin 3 regulates intracellular atp/camp levels and promotes chondrocyte differentiation. *J. Biol. Chem.* **2010**, *285*, 18948–18958. [CrossRef] [PubMed]
5. Ishikawa, M.; Iwamoto, T.; Nakamura, T.; Doyle, A.; Fukumoto, S.; Yamada, Y. Pannexin 3 functions as an er $Ca^{(2+)}$ channel, hemichannel, and gap junction to promote osteoblast differentiation. *J. Cell Biol.* **2011**, *193*, 1257–1274. [CrossRef] [PubMed]
6. Vanden Abeele, F.; Bidaux, G.; Gordienko, D.; Beck, B.; Panchin, Y.V.; Baranova, A.V.; Ivanov, D.V.; Skryma, R.; Prevarskaya, N. Functional implications of calcium permeability of the channel formed by pannexin 1. *J. Cell Boil.* **2006**, *174*, 535–546. [CrossRef] [PubMed]
7. Thompson, R.J. Pannexin channels and ischaemia. *J. Physiol.* **2015**, *593*, 3463–3470. [CrossRef] [PubMed]
8. Pelegrin, P.; Surprenant, A. Pannexin-1 couples to maitotoxin- and nigericin-induced interleukin-1beta release through a dye uptake-independent pathway. *J. Biol. Chem.* **2007**, *282*, 2386–2394. [CrossRef] [PubMed]
9. Baranova, A.; Ivanov, D.; Petrash, N.; Pestova, A.; Skoblov, M.; Kelmanson, I.; Shagin, D.; Nazarenko, S.; Geraymovych, E.; Litvin, O.; et al. The mammalian pannexin family is homologous to the invertebrate innexin gap junction proteins. *Genomics* **2004**, *83*, 706–716. [CrossRef] [PubMed]
10. Le Vasseur, M.; Lelowski, J.; Bechberger, J.F.; Sin, W.C.; Naus, C.C. Pannexin 2 protein expression is not restricted to the cns. *Front. Cell. Neurosci.* **2014**, *8*, 392. [CrossRef] [PubMed]
11. Penuela, S.; Bhalla, R.; Gong, X.-Q.; Cowan, K.N.; Celetti, S.J.; Cowan, B.J.; Bai, D.; Shao, Q.; Laird, D.W. Pannexin 1 and pannexin 3 are glycoproteins that exhibit many distinct characteristics from the connexin family of gap junction proteins. *J. Cell Sci.* **2007**, *120*, 3772–3783. [CrossRef] [PubMed]
12. Celetti, S.J.; Cowan, K.N.; Penuela, S.; Shao, Q.; Churko, J.; Laird, D.W. Implications of pannexin 1 and pannexin 3 for keratinocyte differentiation. *J. Cell Sci.* **2010**, *123*, 1363–1372. [CrossRef] [PubMed]
13. Bond, S.R.; Lau, A.; Penuela, S.; Sampaio, A.V.; Underhill, T.M.; Laird, D.W.; Naus, C.C. Pannexin 3 is a novel target for runx2, expressed by osteoblasts and mature growth plate chondrocytes. *J. Bone Min. Res.* **2011**, *26*, 2911–2922. [CrossRef] [PubMed]
14. Ambrosi, C.; Gassmann, O.; Pranskevich, J.N.; Boassa, D.; Smock, A.; Wang, J.; Dahl, G.; Steinem, C.; Sosinsky, G.E. Pannexin1 and pannexin2 channels show quaternary similarities to connexons and different oligomerization numbers from each other. *J. Biol. Chem.* **2010**, *285*, 24420–24431. [CrossRef] [PubMed]
15. Bruzzone, R.; Hormuzdi, S.G.; Barbe, M.T.; Herb, A.; Monyer, H. Pannexins, a family of gap junction proteins expressed in brain. *Proc. Natl. Acad. Sci. USA* **2003**, *100*, 13644–13649. [CrossRef] [PubMed]
16. Swayne, L.A.; Bennett, S.A. Connexins and pannexins in neuronal development and adult neurogenesis. *BMC Cell Biol.* **2016**, *17* (Suppl. S1), 10. [CrossRef] [PubMed]

17. Swayne, L.A.; Sorbara, C.D.; Bennett, S.A. Pannexin 2 is expressed by postnatal hippocampal neural progenitors and modulates neuronal commitment. *J. Biol. Chem.* **2010**, *285*, 24977–24986. [CrossRef] [PubMed]
18. Vogt, A.; Hormuzdi, S.G.; Monyer, H. Pannexin1 and pannexin2 expression in the developing and mature rat brain. *Brain Res. Mol. Brain Res.* **2005**, *141*, 113–120. [CrossRef] [PubMed]
19. Bargiotas, P.; Krenz, A.; Monyer, H.; Schwaninger, M. Functional outcome of pannexin-deficient mice after cerebral ischemia. *Channels* **2012**, *6*, 453–456. [CrossRef] [PubMed]
20. Blom, N.; Sicheritz-Ponten, T.; Gupta, R.; Gammeltoft, S.; Brunak, S. Prediction of post-translational glycosylation and phosphorylation of proteins from the amino acid sequence. *Proteomics* **2004**, *4*, 1633–1649. [CrossRef] [PubMed]
21. Penuela, S.; Lohman, A.W.; Lai, W.; Gyenis, L.; Litchfield, D.W.; Isakson, B.E.; Laird, D.W. Diverse post-translational modifications of the pannexin family of channel-forming proteins. *Channels* **2014**, *8*, 124–130. [CrossRef] [PubMed]
22. Penuela, S.; Bhalla, R.; Nag, K.; Laird, D.W. Glycosylation regulates pannexin intermixing and cellular localization. *Mol. Boil. Cell* **2009**, *20*, 4313–4323. [CrossRef] [PubMed]
23. Zappalà, A.; Li Volti, G.; Serapide, M.F.; Pellitteri, R.; Falchi, M.; La Delia, F.; Cicirata, V.; Cicirata, F. Expression of pannexin2 protein in healthy and ischemized brain of adult rats. *Neuroscience* **2007**, *148*, 653–667. [CrossRef] [PubMed]
24. Lai, C.P.K.; Bechberger, J.F.; Naus, C.C. Pannexin2 as a novel growth regulator in c6 glioma cells. *Oncogene* **2009**, *28*, 4402–4408. [CrossRef] [PubMed]
25. Wicki-Stordeur, L.E.; Boyce, A.K.J.; Swayne, L.A. Analysis of a pannexin 2-pannexin 1 chimeric protein supports divergent roles for pannexin c-termini in cellular localization. *Cell Commun. Adhes.* **2013**, *20*, 73–79. [CrossRef] [PubMed]
26. Boassa, D.; Nguyen, P.; Hu, J.; Ellisman, M.H.; Sosinsky, G.E. Pannexin2 oligomers localize in the membranes of endosomal vesicles in mammalian cells while pannexin1 channels traffic to the plasma membrane. *Front. Cell. Neurosci.* **2015**, *8*, 15. [CrossRef] [PubMed]
27. Bruzzone, R.; Barbe, M.T.; Jakob, N.J.; Monyer, H. Pharmacological properties of homomeric and heteromeric pannexin hemichannels expressed in xenopus oocytes. *J. Neurochem.* **2005**, *92*, 1033–1043. [CrossRef] [PubMed]
28. Bruzzone, R.; Dermietzel, R. Structure and function of gap junctions in the developing brain. *Cell. Tissue Res.* **2006**, *326*, 239–248. [CrossRef] [PubMed]
29. Dvoriantchikova, G.; Ivanov, D.; Panchin, Y.; Shestopalov, V.I. Expression of pannexin family of proteins in the retina. *FEBS Lett.* **2006**, *580*, 2178–2182. [CrossRef] [PubMed]
30. Tang, W.; Ahmad, S.; Shestopalov, V.I.; Lin, X. Pannexins are new molecular candidates for assembling gap junctions in the cochlea. *Neuroreport* **2008**, *19*, 1253–1257. [CrossRef] [PubMed]
31. Bargiotas, P.; Krenz, A.; Hormuzdi, S.G.; Ridder, D.A.; Herb, A.; Barakat, W.; Penuela, S.; von Engelhardt, J.; Monyer, H.; Schwaninger, M. Pannexins in ischemia-induced neurodegeneration. *Proc. Natl. Acad. Sci. USA* **2011**, *108*, 20772–20777. [CrossRef] [PubMed]
32. Penuela, S.; Celetti, S.J.; Bhalla, R.; Shao, Q.; Laird, D.W. Diverse subcellular distribution profiles of pannexin 1 and pannexin 3. *Cell. Commun. Adhes.* **2008**, *15*, 133–142. [CrossRef] [PubMed]
33. DuBridge, R.B.; Tang, P.; Hsia, H.C.; Leong, P.M.; Miller, J.H.; Calos, M.P. Analysis of mutation in human cells by using an epstein-barr virus shuttle system. *Mol. Cell. Biol.* **1987**, *7*, 379–387. [CrossRef] [PubMed]
34. Penuela, S.; Harland, L.; Simek, J.; Laird, D.W. Pannexin channels and their links to human disease. *Biochem. J.* **2014**, *461*, 371–381. [CrossRef] [PubMed]
35. Bhalla-Gehi, R.; Penuela, S.; Churko, J.M.; Shao, Q.; Laird, D.W. Pannexin1 and pannexin3 delivery, cell surface dynamics, and cytoskeletal interactions. *J. Biol. Chem.* **2010**, *285*, 9147–9160. [CrossRef] [PubMed]
36. Boassa, D.; Ambrosi, C.; Qiu, F.; Dahl, G.; Gaietta, G.; Sosinsky, G. Pannexin1 channels contain a glycosylation site that targets the hexamer to the plasma membrane. *J. Boil. Chem.* **2007**, *282*, 31733–31743. [CrossRef] [PubMed]
37. Boassa, D.; Qiu, F.; Dahl, G.; Sosinsky, G. Trafficking dynamics of glycosylated pannexin 1 proteins. *Cell Commun. Adhes.* **2008**, *15*, 119–132. [CrossRef] [PubMed]

38. Hiramatsu, N.; Joseph, V.T.; Lin, J.H. Monitoring and manipulating mammalian unfolded protein response. *Methods Enzymol.* **2011**, *491*, 183–198. [PubMed]
39. Penuela, S.; Laird, D.W. The cellular life of pannexins. *Wiley Interdiscip. Rev. Membr. Transp. Signal. Banner* **2012**, *1*, 621–632. [CrossRef]
40. Nakamura, N.; Rabouille, C.; Watson, R.; Nilsson, T.; Hui, N.; Slusarewicz, P.; Kreis, T.E.; Warren, G. Characterization of a cis-golgi matrix protein, gm130. *J. Cell Biol.* **1995**, *131*, 1715–1726. [CrossRef] [PubMed]
41. Nakamura, N. Emerging new roles of gm130, a cis-golgi matrix protein, in higher order cell functions. *J. Pharmacol. Sci.* **2010**, *112*, 255–264. [CrossRef] [PubMed]
42. Boyce, A.K.; Prager, R.T.; Wicki-Stordeur, L.E.; Swayne, L.A. Pore positioning: Current concepts in pannexin channel trafficking. *Channels* **2014**, *8*, 110–117. [CrossRef] [PubMed]
43. Chen, B.; Retzlaff, M.; Roos, T.; Frydman, J. Cellular strategies of protein quality control. *Cold Spring Harb. Perspect. Biol.* **2011**, *3*, a004374. [CrossRef] [PubMed]

3

Cellular and Molecular Mechanisms in the Pathogenesis of Classical, Vascular and Hypermobile Ehlers-Danlos Syndromes

Nicola Chiarelli, Marco Ritelli, Nicoletta Zoppi and Marina Colombi *

Division of Biology and Genetics, Department of Molecular and Translational Medicine, University of Brescia, 25121 Brescia, Italy

* Correspondence: marina.colombi@unibs.it

Abstract: The Ehlers-Danlos syndromes (EDS) constitute a heterogenous group of connective tissue disorders characterized by joint hypermobility, skin abnormalities, and vascular fragility. The latest nosology recognizes 13 types caused by pathogenic variants in genes encoding collagens and other molecules involved in collagen processing and extracellular matrix (ECM) biology. Classical (cEDS), vascular (vEDS), and hypermobile (hEDS) EDS are the most frequent types. cEDS and vEDS are caused respectively by defects in collagen V and collagen III, whereas the molecular basis of hEDS is unknown. For these disorders, the molecular pathology remains poorly studied. Herein, we review, expand, and compare our previous transcriptome and protein studies on dermal fibroblasts from cEDS, vEDS, and hEDS patients, offering insights and perspectives in their molecular mechanisms. These cells, though sharing a pathological ECM remodeling, show differences in the underlying pathomechanisms. In cEDS and vEDS fibroblasts, key processes such as collagen biosynthesis/processing, protein folding quality control, endoplasmic reticulum homeostasis, autophagy, and wound healing are perturbed. In hEDS cells, gene expression changes related to cell-matrix interactions, inflammatory/pain responses, and acquisition of an in vitro pro-inflammatory myofibroblast-like phenotype may contribute to the complex pathogenesis of the disorder. Finally, emerging findings from miRNA profiling of hEDS fibroblasts are discussed to add some novel biological aspects about hEDS etiopathogenesis.

Keywords: autophagy; collagen III; collagen V; Ehlers-Danlos syndrome; endoplasmic reticulum; extracellular matrix; fibroblast-to-myofibroblast transition; miRNA; transcriptome; wound healing

---

1. The Extracellular Matrix: An Overview

Connective tissues have an extracellular matrix (ECM) with a specific composition generated during embryogenesis and maintained in adult life. The ECM is a complex network that provides a structural scaffold to the surrounding cells and is a reservoir of bioactive molecules such as cytokines and growth factors that control cell behavior [1]. The main ECM components include proteoglycans, hyaluronic acid, adhesive glycoproteins such as fibronectin and laminins, and fibrous proteins like collagens and elastin [2]. Matricellular proteins such as thrombospondins, osteopontin, periostin, and tenascins are non-structural ECM proteins, primarily acting as mediators of cell–matrix interactions, which are abundantly expressed during embryonic development, wound healing, and tissues renewal [3].

The human matrisome consists of about 300 macromolecules comprising the "core matrisome", which is composed of many different collagens, proteoglycans (e.g., aggrecan, versican, perlecan, and decorin), and glycoproteins (e.g., laminins, elastin, fibronectin, thrombospondins, and tenascins) [4]. Matrisome also includes many matrisome-associated proteins and ECM-regulators, i.e., ECM-cross-linking (e.g., lysyl oxidases, transglutaminases) and ECM-modifying enzymes (e.g., proteases and their inhibitors) together with secreted factors including transforming growth factor β (TGFβ), wingless integrated (Wnt), and multiple cytokines [5].

Collagens represent the major ECM structural components and play a central role in providing the structural integrity of several connective tissues (e.g., cartilage and bone) and various organ systems including skin, lungs, blood vessels, and cornea. Collagens are also involved in cell adhesion, chemotaxis, and migration [1,2]. The dynamic interplay between cells and collagens regulates tissue remodeling during growth, differentiation, morphogenesis, and wound healing [6,7]. The common molecular feature of collagens is their triple helical structure, which consists of three collagenous α-chains with the typical recurring $(Gly\text{-}Xaa\text{-}Yaa)_n$ tripeptide sequence. The presence of glycine residues in the collagenous domain is essential for stability and correct assembly of the triple helix. Collagen biosynthesis, assembly, and maturation require a sequence of well-controlled intracellular and extracellular events (for review see [8,9]). Collagen I is the most abundant type expressed in bone, cornea, dermis, and tendon. Collagen III is primarily present in the tunica media of the blood vessels and hollow organs (e.g., uterus, intestine). Collagen V is widely distributed, especially in dermis, tendons, and muscles, playing a central role in collagen I fibrillogenesis [9]. These fibrillar collagens form structures necessary to ensure the strength and structural integrity of the ECM of all connective tissues and organs of the body [10].

Fibronectin is a dimeric and fibrillar glycoprotein ubiquitously organized in the ECM of all tissues and is also present in soluble form in the plasma. Cellular fibronectin self-assembles in fibers and binds collagens, fibrin, proteoglycans, and cell surface receptors, providing cell growth, adhesion, and migration. During wound healing, it forms a provisional matrix with fibrin and enters in the granulation tissue formation in the late phase of re-epithelization [11].

In addition to ensuring physical support and structural integrity, the proper ECM composition and organization are crucial for cell health. ECM undergoes a continuous turnover either under physiological or in pathological circumstances, and its homeostasis is critical for connective tissues architecture and function [12,13]. Integrins are specific cell surface receptors that mediate the complex cell-matrix interactions. These bridging molecules, which are heterodimeric transmembrane receptors containing α and β subunits, connect ECM to cytoskeleton by interacting via their extracellular domain with collagens and other matrix molecules and via their cytoplasmic tails with cytoskeleton components (e.g., actin, vinculin, talin, paxillin), thus mediating cell adhesion and motility [14,15].

2. Pathological ECM Remodeling and Perturbation of Cellular Homeostasis

Cell-matrix interaction via integrins is crucial for cell survival and tissue homeostasis. Prolonged loss of integrin-mediated cell–ECM adhesion leads to anoikis [16]. Under physiological conditions, ECM detachment triggers anti-apoptotic signals as a cell survival mechanism to delay the onset of anoikis. One of such signaling pathways is autophagy, which is a highly conserved cellular catabolic process that promotes homeostasis and mitigates the stress due to ECM detachment [17]. Autophagy is essential for cellular maintenance and homeostasis by promoting the turnover of macromolecules and organelles via the lysosomal degradative pathway [18]. Physiological and pathological changes in the ECM composition play a crucial role in modulating autophagy activity [19,20]. For instance, deficiency of collagen VI, which is associated with a spectrum of different myopathic conditions, perturbs ECM architecture, impairs the autophagic flux, and activates pro-apoptotic signals [21]. Autophagy, in turn, contributes to the maintenance of endoplasmic reticulum (ER) function by mediating its turnover through the autophagic sequestration of ER fragments into autophagosomes, the so-called ER-phagy process [22].

ECM components also modulate immune cell migration into inflamed tissues and their activation and proliferation [23]. The stimulation of the innate immunity results from the recognition of specific mediators, namely pattern recognition receptors, which, in turn, recognize molecules, referred as danger-associated molecular patterns, which are released from damaged tissues [24]. It is well documented that different ECM components or their fragments including the fibronectin 1 extra domain

A, one of the alternative spliced regions of fibronectin encoding gene, tenascin-C, fibrinogen, and several proteoglycans, serve as danger signals and trigger immune responses following tissue damage or in response to pathological ECM remodeling [24,25]. In fibrotic conditions, increased ECM production, accumulation of ECM fragments, augmented secretion of cytokines, fibroblast-to-myofibroblast transition, and activation of immune responses, dependent on toll-like receptors, occur [26]. The regulation of ECM synthesis and remodeling is central for human health, as recognized in different heritable connective tissue disorders [1,27]. Indeed, molecular defects in a large range of ECM-related genes, including those encoding enzymes involved in biosynthesis or processing of ECM proteins, cause a myriad of connective tissue disorders, e.g., Ehlers–Danlos syndromes, Osteogenesis imperfecta, Marfan syndrome, Loeys–Dietz syndromes, arterial tortuosity syndrome, and numerous skeletal dysplasias [1,27]. These disorders are characterized by a multisystem involvement in terms of cardiovascular, skeletal, and cutaneous features [28], highlighting the functional relevance of the ECM in ensuring the integrity and function of several connective tissues.

The pathological consequences of defects in ECM components depend on the balance between extracellular effects, e.g., reduced protein secretion and export of misfolded proteins, and intracellular consequences such as apoptosis activation, ER dysfunction, and autophagy perturbation that impact in different ways on the molecular pathology and disease severity [27,29–31].

3. Ehlers-Danlos Syndromes

Ehlers-Danlos syndromes (EDS) represent a clinically and genetically heterogeneous group of conditions that share a variable combination of skin hyperextensibility, joint hypermobility, and internal organ and vessel fragility [32]. The 2017 international classification of the Ehlers-Danlos syndromes recognizes 13 subtypes, which are caused by pathogenic variants in 19 different genes, mainly encoding fibrillar collagens and collagens-modifying proteins [32]. EDS types are grouped based on the underlying genetic and pathogenetic mechanisms in disorders related to (i) collagens primary structure and processing (*COL1A1*, *COL1A2*, *COL3A1*, *COL5A1*, *COL5A2* and *ADAMTS2*), (ii) collagens folding and cross-linking (*PLOD1* and *FKBP14*), (iii) structure and function of the myomatrix, i.e., the specialized ECM of muscle (*TNXB* and *COL12A1*), (iv) glycosaminoglycans biosynthesis (*B4GALT7*, *B3GALT6*, *CHST14*, and *DSE*), (v) complement pathway (*C1S* and *C1R*), and (vi) intracellular processes (*SLC39A13*, *ZNF469*, and *PRDM5*). The classical (cEDS), vascular (vEDS) and the molecularly unsolved hypermobile (hEDS) EDS forms account for more than 90% of patients. Recently, a new and very rare EDS variant has been identified that is caused by biallelic mutations in the *AEBP1* gene (Table 1) [33–36].

The new nosology proposed for each subtype a set of major, minor, and minimal criteria addressing clinical suspicion for a specific EDS type and confirmatory molecular testing. For a comprehensive overview of all EDS forms see the landmark work by Malfait and colleagues [32].

The decrease in the tensile strength and integrity of skin, joints, and hollow organs is a common disease mechanism shared by the different EDS types [37]. This mechanical weakness is considered the driving factor of connective tissue fragility, even if it is likely that multiple cell-matrix interplays and involvement of distinct intracellular signaling pathways contribute to the molecular pathology of the different EDS phenotypes [38].

In the following chapters, we will review and expand the results derived from our previous transcriptome and in vitro studies on cEDS, vEDS, and hEDS patients' dermal fibroblasts. Taken together, these studies highlighted that the alteration of the ECM structural integrity is a common disease factor contributing to the pathogenesis of all these conditions.

Table 1. EDS types grouped according to the underlying genetic defect and pathomechanisms.

EDS Type	IP	Gene	Protein
Group A: disorders of collagen primary structure and collagen processing			
Classical EDS (cEDS)	AD	Major: *COL5A1*, *COL5A2* Rare: *COL1A1*	COLLV COLLI
Vascular EDS (vEDS)	AD	*COL3A1*	COLLIII
Arthrochalasia EDS (aEDS)	AD	*COL1A1*, *COL1A2*	COLLI
Dermatosparaxis EDS (dEDS)	AR	*ADAMTS2*	ADAMTS-2
Cardiac-valvular EDS (cvEDS)	AR	*COL1A2*	COLLI
Classical-like 2 EDS [A] (cl2EDS)	AR	*AEBP1*	ACLP
Group B: disorders of collagen folding and collagen cross-linking			
Kyphoscoliotic EDS (kEDS)	AR	*PLOD1* *FKBP14*	LH1 FKBP22
Group C: disorders of structure and function of myomatrix			
Classical-like EDS (clEDS) Myopathic EDS (mEDS)	AR AD/AR	*TNXB* *COL12A1*	Tenascin X COLLXII
Group D: disorders of glycosaminoglycan biosynthesis			
Spondylodysplastic EDS (spEDS)	AR	*B4GALT7* *B3GALT6*	β4GalT7 β3GalT6
Musculocontractural EDS (mcEDS)	AR	*CHST14* *DSE*	D4ST1 DSE
Group E: disorders of complement pathway			
Periodontal EDS (pEDS)	AD	*C1R* *C1S*	C1r C1s
Group F: disorders of intracellular processes			
Spondylodysplastic EDS (spEDS)	AR	*SLC39A13*	ZIP13
Brittle Cornea Syndrome (BCS)	AR	*ZNF469* *PRDM5*	ZNF469 PRDM5
EDS type molecularly unsolved			
Hypermobile EDS (hEDS)	AD	Unknown	Unknown

[A] New EDS variant recently defined in [33–36]. AD: autosomal dominant; AR: autosomal recessive; IP: inheritance pattern.

In cEDS and vEDS fibroblasts, the ECM disarray is a direct consequence of molecular defects in respectively collagen V and collagen III that impair common molecular functions essential to guarantee adequate folding and maturation of proteins and biological processes crucial for cell survival and homeostasis. The ECM disorganization observed in hEDS cells may be a consequence of an excessive pathological turnover, mainly due to ECM-degrading enzymes and other so far unknown factors, which might be primary contributors involved in the transition to a pro-inflammatory myofibroblast-like phenotype. Consistently, the perturbation of distinct transcriptional patterns observed in cEDS, vEDS, and hEDS fibroblasts pointed out different disease mechanisms underlying the pathophysiology of these EDS cell types.

Altogether, these insights represent a starting point for future investigations on the numerous pathobiological aspects underlying these conditions. An overview of the biological findings emerged from transcriptome and in vitro studies on dermal fibroblasts from cEDS, vEDS, and hEDS patients is summarized in Table 2.

Table 2. Overview of the biological processes dysregulated in cEDS, vEDS, and hEDS patients' dermal fibroblasts emerged from transcriptome and in vitro studies.

Insights in the Pathogenesis of cEDS, vEDS, and hEDS	Transcriptome Findings on Patients' Fibroblasts			In Vitro Studies on Patients' Fibroblasts		
Perturbed Biological Processes	**cEDS**	**vEDS**	**hEDS**	**cEDS**	**vEDS**	**hEDS**
ECM disorganization	+	+	+	+	+	+
Altered cell-matrix interactions	−	−	+	+	+	+
Disturbed cell-cell contacts	−	−	+	−	−	+
Fibroblast-to-myofibroblast transition	−	−	+	−	−	+
Altered inflammatory responses	+	−	+	−	na	+
Perturbed cell migration	+	+	−	+	+	+
Defective wound healing	+	+	−	+	na	na
Survival from anoikis	−	−	−	+	+	na
Collagens biosynthesis/processing	+	+	−	na	+	na
ER homeostasis/protein folding	+	+	−	na	+	na

+: detected by transcriptome or in vitro studies, −: not experimentally detected by transcriptome or in vitro studies, na: not ascertained.

4. Classical Ehlers-Danlos Syndrome

Classical EDS (cEDS, OMIM#130000) is characterized by marked skin involvement, generalized joint hypermobility, and abnormal wound healing [32,39]. Most patients harbor point mutations or chromosomal rearrangements in *COL5A1* or *COL5A2* genes encoding the collagen V [40,41]. This collagen is abundantly distributed in a variety of tissues as heterotrimers, which co-assemble with collagen I to form heterotypic fibrils [42].

Collagen V knockout mice synthesize and secrete normal amounts of collagen I, but collagen fibrils are absent, and the animals die at the onset of organogenesis, supporting the crucial role of collagen V for embryonic development [43].

Collagen V haploinsufficiency is the most common molecular defect caused by *COL5A1* null alleles, whereas rare *COL5A1* variants and the majority of *COL5A2* mutations reported so far affect collagen V structural integrity by exerting a dominant negative effect [40,41].

5. Altered ECM Turnover, Wound Healing, and Inflammation in cEDS Fibroblasts

Although the reduced availability of collagen V is crucial in the pathogenesis of cEDS, the molecular aspects contributing to the pathophysiology of the disorder remain poorly characterized. Our in vitro findings demonstrated that cEDS patients' fibroblasts show disassembly of many ECM components, including collagen V and III, fibronectin, and fibrillins, and disorganization of collagen- and fibronectin-specific $\alpha2\beta1$ and $\alpha5\beta1$ integrin receptors [44–47]. cEDS cells also exhibit a reduced in vitro migration capability, an abnormal wound healing response, and a crosstalk involving the $\alpha v\beta3$ integrin and epidermal growth factor (EGF) receptor that rescues them from anoikis [44–50]. In line with these in vitro findings, *Col5a1* and *Col5a2* deficient mice show a defective wound healing response and reduced cell migration [51,52].

Transcriptome profiling of cEDS fibroblasts added new insights into the complex molecular mechanisms involved in the maintenance of ECM homeostasis and proper wound healing, since patients' cells showed the dysregulated expression of many genes encoding matricellular and soluble proteins with prominent functions in cell proliferation and migration, collagen assembly and ECM remodeling during wound healing, i.e., *SPP1*, *POSTN*, *EDIL3*, *IGFBP2*, and *C3* [47]. Wound healing is a highly controlled multistep process involving several growth factors, cytokines, matrix metalloproteases, and cellular receptors, as well as proper crosstalk of different ECM constituents essential for ensuring tissue regeneration [53]. In addition to ECM glycoproteins and collagens, many other matricellular proteins including osteopontin, periostin, and tenascins are required for the formation of a provisional ECM during wound repair [54,55].

Osteopontin encoded by *SPP1*, which shows a decreased expression in patients' cells, is involved in several physiological processes related to inflammation, biomineralization, cell viability, and wound healing [56,57]. Through its interaction with the $\alpha v\beta 3$ integrin, osteopontin facilitates the adhesion of bone cells during bone tissue formation by stimulating a mineralized collagen ECM [58,59]. Finally, the functional role of osteopontin in the ECM reorganization during wound healing is crucial, since *Opn*-deficient mice show ECM disorganization and disassembly of collagen fibrils in the deep layers of wound sites [60].

In cEDS fibroblasts, the decreased expression of periostin encoded by *POSTN* may also contribute to the generalized ECM disarray and in vitro poor wound healing [44,48]. Indeed, periostin plays an important role in ECM structure and organization and particularly in collagen assembly, by acting as a scaffold protein for the bone morphogenetic protein 1, which facilities the proteolytic activation of lysyl oxidase that, in turn, catalyzes the covalent cross-link formation of collagens [61]. Consistently, *Postn*-deficient mice exhibit marked reduction of collagen cross-linking and increased levels of collagen fragments owing to proteolytic digestion [62,63]. Periostin also acts as a pro-survival protein in many cellular circumstances by interacting with $\alpha v\beta 3$ and $\alpha v\beta 5$ integrin receptors and mediating the activation of several intracellular signaling pathways [64]. In wound sites, it promotes activation of fibroblasts during wound contraction and stimulates collagen assembly and ECM reorganization [65,66]. *POSTN* not only shows a diminished expression in vEDS cells but also in dermal fibroblasts from patients with *FKBP14*-kEDS [67], further emphasizing the crucial role of periostin as a scaffold matricellular protein necessary for collagen assembly and ECM stability.

EDIL3 (EGF-like repeat- and discoidin I-like domain-containing protein 3), the most down-regulated transcript in cEDS fibroblasts, encodes an ECM-associated protein that promotes angiogenesis in vitro through binding to $\alpha v\beta 3$ and $\alpha v\beta 5$ integrins [68]. It stimulates cell migration and proliferation, mediates apoptotic cell phagocytosis, regulates neutrophil recruitment to the inflamed tissue, and prevents chondrocyte anoikis through its interaction with the $\alpha v\beta 3$ integrin [69–71].

IGFBP2 (insulin-like growth factor-binding protein 2), the most up-regulated gene in cEDS cells, enhances cell migration in different cell types through its binding to $\alpha v\beta 3$ and $\alpha 5\beta 1$ integrins [72,73]. Its high expression in cEDS cells might represent a transcriptional response in the attempt to counteract, at least in vitro, their reduced migration capability [48,49].

Of note is also the marked up-regulation of the complement factor C3 belonging to a complex network of plasma and membrane proteins involved in the innate immunity [74]. Complement can modulate the inflammatory response during wound healing to restore tissue injury; however, its unbalanced or prolonged activation can exacerbate inflammation, delaying the physiological wound healing [75]. Specifically, C3 functions as a negative regulator of tissue healing, since *C3*-deficient mice exhibit an increased wound healing and angiogenesis [76].

Taken together, these gene expression abnormalities expand the current understanding of altered molecular mechanisms underlying the deficient wound healing response observed in cEDS cells. Additional functional work might help to establish the concrete involvement of these proteins including the $\alpha v\beta 3$ integrin in the impaired wound healing, which likely leads to the cutaneous manifestations of cEDS [39,77].

6. Perturbation of ER Homeostasis and Autophagy in cEDS Fibroblasts

ER is a fundamental cellular organelle involved in the maintenance of numerous aspects of cell health by ensuring folding and exporting of secretory or transmembrane proteins [78]. The biosynthesis, processing, and integrity of collagens and other ECM structural constituents are critical for intracellular proteostasis [79]. To restore intracellular equilibrium, the ER counteracts the accumulation of aggregated or misfolded proteins by means of quality control mechanisms such as unfolded protein response, ER-associated degradation, and autophagy [80].

In cEDS fibroblasts, a possible unbalance of ER homeostasis and autophagy was assumed given the decreased expression of many associated genes such as *DNAJB7*, *ATG10*, *CCPG1*, and *SVIP* [47]. *DNAJB7* encodes a member of the J protein/heat shock protein family acting as ER chaperones in the quality control of aggregate protein [81]. *ATG10* is a member of the autophagy related proteins family that participates to the generation and expansion of autophagosomes [22]. The protein encoded by *CCPG1* acts as an ER-phagy cargo receptor facilitating the attachment to growing autophagosomes of the microtubule-associated LC3 protein that is crucial for autophagosome maturation [22,78,82].

CCPG1 plays a key role in the ER proteostasis, since its deficiency causes accumulated insoluble proteins and consequent ER dilation [83]. A recent study reported the contribution of ER-phagy in the selective degradation of misfolded procollagen I molecules via a calnexin-FAM134B complex [84]. Furthermore, inefficient procollagen folding in the ER may induce autophagy as a cytoprotective mechanism [85]. Based on these findings, it is reasonable to speculate a possible role of CCPG1 in this autophagy-dependent mechanism and that its decreased expression in cEDS fibroblasts might impair the ER quality control. The disturbance of ER homeostasis in cEDS is also suggested by the decreased transcription of the small VCP/p97-interacting protein (SVIP), which is a modulator of the ER-associated degradation pathway [86,87]. Previous and recent data highlighted the contribution of SVIP in the regulation of autophagy, since its overexpression is associated with increased LC3 lipidation and attenuation of hepatic fibrosis by the induction of the autophagic flux [88,89].

The impairment of ECM organization, matrix-cell interactions, and the activation of ECM-dependent intracellular signaling may elicit autophagy [18,19]. Cell detachment from the ECM activates the autophagy pathway that, in turn, protects cells from anoikis [90]. Moreover, depletion of autophagy regulators is associated with induction of pro-apoptotic signals, decrease of collagen degradation via lysosome pathway, and regulation of cell adhesion [90,91]. In line with these observations, the aberrant expression of collagen V and defective remodeling of ECM in cEDS cells might affect ER homeostasis and autophagy, and consequently activate a pro-survival mechanism mediated by a crosstalk between $\alpha v\beta 3$ integrin and EGF receptor [45,50]. Additional studies are needed to better elucidate the contribution of these processes in the molecular pathology of cEDS.

7. Vascular Ehlers-Danlos Syndrome

Among the different EDS forms, vascular EDS (vEDS, OMIM#130050) is the most severe type and is primarily characterized by life-threatening features of tissue fragility leading to arterial dissection or aneurysm, gastrointestinal ruptures, and pregnancy complications at a young age [92,93].

vEDS is caused by mutations in *COL3A1* encoding collagen III that shows a predominant expression in blood vessels and hollow organs [94]. Most disease-causing variants in *COL3A1* are glycine substitutions that destroy the triple helical winding, thus altering the structural integrity of collagen III due to misfolded procollagen III in the ER, and thereby impairing the secretion and deposition into the ECM of functionally mature molecules [95,96].

Col3a1 deficient mice show a reduced lifespan mainly due to arterial ruptures and abnormalities of collagen fibril organization in several collagen-rich organs, i.e., aorta, skin, lung, and bowel [10].

Our previous protein findings on cultured patients' fibroblasts showed that dominant negative mutations in *COL3A1* lead to the reduced secretion of collagen I into the ECM [44], consistent with the known regulatory role of collagen III in synthesis and deposition of heterotypic fibrils that largely contain collagen I [96].

8. Disturbance of ECM Organization, Collagens Processing, and ER Homeostasis in vEDS Fibroblasts

Although it is well known that the disruption of the collagen III triple helical structure leads to abnormal protein folding, different biological aspects of the vEDS pathogenesis are not yet fully studied. In line with cEDS and hEDS transcriptome profiling, vEDS fibroblasts show the differential expression of several genes encoding structural constituents of the ECM, further supporting the notion that abnormal ECM remodeling is a common denominator of these conditions [50,97].

vEDS cells showed a marked decrease in expression of the fibrillin 2 encoding gene (*FBN2*). Fibrillins are essential structural ECM components involved in the organization of blood vessels and dermis, and in combination with elastic fibers they act as scaffold to ensure tissue elasticity [98]. Moreover, fibrillins interact with elastin microfibril interface-located proteins (EMILINs) and facilitate their incorporation into the dermal ECM [99].

Fibrillins also regulate the bioavailability of the TFGβ through the interaction with latent TFGβ binding proteins [99]. Specifically, fibrillin 2 plays a role in bone and soft connective tissue morphology by influencing the collagen cross-linking [100].

Besides its role in elastogenesis and ECM stability, fibrillin 2 also has a role during wound healing [101]. About this, vEDS fibroblasts share with cEDS cells the decreased expression of the related periostin-encoding gene and show reduced migration capability [49]. Consistently, both altered wound healing and reduced total collagen content were reported in a *Col3a1* transgenic mouse model [102].

Our protein findings confirmed the pathological ECM remodeling of vEDS fibroblasts, as a generalized fibrillin disarray in combination with the disassembly of EMILINs and elastin network was revealed, consistent with the extreme vascular fragility observed in vEDS patients [97]. The disorganization of core proteins of the proteoglycans perlecan, versican, and decorin, which are involved in the formation of collagen fibrils, further emphasizes the widespread ECM disarray and altered collagens biosynthesis/secretion of vEDS cells that are consequent to collagen III defect [97].

The biosynthetic pathway of fibrillar collagens is a highly regulated process involving folding enzymes, molecular chaperones, and post-translational modifications essential for proper protein assembly, stability of collagen fibrils, and their transport to the cell surface [8,9]. In vEDS cells, this complex machinery seems to be perturbed given the reduced expression of many ER-resident enzymes involved in different steps of collagen biosynthesis, i.e., *P4HA2, P4HA3, LOXL3,* and *FKBP14.*

P4HA2 and *P4HA3* encode the α-subunit of the collagen prolyl-4-hydroxylase, which catalyzes the hydroxylation of collagen prolyl residues necessary to provide thermal stability to the collagen triple helix. Lysyl oxidase-like 3 (*LOXL3*) stabilizes the formation of intra- and intermolecular crosslinks during assembly of collagen and elastin fibrils. *FKBP14* encodes a peptidyl-prolyl cis-trans isomerase (FKBP22) that catalyzes in the ER lumen collagen folding and it functions as a molecular chaperone for different collagens including collagen III [8,103]. Dermal fibroblasts of *FKBP14*-deficient patients show a generalized perturbation of protein folding and a consequent enlargement of ER cisternae [104]. The marked decrease of FKBP22 protein levels observed in vEDS cells suggests an ER accumulation of misfolded proteins, consistent with the possible dilation of ER cisternae evinced by immunofluorescence analysis with the ER marker PDI [97].

Structural mutations in different collagen types disturb the assembly into hetero- or homotrimers or lead to abnormal triple helix folding. The consequent accumulation of misfolded collagen molecules into the ER lumen activates the proteasomal degradation system to re-establish ER proteostasis [27]. In vEDS cells, this quality control machinery might not work properly, given the decreased transcription of several genes encoding different catalytic and non-catalytic subunits of the proteasome complex, such as *PSMA6, PSMB6, PSMC3,* and *PSMD2.* In addition, the reduced transcription of members belonging to the DnaJ heat shock protein family, i.e., *DNAJB7, DNAJB11, DNAJC3, DNAJC10,* and *DNAJC24,* and to the thioredoxin superfamily, i.e., *TXN, PDIA4, PDIA5,* and *PDIA6,* which all act as intracellular mediators for correct protein folding and intracellular redox balance [105], further corroborates a perturbed ER proteostasis in vEDS fibroblasts.

This imbalance can be overcome by the activation of stress-related pathways, such as unfolded protein response and autophagy to restore basal cellular equilibrium [80]. The alteration of the ER redox state may also trigger pro-death signals through the regulation of members of the Bcl-2 family and activation of caspase-dependent apoptosis [106,107]. Consistently, we previously demonstrated that vEDS fibroblasts are in a pre-apoptotic state, due to downregulation of the Bcl-2 anti-apoptotic protein and increased levels of caspase enzymes, and activate a cell survival mechanism through an $\alpha v\beta 3$-EGFR crosstalk [45,50]. However, in vEDS cells an enhanced expression of unfolded protein response-related genes was not identified, consistent with the recent findings on cultured dermal fibroblasts from *Col3a1* transgenic mice that did not show elevated levels of the unfolded protein response markers *Bip* and *Chop* [102]. In line with this evidence, a recent transcriptome analysis of dermal fibroblasts from *FKBP14*-kEDS patients did not reveal a high expression of genes associated with ER stress and unfolded protein response activation [67], though early data on this EDS cell type suggested an enlargement of ER [104]. Nevertheless, given that different reports highlighted the role of ER stress in the pathogenesis of several collagenopathies [27,108,109], further work is warranted to explore the possible ER perturbation as a disease mechanism of vEDS to identify novel potential therapeutic targets.

9. Hypermobile Ehlers-Danlos Syndrome

Hypermobile EDS (hEDS, OMIM#130020), mainly characterized by generalized joint hypermobility and its complications, minor skin changes, and apparently segregating with an autosomal dominant pattern, is still without a known molecular basis. The phenotypic spectrum of hEDS is wide-ranging and heterogeneous and further complicated by multiple associated symptoms shared with other heritable or acquired (autoimmune) connective tissue disorders and chronic inflammatory systemic diseases [32,110,111].

Despite the significant advances in molecular genetic techniques, attempts to disclose the genetic cause(s) of hEDS have been so far inconclusive. Several studies struggled to define its genetic etiology but without compelling evidence, corroborating the hypothesis of a high genetic heterogeneity of the condition [112–115]. The introduction of more selective clinical criteria for hEDS in the novel classification aimed to minimize heterogeneity allows for the formation of homogeneous cohorts to facilitate scientific research to discover the underlying genetic cause(s) of the condition [32]. Nowadays, hEDS is considered at one end of a continuous spectrum of phenotypes, which originates from isolated non-syndromic joint hypermobility and passing through the recently defined hypermobility spectrum disorders (HSD) [111]. HSD refers to patients who present symptomatic joint hypermobility but do not fulfill the new diagnostic criteria of hEDS. Recently, given the clinical continuity between hEDS and HSD and our data on patients' dermal fibroblasts [49], it was proposed that these disorders might be considered as a single entity, referred to as hEDS/HSD [116], as already occurred for the hypermobility type of EDS and joint hypermobility syndrome [117]. Until now, no validated biological biomarkers have been identified for recognizing hEDS/HSD, which are dominated by extremely variable phenotypes and chronic disability affecting patients' quality of life [111,116].

In this intricate scenario, the integration of various biological knowledge could be an effective strategy to delineate molecular mechanisms contributing to the disease pathophysiology. Transcriptome and proteome profiling can be useful to reveal specific biological signatures, thus providing insights not only for the understanding of the pathomechanisms but also for the identification of reliable tools for therapeutic options [118–122].

Previous findings based on transcriptome and protein studies on a cohort of hEDS/HSD patient-derived dermal fibroblasts represent up to now the main effort to unravel their complex etiopathogenesis [48,123]. Proteome profiling of patients' cells is currently ongoing to corroborate these data, since the gene expression profiling and cellular studies on patients' fibroblasts provided significant clues that are likely relevant for the disease pathogenesis. In the following paragraphs we review our past findings and discuss some novel emerging aspects, offering future perspectives for molecular research in this field.

10. Pathological ECM Remodeling and Defective Cell-Cell Interactions in hEDS/HSD Cells

Although hEDS/HSD etiology remains elusive, patients' skin fibroblasts show a disorganization of the ECM like that observed in cells derived from the other EDS types. In particular, hEDS/HSD, cEDS, and vEDS fibroblasts exhibit a marked disorganization of collagen and fibronectin ECM and their specific α2β1 and α5β1 integrin receptors and showed the preferential expression of the αvβ3 integrin [44,49,50,123].

Transcriptome of hEDS/HSD fibroblasts revealed the dysregulated expression of several genes encoding either ECM glycoproteins such as elastin (*ELN*) and sparc/osteonectin (*SPOCK*), ECM regulators, i.e., metalloproteinases (*MMP16*, *PAPPA2*) and transglutaminase (*TGM2*), or ECM associated secreted factors such as secreted frizzled-related protein 2 (*SFRP2*) and transforming growth factor alpha (*TGFA*). This ECM signature is in common with cEDS and vEDS cells, underlining that the matrix perturbation may act as a key driving factor for the EDS pathogenesis, irrespective of the underlying molecular defects [50].

Cells sense the intrinsic mechanical properties of the ECM and convert these stimuli into intracellular signals [124]. In addition to integrins that primarily mediate this cell response, intracellular signals may be triggered also through the cadherin superfamily, which are calcium-dependent transmembrane proteins forming complex adhesions and connect to the actin cytoskeleton via numerous proteins [125,126]. Interestingly, transcriptome profiling of hEDS/HSD cells revealed a differential expression of many adhesion molecule-encoding genes including members of cadherins and protocadherins, i.e., *CDH2*, *CDH10*, *PCDH9*, *PCDHB16*, *PCDHB18*, claudins (*CLDN11*), and desmosomes (desmoplakin, *DSP*), which are involved in the formation of specialized cell-cell junction complexes essential for maintaining epithelial integrity, morphogenesis, and tissue architecture [127,128]. Since these adhesion proteins can act as signaling modulators of intracellular pathways, such as Wnt, Hippo, NF-kB, JAK-STAT that are crucial for development and organogenesis [128], their altered expression could impact on multiple biological processes essential for embryogenesis and tissue homeostasis.

These transcriptional changes suggested a fibroblast-to-myofibroblast transition of hEDS/HSD cells. This phenomenon induces the formation of cells with muscle-like features that are characterized by increased cell contractility, formation of alpha smooth muscle actin (α-SMA)-stress fibers, together with the reorganization of cell-matrix and cell-cell contacts and cytoskeletal architecture [127,129–131]. Our in vitro studies confirmed the phenotypic conversion of hEDS/HSD fibroblasts into migrating myofibroblast-like cells, since they express the typical markers α-SMA and cadherin-11 and show augmented levels of the protease MMP9 and an altered expression of the inflammation mediators CYR61 and CTGF [49]. This phenotypic switch is elicited by a signal transduction pathway involving the αvβ3 integrin that signals through the integrin linked kinase (ILK) and the transcription factor Snail1 [49,50]. This myofibroblast-like phenotype observed in vitro might reflect a persistent in vivo inflammatory-like condition consistent with the patients' systemic clinical manifestations, comprising gastrointestinal dysfunction, increased susceptibility to osteoarthritis, chronic generalized musculoskeletal pain, inflammatory soft-tissue lesions, and neurological features [110,111].

Activation of myofibroblasts is itself part of physiological wound repair following tissue injury, whereas in chronic injury and inflammatory fibrotic conditions their persistent activation exacerbates the disease progression [132–135]. During fibroblast-to-myofibroblast transition, a complex mechanochemical signaling is activated involving profibrotic secreted factors such as TGFβ and Wnt and ECM-degrading enzymes and intracellular effectors required for stress fiber contractility [127,131]. At molecular level, the cytokine TGFβ is considered the master regulator of profibrotic processes. A growing body of evidence has highlighted the regulation of the Wnt/β-catenin pathway by TGFβ as well as the involvement of their downstream molecular effectors in the fibroblast-to-myofibroblast transition and fibrotic responses [136].

As revealed by transcriptome analysis, several signaling pathways essential for cell growth and proliferation were found to be likely perturbed in hEDS/HSD fibroblasts, i.e., TGFβ, TNF, Jak-STAT, and PI3K-Akt [123]. Transcriptomics data also suggested the differential expression of different Wnt-related genes including the up-regulated frizzled receptor 3 (*FZD3*) and the down-regulated Wnt negative regulators *PRICKLE1* and *SFRP2*. *SFRP2*, the most down-regulated transcript in patients' cells, acts as a critical Wnt modulator, since it directly binds to Wnt proteins and prevents their interactions with FZD receptors [137].

The synergistic crosstalk between TGFβ and Wnt signaling in the myofibroblast activation is documented as well as the inhibitory role of SFRP2 in the TGFβ-dependent myofibroblast formation and post-inflammatory fibrosis [138,139]. In this view, a possible involvement of these signaling pathways in the pathomechanisms of hEDS/HSD can be envisaged. Our findings may offer further clues to address important questions concerning the activation of these pathological mechanisms, and it remains to be clarified which growth factors, i.e., TGFβ, CTGF, and key regulatory pathways sustain the fibroblast-to-myofibroblast transition of hEDS/HSD cells.

11. Differential Expression of Genes Involved in Inflammatory, Immune, and Pain Response in hEDS/HSD Cells

Over the past few years, clinical research described the presence of comorbidities in hEDS/HSD patients, such as functional gastrointestinal and eosinophilic disorders [140,141], increased prevalence of asthma [142], and chronic pain syndromes, i.e., chronic fatigue, fibromyalgia, irritable bowel disease, and inflammatory joints conditions [111,143], though specific underlying causes and mechanisms remain to be explored. In this regard, transcriptome of hEDS/HSD cells revealed the aberrant transcription of a range of genes related to inflammation, pain, and immune responses, i.e., *AQP9*, *CFD*, *SPON2*, *PRLR*, and *NR4A* receptors, which might impair biological functions and molecular pathways with a potential role in the disease's pathogenesis. Among them, patients' cells showed the enhanced expression of *AQP9*, a member of the family of water-selective membrane channels that play a role both in antimicrobial defense and skin barrier permeability [144]. A high expression of this transporter was detected in synovial tissues and fibroblast-like synoviocytes from osteoarthritis and rheumatoid arthritis patients and may have a role in the pathogenesis of inflammatory synovitis [145,146].

In line with this finding, patients' cells also showed increased mRNA levels of complement factor D (*CFD*), a component of the alternative complement pathway [147], which is involved in pathophysiological mechanisms of osteoarthritis and is considered as a potential predictive biomarker of joint pain in patients with hip and knee osteoarthritis [148–150].

In hEDS/HSD no reliable biomarkers have been identified. A previous study identified elevated basal serum tryptase levels due to increased *TPSAB1* copy number associated with hereditary alpha tryptasemia in individuals with multisystem complaints, i.e., joint hypermobility, sleep disruption, irritable bowel syndrome, body pain, headache, arthralgia, and chronic gastroesophageal reflux, partly overlapping with those frequently observed in hEDS/HSD patients [151]. In our hEDS/HSD patients, no elevated basal serum tryptase level was observed, suggesting the absence of the association between their clinical features and copy number variations in the *TPSAB1* gene.

Other inflammation-related genes dysregulated in hEDS/HSD include *SPON2*, up-regulated in patients' cells, which encodes an ECM protein with multifunctional properties in the innate immune system and inflammatory cell recruitment [152–154], and *PRLR*, showing a decreased expression in hEDS/HSD cells, which encode the prolactin receptor implicated in inflammatory responses and immune cells regulation [155,156]. The prolactin-PRLR axis contributes to the activation of pain-related pathways through the sensitization of transient receptor potential channels that promote painful sensations [157,158]. Chronic pain represents a common complaint among hEDS/HSD patients affecting their quality of life [111,116], though specific molecular pathways or mediators of pain are still unknown.

As further evidence of unbalanced inflammatory responses in patients' cells, transcriptome revealed a decreased expression of the *NR4A* nuclear receptors (*NR4A1*, *NR4A2*, *NR4A3*), which act as transcriptional regulators of inflammatory responses mediated by NF-kB signaling [159–161]. These receptors attenuate inflammatory events through inhibition of the NF-kB nuclear translocation and induction of the expression of its inhibitor NFKBIA, which, in turn, blocks the NF-kB nuclear localizing sequence [159]. The concomitant decreased mRNA levels of *NR4A1* and *NFKBIA* in patients' cells may be related to aberrant NF-kB signaling.

Despite additional work being required to support these hypotheses, our findings depict the complex sequence of transcriptional events that should stimulate more investigations to provide new insights into the pathomechanisms underlying the molecular networks related to aberrant inflammatory responses associated with hEDS/HSD.

12. Emerging Aspects of hEDS/HSD Pathophysiology by microRNAs Profiling

Transcriptome analysis may be a valuable strategy also to delineate distinct molecular signatures related to the differential expression of microRNAs (miRNAs). miRNAs are small non-coding RNA molecules ranging from 20–25 nucleotides in length that act mainly as negative regulators of gene expression by promoting the degradation of target mRNAs or repressing their translation [162,163]. Aberrant miRNA expression has been reported in several pathological conditions including cancer, musculoskeletal disorders, painful peripheral neuropathies, and fibromyalgia [164–166].

Our previous expression profiling of hEDS/HSD fibroblasts identified 19 dysregulated miRNAs [123]. Here, we report some examples that might offer interesting clues about the possible involvement of miRNAs in the regulation of potential targets and molecular pathways related to inflammation and Wnt signaling that seem to have a role in the disease pathogenesis.

The most overexpressed miRNA in patients' cells was the miR-378-3p, which is considered a modulator of the epithelial-to-mesenchymal transition and is associated with inflammation and fibrosis through the positive modulation of NF-kB and TNFα pathways [167,168]. miRNA-224, which is also up-regulated in hEDS/HSD cells, is associated with the activation of the Wnt/β-catenin signaling through the inhibition of the expression of glycogen synthase kinase 3β and SFRP2, which are known Wnt suppressors [169]. Therefore, it is likely reasonable to assume that the enhanced expression of this miRNA may contribute to the decreased mRNA level of *SFRP2* observed in hEDS/HSD cells, supporting the hypothesis that the aberrant signaling of the Wnt/β-catenin axis might play a role in the disease mechanisms of hEDS/HSD.

We previously demonstrated the involvement of the ILK in the fibroblast-to-myofibroblast switch of hEDS/HSD cells. The ILK acts downstream of the phosphatidylinositol 3-kinase signaling pathway and negatively regulates the action of the glycogen synthase kinase 3β by phosphorylation of a specific serine residue, further strengthening our assumption that Wnt/β-catenin signaling is involved in hEDS/HSD pathogenesis [49,50]. Consistently, patients' fibroblasts show a reduced expression of the miRNA-23a, which is implicated in the Wnt pathway regulation as well, by inhibiting the expression of FDZ5 and FDZ7 receptors [170]. Decreased levels of this miRNA were also found in cerebrospinal fluid and serum of patients with fibromyalgia [171], a painful disorder in differential diagnosis with hEDS/HSD [172], which might suggest a possible involvement of specific miRNA signatures or a common disease pattern in both conditions. In addition, the altered expression of this miRNA in synovial fibroblasts of psoriatic arthritis patients, results in the enhanced expression of pro-inflammatory mediators and matrix degrading enzymes, further promoting joint degeneration and synovial inflammation [173].

Several studies highlighted the contribution of miRNAs in the modulation of the expression of ECM structural proteins and related signaling molecules, thus emphasizing the close relationship between ECM homeostasis and inflammatory pain related conditions [174–176].

As the expression of miRNAs can be modulated to mediate the expression of their target genes, in-depth in vitro studies on a large cohort of patients' cells could provide further evidence on mechanisms of action of miRNAs and their impact on diverse target genes and altered pathways relevant for the pathophysiology of hEDS/HSD, thus offering new perspectives to identify potential molecular therapeutic targets.

13. Conclusions and Perspectives

Transcriptome and in vitro analyses on cEDS, vEDS, and hEDS/HSD dermal fibroblasts expanded the knowledge about molecular mechanisms involved in the pathophysiology of these connective tissue disorders (Figure 1).

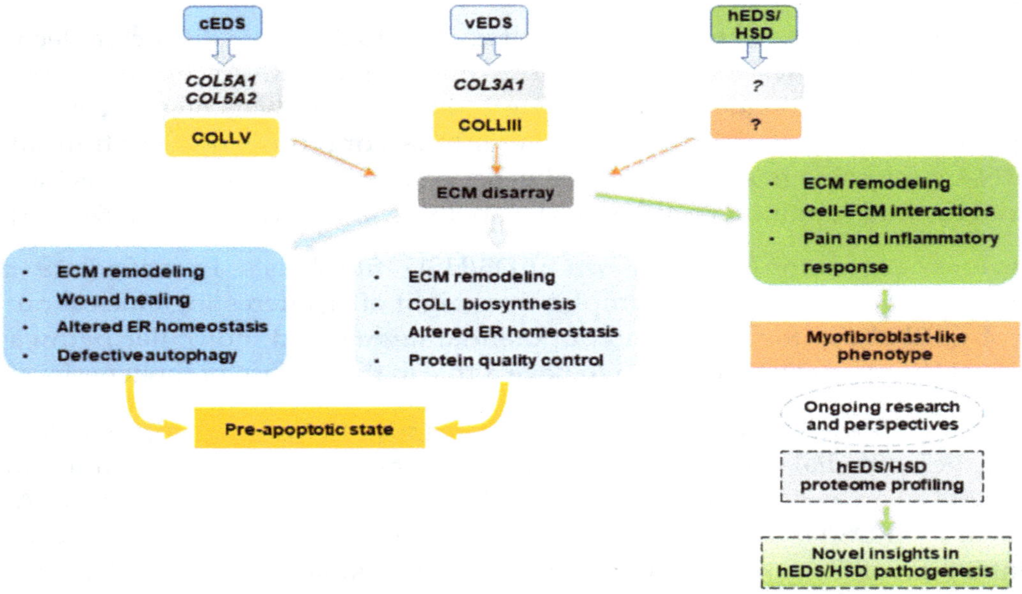

Figure 1. Schematic illustration summarizing the processes likely involved in the pathogenesis of cEDS, vEDS, and hEDS/HSD derived from transcriptome and in vitro studies of patients' skin fibroblasts.

Our findings indicate that these cells share a deregulated expression of many matrix-related genes and a widespread disarray of several ECM structural constituents, thus highlighting the functional relevance of a proper organization and function of the ECM in providing stability to connective tissues. In cEDS and vEDS dermal fibroblasts, the pathological ECM turnover is directly caused by the underlying molecular defect causing abnormal expression of collagen V and collagen III, which, in turn, perturbs key physiological processes critical for collagen processing itself and to maintain cell homeostasis. In the absence of a known genetic etiology, the abnormal ECM organization present in hEDS/HSD cells may be a functional consequence of excessive remodeling due to increased levels of ECM-degrading enzymes and concomitant acquisition of a pro-inflammatory myofibroblast-like phenotype. hEDS/HSD transcriptome profiling for the first time has shed light on different pathobiological aspects of the disease. The dysregulated expression of genes involved in cell-matrix interactions and specific intracellular signaling pathways may have a role in the phenotypic switch of hEDS/HSD cells. Transcriptional changes of different genes and miRNAs involved in molecular pathways related to pain and inflammatory response might provide further clues to dissect the intricate biological events involved in chronic and musculoskeletal pain affecting hEDS/HSD patients. To deepen the knowledge on hEDS/HSD pathophysiology, proteome profiling of patients' cells is currently ongoing to decipher the complex protein network and identify potential bioactive molecules involved in the disease pathogenesis to offer therapeutic options for hEDS/HSD patients.

Author Contributions: Conceptualization: N.C., M.R., M.C.; writing and original draft preparation: N.C., M.R., M.C.; writing, review and editing: N.C., M.R., N.Z., M.C.; supervision: M.C.

Acknowledgments: The authors wish to thank the patients for their kind availability for these studies and the Fazzo Cusan family for its generous support.

References

1. Theocharis, A.D.; Manou, D.; Karamanos, N.K. The extracellular matrix as a multitasking player in disease. *FEBS J.* **2019**. [CrossRef] [PubMed]
2. Arseni, L.; Lombardi, A.; Orioli, D. From Structure to Phenotype: Impact of Collagen Alterations on Human Health. *Int. J. Mol. Sci.* **2018**, *19*, 5. [CrossRef] [PubMed]
3. Murphy-Ullrich, J.E.; Sage, E.H. Revisiting the matricellular concept. *Matrix Biol.* **2014**, *37*, 1–14. [CrossRef] [PubMed]
4. Hynes, R.O.; Naba, A. Overview of the matrisome—An inventory of extracellular matrix constituents and functions. *Cold Spring Harb. Perspect. Biol.* **2012**, *4*, a004903. [CrossRef] [PubMed]
5. Naba, A.; Clauser, K.R.; Ding, H.; Whittaker, C.A.; Carr, S.A.; Hynes, R.O. The extracellular matrix: Tools and insights for the "omics" era. *Matrix Biol.* **2016**, *49*, 10–24. [CrossRef] [PubMed]
6. Myllyharju, J.; Kivirikko, K.I. Collagens, modifying enzymes and their mutations in humans, flies and worms. *Trends Genet.* **2004**, *20*, 33–43. [CrossRef] [PubMed]
7. Nyström, A.; Bruckner-Tuderman, L. Matrix molecules and skin biology. *Semin. Cell Dev. Biol.* **2019**, *89*, 136–146. [CrossRef] [PubMed]
8. Gjaltema, R.A.; Bank, R.A. Molecular insights into prolyl and lysyl hydroxylation of fibrillar collagens in health and disease. *Crit. Rev. Biochem. Mol. Biol.* **2017**, *52*, 74–95. [CrossRef] [PubMed]
9. Sorushanova, A.; Delgado, L.M.; Wu, Z.; Shologu, N.; Kshirsagar, A.; Raghunath, R.; Mullen, A.M.; Bayon, Y.; Pandit, A.; Raghunath, M.; et al. The Collagen Suprafamily: From Biosynthesis to Advanced Biomaterial Development. *Adv. Mater.* **2019**, *31*, e1801651. [CrossRef] [PubMed]
10. Malfait, F. Vascular aspects of the Ehlers-Danlos Syndromes. *Matrix Biol.* **2018**, *71–72*, 380–395. [CrossRef] [PubMed]
11. Lenselink, E.A. Role of fibronectin in normal wound healing. *Int. Wound J.* **2015**, *12*, 313–316. [CrossRef] [PubMed]
12. Iozzo, R.V.; Gubbiotti, M.A. Extracellular matrix: The driving force of mammalian diseases. *Matrix Biol.* **2018**, *71–72*, 1–9. [CrossRef] [PubMed]
13. Karamanos, N.K.; Theocharis, A.D.; Neill, T.; Iozzo, R.V. Matrix modeling and remodeling: A biological interplay regulating tissue homeostasis and diseases. *Matrix Biol.* **2019**, *75–76*, 1–11. [CrossRef] [PubMed]
14. Schwartz, M.A. Integrins and extracellular matrix in mechanotransduction. *Cold Spring Harb. Perspect. Biol.* **2010**, *2*, a005066. [CrossRef] [PubMed]
15. Campbell, I.D.; Humphries, M.J. Integrin structure, activation, and interactions. *Cold Spring Harb. Perspect. Biol.* **2011**, *3*, a004994. [CrossRef] [PubMed]
16. Frisch, S.M.; Francis, H. Disruption of epithelial cell matrix interactions induces apoptosis. *J. Cell Biol.* **1994**, *124*, 619–626. [CrossRef] [PubMed]
17. Vlahakis, A.; Debnath, J. The Interconnections between Autophagy and Integrin-Mediated Cell Adhesion. *J. Mol. Biol.* **2017**, *429*, 515–530. [CrossRef]
18. Lock, R.; Debnath, J. Extracellular matrix regulation of autophagy. *Curr. Opin. Cell Biol.* **2008**, *20*, 583–588. [CrossRef]
19. Neill, T.; Schaefer, L.; Iozzo, R.V. Instructive roles of extracellular matrix on autophagy. *Am. J. Pathol.* **2014**, *184*, 2146–2153. [CrossRef]
20. Settembre, C.; Cinque, L.; Bartolomeo, R.; Di Malta, C.; De Leonibus, C.; Forrester, A. Defective collagen proteostasis and matrix formation in the pathogenesis of lysosomal storage disorders. *Matrix Biol.* **2018**, *71–72*, 283–293. [CrossRef]
21. Lamandé, S.R.; Bateman, J.F. Collagen VI disorders: Insights on form and function in the extracellular matrix and beyond. *Matrix Biol.* **2018**, *71–72*, 348–367. [CrossRef]
22. Wilkinson, S. Emerging Principles of Selective ER Autophagy. *J. Mol. Biol.* **2019**. [CrossRef]
23. Bonnans, C.; Chou, J.; Werb, Z. Remodelling the extracellular matrix in development and disease. *Nat. Rev. Mol. Cell Biol.* **2014**, *15*, 786–801. [CrossRef]
24. Frevert, C.W.; Felgenhauer, J.; Wygrecka, M.; Nastase, M.V.; Schaefer, L. Danger-Associated Molecular Patterns Derived From the Extracellular Matrix Provide Temporal Control of Innate Immunity. *J. Histochem. Cytochem.* **2018**, *66*, 213–227. [CrossRef]

25. Genovese, F.; Karsdal, M.A. Protein degradation fragments as diagnostic and prognostic biomarkers of connective tissue diseases: Understanding the extracellular matrix message and implication for current and future serological biomarkers. *Expert Rev. Proteom.* **2016**, *13*, 213–225. [CrossRef]
26. Bhattacharyya, S.; Midwood, K.S.; Yin, H.; Varga, J. Toll-Like Receptor-4 Signaling Drives Persistent Fibroblast Activation and Prevents Fibrosis Resolution in Scleroderma. *Adv. Wound Care* **2017**, *6*, 356–369. [CrossRef]
27. Lamandé, S.R.; Bateman, J.F. Genetic Disorders of the Extracellular Matrix. *Anat. Rec.* **2019**. [CrossRef]
28. Colombi, M.; Dordoni, C.; Chiarelli, N.; Ritelli, M. Differential diagnosis and diagnostic flow chart of joint hypermobility syndrome/Ehlers-Danlos syndrome hypermobility type compared to other heritable connective tissue disorders. *Am. J. Med. Genet. Part C* **2015**, *169*, 6–22. [CrossRef]
29. Bateman, J.F.; Boot-Handford, R.P.; Lamande, S.R. Genetic diseases of connective tissues: Cellular and extra cellular effects of ECM mutations. *Nat. Rev. Genet.* **2009**, *10*, 173–183. [CrossRef]
30. Lu, P.; Takai, K.; Weaver, V.M.; Werb, Z. Extracellular matrix degradation and remodeling in development and disease. *Cold Spring Harb. Perspect. Biol.* **2011**, *3*, a005058. [CrossRef]
31. Karsdal, M.A.; Nielsen, M.J.; Sand, J.M.; Henriksen, K.; Genovese, F.; Bay-Jensen, A.C.; Smith, V.; Adamkewicz, J.I.; Christiansen, C.; Leeming, D.J. Extracellular matrix remodeling: The common denominator in connective tissue diseases. Possibilities for evaluation and current understanding of the matrix as more than a passive architecture, but a key player in tissue failure. *ASSAY Drug Dev. Technol.* **2013**, *11*, 70–92. [CrossRef]
32. Malfait, F.; Francomano, C.; Byers, P.; Belmont, J.; Berglund, B.; Black, J.; Bloom, L.; Bowen, J.M.; Brady, A.F.; Burrows, N.P.; et al. The 2017 international classification of the Ehlers-Danlos syndromes. *Am. J. Med. Genet. C Semin. Med. Genet.* **2017**, *175*, 8–26. [CrossRef]
33. Blackburn, P.R.; Xu, Z.; Tumelty, K.E.; Zhao, R.W.; Monis, W.J.; Harris, K.G.; Gass, J.M.; Cousin, M.A.; Boczek, N.J.; Mitkov, M.V.; et al. Bi-allelic alterations in AEBP1 lead to defective collagen assembly and connective tissue structure resulting in a variant of Ehlers-Danlos syndrome. *Am. J. Hum. Genet.* **2018**, *102*, 696–705. [CrossRef]
34. Hebebrand, M.; Vasileiou, G.; Krumbiegel, M.; Kraus, C.; Uebe, S.; Ekici, A.B.; Thiel, C.T.; Reis, A.; Popp, B. A biallelic truncating AEBP1 variant causes connective tissue disorder in two siblings. *Am. J. Med. Genet. A* **2019**, *179*, 50–56. [CrossRef]
35. Syx, D.; De Wandele, I.; Symoens, S.; De Rycke, R.; Hougrand, O.; Voermans, N.; De Paepe, A.; Malfait, F. Bi-allelic AEBP1 mutations in two patients with Ehlers-Danlos syndrome. *Hum. Mol. Genet.* **2019**, *28*, 1853–1864. [CrossRef]
36. Ritelli, M.; Cinquina, V.; Venturini, M.; Pezzaioli, L.; Formenti, A.M.; Chiarelli, N.; Colombi, M. Expanding the Clinical and Mutational Spectrum of Recessive AEBP1-Related Classical-Like Ehlers-Danlos Syndrome. *Genes.* **2019**, *10*, 135. [CrossRef]
37. Maugeri, A.; De Paepe, A.; Malfait, F. Genetics and testing of Ehlers-Danlos syndrome and of differential diagnostic diseases. In *Ehlers-Danlos Syndrome: A Multidisciplinary Approach*, 1st ed.; Jacobs, J.W.G., Cornelissens, L.J.M., Eds.; IOS Press BV: Amsterdam, The Netherlands, 2018; Chapter 3, pp. 33–46.
38. Damme, T.M.; Syx, D.; Coucke, P.; Symoens, S.; De Paepe, A.; Malfait, F. Genetics of the Ehlers–Danlos syndrome: More than collagen disorders. *Expert Opin. Orphan Drugs* **2015**, *3*, 379–392. [CrossRef]
39. Bowen, J.M.; Sobey, G.J.; Burrows, N.P.; Colombi, M.; Lavallee, M.E.; Malfait, F.; Francomano, C.A. Ehlers-Danlos syndrome, classical type. *Am. J. Med. Genet. C Semin. Med. Genet.* **2017**, *75*, 27–39. [CrossRef]
40. Symoens, S.; Syx, D.; Malfait, F.; Callewaert, B.; De Backer, J.; Vanakker, O.; Coucke, P.; De Paepe, A. Comprehensive molecular analysis demonstrates type V collagen mutations in over 90% of patients with classic EDS and allows to refine diagnostic criteria. *Hum. Mutat.* **2012**, *33*, 1485–1493. [CrossRef]
41. Ritelli, M.; Dordoni, C.; Venturini, M.; Chiarelli, N.; Quinzani, S.; Traversa, M.; Zoppi, N.; Vascellaro, A.; Wischmeijer, A.; Manfredini, E.; et al. Clinical and molecular characterization of 40 patients with classic Ehlers-Danlos syndrome: Identification of 18 COL5A1 and 2 COL5A2 novel mutations. *Orphanet J. Rare Dis.* **2013**, *8*, 58. [CrossRef]
42. Wenstrup, R.J.; Florer, J.B.; Brunskill, E.W.; Bell, S.M.; Chervoneva, I.; Birk, D.E. Type V collagen controls the initiation of collagen fibril assembly. *J. Biol. Chem.* **2004**, *279*, 53331–53337. [CrossRef]
43. Mak, K.M.; Png, C.Y.; Lee, D.J. Type V Collagen in Health, Disease, and Fibrosis. *Anat. Rec.* **2016**, *299*, 613–629. [CrossRef]

44. Zoppi, N.; Gardella, R.; De Paepe, A.; Barlati, S.; Colombi, M. Human fibroblasts with mutations in COL5A1 and COL3A1 genes do not organize collagens and fibronectin in the extracellular matrix, down-regulate $\alpha2\beta1$ integrin, and recruit $\alpha v\beta3$ instead of $\alpha5\beta1$ integrin. *J. Biol. Chem.* **2004**, *30*, 18157–18168. [CrossRef]
45. Zoppi, N.; Barlati, S.; Colombi, M. FAK-independent $\alpha v\beta3$ integrin-EGFR complexes rescue from anoikis matrix-defective fibroblasts. *Biochim. Biophys. Acta* **2008**, *1783*, 1177–1188. [CrossRef]
46. Zoppi, N.; Ritelli, M.; Colombi, M. Type III and V collagens modulate the expression and assembly of EDA+fibronectin in the extracellular matrix of defective Ehlers-Danlos syndrome fibroblasts. *Biochim. Biophys. Acta* **2012**, *1820*, 1576–1587. [CrossRef]
47. Chiarelli, N.; Carini, G.; Zoppi, N.; Ritelli, M.; Colombi, M. Molecular insights in the pathogenesis of classical Ehlers-Danlos syndrome from transcriptome-wide expression profiling of patients' skin fibroblasts. *PLoS ONE* **2019**, *14*, e0211647. [CrossRef]
48. Viglio, S.; Zoppi, N.; Sangalli, A.; Gallanti, A.; Barlati, S.; Mottes, M.; Colombi, M.; Valli, M. Rescue of migratory defects of Ehlers-Danlos syndrome fibroblasts in vitro by type V collagen but not insulin-like binding protein-1. *J. Investig. Dermatol.* **2008**, *128*, 1915–1919. [CrossRef]
49. Zoppi, N.; Chiarelli, N.; Binetti, S.; Ritelli, M.; Colombi, M. Dermal fibroblast-to-myofibroblast transition sustained by $\alpha v\beta3$ integrin-ILK-Snail1/Slug signaling is a common feature for hypermobile Ehlers-Danlos syndrome and hypermobility spectrum disorders. *Biochim. Biophys. Acta* **2018**, *1864*, 1010–1023. [CrossRef]
50. Zoppi, N.; Chiarelli, N.; Ritelli, M.; Colombi, M. Multifaced Roles of the $\alpha v\beta3$ Integrin in Ehlers-Danlos and Arterial Tortuosity Syndromes' Dermal Fibroblasts. *Int. J. Mol. Sci.* **2018**, *19*, 982. [CrossRef]
51. DeNigris, J.; Yao, Q.; Birk, E.K.; Birk, D.E. Altered dermal fibroblast behavior in a collagen V haploinsufficient murine model of classic Ehlers-Danlos syndrome. *Connect. Tissue Res.* **2016**, *57*, 1–9. [CrossRef]
52. Park, A.C.; Phan, N.; Massoudi, D.; Liu, Z.; Kernien, J.F.; Adams, S.M.; Davidson, J.M.; Birk, D.E.; Liu, B.; Greenspan, D.S. Deficits in Col5a2 Expression Result in Novel Skin and Adipose Abnormalities and Predisposition to Aortic Aneurysms and Dissections. *Am. J. Pathol.* **2017**, *187*, 2300–2311. [CrossRef]
53. Rousselle, P.; Montmasson, M.; Garnier, C. Extracellular matrix contribution to skin wound re-epithelialization. *Matrix Biol.* **2019**, *75–76*, 12–26. [CrossRef]
54. Tracy, L.E.; Minasian, R.A.; Caterson, E.J. Extracellular Matrix and Dermal Fibroblast Function in the Healing Wound. *Adv. Wound Care* **2016**, *5*, 119–136. [CrossRef]
55. Chester, D.; Brown, A.C. The role of biophysical properties of provisional matrix proteins in wound repair. *Matrix Biol.* **2017**, *60–61*, 124–140. [CrossRef]
56. Wang, W.; Li, P.; Li, W.; Jiang, J.; Cui, Y.; Li, S.; Wang, Z. Osteopontin activates mesenchymal stem cells to repair skin wound. *PLoS ONE* **2017**, *12*, e0185346. [CrossRef]
57. Icer, M.A.; Gezmen-Karadag, M. The multiple functions and mechanisms of osteopontin. *Clin. Biochem.* **2018**, *59*, 17–24. [CrossRef]
58. Ross, F.P.; Chappel, J.; Alvarez, J.; Sander, D.; Butler, W.; Farach-Carson, M.; Mintz, K.; Robey, P.G.; Teitelbaum, S.; Cheresh, D. Interactions between the bone matrix proteins osteopontin and bone sialoprotein and the osteoclast integrin alpha v beta 3 potentiate bone resorption. *J. Biol. Chem.* **1993**, *268*, 9901–9907.
59. Giachelli, C.M.; Steitz, S. Osteopontin: A versatile regulator of inflammation and biomineralization. *Matrix Biol.* **2000**, *19*, 615–622. [CrossRef]
60. Liaw, L.; Birk, D.E.; Ballas, C.B.; Whitsitt, J.S.; Davidson, J.M.; Hogan, B.L. Altered wound healing in mice lacking a functional osteopontin gene (spp1). *J. Clin. Investig.* **1998**, *101*, 1468–1478. [CrossRef]
61. Maruhashi, T. Interaction between periostin and BMP-1 promotes proteolytic activation of lysyl oxidase. *J. Biol. Chem.* **2010**, *285*, 13294–13303. [CrossRef]
62. Egbert, M.; Ruetze, M.; Sattler, M.; Wenck, H.; Gallinat, S.; Lucius, R.; Weise, J.M. The matricellular protein periostin contributes to proper collagen function and is downregulated during skin aging. *J. Dermatol. Sci.* **2014**, *73*, 40–48. [CrossRef]
63. González-González, L.; Alonso, J. Periostin: A Matricellular Protein with Multiple Functions in Cancer Development and Progression. *Front. Oncol.* **2018**, *8*, 225. [CrossRef]
64. Li, G.; Jin, R.; Norris, R.A.; Zhang, L.; Yu, S.; Wu, F.; Markwald, R.R.; Nanda, A.; Conway, S.J.; Smyth, S.S.; et al. Periostin mediates vascular smooth muscle cell migration through the integrins alphavbeta3 and alphavbeta5 and focal adhesion kinase (FAK) pathway. *Atherosclerosis* **2010**, *208*, 358–365. [CrossRef]
65. Walker, J.T.; McLeod, K.; Kim, S.; Conway, S.J.; Hamilton, D.W. Periostin as a multifunctional modulator of the wound healing response. *Cell Tissue Res.* **2016**, *365*, 453–465. [CrossRef]

66. Nunomura, S.; Nanri, Y.; Ogawa, M.; Arima, K.; Mitamura, Y.; Yoshihara, T.; Hasuwa, H.; Conway, S.J.; Izuhara, K. Constitutive overexpression of periostin delays wound healing in mouse skin. *Wound Repair Regen.* **2018**, *26*, 6–15. [CrossRef]
67. Lim, P.J.; Lindert, U.; Opitz, L.; Hausser, I.; Rohrbach, M.; Giunta, C. Transcriptome Profiling of Primary Skin Fibroblasts Reveal Distinct Molecular Features Between PLOD1-and FKBP14-Kyphoscoliotic Ehlers-Danlos Syndrome. *Genes* **2019**, *10*, 517. [CrossRef]
68. Penta, K.; Varner, J.A.; Liaw, L.; Hidai, C.; Schatzman, R.; Quertermous, T. Del1 induces integrin signaling and angiogenesis by ligation of alphaVbeta3. *J. Biol. Chem.* **1999**, *274*, 11101–11109. [CrossRef]
69. Shen, W.; Zhu, S.; Qin, H.; Zhong, M.; Wu, J.; Zhang, R.; Song, H. EDIL3 knockdown inhibits retinal angiogenesis through the induction of cell cycle arrest in vitro. *Mol. Med. Rep.* **2017**, *16*, 4054–4060. [CrossRef]
70. Wang, Z.; Boyko, T.; Tran, M.C.; LaRussa, M.; Bhatia, N.; Rashidi, V.; Longaker, M.T.; Yang, G.P. DEL1 protects against chondrocyte apoptosis through integrin binding. *J. Surg. Res.* **2018**, *231*, 1–9. [CrossRef]
71. Hajishengallis, G.; Chavakis, T. DEL-1-Regulated Immune Plasticity and Inflammatory Disorders. *Trends Mol. Med.* **2019**, *25*, 444–459. [CrossRef]
72. Brandt, K.; Grunler, J.; Brismar, K.; Wang, J. Effects of IGFBP-1 and IGFBP-2 and their fragments on migration and IGF-induced proliferation of human dermal fibroblasts. *Growth Horm. IGF Res.* **2015**, *25*, 34–40. [CrossRef]
73. Katayama, H.; Tamai, K.; Shibuya, R.; Nakamura, M.; Mochizuki, M.; Yamaguchi, K.; Kawamura, S.; Tochigi, T.; Sato, I.; Okanishi, T.; et al. Long non-coding RNA HOTAIR promotes cell migration by upregulating insulin growth factor-binding protein 2 in renal cell carcinoma. *Sci. Rep.* **2017**, *7*, 12016. [CrossRef]
74. Ahmad, S.; Bhatia, K.; Kindelin, A.; Ducruet, A.F. The Role of Complement C3a Receptor in Stroke. *Neuromol. Med.* **2019**. [CrossRef]
75. Korkmaz, H.I.; Krijnen, P.A.J.; Ulrich, M.M.W.; de Jong, E.; van Zuijlen, P.P.M.; Niessen, H.W.M. The role of complement in the acute phase response after burns. *Burns* **2017**, *43*, 1390–1399. [CrossRef]
76. Rafail, S.; Kourtzelis, I.; Foukas, P.G.; Markiewski, M.M.; DeAngelis, R.A.; Guariento, M.; Ricklin, D.; Grice, E.A.; Lambris, J.D. Complement deficiency promotes cutaneous wound healing in mice. *J. Immunol.* **2015**, *194*, 1285–1291. [CrossRef]
77. Colombi, M.; Dordoni, C.; Venturini, M.; Ciaccio, C.; Morlino, S.; Chiarelli, N.; Zanca, A.; Calzavara-Pinton, P.; Zoppi, N.; Castori, M.; et al. Spectrum of mucocutaneous, ocular and facial features and delineation of novel presentations in 62 classical Ehlers-Danlos syndrome patients. *Clin. Genet.* **2017**, *92*, 624–631. [CrossRef]
78. Smith, M.; Wilkinson, S. ER homeostasis and autophagy. *Essays Biochem.* **2017**, *61*, 625–635. [CrossRef]
79. Wong, M.Y.; Shoulders, M.D. Targeting defective proteostasis in the collagenopathies. *Curr. Opin. Chem. Biol.* **2019**, *50*, 80–88. [CrossRef]
80. Moon, H.W.; Han, H.G.; Jeon, Y.J. Protein Quality Control in the Endoplasmic Reticulum and Cancer. *Int. J. Mol. Sci.* **2018**, *19*, 3020. [CrossRef]
81. Mogk, A.; Bukau, B.; Kampinga, H.H. Cellular Handling of Protein Aggregates by Disaggregation Machines. *Mol. Cell* **2018**, *69*, 214–226. [CrossRef]
82. Wilkinson, S. ER-phagy: Shaping up and destressing the endoplasmic reticulum. *FEBS J.* **2019**. [CrossRef]
83. Smith, M.D.; Harley, M.E.; Kemp, A.J.; Wills, J.; Lee, M.; Arends, M.; von Kriegsheim, A.; Behrends, C.; Wilkinson, S. CCPG1 is a non-canonical autophagy cargo receptor essential for ER-phagy and pancreatic ER proteostasis. *Dev. Cell* **2018**, *44*, 217–232. [CrossRef]
84. Forrester, A.; De Leonibus, C.; Grumati, P.; Fasana, E.; Piemontese, M.; Staiano, L.; Fregno, I.; Raimondi, A.; Marazza, A.; Bruno, G.; et al. A selective ER-phagy exerts procollagen quality control via a Calnexin-FAM134B complex. *EMBO J.* **2019**, *38*, e99847. [CrossRef]
85. Ishida, Y.; Yamamoto, A.; Kitamura, A.; Lamandé, S.R.; Yoshimori, T.; Bateman, J.F.; Kubota, H.; Nagata, K. Autophagic elimination of misfolded procollagen aggregates in the endoplasmic reticulum as a means of cell protection. *Mol. Biol. Cell* **2009**, *20*, 2744–2754. [CrossRef]
86. Nagahama, M.; Suzuki, M.; Hamada, Y.; Hatsuzawa, K.; Tani, K.; Yamamoto, A.; Tagaya, M. SVIP is a novel VCP/p97-interacting protein whose expression causes cell vacuolation. *Mol. Biol. Cell* **2003**, *14*, 262–273. [CrossRef]
87. Ballar, P.; Zhong, Y.; Nagahama, M.; Tagaya, M.; Shen, Y.; Fang, S. Identification of SVIP as an endogenous inhibitor of endoplasmic reticulum-associated degradation. *J. Biol. Chem.* **2007**, *282*, 33908–33914. [CrossRef]

88. Wang, Y.; Ballar, P.; Zhong, Y.; Zhang, X.; Liu, C.; Zhang, Y.J.; Monteiro, M.J.; Li, J.; Fang, S. SVIP induces localization of p97/VCP to the plasma and lysosomal membranes and regulates autophagy. *PLoS ONE* **2011**, *6*, e24478. [CrossRef]
89. Jia, D.; Wang, Y.Y.; Wang, P.; Huang, Y.; Liang, D.Y.; Wang, D.; Cheng, C.; Zhang, C.; Guo, L.; Liang, P.; et al. SVIP alleviates CCl4-induced liver fibrosis via activating autophagy and protecting hepatocytes. *Cell Death Dis.* **2019**, *10*, 71. [CrossRef]
90. Fung, C.; Lock, R.; Gao, S.; Salas, E.; Debnath, J. Induction of autophagy during extracellular matrix detachment promotes cell survival. *Mol. Biol. Cell* **2008**, *19*, 797–806. [CrossRef]
91. Kawano, S.; Torisu, T.; Esaki, M.; Torisu, K.; Matsuno, Y.; Kitazono, T. Autophagy promotes degradation of internalized collagen and regulates distribution of focal adhesions to suppress cell adhesion. *Biol. Open* **2017**, *6*, 1644–1653. [CrossRef]
92. Byers, P.H.; Belmont, J.; Black, J.; De Backer, J.; Frank, M.; Jeunemaitre, X.; Johnson, D.; Pepin, M.; Robert, L.; Sanders, L.; et al. Diagnosis, natural history, and management in vascular Ehlers-Danlos syndrome. *Am. J. Med. Genet. C Semin. Med. Genet.* **2017**, *175*, 40–47. [CrossRef]
93. Ritelli, M.; Rovati, C.; Venturini, M.; Chiarelli, N.; Cinquina, V.; Castori, M.; Colombi, M. Application of the 2017 criteria for vascular Ehlers-Danlos syndrome in 50 patients ascertained according to the Villefranche nosology. *Clin. Genet.* under review.
94. Pepin, M.; Schwarze, U.; Superti-Furga, A.; Byers, P.H. Clinical and genetic features of Ehlers-Danlos syndrome type IV, the vascular type. *N. Engl. J. Med.* **2000**, *342*, 673–680. [CrossRef]
95. Smith, L.T.; Schwarze, U.; Goldstein, J.; Byers, P.H. Mutations in the COL3A1 gene result in the Ehlers-Danlos syndrome type IV and alterations in the size and distribution of the major collagen fibrils of the dermis. *J. Investig. Dermatol.* **1997**, *108*, 241–247. [CrossRef]
96. Liu, X.; Wu, H.; Byrne, M.; Krane, S.; Jaenisch, R. Type III collagen is crucial for collagen I fibrillogenesis and for normal cardiovascular development. *Proc. Natl. Acad. Sci. USA* **1997**, *94*, 1852–1856. [CrossRef]
97. Chiarelli, N.; Carini, G.; Zoppi, N.; Ritelli, M.; Colombi, M. Transcriptome analysis of skin fibroblasts with dominant negative COL3A1 mutations provides molecular insights into the etiopathology of vascular Ehlers-Danlos syndrome. *PLoS ONE* **2018**, *13*, e0191220. [CrossRef]
98. Sengle, G.; Sakai, L.Y. The fibrillin microfibril scaffold: A niche for growth factors and mechanosensation? *Matrix Biol.* **2015**, *47*, 3–12. [CrossRef]
99. Schiavinato, A.; Keene, D.R.; Wohl, A.P.; Corallo, D.; Colombatti, A.; Wagener, R.; Paulsson, M.; Bonaldo, P.; Sengle, G. Targeting of EMILIN-1 and EMILIN-2 to fibrillin microfibrils facilitates their incorporation into the extracellular matrix. *J. Investig. Dermatol.* **2016**, *136*, 1150–1160. [CrossRef]
100. Boregowda, R.; Paul, E.; White, J.; Ritty, T.M. Bone and soft connective tissue alterations result from loss of fibrillin-2 expression. *Matrix Biol.* **2008**, *27*, 661–666. [CrossRef]
101. Brinckmann, J.; Hunzelmann, N.; Kahle, B.; Rohwedel, J.; Kramer, J.; Gibson, M.A.; Hubmacher, D.; Reinhardt, D.P. Enhanced fibrillin-2 expression is a general feature of wound healing and sclerosis: Potential alteration of cell attachment and storage of TGF-beta. *Lab. Investig.* **2010**, *90*, 739–752. [CrossRef]
102. D'Hondt, S.; Guillemyn, B.; Syx, D.; Symoens, S.; De Rycke, R.; Vanhoutte, L.; Toussaint, W.; Lambrecht, B.N.; De Paepe, A.; Keene, D.R.; et al. Type III collagen affects dermal and vascular collagen fibrillogenesis and tissue integrity in a mutant Col3a1 transgenic mouse model. *Matrix Biol.* **2018**, *70*, 72–83. [CrossRef]
103. Ishikawa, Y.; Bächinger, H.P. A substrate preference for the rough endoplasmic reticulum resident protein FKBP22 during collagen biosynthesis. *J. Biol. Chem.* **2014**, *289*, 18189–18201. [CrossRef]
104. Baumann, M.; Giunta, C.; Krabichler, B.; Rüschendorf, F.; Zoppi, N.; Colombi, M.; Bittner, R.E.; Quijano-Roy, S.; Muntoni, F.; Cirak, S.; et al. Mutations in FKBP14 cause a variant of Ehlers-Danlos syndrome with progressive kyphoscoliosis, myopathy, and hearing loss. *Am. J. Hum. Genet.* **2012**, *90*, 201–216. [CrossRef]
105. Soares Moretti, A.; Martins Laurindo, F.R. Protein disulfide isomerases: Redox connections in and out of the endoplasmic reticulum. *Arch. Biochem. Biophys.* **2017**, *617*, 106–119. [CrossRef]
106. Szegezdi, E.; Macdonald, D.C.; Ni Chonghaile, T.; Gupta, S.; Samali, A. Bcl-2 family on guard at the ER. *Am. J. Physiol.-Cell Physiol.* **2009**, *296*, C941–C953. [CrossRef]
107. Sisinni, L.; Pietrafesa, M.; Lepore, S.; Maddalena, F.; Condelli, V.; Esposito, F.; Landriscina, M. Endoplasmic Reticulum Stress and Unfolded Protein Response in Breast Cancer: The Balance between Apoptosis and Autophagy and Its Role in Drug Resistance. *Int. J. Mol. Sci.* **2019**, *20*, 857. [CrossRef]

108. Boot-Handford, R.P.; Briggs, M.D. The unfolded protein response and its relevance to connective tissue diseases. *Cell Tissue Res.* **2010**, *339*, 197–211. [CrossRef]
109. Hughes, A.; Oxford, A.E.; Tawara, K.; Jorcyk, C.L.; Oxford, J.T. Endoplasmic Reticulum Stress and Unfolded Protein Response in Cartilage Pathophysiology; Contributing Factors to Apoptosis and Osteoarthritis. *Int. J. Mol. Sci.* **2017**, *18*, 665. [CrossRef]
110. Tinkle, B.; Castori, M.; Berglund, B.; Cohen, H.; Grahame, R.; Kazkaz, H.; Levy, H. Hypermobile Ehlers-Danlos syndrome (a.k.a. Ehlers-Danlos syndrome type III and Ehlers-Danlos syndrome hypermobility type): Clinical description and natural history. *Am. J. Med. Genet. C Semin. Med. Genet.* **2017**, *175*, 48–69. [CrossRef]
111. Castori, M.; Tinkle, B.; Levy, H.; Grahame, R.; Malfait, F.; Hakim, A. A framework for the classification of joint hypermobility and related conditions. *Am. J. Med. Genet. C Semin. Med. Genet.* **2017**, *175*, 148–157. [CrossRef]
112. Schalkwijk, J.; Zweers, M.C.; Steijlen, P.M.; Dean, W.B.; Taylor, G.; van Vlijmen, I.M.; van Haren, B.; Miller, W.L.; Bristow, J. A recessive form of the Ehlers-Danlos syndrome caused by tenascin-X deficiency. *N. Engl. J. Med.* **2001**, *345*, 1167–1175. [CrossRef]
113. Merke, D.P.; Chen, W.; Morissette, R.; Xu, Z.; Van Ryzin, C.; Sachdev, V.; Hannoush, H.; Shanbhag, S.M.; Acevedo, A.T.; Nishitani, M.; et al. Tenascin-X haploinsufficiency associated with Ehlers-Danlos syndrome in patients with congenital adrenal hyperplasia. *J. Clin. Endocrinol. Metab.* **2013**, *98*, 379–387. [CrossRef]
114. Morissette, R.; Chen, W.; Perritt, A.F.; Dreiling, J.L.; Arai, A.E.; Sachdev, V.; Hannoush, H.; Mallappa, A.; Xu, Z.; McDonnell, N.B.; et al. Broadening the Spectrum of Ehlers Danlos Syndrome in Patients with Congenital Adrenal Hyperplasia. *J. Clin. Endocrinol. Metab.* **2015**, *100*, 1143–1152. [CrossRef]
115. Syx, D.; Symoens, S.; Steyaert, W.; De Paepe, A.; Coucke, P.J.; Malfait, F. Ehlers-Danlos Syndrome, Hypermobility Type, Is Linked to Chromosome 8p22-8p21.1 in an Extended Belgian Family. *Dis. Markers* **2015**, *2015*, 828970. [CrossRef]
116. Copetti, M.; Morlino, S.; Colombi, M.; Grammatico, P.; Fontana, A.; Castori, M. Severity classes in adults with hypermobile Ehlers-Danlos syndrome/hypermobility spectrum disorders: A pilot study of 105 Italian patients. *Rheumatology* **2019**, kez029. [CrossRef]
117. Castori, M.; Dordoni, C.; Valiante, M.; Sperduti, I.; Ritelli, M.; Morlino, S.; Chiarelli, N.; Celletti, C.; Venturini, M.; Camerota, F.; et al. Nosology and inheritance pattern(s) of joint hypermobility syndrome and Ehlers-Danlos syndrome, hypermobility type: A study of intrafamilial and interfamilial variability in 23 Italian pedigrees. *Am. J. Med. Genet. A* **2014**, *164*, 3010–3020. [CrossRef]
118. Ritelli, M.; Chiarelli, N.; Zoppi, N.; Dordoni, C.; Quinzani, S.; Traversa, M.; Venturini, M.; Calzavara-Pinton, P.; Colombi, M. Insights in the etiopathology of galactosyltransferase II (GalT-II) deficiency from transcriptome-wide expression profiling of skin fibroblasts of two sisters with compound heterozygosity for two novel B3GALT6 mutations. *Mol. Genet. Metab. Rep.* **2014**, *20*, 1–15. [CrossRef]
119. Zoppi, N.; Chiarelli, N.; Cinquina, V.; Ritelli, M.; Colombi, M. GLUT10 deficiency leads to oxidative stress and non-canonical $\alpha v \beta 3$ integrin-mediated TGFβ signaling associated with extracellular matrix disarray in arterial tortuosity syndrome skin fibroblasts. *Hum. Mol. Genet.* **2015**, *24*, 6769–6787. [CrossRef]
120. Manzoni, C.; Kia, D.A.; Vandrovcova, J.; Hardy, J.; Wood, N.W.; Lewis, P.A.; Ferrari, R. Genome, transcriptome and proteome: The rise of omics data and their integration in biomedical sciences. *Brief. Bioinform.* **2018**, *19*, 286–302. [CrossRef]
121. Casamassimi, A.; Federico, A.; Rienzo, M.; Esposito, S.; Ciccodicola, A. Transcriptome Profiling in Human Diseases: New Advances and Perspectives. *Int. J. Mol. Sci.* **2017**, *18*, 1652. [CrossRef]
122. Ideozu, J.E.; Zhang, X.; McColley, S.; Levy, H. Transcriptome Profiling and Molecular Therapeutic Advances in Cystic Fibrosis: Recent Insights. *Genes* **2019**, *10*, 180. [CrossRef]
123. Chiarelli, N.; Carini, G.; Zoppi, N.; Dordoni, C.; Ritelli, M.; Venturini, M.; Castori, M.; Colombi, M. Transcriptome-wide expression profiling in skin fibroblasts of patients with joint hypermobility syndrome/Ehlers-Danlos syndrome hypermobility type. *PLoS ONE* **2016**, *11*, e0161347. [CrossRef]
124. Jansen, K.A.; Atherton, P.; Ballestrem, C. Mechanotransduction at the cell-matrix interface. *Semin. Cell Dev. Biol.* **2017**, *71*, 75–83. [CrossRef]
125. Freedman, B.R.; Bade, N.D.; Riggin, C.N.; Zhang, S.; Haines, P.G.; Ong, K.L.; Janmey, P.A. The (dys) functional extracellular matrix. *Biochim. Biophys. Acta* **2015**, *1853*, 3153–3164. [CrossRef]
126. Kalluri, R.; Neilson, E.R. Epithelial-mesenchymal transition and its implications for fibrosis. *J. Clin. Investig.* **2003**, *112*, 1776–1784. [CrossRef]

127. Lamouille, S.; Xu, J.; Derynck, R. Molecular mechanisms of epithelial-mesenchymal transition. *Nat. Rev. Mol. Cell Biol.* **2014**, *15*, 178–196. [CrossRef]
128. McCrea, P.D.; Maher, M.T.; Gottardi, C.J. Nuclear signaling from cadherin adhesion complexes. *Curr. Top. Dev. Biol.* **2015**, *112*, 129–196.
129. Hinz, B.; Gabbiani, G. Cell-matrix and cell-cell contacts of myofibroblasts: Role in connective tissue remodeling. *Thromb. Haemost.* **2003**, *90*, 993–1002.
130. Michalik, M.; Wójcik-Pszczoła, K.; Paw, M.; Wnuk, D.; Koczurkiewicz, P.; Sanak, M.; Pękala, E.; Madeja, Z. Fibroblast-to-myofibroblast transition in bronchial asthma. *Cell. Mol. Life Sci.* **2018**, *75*, 3943–3961. [CrossRef]
131. Hinz, B.; McCulloch, C.A.; Coelho, N.M. Mechanical regulation of myofibroblast phenoconversion and collagen contraction. *Exp. Cell Res.* **2019**, *379*, 119–128. [CrossRef]
132. Pakshir, P.; Hinz, B. The big five in fibrosis: Macrophages, myofibroblasts, matrix, mechanics, and miscommunication. *Matrix Biol.* **2018**, *68–69*, 81–93. [CrossRef]
133. Mullenbrock, S.; Liu, F.; Szak, S.; Hronowski, X.; Gao, B.; Juhasz, P.; Sun, C.; Liu, M.; McLaughlin, H.; Xiao, Q.; et al. Systems Analysis of Transcriptomic and Proteomic Profiles Identifies Novel Regulation of Fibrotic Programs by miRNAs in Pulmonary Fibrosis Fibroblasts. *Genes* **2018**, *9*, 588. [CrossRef]
134. Van Caam, A.; Vonk, M.; van den Hoogen, F.; van Lent, P.; van der Kraan, P. Unraveling SSc Pathophysiology; The Myofibroblast. *Front. Immunol.* **2018**, *9*, 2452. [CrossRef]
135. Watanabe, T.; Baker Frost, D.A.; Mlakar, L.; Heywood, J.; da Silveira, W.A.; Hardiman, G.; Feghali-Bostwick, C. A Human Skin Model Recapitulates Systemic Sclerosis Dermal Fibrosis and Identifies COL22A1 as a TGFβ Early Response Gene that Mediates Fibroblast to Myofibroblast Transition. *Genes* **2019**, *10*, 75. [CrossRef]
136. Działo, E.; Tkacz, K.; Błyszczuk, P. Crosstalk between the TGF-β and WNT signalling pathways during cardiac fibrogenesis. *Acta Biochim. Pol.* **2018**, *65*, 341–349. [CrossRef]
137. Cruciat, C.M.; Niehrs, C. Secreted and transmembrane wnt inhibitors and activators. *Cold Spring Harb. Perspect. Biol.* **2013**, *5*, a015081. [CrossRef]
138. Carthy, J.M.; Garmaroudi, F.S.; Luo, Z.; McManus, B.M. Wnt3a induces myofibroblast differentiation by upregulating TGF-β signaling through SMAD2 in a β-catenin-dependent manner. *PLoS ONE* **2011**, *6*, e19809. [CrossRef]
139. Blyszczuk, P.; Müller-Edenborn, B.; Valenta, T.; Osto, E.; Stellato, M.; Behnke, S.; Glatz, K.; Basler, K.; Lüscher, T.F.; Distler, O.; et al. Transforming growth factor-β-dependent Wnt secretion controls myofibroblast formation and myocardial fibrosis progression in experimental autoimmune myocarditis. *Eur. Heart J.* **2017**, *38*, 1413–1425. [CrossRef]
140. Abonia, J.P.; Wen, T.; Stucke, E.M.; Grotjan, T.; Griffith, M.S.; Kemme, K.A.; Collins, M.H.; Putnam, P.E.; Franciosi, J.P.; Von Tiehl, K.F.; et al. High prevalence of eosinophilic esophagitis in patients with inherited connective tissue disorders. *J. Allergy Clin. Immunol.* **2013**, *132*, 378–386. [CrossRef]
141. Fikree, A.; Grahame, R.; Aktar, R.; Farmer, A.D.; Hakim, A.J.; Morris, J.K.; Knowles, C.H.; Aziz, Q. A prospective evaluation of undiagnosed joint hypermobility syndrome in patients with gastrointestinal symptoms. *Clin. Gastroenterol. Hepatol.* **2013**, *27*, 569–579. [CrossRef]
142. Morgan, A.W.; Pearson, S.B.; Davies, S.; Gooi, H.C.; Bird, H.A. Asthma and airway collapse in two heritable disorders of connective tissue. *Ann. Rheum. Dis.* **2007**, *66*, 1369–1373. [CrossRef]
143. Rodgers, K.R.; Gui, J.; Dinulos, M.B.; Chou, R.C. Ehlers-Danlos syndrome hypermobility type is associated with rheumatic diseases. *Sci. Rep.* **2017**, *7*, 39636. [CrossRef]
144. Grether-Beck, S.; Felsner, I.; Brenden, H.; Kohne, Z.; Majora, M.; Marini, A.; Jaenicke, T.; Rodriguez-Martin, M.; Trullas, C.; Hupe, M.; et al. Urea uptake enhances barrier function and antimicrobial defense in humans by regulating epidermal gene expression. *J. Investig. Dermatol.* **2012**, *132*, 1561–1572. [CrossRef]
145. Nagahara, M.; Waguri-Nagaya, Y.; Yamagami, T.; Aoyama, M.; Tada, T.; Inoue, K.; Asai, K.; Otsuka, T. TNF-alpha-induced aquaporin 9 in synoviocytes from patients with OA and RA. *Rheumatology* **2010**, *49*, 898–906. [CrossRef]
146. Takeuchi, K.; Hayashi, S.; Matumoto, T.; Hashimoto, S.; Takayama, K.; Chinzei, N.; Kihara, S.; Haneda, M.; Kirizuki, S.; Kuroda, Y.; et al. Downregulation of aquaporin 9 decreases catabolic factor expression through nuclear factor-κB signaling in chondrocytes. *Int. J. Mol. Med.* **2018**, *42*, 1548–1558. [CrossRef]
147. Xu, Y.; Ma, M.; Ippolito, G.C.; Schroeder, H.W.; Carroll, M.C.; Volanakis, J.E. Complement activation in factor D-deficient mice. *Proc. Natl. Acad. Sci. USA* **2001**, *98*, 14577–14582. [CrossRef]

148. Kluzek, S.; Arden, N.K.; Newton, J. Adipokines as potential prognostic biomarkers in patients with acute knee injury. *Biomarkers* **2015**, *20*, 519–525. [CrossRef]
149. Martel-Pelletier, J.; Raynauld, J.P.; Dorais, M.; Abram, F.; Pelletier, J.P. The levels of the adipokines adipsin and leptin are associated with knee osteoarthritis progression as assessed by MRI and incidence of total knee replacement in symptomatic osteoarthritis patients: A post hoc analysis. *Rheumatology* **2016**, *55*, 680–688. [CrossRef]
150. Chandran, V.; Abji, F.; Perruccio, A.V.; Gandhi, R.; Li, S.; Cook, R.J.; Gladman, D.D. Serum-based soluble markers differentiate psoriatic arthritis from osteoarthritis. *Ann. Rheum. Dis.* **2019**, *78*, 796–801. [CrossRef]
151. Lyons, J.J.; Yu, X.; Hughes, J.D.; Le, Q.T.; Jamil, A.; Bai, Y.; Ho, N.; Zhao, M.; Liu, Y.; O'Connell, M.P.; et al. Elevated basal serum tryptase identifies a multisystem disorder associated with increased TPSAB1 copy number. *Nat. Genet.* **2016**, *48*, 1564–1569. [CrossRef]
152. He, Y.W.; Li, H.; Zhang, J.; Hsu, C.L.; Lin, E.; Zhang, N.; Guo, J.; Forbush, K.A.; Bevan, M.J. The extracellular matrix protein mindin is a pattern-recognition molecule for microbial pathogens. *Nat. Immunol.* **2004**, *5*, 88–97. [CrossRef]
153. Jia, W.; Li, H.; He, Y.W. The extracellular matrix protein mindin serves as an integrin ligand and is critical for inflammatory cell recruitment. *Blood* **2005**, *106*, 3854–3859. [CrossRef]
154. Liu, Y.S.; Wang, L.F.; Cheng, X.S.; Huo, Y.N.; Ouyang, X.M.; Liang, L.Y.; Lin, Y.; Wu, J.F.; Ren, J.L.; Guleng, B. The pattern-recognition molecule mindin binds integrin Mac-1 to promote macrophage phagocytosis via Syk activation and NF-κB p65 translocation. *J. Cell. Mol. Med.* **2019**, *23*, 3402–3416. [CrossRef]
155. Clapp, C.; Adán, N.; Ledesma-Colunga, M.G.; Solís-Gutiérrez, M.; Triebel, J.; Martínez de la Escalera, G. The role of the prolactin/vasoinhibin axis in rheumatoid arthritis: An integrative overview. *Cell. Mol. Life Sci.* **2016**, *73*, 2929–2948. [CrossRef]
156. Ledesma-Colunga, M.G.; Adán, N.; Ortiz, G.; Solís-Gutiérrez, M.; López-Barrera, F.; Martínez de la Escalera, G.; Clapp, C. Prolactin blocks the expression of receptor activator of nuclear factor κB ligand and reduces osteoclastogenesis and bone loss in murine inflammatory arthritis. *Arthritis Res. Ther.* **2017**, *19*, 93. [CrossRef]
157. Patil, M.J.; Ruparel, S.B.; Henry, M.A.; Akopian, A.N. Prolactin regulates TRPV1, TRPA1, and TRPM8 in sensory neurons in a sex-dependent manner: Contribution of prolactin receptor to inflammatory pain. *Am. J. Physiol. Endocrinol. Metab.* **2013**, *305*, E1154–E1164. [CrossRef]
158. Basso, L.; Altier, C. Transient Receptor Potential Channels in neuropathic pain. *Curr. Opin. Pharmacol.* **2017**, *32*, 9–15. [CrossRef]
159. Rodríguez-Calvo, R.; Tajes, M.; Vázquez-Carrera, M. The NR4A subfamily of nuclear receptors: Potential new therapeutic targets for the treatment of inflammatory diseases. *Expert Opin. Ther. Targets* **2017**, *21*, 291–304. [CrossRef]
160. Murphy, E.P.; Crean, D. Molecular Interactions between NR4A Orphan Nuclear Receptors and NF-Kb Are Required for Appropriate Inflammatory Responses and Immune Cell Homeostasis. *Biomolecules* **2015**, *5*, 1302–1318. [CrossRef]
161. Banno, A.; Lakshmi, S.P.; Reddy, A.T.; Kim, S.C.; Reddy, R.C. Key Functions and Therapeutic Prospects of Nur77 in Inflammation Related Lung Diseases. *Am. J. Pathol.* **2019**, *189*, 482–491. [CrossRef]
162. Fernandes, J.C.R.; Acuña, S.M.; Aoki, J.I.; Floeter-Winter, L.M.; Muxel, S.M. Long Non-Coding RNAs in the Regulation of Gene Expression: Physiology and Disease. *Noncoding RNA* **2019**, *5*, 17. [CrossRef]
163. Filipowicz, W.; Bhattacharyya, S.N.; Sonenberg, N. Mechanisms of post-transcriptional regulation by microRNAs: Are the answers insight? *Nat. Rev. Genet* **2008**, *9*, 102–114. [CrossRef]
164. Leinders, M.; Üçeyler, N.; Thomann, A.; Sommer, C. Aberrant microRNA expression in patients with painful peripheral neuropathies. *J. Neurol. Sci.* **2017**, *380*, 242–249. [CrossRef]
165. Greco, S.; Cardinali, B.; Falcone, G.; Martelli, F. Circular RNAs in Muscle Function and Disease. *Int. J. Mol. Sci.* **2018**, *19*, 3454. [CrossRef]
166. D'Agnelli, S.; Arendt-Nielsen, L.; Gerra, M.C.; Zatorri, K.; Boggiani, L.; Baciarello, M.; Bignami, E. Fibromyalgia: Genetics and epigenetics insights may provide the basis for the development of diagnostic biomarkers. *Mol. Pain* **2019**, *15*, 1744806918819944. [CrossRef]
167. Kim, J.; Hyun, J.; Wang, S.; Lee, C.; Jung, Y. MicroRNA-378 is involved in hedgehog-driven epithelial-to-mesenchymal transition in hepatocytes of regenerating liver. *Cell Death Dis.* **2018**, *9*, 721. [CrossRef]

168. Zhang, T.; Hu, J.; Wang, X.; Zhao, X.; Li, Z.; Niu, J.; Steer, C.J.; Zheng, G.; Song, G. MicroRNA-378 promotes hepatic inflammation and fibrosis via modulation of the NF-κB-TNFα pathway. *J. Hepatol.* **2019**, *70*, 87–96. [CrossRef]
169. Xiao, Z.; Deng, D.; He, L.; Jiao, H.; Ye, Y.; Liang, L.; Ding, Y.; Liao, W. MicroRNA-224 sustains Wnt/β-catenin signaling and promotes aggressive phenotype of colorectal cancer. *J. Exp. Clin. Cancer Res.* **2016**, *35*, 21.
170. Peng, Y.; Zhang, X.; Feng, X.; Fan, X.; Jin, Z. The crosstalk between microRNAs and the Wnt/β-catenin signaling pathway in cancer. *Oncotarget* **2017**, *8*, 14089–14106. [CrossRef]
171. Bjersing, J.L.; Lundborg, C.; Bokarewa, M.I.; Mannerkorpi, K. Profile of cerebrospinal microRNAs in fibromyalgia. *PLoS ONE* **2013**, *8*, e78762. [CrossRef]
172. Chopra, P.; Tinkle, B.; Hamonet, C.; Brock, I.; Gompel, A.; Bulbena, A.; Francomano, C. Pain management in the Ehlers-Danlos syndromes. *Am. J. Med. Genet. C Semin. Med. Genet.* **2017**, *175*, 212–219. [CrossRef]
173. Wade, S.M.; Trenkmann, M.; McGarry, T.; Canavan, M.; Marzaioli, V.; Wade, S.C.; Veale, D.J.; Fearon, U. Altered expression of microRNA-23a in psoriatic arthritis modulates synovial fibroblast pro-inflammatory mechanisms via phosphodiesterase 4B. *J. Autoimmun.* **2019**, *96*, 86–93. [CrossRef]
174. Tajerian, M.; Clark, J.D. The role of the extracellular matrix in chronic pain following injury. *Pain* **2015**, *156*, 366–370. [CrossRef]
175. Parisien, M.; Samoshkin, A.; Tansley, S.N.; Piltonen, M.H.; Martin, L.J.; El-Hachem, N.; Dagostino, C.; Allegri, M.; Mogil, J.S.; Khoutorsky, A.; et al. Genetic pathway analysis reveals a major role for extracellular matrix organization in inflammatory and neuropathic pain. *Pain* **2019**, *60*, 932–944. [CrossRef]
176. Andersen, H.H.; Duroux, M.; Gazerani, P. MicroRNA as modulators and biomarkers of inflammatory and neuropathic pain conditions. *Neurobiol. Dis.* **2014**, *71*, 159–168. [CrossRef]

4

Autophagy: Dual Response in the Development of Hepatocellular Carcinoma

Hamza O. Yazdani [1], Hai Huang [2] and Allan Tsung [2,*]

1 Department of Surgery, University of Pittsburgh, Pittsburg, PA 15213-2582, USA; obaidh3@upmc.edu
2 Division of Surgical Oncology, Department of Surgery, The Ohio State University Wexner Medical Center, N924 Doan Hall, 410 West 10th Ave., Columbus, OH 43210, USA; huang.3900@osu.edu
* Correspondence: Allan.Tsung@osumc.edu

Abstract: Autophagy is an evolutionary conserved intracellular mechanism which helps eukaryotic cells in maintaining their metabolic state to afford high-efficiency energy requirements. In the physiology of a normal liver and the pathogenesis of liver diseases, autophagy plays a crucial role. Autophagy has been found to be both upregulated and downregulated in different cancers providing the evidence that autophagy plays a dual role in suppressing and promoting cell survival. Hepatocellular carcinoma (HCC) is the most common primary liver cancer and the major leading cause of cancer mortality worldwide. In light of its high complexity and poor prognosis, it is essential to improve our understanding of autophagy's role in HCC. In this review, we summarize the dual mechanism of autophagy in the development of HCC and elucidate the currently used therapeutic strategies for anti-HCC therapy.

Keywords: hepatocellular carcinoma; inflammation; mitophagy; oxidative stress; HCC therapy

1. Introduction

Autophagy (macroautophagy) is the fundamental cellular process in maintaining cell homeostasis by targeting damaged intracellular organelles and misfolded proteins to lysosomal degradation [1]. It is a conserved evolutionary process that takes part in all mammalian cells under basal conditions and generates building block molecules to support essential cellular processes [2]. Autophagy is a multistep process including membrane rearrangement in forming a double-membrane bond structure known as autophagosomes. The vesicle fusion of these autophagosomes with lytic compartments generates autolysosomes where lysosomal enzymatic degradation of contents is recycled and releases nucleotides, fatty acids, and amino acids to refuel the cells with energy to maintain necessary molecular synthesis [2].

The role of autophagy is complex and differs from organ to organ. An organ such as muscles and the liver requires autophagy to remove excessive protein aggregation, lipid accumulation, and damaged mitochondria to prevent excessive ROS generation leading to oxidative stress [3,4]. Defects in autophagy have shown to contributes in several pathogeneses of human diseases ranging from neurodegenerative and metabolic diseases to cancers [5]. The dysregulation of autophagy has been increasingly indicated to play a role in liver diseases such as alcoholic liver disease, non-alcoholic fatty liver disease (NAFLD), hepatosteatosis, hepatomegaly, and primary liver malignancies such as hepatocellular carcinoma (HCC) [6,7].

Hepatocellular carcinoma is a serious threat towards human health. It is the sixth most malignant cancer worldwide and the fifth most common malignancy in men [8]. Despite recent advances in treatments and surgical resection, the five-year survival rate remains unsatisfactory [9]. The most common identified risk factors for HCC development are the consequences of unresolved oxidative stress, persistent inflammation, viral infections, metabolic dysfunction, liver alcohol disease, and fatty liver disease. Autophagy may serve as a protective mechanism against the initial and persistent liver injury in these disease states but autophagy may also play a significant role in the development and growth of hepatic tumor cells in this inflammatory environment [10,11]. The link between autophagy and cancer has been long proposed. The underlying mechanisms regulating the autophagic response in HCC requires further understanding to develop effective treatment strategies.

2. Role of Autophagy in Normal Liver Homeostasis

Autophagy is involved in diverse physiology and pathophysiology of the liver. The liver displays a complex metabolism with a variety of functions including protein and lipid synthesis and secretion of bile acid. Increased accumulation of ubiquitin proteins aggregation observed in the liver-specific Atg7 knockout mice suggested a basal function of autophagy in continuous turnover of the cytoplasmic proteins [12,13]. Disturbance in the basal autophagy of the liver can lead to the accumulation of elementary bodies, damaged mitochondria, deformed peroxisomes, and abnormal membrane structures resulting in liver injury. Autophagy can be general and nonselective, involving the degradation of a bulk cytoplasmic portion or organelle-specific degradation. The cell can undergo different forms of autophagy which include xenophagy (degradation of viruses), lipophagy (degradation of lipid droplets), ribophagy (degradation of ribosomes), pexophagy (degradation of peroxisomes), reticulophagy (degradation of ER), and mitophagy (degradation of mitochondria). Of these, mitophagy is one of the most well characterized since hepatocytes contain numerous mitochondria to provide the high energy demand for metabolism. Liver specific autophagy deficient mice provide evidence for swollen mitochondria and increased ROS formation [14]. Liver injury is also associated with mitochondrial membrane permeabilization which can activate a mitochondrial apoptotic pathway regulating BAX and Bad (BCL2 family) mediated cell death [15]. The different forms and role of autophagy in the healthy liver are best described in detail by Takashi U Eno et al. [16].

Hepatocytes are primarily dependent on autophagy degradation due to its intense metabolism and high energy demand to maintain proper functioning. The defect in any of the forms of autophagy can contribute to severe liver functional damage such as hepatitis, fibrosis, cirrhosis, and HCC development [17,18]. One of the most common causes of acute and chronic liver disease is the infection of the liver with hepatotropic viruses. Hepatitis B and C viruses are both linked to the autophagy. It has been shown that the X protein of the HBV (HBx) can induce autophagy due to its ability to bind to the PI3k autophagic molecule. On the other hand, the Hepatitis C virus (HCV) can adapt autophagy content to enhance its replication by inhibiting the maturation of autophagosome into autophagolysosomes. Both these viruses are shown to induce autophagy by transcriptional upregulation of Beclin1 [19].

Autophagy also plays a role in lipid metabolism and thus can influence the development of fatty liver disease, a rapidly increasing cause of chronic liver disease in the world. Hepatocytes are the main source for natural lipids stored in the form of triglycerides (TGs) and lipid droplets (LDs). Interestingly, the first degradation of lipid droplets through lipophagy was observed in mouse liver. It has been shown that ATg7 knockout mice showed significant increase levels of TGs and LDs in the hepatocytes leading to a decrease in the levels of free fatty acids (FFAs), necessary for ATP generation [20]. Another study illustrates the formation of hepatic steatosis in mice due to the consumption of a high-fat diet. This process occurs through autophagy activation in hepatic stellate cells and is due to the suppression of mTOR phosphorylation which increased expression of Sirt1 through the AMPK pathway [21].

3. Role of Autophagy in Hepatocellular Carcinoma

Hepatocellular carcinoma is one of the most common primary cancer and a major leading cause of death worldwide [22]. An estimation of 30,200 deaths is predicted this year [23]. The high proliferative capability of HCC cells has been linked to persistent inflammation and increased oxidative stress. Autophagy has been shown to play a dual role in cancer. Autophagy could be either tumor suppressive or tumor promoting. Here we review both the pro- and anti-tumor mechanism of autophagy that take place during the development and growth of HCC.

3.1. Tumor-Suppressive Role of Autophagy

Inflammation is recognized as a hallmark of cancer in promoting tumor growth and is associated with the poor prognosis of many solid tumors [24]. It is well known that HCC progression is highly correlated with the persistent inflammatory stimulation [25]. Autophagy has been suggested to prevent cancer progression by suppressing inflammation [26–29] while inhibition of autophagy can lead to a sustained and elevated level of inflammation [30,31]. Inflammasomes are the major drivers for chronic inflammation in the liver [32,33]. Interestingly, the capability of cells to suppress inflammation through autophagy was first observed in autophagic inhibited mice. Lack of autophagic responses in ATG16L1 knockout mice undergoing septic shock revealed an elevated level of inflammasome associated IL-1β and IL-18 cytokine production compared to wild-type controls [28]. Further studies showed that depletion of the autophagic proteins, LC3B and Beclin1, enhanced Caspase-1 activation which was NALP3 inflammasomes dependent. Mice lacking LC3B protein were more susceptible to LPS induced mortality [34]. In addition, a recent study showed the effect of chemokine (C-X-C motif) ligand 17 (CXCL17) in suppressing autophagy [35]. In human HCC tissues, elevated expression of CXCL17 has been observed which can also promote cell proliferation and migration when treated invitro. Silencing of this induced autophagy which is due to the enhanced nuclear translocation of liver kinase b1 (LKB1) that phosphorylates and activates AMPK. This lead to decrease in tumor volume and proliferation.

Beclin1, an important autophagic protein, has been shown to be associated with HCC tumors. The decreased Beclin1 expression observed in human HCC tissues correlated with tumor recurrence and disease-free survival [36]. Studies have also shown that knocking out Beclin1 in mice is embryonically lethal whereas heterogeneous Beclin1 mice developed spontaneous HCC [37]. In addition, normal hepatocytes show higher expression and activity of autophagic-associated proteins compared with HCC cell lines providing evidence that autophagy plays a tumor suppressive role [14]. A recent study demonstrated the effect of adrenaline in promoting hepatocarcinogenesis [38]. Treatment of adrenaline in DEN-induced HCC mice showed a remarkable increase in liver injury along with increased tumor number and tumor size. Mechanistically, increase in adrenaline activated the adrenergic receptors ADRB2 which inhibited autophagy activation by disrupting the Beclin1/VPS34/ATg14 complex.

Since autophagy plays a vital role in suppressing cancer inflammation, inhibition of autophagy has also been shown to result in an excessive accumulation of p62 protein [39]. P62 is an autophagic substrate which is used in measuring autophagic activity [40,41]. Transgenic P62 knockout animals displayed irregular cell mitotic activity with an increased expression of insulin-like growth factor 2 (IGF2) in their HCC tumors [42]. It has been reported that p62 is necessary for the HCC initiation by maintaining metabolic homeostasis through the mTOR pathway [43] and ablation of p62 inhibits growth and proliferation [14]. In a study, 90 HCC-resected tumors were analyzed for the accumulation of intracellular hyaline bodies (IHB) which are cytoplasmic inclusions consisting of p62. Patients with increased IHB were shown to be associated with significantly shorter overall survival [44]. Moreover. P62 is also known to interact with tumor necrosis factor receptor-associated factor 6 (TRAF6) that induces nuclear factor (NF-kB) activation [45]. Zhang et al. [46] have shown that DEAD-box protein 5 (DDX5), a tumor suppressor protein in the liver [47], binds to p62 and interferes with P62/TRAF6 interaction. This results in autophagy induction. However, the expression of DDX5 in the human HCC tumor tissues is relatively lower when compared to its non-tumor counterpart. Autophagy has also been shown to contribute to the anti-proliferative activity of interferon gamma (IFN-gamma), a pleiotropic cytokine that facilitates anti-viral and anti-proliferative effects in cancer cells. In HCC cell lines, stimulated autophagosome formation inhibited cell growth. Silencing of autophagy in these cells abolished the inhibitory effect, suggesting an essential anti-tumorigenic activity [48].

Similarly, multiple miRNAs which are found to target autophagic comprised genes for autophagy modulation [49–51] may also play a part in HCC growth and inhibition. miR-7 is a well acknowledged tumor suppressive microRNA in cancers. In HCC tumors, levels of miR-7 are significantly downregulated. It has been shown that upregulation of miR-7 in HCC cell lines increases autophagic activity by targeting the mTOR pathway, leading to a decrease in cancer cell proliferation [52]. miR-85 is an essential component during liver development and has also been linked as a tumor suppressor in HCC. In human HCC cell line HepG2, transfection of miR-85 upregulated autophagic activity which resulted in cell cycle arrest [53]. Our group has also previously shown that miR-375 is downregulated in HCC cell lines and tissues [54]. We found that miR-375 inhibits autophagy by suppressing the conversion of LC3I to LC3II by downregulating ATG7. Inoculating miR-375 overexpressed cells in nude mice showed significantly decreased tumor growth [51].

3.2. *Tumor-Promoting Role of Autophagy*

Hypoxia-induced oxidative stress is one of the most prominent features in all solid tumors [55,56] due to the inadequate blood supply that tumors experience as they grow. Under oxygen deprivation, cells respond by regulating their metabolic and bioenergetics demands to overcome the hypoxic resistance [57–59]. Hypoxia-induced autophagy in hepatocytes and HCC tumor cells relies upon the stabilization of hypoxia-inducible factor (HIF1α). HIF is the important regulator that maintains oxygen homeostasis. It has been shown that HIF1-α upregulates BNIP3 and BNIP3L proteins which binds to the BCL-2 protein. This process inhibits the disruptive interaction between BCL-2 and Beclin1 [60] to induce autophagy for cellular survival in hypoxic conditions. In addition, hypoxia is also shown to upregulate early growth response gene-1 (Egr-1) expression. Egr-1 is a zinc finger nuclear protein and functions as a transcriptional regulator [61]. Upregulation of hypoxia induced Egr-1 has shown to induce autophagy in HCC cell lines promoting migration. Inhibiting Egr-1 function by Ad-DN-Egr-1 revealed the attenuated autophagosome formation due to inhibited binding of Egr-1 at LC3 promoter region (-233 to -214) [62].

The extensive reactive oxygen species generation during the developing tumor is the primary outcome of hypoxic stress. Increased ROS levels are shown to oxidize cellular components such as DNA, lipids, and proteins [63,64]. ROS can be generated by the NADPH oxidase complexes in the cell membrane, endoplasmic reticulum, peroxisomes, and mitochondria [65,66]. Tumors adapt different mechanisms to eliminates intracellular ROS, one of which is by the upregulation of anti-oxidant proteins NRF2 [67]. NRF2 is a cytoplasmic protein which translocates to the nucleus for the transcription of redox-balancing proteins and β-oxidant enzymes and is upregulated by autophagy. The autophagic protein p62 has been shown to interact with NRF2 [68]. Phosphorylated p62 binds with Keap1 (NRF2 inhibitory protein) allowing NRF2 release and cytosolic stabilization [69,70]. The clinical implication of NRF2 was elucidated in 107 HCC patients where patients that expressed higher levels of pNRF2 were significantly associated with worst disease-free survival and poor overall survival [71]. Thus, p62 induces the antioxidant activation pathway to prevent extreme organelle injury leading to tumor cell death.

Another important mechanism to control excess ROS production is by the removal of damaged organelles from the cell. Injured and non-functional mitochondria are the major source of cellular ROS production and the induction of mitophagy helps clear these damaged mitochondria to maintain cell function and bioenergetics [72,73]. Mitochondrial ROS is eliminated regularly by the superoxide dismutase within the cytosol [74,75] which is also activated by the NRF2 protein [76]. Depolarized mitochondria cleared via mitophagy are regulated by PINK1 and Parkin1 [77]. It is reported that mitophagy can degrade tumor suppressor p53 once localized to mitochondria and inhibit its subcellular localization. Mitophagy impairment results in p53 accumulation and its phosphorylation by PINK1 prevent hepatic cancer cell stemness [78]. However, excessive induction of mitophagy can also inhibit HCC migration. When yes-activated protein (Yap), a highly upregulated protein in HCC, is depleted, mitophagy is overactivated leading to cellular energy deprivation [79]. In contrast, the excessive activation of autophagy may also lead to autophagic cell death [80,81]. This process requires an additional cell death signaling, including the phosphorylation of c-Jun N-terminal kinase (JNK) [82]. Interestingly, the pro-apoptotic (Bax/Bak) deficient cells showed an autophagic cell death when exposed to apoptotic stimuli. This was driven through the increase in the level of JNK phosphorylation. However, treatment with the JNK inhibitor further revealed that a simultaneous activation of autophagy and JNK is required for the autophagic cell death. Numerous other cell death and tumor suppressor-related proteins are shown to trigger autophagic cell death in the literature [83–85].

Autophagy can also regulate inflammatory immune response by the release and degradation of damage associated molecular patterns (DAMPS) including high mobility group box 1 (HMGB1), histones, ATP, mitochondrial (mt)DNA, and mitochondrial transcription factor A (TFAM). HMGB1 is a well-characterized DAMP which can be released from necrotic or apoptotic hepatocytes [86,87]. Interestingly, autophagy-mediated intracellular mobilization of HMGB1 enables tumor growth by inducing cell survival and apoptosis [88,89]. We have previously shown that under hypoxic stress, HMGB1 translocates from nucleus to cytoplasm in HCC cells. Intracellular translocation of HMGB1 facilitates its interaction with mtDNA in the cytosol where together they activate TLR9 signaling pathways to enhance tumor growth [90].

3.3. Autophagy in HCC Metastasis

Autophagy, due to its tumor promoting role, also plays a part in tumor metastasis. Increasing evidence suggests the upregulation of autophagy during the process of tumor metastasis [91,92]. As the primary tumor grows and encounter harsh microenvironment, part of it escapes and intravasates within the circulatory and lymphatic system, localizing at distal organs [93]. Cell detachment from the extracellular matrix (ECM) has demonstrated to trigger autophagy which then protects it from anoikis, a type of cell death induced in response to ECM detachment [94]. In addition, Autophagy can also induce changes in the cell adhesion signaling that facilitates invasion and migration [95].

Autophagy in hepatocellular carcinoma has shown to facilitate metastasis by upregulating the expression of epithelial–mesenchymal transition (EMT). Induction of autophagy in the starved cells inhibited the expression of epithelial markers and induced mesenchymal expression along with cell invasion marker matrix metalloproteinase-9 (MMP9) [96]. These changes were regulated by the activation of TGF-beta and phosphorylation of Smad3 signaling pathway. In another study, inhibition of autophagy via silencing Beclin1 and ATG5 in HCC lung metastasis model markedly decreased distal metastasis to the lungs [97]. This effect is observed due to the impaired anoikis resistance that can suppress the colonization of HCC cells. However, silencing of autophagy mediators showed no effect in the expression of cell migration and invasion regulators.

Autophagy-mediated cancer cell metastasis can be stimulated by numerous stress factors persisting within the tumor microenvironment. One of which is the fluid shear stress (FSS). Wang et al. [98] showed that HCC cells, when exposed to 1.4 dyn/cm^2 of FSS, induce autophagy in a time-dependent manner. Furthermore, inhibition of autophagy attenuated cells to migrate and downregulate the expression of PI3K/FAK/Rho GTPase pathway. This suggests that the activation of autophagy via FSS is a PI3K/FAK/Rho GTPase-dependent pathway.

4. Autophagy in HCC Therapy

As described above, autophagy can be either be pro- or anti-tumorigenic for HCC. Therefore, modulation of autophagy-based HCC therapy is very complex and will vary depending on the setting. Autophagy can suppress liver inflammation and thus decrease the carcinogenic environment in the liver but it can also promote and maintain tumor cell homeostasis by inducing mitophagy in growing HCC tumors. In addition, both the induction and inhibition of autophagy has been investigated to induce tumor cell death [99,100]. Currently, there are a variety of therapeutic agents that are being used either individually or in combination with other agents for anti-HCC therapy. The current agents used to selectively target autophagy to induce HCC cell death are described in Table 1.

4.1. Autophagy Inducers

The autophagy inducer sorafenib is the first-line drug used for the treatment of advanced HCC [101]. Currently, sorafenib is the only drug that has been shown to improve HCC patient survival [102]. In a randomized controlled trial, patients with advanced HCC treated with sorafenib had an improved rate of overall survival compared to patients given placebo. Sorafenib has been shown to promote cell death through the upregulation of autophagy via myeloid cell leukemia-1 (Mcl-1) signaling pathway [103]. In addition, sorafenib can also inhibit tumor growth by targeting the RAF/MEK/ERK pathway to induce cell cycle arrest [104]. Besides Mcl-1 and ERK pathways, sorafenib can also inhibit the activation of PI3K/AKT/mTOR pathways which initiates a signaling cascade for autophagy induction [105,106]. In a recent study, sorafenib is also shown to regulate cell endoplasmic reticulum (ER) stress, JNK, Akt, and AMPK pathway leading to elevated autophagy which later shifts towards apoptosis [107]. At an early time point (3–12 h) sorafenib increases ER stress which is shown to induce the autophagic survival process in HCC cell line by regulating JNK/AMPK signaling pathway. At a later stage (24 h), a significant increase in the ER stress and PERK-CHOP dependent rise of Bim shifted autophagy to apoptosis cell death.

Besides its tumor suppressing function, long term sorafenib treatment has also shown to trigger chemo-resistance in HCC cells [108]. Thus, the combination of sorafenib with SAHA, another autophagy-inducer, has been used to improve responses against HCC compared to treating with sorafenib alone [109]. Sustained treatment of sorafenib has also shown to increase tumor hypoxic environment that leads to decrease treatment efficiency [110]. Combination of melatonin with sorafenib has shown to enhance sorafenib's cytotoxicity against human HCC cells by decreasing hypoxic resistance [111]. Co-administration diminished the expression of BNIP3 and NIX, hypoxia induced mitophagy mediators. Due to the common occurrence of tumor resistance, the combinations of different drugs with sorafenib are currently being studied to increase chemo-sensitivity and decrease tumor growth. A detailed combination of reagents with sorafenib are extensively reviewed elsewhere [112].

4.2. Autophagy Inhibitors

Since autophagy can be utilized by the growing cancer cells for its survival and add resistance towards chemotherapeutic reagents, inhibiting autophagy can also be a promising strategy against cancer therapy. At present chloroquine (CQ), an anti-malarial drug, can be used for the inhibition of autophagy through the suppression of lysosomes. Treatment with CQ neutralizes the pH levels of lysosomes required in the final stages of autophagy for degradation [113]. CQ is being effectively used in patients with the combination of drugs capable of inducing cell apoptosis such as oxaliplatin [114]. It is reported that co-treatment of proliferative HCC cell lines with CQ and sorafenib can lead to a marked suppression of its growth [105]. In a liver xenograft tumor model, nude mice treated with CQ and sorafenib combined achieved a higher level of tumor regression compared to treatment with sorafenib alone. In addition, 3-methyladenine (3-MA) which inhibits the interaction of autophagosomes and lysosomes can enhance anti-HCC therapy when combined with cisplatin, doxorubicin, and sorafenib [115]. Similarly, suppression of autophagy by administration of 3-MA and inactive ATg4B suppresses the proliferation of Huh7 cells [116]. Hence, inhibition of autophagy can promote the death of HCC cells but these treatments with their known side effects highlight a major risk in triggering the neoplasticism within the normal hepatocytes.

Table 1. Therapeutic reagents modulating autophagy in anti-HCC treatment.

Reagents	Autophagy Target	Cells Treated	Result	Ref.
Sirolimus (Rapamycin)	mTOR	HepG2	Upregulation of autophagy-cell death	[117,118]
Temsirolimus (CCI-779)	mTOR	HepG2, Huh7	Upregulation of autophagy-cell death	[119]
Everolimus (RAD001)	mTOR	Hep3B, HepG2, Huh7	Upregulation of autophagy-cell death	[120]
Pemetrexed	mTORC1	HepG2	Upregulation of autophagy-cell death	[121]
SC-59	mTORC1	PLC5, Sk-Hep1, HepG2 and Hep3B	Upregulation of autophagy-cell death	[122,123]
BEZ235	PI3K/mTOR	Hep3B, PLC/PRF/5	Upregulation of autophagy-cell death	[124]
MK-2206	AKT	SNU449, SNU378, SNU475	Upregulation of autophagy-cell death	[125]
SB203580	MAPK	HepG2, Hep3B, PLC/PRF/5, Huh-7	Upregulation of autophagy-cell death	[126]
Regorafenib	Tyrosine-kinase inhibitor	HepG2 and Hep3B	Upregulation of autophagy-cell death	[127]
Sorafenib	Tyrosine-kinase inhibitor	Hep3B, HepG2, Huh7	Upregulation of autophagy-cell death	[105,112]
Nilotinib	Tyrosine kinase inhibitor	PLC5, Huh-7, Hep3B	Upregulation of autophagy-cell death	[128]
ABT-737	JNK pathway	Huh7, HepG2	Upregulation of autophagy-cell death	[129]
OSU-03012	PDK1/AKT	Huh7, Hep3B, and HepG2	Upregulation of autophagy-cell death	[130]
5-FU	Induce ER stress	HepG2, SMMC-7721, Hep3B, BEL-7402	Upregulation of autophagy-cell survival	[114]
Bortezomib	Proteasome inhibitor	Huh7, HepG2, HuH7, human hepatocytes, rat hepatocytes	Upregulation of autophagy-cell death	[131]
Chloroquine	Lysosome	HepG2, Huh7, HA22T/VGH, Mahlavu	Downregulation of autophagy-cell death	[132,133]
3-MA	PI3K III	H22, HepG2, PLC/PRF/5, SMMC7721	Downregulation of autophagy-cell death and cell survival	[134,135]
Bafilomycin A1	Lysosome	BEL7402, HepG2, Huh7, SMMC-7721	Downregulation of autophagy-cell death	[136]

5. Concluding Remarks

Autophagy is the vital response for hepatocytes undergoing stress in the maintenance of cellular homeostasis and quality control. As we outlined in this review, evidence supports a dual role of autophagy in the progression of HCC (Figure 1). Targeting autophagy can be used to treat liver cancer. However, caution should be noted as autophagy can inhibit the development of HCC but also act as a tumor promoter resulting resistance to HCC tumor therapy [137]. Multiple direct and indirect interactions including complex mechanistic overlap between apoptotic and autophagic cell death have been studied [138,139]. Many studies indicate that the apoptotic events alter autophagy. However, the molecular role of autophagy controlling apoptosis requires further investigation. In the developing tumor microenvironment, hypoxia is a common stimulus in many cancers and hepatotropic viruses can induce a hypoxic environment initiating hypoxic oxidative and inflammatory responses [140]. Thus improving tumor oxygenation or suppressing hypoxia-induced autophagy signaling could be a potential future therapeutic pathway to target. We currently have a minimal understanding regarding the stress signaling that takes part in the complex coordination of autophagy to respond during different intracellular and extracellular stimuli in HCC. Additional studies are necessary to further elucidate the mechanisms underlying autophagy's role in HCC.

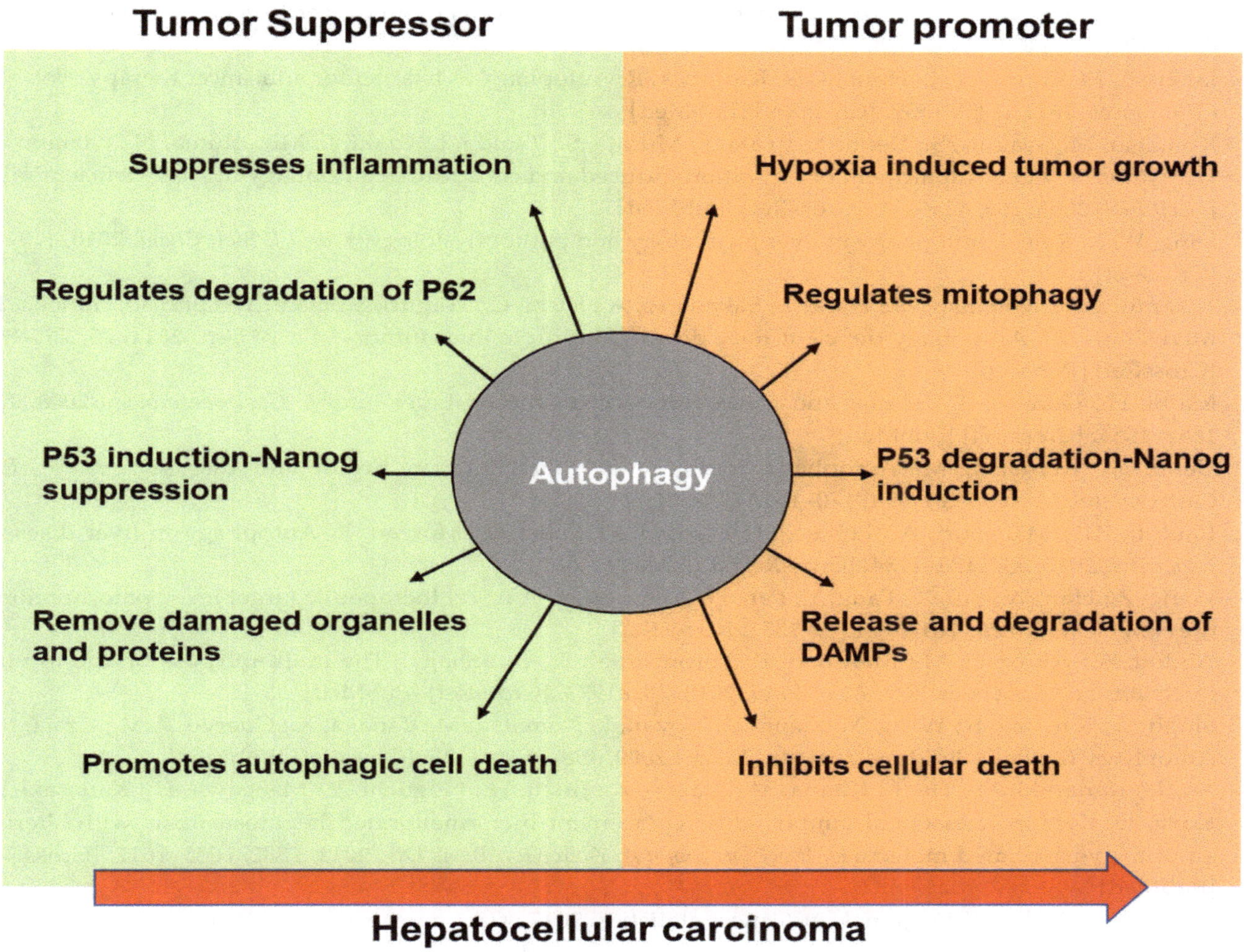

Figure 1. Schematic diagram illustrating the proposed role of autophagy during the development of hepatocellular carcinoma.

Acknowledgments: We thank Jannat Malik for linguistic revision.

References

1. Xie, Z.; Klionsky, D.J. Autophagosome formation: Core machinery and adaptations. *Nat. Cell Biol.* **2007**, *9*, 1102–1109. [CrossRef] [PubMed]
2. Devenish, R.J.; Klionsky, D.J. Autophagy: Mechanism and physiological relevance "brewed" from yeast studies. *Front. Biosci.* **2012**, *54*, 1354–1363. [CrossRef]
3. White, E. The role for autophagy in cancer. *J. Clin. Investig.* **2015**, *125*, 42–46. [CrossRef] [PubMed]
4. Mizushima, N.; Komatsu, M. Autophagy: Renovation of Cells and Tissues. *Cell* **2011**, *147*, 728–741. [CrossRef] [PubMed]
5. Huang, J.; Klionsky, D.J. Autophagy and human disease. *Cell Cycle* **2007**, *6*, 1837–1849. [CrossRef] [PubMed]
6. Yorimitsu, T.; Klionsky, D.J. Autophagy: Molecular machinery for self-eating. *Cell Death Differ.* **2005**, *12*, 1542–1552. [CrossRef] [PubMed]
7. Kwanten, W.J.; Martinet, W.; Michielsen, P.P.; Francque, S.M. Role of autophagy in the pathophysiology of nonalcoholic fatty liver disease: A controversial issue. *World J. Gastroenterol.* **2014**, *20*, 7325–7338. [CrossRef]
8. Cui, J.; Gong, Z.; Shen, H.-M. The role of autophagy in liver cancer: Molecular mechanisms and potential therapeutic targets. *Biochim. Biophys. Acta Rev. Cancer* **2013**, *1836*, 15–26. [CrossRef]

9. Portolani, N.; Coniglio, A.; Ghidoni, S.; Giovanelli, M.; Benetti, A.; Tiberio, G.A.M.; Giulini, S.M. Early and Late Recurrence after Liver Resection for Hepatocellular Carcinoma. *Ann. Surg.* **2006**, *243*, 229–235. [CrossRef]
10. White, E. Deconvoluting the context-dependent role for autophagy in cancer. *Nat. Rev. Cancer* **2012**, *12*, 401–410. [CrossRef]
11. Janku, F.; McConkey, D.J.; Hong, D.S.; Kurzrock, R. Autophagy as a target for anticancer therapy. *Nat. Rev. Clin. Oncol.* **2011**, *8*, 528–539. [CrossRef] [PubMed]
12. Komatsu, M.; Waguri, S.; Ueno, T.; Iwata, J.; Murata, S.; Tanida, I.; Ezaki, J.; Mizushima, N.; Ohsumi, Y.; Uchiyama, Y.; et al. Impairment of starvation-induced and constitutive autophagy in Atg7-deficient mice. *J. Cell Biol.* **2005**, *169*, 425–434. [CrossRef] [PubMed]
13. Ding, W.-X. Role of autophagy in liver physiology and pathophysiology. *World J. Biol. Chem.* **2010**, *1*, 3–12. [CrossRef]
14. Takamura, A.; Komatsu, M.; Hara, T.; Sakamoto, A.; Kishi, C.; Waguri, S.; Eishi, Y.; Hino, O.; Tanaka, K.; Mizushima, N. Autophagy-deficient mice develop multiple liver tumors. *Genes Dev.* **2011**, *25*, 795–800. [CrossRef] [PubMed]
15. Malhi, H.; Gores, G.J. Cellular and Molecular Mechanisms of Liver Injury. *Gastroenterology* **2008**, *134*, 1641–1654. [CrossRef] [PubMed]
16. Ueno, T.; Komatsu, M. Autophagy in the liver: Functions in health and disease. *Nat. Rev. Gastroenterol. Hepatol.* **2017**, *14*, 170–184. [CrossRef]
17. Rautou, P.E.; Mansouri, A.; Lebrec, D.; Durand, F.; Valla, D.; Moreau, R. Autophagy in liver diseases. *J. Hepatol.* **2010**, *53*, 1123–1134. [CrossRef] [PubMed]
18. Wang, Z.; Han, W.; Sui, X.; Fang, Y.; Pan, H. Autophagy: A novel therapeutic target for hepatocarcinoma (Review). *Oncol. Lett.* **2014**, *7*, 1345–1351. [CrossRef]
19. Abdoli, A.; Alirezaei, M.; Mehrbod, P.; Forouzanfar, F. Autophagy: The multi-purpose bridge in viral infections and host cells. *Rev. Med. Virol.* **2018**, *28*, e1973. [CrossRef] [PubMed]
20. Singh, R.; Kaushik, S.; Wang, Y.; Xiang, Y.; Novak, I.; Komatsu, M.; Tanaka, K.; Cuervo, A.M.; Czaja, M.J. Autophagy regulates lipid metabolism. *Nature* **2009**, *458*, 1131–1135. [CrossRef] [PubMed]
21. Xu, L.; Kanasaki, M.; He, J.; Kitada, M.; Nagao, K.; Jinzu, H.; Noguchi, Y.; Maegawa, H.; Kanasaki, K.; Koya, D. Ketogenic essential amino acids replacement diet ameliorated hepatosteatosis with altering autophagy-associated molecules. *Biochim. Biophys. Acta Mol. Basis Dis.* **2013**, *1832*, 1605–1612. [CrossRef] [PubMed]
22. Siegel, R.L.; Miller, K.D.; Jemal, A. Cancer statistics, 2017. *CA Cancer J. Clin.* **2017**, *67*, 7–30. [CrossRef] [PubMed]
23. Auld, S.K.J.R.; Scholefield, J.A.; Little, T.J. Genetic variation in the cellular response of Daphnia magna (Crustacea: Cladocera) to its bacterial parasite. *Proc. Biol. Sci.* **2010**, *277*, 3291–3297. [CrossRef] [PubMed]
24. Zhong, J.-H.; Huang, D.-H.; Chen, Z.-Y. Prognostic role of systemic immune-inflammation index in solid tumors: A systematic review and meta-analysis. *Oncotarget* **2017**, *8*, 75381–75388. [CrossRef] [PubMed]
25. Arzumanyan, A.; Reis, H.M.; Feitelson, M.A. Pathogenic mechanisms in HBV- and HCV-associated hepatocellular carcinoma. *Nat. Rev. Cancer* **2013**, *13*, 123–135. [CrossRef] [PubMed]
26. Zhang, L.; Sung, J.J.Y.; Yu, J.; Ng, S.C.; Wong, S.H.; Cho, C.H.; Ng, S.S.M.; Chan, F.K.L.; Wu, W.K.K. Xenophagy in Helicobacter pylori- and Epstein-Barr virus-induced gastric cancer. *J. Pathol.* **2014**, *233*, 103–112. [CrossRef] [PubMed]
27. Shibutani, S.T.; Saitoh, T.; Nowag, H.; Münz, C.; Yoshimori, T. Autophagy and autophagy-related proteins in the immune system. *Nat. Immunol.* **2015**, *16*, 1014–1024. [CrossRef] [PubMed]
28. Saitoh, T.; Fujita, N.; Jang, M.H.; Uematsu, S.; Yang, B.-G.; Satoh, T.; Omori, H.; Noda, T.; Yamamoto, N.; Komatsu, M.; et al. Loss of the autophagy protein Atg16L1 enhances endotoxin-induced IL-1β production. *Nature* **2008**, *456*, 264–268. [CrossRef]
29. Zhou, R.; Yazdi, A.S.; Menu, P.; Tschopp, J. A role for mitochondria in NLRP3 inflammasome activation. *Nature* **2011**, *469*, 221–225. [CrossRef]
30. Bujak, A.L.; Crane, J.D.; Lally, J.S.; Ford, R.J.; Kang, S.J.; Rebalka, I.A.; Green, A.E.; Kemp, B.E.; Hawke, T.J.; Schertzer, J.D.; et al. AMPK activation of muscle autophagy prevents fasting-induced hypoglycemia and myopathy during aging. *Cell Metab.* **2015**, *21*, 883–890. [CrossRef]

31. Zhong, Z.; Sanchez-Lopez, E.; Karin, M. Autophagy, Inflammation, and Immunity: A Troika Governing Cancer and Its Treatment. *Cell* **2016**, *166*, 288–298. [CrossRef] [PubMed]
32. Mridha, A.R.; Wree, A.; Robertson, A.A.B.; Yeh, M.M.; Johnson, C.D.; Van Rooyen, D.M.; Haczeyni, F.; Teoh, N.C.H.; Savard, C.; Ioannou, G.N.; et al. NLRP3 inflammasome blockade reduces liver inflammation and fibrosis in experimental NASH in mice. *J. Hepatol.* **2017**, *66*, 1037–1046. [CrossRef] [PubMed]
33. Petrasek, J.; Bala, S.; Csak, T.; Lippai, D.; Kodys, K.; Menashy, V.; Barrieau, M.; Min, S.-Y.; Kurt-Jones, E.A.; Szabo, G. IL-1 receptor antagonist ameliorates inflammasome-dependent alcoholic steatohepatitis in mice. *J. Clin. Investig.* **2012**, *122*, 3476–3489. [CrossRef] [PubMed]
34. Nakahira, K.; Haspel, J.A.; Rathinam, V.A.K.; Lee, S.-J.; Dolinay, T.; Lam, H.C.; Englert, J.A.; Rabinovitch, M.; Cernadas, M.; Kim, H.P.; et al. Autophagy proteins regulate innate immune responses by inhibiting the release of mitochondrial DNA mediated by the NALP3 inflammasome. *Nat. Immunol.* **2011**, *12*, 222–230. [CrossRef] [PubMed]
35. Wang, L.; Li, H.; Zhen, Z.; Ma, X.; Yu, W.; Zeng, H.; Li, L. CXCL17 promotes cell metastasis and inhibits autophagy via the LKB1-AMPK pathway in hepatocellular carcinoma. *Gene* **2019**, *690*, 129–136. [CrossRef]
36. Kotsafti, A.; Farinati, F.; Cardin, R.; Cillo, U.; Nitti, D.; Bortolami, M. Autophagy and apoptosis-related genes in chronic liver disease and hepatocellular carcinoma. *BMC Gastroenterol.* **2012**, *12*, 118. [CrossRef]
37. Yue, Z.; Jin, S.; Yang, C.; Levine, A.J.; Heintz, N. Beclin 1, an autophagy gene essential for early embryonic development, is a haploinsufficient tumor suppressor. *Proc. Natl. Acad. Sci. USA* **2003**, *100*, 15077–15082. [CrossRef]
38. Wu, F.-Q.; Fang, T.; Yu, L.-X.; Lv, G.-S.; Lv, H.-W.; Liang, D.; Li, T.; Wang, C.-Z.; Tan, Y.-X.; Ding, J.; et al. ADRB2 signaling promotes HCC progression and sorafenib resistance by inhibiting autophagic degradation of HIF1α. *J. Hepatol.* **2016**, *65*, 314–324. [CrossRef]
39. Pursiheimo, J.-P.; Rantanen, K.; Heikkinen, P.T.; Johansen, T.; Jaakkola, P.M. Hypoxia-activated autophagy accelerates degradation of SQSTM1/p62. *Oncogene* **2009**, *28*, 334–344. [CrossRef]
40. Komatsu, M.; Waguri, S.; Koike, M.; Sou, Y.; Ueno, T.; Hara, T.; Mizushima, N.; Iwata, J.; Ezaki, J.; Murata, S.; et al. Homeostatic Levels of p62 Control Cytoplasmic Inclusion Body Formation in Autophagy-Deficient Mice. *Cell* **2007**, *131*, 1149–1163. [CrossRef]
41. Yoshii, S.R.; Mizushima, N. Monitoring and Measuring Autophagy. *Int. J. Mol. Sci.* **2017**, *18*, 1865. [CrossRef] [PubMed]
42. Kessler, S.M.; Laggai, S.; Barghash, A.; Schultheiss, C.S.; Lederer, E.; Artl, M.; Helms, V.; Haybaeck, J.; Kiemer, A.K. IMP2/p62 induces genomic instability and an aggressive hepatocellular carcinoma phenotype. *Cell Death Dis.* **2015**, *6*, e1894. [CrossRef] [PubMed]
43. Umemura, A.; He, F.; Taniguchi, K.; Nakagawa, H.; Yamachika, S.; Font-Burgada, J.; Zhong, Z.; Subramaniam, S.; Raghunandan, S.; Duran, A.; et al. p62, Upregulated during Preneoplasia, Induces Hepatocellular Carcinogenesis by Maintaining Survival of Stressed HCC-Initiating Cells. *Cancer Cell* **2016**, *29*, 935–948. [CrossRef] [PubMed]
44. Aigelsreiter, A.; Neumann, J.; Pichler, M.; Halasz, J.; Zatloukal, K.; Berghold, A.; Douschan, P.; Rainer, F.; Stauber, R.; Haybaeck, J.; et al. Hepatocellular carcinomas with intracellular hyaline bodies have a poor prognosis. *Liver Int.* **2017**, *37*, 600–610. [CrossRef]
45. Moscat, J.; Diaz-Meco, M.T. p62 at the Crossroads of Autophagy, Apoptosis, and Cancer. *Cell* **2009**, *137*, 1001–1004. [CrossRef] [PubMed]
46. Zhang, H.; Zhang, Y.; Zhu, X.; Chen, C.; Zhang, C.; Xia, Y.; Zhao, Y.; Andrisani, O.; Kong, L. DEAD Box Protein 5 Inhibits Liver Tumorigenesis by Stimulating Autophagy via Interaction with p62/SQSTM1. *Hepatology* **2018**. [CrossRef] [PubMed]
47. Nicol, S.M.; Bray, S.E.; Derek Black, H.; Lorimore, S.A.; Wright, E.G.; Lane, D.P.; Meek, D.W.; Coates, P.J.; Fuller-Pace, F.V. The RNA helicase p68 (DDX5) is selectively required for the induction of p53-dependent p21 expression and cell-cycle arrest after DNA damage. *Oncogene* **2013**, *32*, 3461–3469. [CrossRef] [PubMed]
48. Li, P.; Du, Q.; Cao, Z.; Guo, Z.; Evankovich, J.; Yan, W.; Chang, Y.; Shao, L.; Stolz, D.B.; Tsung, A.; et al. Interferon-gamma induces autophagy with growth inhibition and cell death in human hepatocellular carcinoma (HCC) cells through interferon-regulatory factor-1 (IRF-1). *Cancer Lett.* **2012**, *314*, 213–222. [CrossRef] [PubMed]
49. Zhu, H.; Wu, H.; Liu, X.; Li, B.; Chen, Y.; Ren, X.; Liu, C.-G.; Yang, J.-M. Regulation of autophagy by a beclin 1-targeted microRNA, miR-30a, in cancer cells. *Autophagy* **2009**, *5*, 816–823. [CrossRef] [PubMed]

50. Frankel, L.B.; Wen, J.; Lees, M.; Høyer-Hansen, M.; Farkas, T.; Krogh, A.; Jäättelä, M.; Lund, A.H. microRNA-101 is a potent inhibitor of autophagy. *EMBO J.* **2011**, *30*, 4628–4641. [CrossRef]
51. Chang, Y.; Yan, W.; He, X.; Zhang, L.; Li, C.; Huang, H.; Nace, G.; Geller, D.A.; Lin, J.; Tsung, A. MiR-375 inhibits autophagy and reduces viability of hepatocellular carcinoma cells under hypoxic conditions. *Gastroenterology* **2012**, *143*, 177–187. [CrossRef]
52. Wang, Y.; Wang, Q.; Song, J. Inhibition of autophagy potentiates the proliferation inhibition activity of microRNA-7 in human hepatocellular carcinoma cells. *Oncol. Lett.* **2017**, *14*, 3566–3572. [CrossRef] [PubMed]
53. Zhou, L.; Liu, S.; Han, M.; Feng, S.; Liang, J.; Li, Z.; Li, Y.; Lu, H.; Liu, T.; Ma, Y.; et al. MicroRNA-185 induces potent autophagy via AKT signaling in hepatocellular carcinoma. *Tumour Biol.* **2017**, *39*, 1010428317694313. [CrossRef] [PubMed]
54. Chang, Y.; Lin, J.; Tsung, A. Manipulation of autophagy by MIR375 generates antitumor effects in liver cancer. *Autophagy* **2012**, *8*, 1833–1834. [CrossRef] [PubMed]
55. Wong, C.C.-L.; Kai, A.K.-L.; Ng, I.O.-L. The impact of hypoxia in hepatocellular carcinoma metastasis. *Front. Med.* **2014**, *8*, 33–41. [CrossRef] [PubMed]
56. Wilson, G.K.; Tennant, D.A.; McKeating, J.A. Hypoxia inducible factors in liver disease and hepatocellular carcinoma: Current understanding and future directions. *J. Hepatol.* **2014**, *61*, 1397–1406. [CrossRef] [PubMed]
57. Eales, K.L.; Hollinshead, K.E.R.; Tennant, D.A. Hypoxia and metabolic adaptation of cancer cells. *Oncogenesis* **2016**, *61*, 1397–1406. [CrossRef]
58. Tohme, S.; Yazdani, H.O.; Liu, Y.; Loughran, P.; van der Windt, D.J.; Huang, H.; Simmons, R.L.; Shiva, S.; Tai, S.; Tsung, A. Hypoxia mediates mitochondrial biogenesis in hepatocellular carcinoma to promote tumor growth through HMGB1 and TLR9 interaction. *Hepatology* **2017**, *66*, 182–197. [CrossRef]
59. Schito, L.; Rey, S. Cell-Autonomous Metabolic Reprogramming in Hypoxia. *Trends Cell Biol.* **2018**, *28*, 128–142. [CrossRef]
60. Bellot, G.; Garcia-Medina, R.; Gounon, P.; Chiche, J.; Roux, D.; Pouyssegur, J.; Mazure, N.M. Hypoxia-Induced Autophagy Is Mediated through Hypoxia-Inducible Factor Induction of BNIP3 and BNIP3L via Their BH3 Domains. *Mol. Cell. Biol.* **2009**, *29*, 2570–2581. [CrossRef]
61. Sijtsema, W.Y. Sport voor mensen met een handicap. *Tijdschrift voor Ziekenverpleging* **1977**, *30*, 115–125. [PubMed]
62. Peng, W.X.; Xiong, E.M.; Ge, L.; Wan, Y.Y.; Zhang, C.L.; Du, F.Y.; Xu, M.; Bhat, R.A.; Jin, J.; Gong, A.H. Egr-1 promotes hypoxia-induced autophagy to enhance chemo-resistance of hepatocellular carcinoma cells. *Exp. Cell Res.* **2016**, *340*, 62–70. [CrossRef] [PubMed]
63. Bjelland, S.; Seeberg, E. Mutagenicity, toxicity and repair of DNA base damage induced by oxidation. *Mutat. Res.* **2003**, *531*, 37–80. [CrossRef]
64. Scherz-Shouval, R.; Elazar, Z. ROS, mitochondria and the regulation of autophagy. *Trends Cell Biol.* **2007**, *17*, 422–427. [CrossRef] [PubMed]
65. Han, D.; Williams, E.; Cadenas, E. Mitochondrial respiratory chain-dependent generation of superoxide anion and its release into the intermembrane space. *Biochem. J.* **2001**, *353*, 411–416. [CrossRef]
66. Muller, F. The nature and mechanism of superoxide production by the electron transport chain: Its relevance to aging. *Age* **2000**, *23*, 227–253. [CrossRef] [PubMed]
67. Jain, A.; Lamark, T.; Sjøttem, E.; Larsen, K.B.; Awuh, J.A.; Øvervatn, A.; McMahon, M.; Hayes, J.D.; Johansen, T. p62/SQSTM1 is a target gene for transcription factor NRF2 and creates a positive feedback loop by inducing antioxidant response element-driven gene transcription. *J. Biol. Chem.* **2010**, *285*, 22576–22591. [CrossRef] [PubMed]
68. Copple, I.M.; Lister, A.; Obeng, A.D.; Kitteringham, N.R.; Jenkins, R.E.; Layfield, R.; Foster, B.J.; Goldring, C.E.; Park, B.K. Physical and functional interaction of sequestosome 1 with Keap1 regulates the Keap1-Nrf2 cell defense pathway. *J. Biol. Chem.* **2010**, *285*, 16782–16788. [CrossRef] [PubMed]
69. Katsuragi, Y.; Ichimura, Y.; Komatsu, M. Regulation of the Keap1–Nrf2 pathway by p62/SQSTM1. *Curr. Opin. Toxicol.* **2016**, *1*, 54–61. [CrossRef]
70. Bartolini, D.; Dallaglio, K.; Torquato, P.; Piroddi, M.; Galli, F. Nrf2-p62 autophagy pathway and its response to oxidative stress in hepatocellular carcinoma. *Transl. Res.* **2018**, *193*, 54–71. [CrossRef] [PubMed]

71. Chen, J.; Yu, Y.; Ji, T.; Ma, R.; Chen, M.; Li, G.; Li, F.; Ding, Q.; Kang, Q.; Huang, D.; et al. Clinical implication of Keap1 and phosphorylated Nrf2 expression in hepatocellular carcinoma. *Cancer Med.* **2016**, *5*, 2678–2687. [CrossRef] [PubMed]
72. Lemasters, J.J. Selective Mitochondrial Autophagy, or Mitophagy, as a Targeted Defense against Oxidative Stress, Mitochondrial Dysfunction, and Aging. *Rejuv. Res.* **2005**, *8*, 3–5. [CrossRef] [PubMed]
73. Wild, P.; Dikic, I. Mitochondria get a Parkin' ticket. *Nat. Cell Biol.* **2010**, *12*, 104–106. [CrossRef] [PubMed]
74. Bedard, K.; Krause, K.-H. The NOX Family of ROS-Generating NADPH Oxidases: Physiology and Pathophysiology. *Physiol. Rev.* **2007**, *87*, 245–313. [CrossRef] [PubMed]
75. Lambeth, J.D. NOX enzymes and the biology of reactive oxygen. *Nat. Rev. Immunol.* **2004**, *4*, 181–189. [CrossRef] [PubMed]
76. Ma, Q. Role of Nrf2 in Oxidative Stress and Toxicity. *Annu. Rev. Pharmacol. Toxicol.* **2013**, *53*, 401–426. [CrossRef] [PubMed]
77. Twig, G.; Elorza, A.; Molina, A.J.A.; Mohamed, H.; Wikstrom, J.D.; Walzer, G.; Stiles, L.; Haigh, S.E.; Katz, S.; Las, G.; et al. Fission and selective fusion govern mitochondrial segregation and elimination by autophagy. *EMBO J.* **2008**, *27*, 433–446. [CrossRef]
78. Liu, K.; Lee, J.; Kim, J.Y.; Wang, L.; Tian, Y.; Chan, S.T.; Cho, C.; Machida, K.; Chen, D.; Ou, J.-H.J. Mitophagy Controls the Activities of Tumor Suppressor p53 to Regulate Hepatic Cancer Stem Cells. *Mol. Cell* **2017**, *68*, 281–292. [CrossRef] [PubMed]
79. Shi, C.; Cai, Y.; Li, Y.; Li, Y.; Hu, N.; Ma, S.; Hu, S.; Zhu, P.; Wang, W.; Zhou, H. Yap promotes hepatocellular carcinoma metastasis and mobilization via governing cofilin/F-actin/lamellipodium axis by regulation of JNK/Bnip3/SERCA/CaMKII pathways. *Redox Biol.* **2018**, *14*, 59–71. [CrossRef]
80. Inbal, B.; Bialik, S.; Sabanay, I.; Shani, G.; Kimchi, A. DAP kinase and DRP-1 mediate membrane blebbing and the formation of autophagic vesicles during programmed cell death. *J. Cell Biol.* **2002**, *157*, 455–468. [CrossRef] [PubMed]
81. Dasari, S.K.; Bialik, S.; Levin-Zaidman, S.; Levin-Salomon, V.; Merrill, A.H.; Futerman, A.H.; Kimchi, A. Signalome-wide RNAi screen identifies GBA1 as a positive mediator of autophagic cell death. *Cell Death Differ.* **2017**, *24*, 1288–1302. [CrossRef] [PubMed]
82. Shimizu, S.; Konishi, A.; Nishida, Y.; Mizuta, T.; Nishina, H.; Yamamoto, A.; Tsujimoto, Y. Involvement of JNK in the regulation of autophagic cell death. *Oncogene* **2010**, *29*, 2070–2082. [CrossRef] [PubMed]
83. Arakawa, S.; Tsujioka, M.; Yoshida, T.; Tajima-Sakurai, H.; Nishida, Y.; Matsuoka, Y.; Yoshino, I.; Tsujimoto, Y.; Shimizu, S. Role of Atg5-dependent cell death in the embryonic development of Bax/Bak double-knockout mice. *Cell Death Differ.* **2017**, *24*, 1598–1608. [CrossRef] [PubMed]
84. Reef, S.; Zalckvar, E.; Shifman, O.; Bialik, S.; Sabanay, H.; Oren, M.; Kimchi, A. A short mitochondrial form of p19ARF induces autophagy and caspase-independent cell death. *Mol. Cell* **2006**, *22*, 463–475. [CrossRef] [PubMed]
85. Yanagisawa, H.; Miyashita, T.; Nakano, Y.; Yamamoto, D. HSpin1, a transmembrane protein interacting with Bcl-2/Bcl-xL, induces a caspase-independent autophagic cell death. *Cell Death Differ.* **2003**, *10*, 798–807. [CrossRef] [PubMed]
86. Chen, M.; Liu, Y.; Varley, P.; Chang, Y.; He, X.X.; Huang, H.; Tang, D.; Lotze, M.T.; Lin, J.; Tsung, A. High-mobility group box 1 promotes hepatocellular carcinoma progression through MIR-21-mediated matrix metalloproteinase activity. *Cancer Res.* **2015**, *75*, 1645–1656. [CrossRef] [PubMed]
87. Huang, H.; Nace, G.W.; McDonald, K.-A.; Tai, S.; Klune, J.R.; Rosborough, B.R.; Ding, Q.; Loughran, P.; Zhu, X.; Beer-Stolz, D.; et al. Hepatocyte-specific high-mobility group box 1 deletion worsens the injury in liver ischemia/reperfusion: A role for intracellular high-mobility group box 1 in cellular protection. *Hepatology* **2014**, *59*, 1984–1997. [CrossRef]
88. Pan, B.; Chen, D.; Huang, J.; Wang, R.; Feng, B.; Song, H.; Chen, L. HMGB1-mediated autophagy promotes docetaxel resistance in human lung adenocarcinoma. *Mol. Cancer* **2014**, *13*, 165. [CrossRef] [PubMed]
89. Zhao, M.; Yang, M.; Yang, L.; Yu, Y.; Xie, M.; Zhu, S.; Kang, R.; Tang, D.; Jiang, Z.; Yuan, W.; et al. HMGB1 regulates autophagy through increasing transcriptional activities of JNK and ERK in human myeloid leukemia cells. *BMB Rep.* **2011**, *44*, 601–606. [CrossRef]
90. Liu, Y.; Yan, W.; Tohme, S.; Chen, M.; Fu, Y.; Tian, D.; Lotze, M.; Tang, D.; Tsung, A. Hypoxia induced HMGB1 and mitochondrial DNA interactions mediate tumor growth in hepatocellular carcinoma through Toll-like receptor 9. *J. Hepatol.* **2015**, *63*, 114–121. [CrossRef] [PubMed]

91. Debnath, J. Detachment-induced autophagy during anoikis and lumen formation in epithelial acini. *Autophagy* **2008**, *4*, 351–353. [CrossRef] [PubMed]
92. Peng, Y.-F.; Shi, Y.-H.; Shen, Y.-H.; Ding, Z.-B.; Ke, A.-W.; Zhou, J.; Qiu, S.-J.; Fan, J. Promoting colonization in metastatic HCC cells by modulation of autophagy. *PLoS ONE* **2013**, *8*, e74407. [CrossRef] [PubMed]
93. Seyfried, T.N.; Huysentruyt, L.C. On the Origin of Cancer Metastasis. *Crit. Rev. Oncog.* **2013**, *18*, 43–73. [CrossRef] [PubMed]
94. Avivar-Valderas, A.; Salas, E.; Bobrovnikova-Marjon, E.; Diehl, J.A.; Nagi, C.; Debnath, J.; Aguirre-Ghiso, J.A. PERK Integrates Autophagy and Oxidative Stress Responses To Promote Survival during Extracellular Matrix Detachment. *Mol. Cell. Biol.* **2011**, *31*, 3616–3629. [CrossRef] [PubMed]
95. Sharifi, M.N.; Mowers, E.E.; Drake, L.E.; Collier, C.; Chen, H.; Zamora, M.; Mui, S.; Macleod, K.F. Autophagy Promotes Focal Adhesion Disassembly and Cell Motility of Metastatic Tumor Cells through the Direct Interaction of Paxillin with LC3. *Cell Rep.* **2016**, *15*, 1660–1672. [CrossRef]
96. Li, J.; Yang, B.; Zhou, Q.; Wu, Y.; Shang, D.; Guo, Y.; Song, Z.; Zheng, Q.; Xiong, J. Autophagy promotes hepatocellular carcinoma cell invasion through activation of epithelial–mesenchymal transition. *Carcinogenesis* **2013**, *34*, 1343–1351. [CrossRef]
97. Peng, Y.F.; Shi, Y.H.; Ding, Z.B; Ke, A.W.; Gu, C.Y.; Hui, B.; Zhou, J.; Qiu, S.J.; Dai, Z.; Fan, J. Autophagy inhibition suppresses pulmonary metastasis of HCC in mice via impairing anoikis resistance and colonization of HCC cells. *Autophagy* **2013**, *9*, 2056–2068. [CrossRef]
98. Wang, X.; Zhang, Y.; Feng, T.; Su, G.; He, J.; Gao, W.; Shen, Y.; Liu, X. Fluid shear stress promotes autophagy in hepatocellular carcinoma cells. *Int. J. Biol. Sci.* **2018**, *14*, 1277–1290. [CrossRef]
99. Shen, H.-M.; Codogno, P. Autophagic cell death: Loch Ness monster or endangered species? *Autophagy* **2011**, *7*, 457–465. [CrossRef]
100. Boya, P.; Gonzalez-Polo, R.-A.; Casares, N.; Perfettini, J.-L.; Dessen, P.; Larochette, N.; Metivier, D.; Meley, D.; Souquere, S.; Yoshimori, T.; et al. Inhibition of Macroautophagy Triggers Apoptosis. *Mol. Cell. Biol.* **2005**, *25*, 1025–1040. [CrossRef]
101. Cheng, A.-L.; Kang, Y.-K.; Chen, Z.; Tsao, C.-J.; Qin, S.; Kim, J.S.; Luo, R.; Feng, J.; Ye, S.; Yang, T.-S.; et al. Efficacy and safety of sorafenib in patients in the Asia-Pacific region with advanced hepatocellular carcinoma: A phase III randomised, double-blind, placebo-controlled trial. *Lancet Oncol.* **2009**, *10*, 25–34. [CrossRef]
102. Abdel-Rahman, O.; Fouad, M. Sorafenib-based combination as a first line treatment for advanced hepatocellular carcinoma: A systematic review of the literature. *Crit. Rev. Oncol. Hematol.* **2014**, *91*, 1–8. [CrossRef] [PubMed]
103. Decaens, T.; Luciani, A.; Itti, E.; Hulin, A.; Roudot-Thoraval, F.; Laurent, A.; Zafrani, E.S.; Mallat, A.; Duvoux, C. Phase II study of sirolimus in treatment-naive patients with advanced hepatocellular carcinoma. *Dig. Liver Dis.* **2012**, *44*, 610–616. [CrossRef]
104. Adnane, L.; Trail, P.A.; Taylor, I.; Wilhelm, S.M. Sorafenib (BAY 43-9006, Nexavar®), a Dual-Action Inhibitor That Targets RAF/MEK/ERK Pathway in Tumor Cells and Tyrosine Kinases VEGFR/PDGFR in Tumor Vasculature. *Methods Enzymol.* **2006**, *407*, 597–612. [PubMed]
105. Shimizu, S.; Takehara, T.; Hikita, H.; Kodama, T.; Tsunematsu, H.; Miyagi, T.; Hosui, A.; Ishida, H.; Tatsumi, T.; Kanto, T.; et al. Inhibition of autophagy potentiates the antitumor effect of the multikinase inhibitor sorafenib in hepatocellular carcinoma. *Int. J. Cancer* **2012**, *131*, 548–557. [CrossRef] [PubMed]
106. Gedaly, R.; Angulo, P.; Hundley, J.; Daily, M.F.; Chen, C.; Evers, B.M. PKI-587 and sorafenib targeting PI3K/AKT/mTOR and Ras/Raf/MAPK pathways synergistically inhibit HCC cell proliferation. *J. Surg. Res.* **2012**, *176*, 542–548. [CrossRef] [PubMed]
107. Rodríguez-Hernández, M.A.; González, R.; de la Rosa, Á.J.; Gallego, P.; Ordóñez, R.; Navarro-Villarán, E.; Contreras, L.; Rodríguez-Arribas, M.; González-Gallego, J.; Álamo-Martínez, J.M.; et al. Molecular characterization of autophagic and apoptotic signaling induced by sorafenib in liver cancer cells. *J. Cell. Physiol.* **2019**, *234*, 692–708. [CrossRef] [PubMed]
108. Nishida, N.; Kitano, M.; Sakurai, T.; Kudo, M. Molecular Mechanism and Prediction of Sorafenib Chemoresistance in Human Hepatocellular Carcinoma. *Dig. Dis.* **2015**, *33*, 771–779. [CrossRef]
109. Lachenmayer, A.; Toffanin, S.; Cabellos, L.; Alsinet, C.; Hoshida, Y.; Villanueva, A.; Minguez, B.; Tsai, H.W.; Ward, S.C.; Thung, S.; et al. Combination therapy for hepatocellular carcinoma: Additive preclinical efficacy of the HDAC inhibitor panobinostat with sorafenib. *J. Hepatol.* **2012**, *56*, 1343–1350. [CrossRef]

110. Liang, Y.; Zheng, T.; Song, R.; Wang, J.; Yin, D.; Wang, L.; Liu, H.; Tian, L.; Fang, X.; Meng, X.; et al. Hypoxia-mediated sorafenib resistance can be overcome by EF24 through Von Hippel-Lindau tumor suppressor-dependent HIF-1α inhibition in hepatocellular carcinoma. *Hepatology* **2013**, *57*, 1847–1857. [CrossRef]
111. Prieto-Domínguez, N.; Méndez-Blanco, C.; Carbajo-Pescador, S.; Fondevila, F.; García-Palomo, A.; González-Gallego, J.; Mauriz, J.L. Melatonin enhances sorafenib actions in human hepatocarcinoma cells by inhibiting mTORC1/p70S6K/HIF-1α and hypoxia-mediated mitophagy. *Oncotarget* **2017**, *8*, 91402–91414. [CrossRef] [PubMed]
112. Prieto-Domínguez, N.; Ordóñez, R.; Fernández, A.; García-Palomo, A.; Muntané, J.; González-Gallego, J.; Mauriz, J.L. Modulation of Autophagy by Sorafenib: Effects on Treatment Response. *Front. Pharmacol.* **2016**, *7*, 151. [CrossRef] [PubMed]
113. Zhi, X.; Zhong, Q. Autophagy in cancer. *F1000Prime Rep.* **2015**, *7*, 18. [CrossRef] [PubMed]
114. Ding, Z.-B.; Hui, B.; Shi, Y.-H.; Zhou, J.; Peng, Y.-F.; Gu, C.-Y.; Yang, H.; Shi, G.-M.; Ke, A.-W.; Wang, X.-Y.; et al. Autophagy Activation in Hepatocellular Carcinoma Contributes to the Tolerance of Oxaliplatin via Reactive Oxygen Species Modulation. *Clin. Cancer Res.* **2011**, *17*, 6229–6238. [CrossRef] [PubMed]
115. Sheng, J.; Qin, H.; Zhang, K.; Li, B.; Zhang, X. Targeting autophagy in chemotherapy-resistant of hepatocellular carcinoma. *Am. J. Cancer Res.* **2018**, *8*, 354–365. [PubMed]
116. Toshima, T.; Shirabe, K.; Matsumoto, Y.; Yoshiya, S.; Ikegami, T.; Yoshizumi, T.; Soejima, Y.; Ikeda, T.; Maehara, Y. Autophagy enhances hepatocellular carcinoma progression by activation of mitochondrial β-oxidation. *J. Gastroenterol.* **2014**, *49*, 907–916. [CrossRef] [PubMed]
117. Hu, P.; Cheng, B.; He, Y.; Wei, Z.; Wu, D.; Meng, Z. Autophagy suppresses proliferation of HepG2 cells via inhibiting glypican-3/wnt/β-catenin signaling. *Oncotargets Ther.* **2018**, *11*, 193–200. [CrossRef]
118. Da Silva, E.F.G.; Krause, G.C.; Lima, K.G.; Haute, G.V.; Pedrazza, L.; Mesquita, F.C.; Basso, B.S.; Velasquez, A.C.; Nunes, F.B.; De Oliveira, J.R. Rapamycin and fructose-1,6-bisphosphate reduce the HEPG2 cell proliferation via increase of free radicals and apoptosis. *Oncol. Rep.* **2016**, *36*, 2647–2652. [CrossRef]
119. Engl, T.; Rutz, J.; Maxeiner, S.; Juengel, E.; Roos, F.; Khoder, W.; Bechstein, W.O.; Nelson, K.; Tsaur, I.; Haferkamp, A.; et al. mTOR inhibition reduces growth and adhesion of hepatocellular carcinoma cells in vitro. *Mol. Med. Rep.* **2017**, *16*, 7064–7071. [CrossRef]
120. Kim, J.-O.; Kim, K.-H.; Song, I.S.; Cheon, K.-S.; Kim, O.-H.; Lee, S.C.; Lee, S.K.; Kim, S.-J. Potentiation of the anticancer effects of everolimus using a dual mTORC1/2 inhibitor in hepatocellular carcinoma cells. *Oncotarget* **2017**, *8*, 2936–2948. [CrossRef]
121. Tong, Y.; Huang, H.; Pan, H. Inhibition of MEK/ERK activation attenuates autophagy and potentiates pemetrexed-induced activity against HepG2 hepatocellular carcinoma cells. *Biochem. Biophys. Res. Commun.* **2015**, *456*, 86–91. [CrossRef] [PubMed]
122. Huang, C.-Y.; Tai, W.-T.; Hsieh, C.-Y.; Hsu, W.-M.; Lai, Y.-J.; Chen, L.-J.; Shiau, C.-W.; Chen, K.-F. A sorafenib derivative and novel SHP-1 agonist, SC-59, acts synergistically with radiotherapy in hepatocellular carcinoma cells through inhibition of STAT3. *Cancer Lett.* **2014**, *349*, 136–143. [CrossRef] [PubMed]
123. Tai, W.-T.; Shiau, C.-W.; Chen, H.-L.; Liu, C.-Y.; Lin, C.-S.; Cheng, A.-L.; Chen, P.-J.; Chen, K.-F. Mcl-1-dependent activation of Beclin 1 mediates autophagic cell death induced by sorafenib and SC-59 in hepatocellular carcinoma cells. *Cell Death Dis.* **2013**, *4*, e485. [CrossRef] [PubMed]
124. Chang, Z.; Shi, G.; Jin, J.; Guo, H.; Guo, X.; Luo, F.; Song, Y.; Jia, X. Dual PI3K/mTOR inhibitor NVP-BEZ235-induced apoptosis of hepatocellular carcinoma cell lines is enhanced by inhibitors of autophagy. *Int. J. Mol. Med.* **2013**, *31*, 1449–1456. [CrossRef] [PubMed]
125. Simioni, C.; Martelli, A.M.; Cani, A.; Cetin-Atalay, R.; McCubrey, J.A.; Capitani, S.; Neri, L.M. The AKT Inhibitor MK-2206 is Cytotoxic in Hepatocarcinoma Cells Displaying Hyperphosphorylated AKT-1 and Synergizes with Conventional Chemotherapy. *Oncotarget* **2013**, *4*, 1496–1506. [CrossRef] [PubMed]
126. Zhang, H.; Chen, G.G.; Zhang, Z.; Chun, S.; Leung, B.C.S.; Lai, P.B.S. Induction of autophagy in hepatocellular carcinoma cells by SB203580 requires activation of AMPK and DAPK but not p38 MAPK. *Apoptosis* **2012**, *17*, 325–334. [CrossRef] [PubMed]
127. D'Alessandro, R.; Refolo, M.G.; Lippolis, C.; Messa, C.; Cavallini, A.; Rossi, R.; Resta, L.; Di Carlo, A.; Carr, B.I. Reversibility of regorafenib effects in hepatocellular carcinoma cells. *Cancer Chemother. Pharmacol.* **2013**, *72*, 869–877. [CrossRef] [PubMed]

128. Yu, H.C.; Lin, C.S.; Tai, W.T.; Liu, C.Y.; Shiau, C.W.; Chen, K.F. Nilotinib induces autophagy in hepatocellular carcinoma through AMPK activation. *J. Biol. Chem.* **2013**, *288*, 18249–18259. [CrossRef]
129. Ni, Z.; Wang, B.; Dai, X.; Ding, W.; Yang, T.; Li, X.; Lewin, S.; Xu, L.; Lian, J.; He, F. HCC cells with high levels of Bcl-2 are resistant to ABT-737 via activation of the ROS-JNK-autophagy pathway. *Free Radic. Biol. Med.* **2014**, *70*, 194–203. [CrossRef]
130. Gao, M.; Yeh, P.Y.; Lu, Y.S.; Hsu, C.H.; Chen, K.F.; Lee, W.C.; Feng, W.C.; Chen, C.S.; Kuo, M.L.; Cheng, A.L. OSU-03012, a novel celecoxib derivative, induces reactive oxygen species-related autophagy in hepatocellular carcinoma. *Cancer Res.* **2008**, *68*, 9348–9357. [CrossRef]
131. Saeki, I.; Terai, S.; Fujisawa, K.; Takami, T.; Yamamoto, N.; Matsumoto, T.; Hirose, Y.; Murata, Y.; Yamasaki, T.; Sakaida, I. Bortezomib induces tumor-specific cell death and growth inhibition in hepatocellular carcinoma and improves liver fibrosis. *J. Gastroenterol.* **2013**, *48*, 738–750. [CrossRef] [PubMed]
132. Du, H.; Yang, W.; Chen, L.; Shi, M.; Seewoo, V.; Wang, J.; Lin, A.; Liu, Z.; Qiu, W. Role of autophagy in resistance to oxaliplatin in hepatocellular carcinoma cells. *Oncol. Rep.* **2012**, *27*, 143–150. [PubMed]
133. Chen, L.H.; Loong, C.C.; Su, T.L.; Lee, Y.J.; Chu, P.M.; Tsai, M.L.; Tsai, P.H.; Tu, P.H.; Chi, C.W.; Lee, H.C.; et al. Autophagy inhibition enhances apoptosis triggered by BO-1051, an N-mustard derivative, and involves the ATM signaling pathway. *Biochem. Pharmacol.* **2011**, *81*, 594–605. [CrossRef] [PubMed]
134. Hou, Y.J.; Dong, L.W.; Tan, Y.X.; Yang, G.Z.; Pan, Y.F.; Li, Z.; Tang, L.; Wang, M.; Wang, Q.; Wang, H.Y. Inhibition of active autophagy induces apoptosis and increases chemosensitivity in cholangiocarcinoma. *Lab. Invest.* **2011**, *91*, 1146–1157. [CrossRef] [PubMed]
135. Rong, L.-W.; Wang, R.-X.; Zheng, X.-L.; Feng, X.-Q.; Zhang, L.; Zhang, L.; Lin, Y.; Li, Z.-P.; Wang, X. Combination of wogonin and sorafenib effectively kills human hepatocellular carcinoma cells through apoptosis potentiation and autophagy inhibition. *Oncol. Lett.* **2017**, *13*, 5028–5034. [CrossRef] [PubMed]
136. Yan, Y.; Jiang, K.; Liu, P.; Zhang, X.; Dong, X.; Gao, J.; Liu, Q.; Barr, M.P.; Zhang, Q.; Hou, X.; et al. Bafilomycin A1 induces caspase-independent cell death in hepatocellular carcinoma cells via targeting of autophagy and MAPK pathways. *Sci. Rep.* **2016**, *6*, 37052. [CrossRef] [PubMed]
137. Thoen, L.F.R.; Guimarães, E.L.M.; Dollé, L.; Mannaerts, I.; Najimi, M.; Sokal, E.; van Grunsven, L.A. A role for autophagy during hepatic stellate cell activation. *J. Hepatol.* **2011**, *55*, 1353–1360. [CrossRef] [PubMed]
138. Eisenberg-Lerner, A.; Bialik, S.; Simon, H.-U.; Kimchi, A. Life and death partners: Apoptosis, autophagy and the cross-talk between them. *Cell Death Differ.* **2009**, *16*, 966–975. [CrossRef]
139. Booth, L.A.; Tavallai, S.; Hamed, H.A.; Cruickshanks, N.; Dent, P. The role of cell signalling in the crosstalk between autophagy and apoptosis. *Cell. Signal.* **2014**, *26*, 549–555. [CrossRef] [PubMed]
140. McFarlane, S.; Nicholl, M.J.; Sutherland, J.S.; Preston, C.M. Interaction of the human cytomegalovirus particle with the host cell induces hypoxia-inducible factor 1 alpha. *Virology* **2011**, *414*, 83–90. [CrossRef]

5

Irradiation-Induced Cardiac Connexin-43 and miR-21 Responses are Hampered by Treatment with Atorvastatin and Aspirin

Csilla Viczenczova [1], Branislav Kura [1], Tamara Egan Benova [1], Chang Yin [2], Rakesh C. Kukreja [2], Jan Slezak [1], Narcis Tribulova [1] and Barbara Szeiffova Bacova [1,*]

[1] Institute for Heart Research, Center of Experimental Medicine, Slovak Academy of Sciences, Bratislava 841 04, Slovak Republic; viczencz.csilla@gmail.com (C.V.); branislav.kura@savba.sk (B.K.); tamara.benova@savba.sk (T.E.B.); jan.slezak@savba.sk (J.S.); narcisa.tribulova@savba.sk (N.T.)

[2] Division of Cardiology, Medical College of Virginia, Virginia Commonwealth University, Richmond, VA 23298, USA; rakesh@vcu.edu (C.Y.); rakesh.kukreja@vcuhealth.org (R.C.K.)

* Correspondence: barbara.bacova@savba.sk

Abstract: Radiation of the chest during cancer therapy is deleterious to the heart, mostly due to oxidative stress and inflammation related injury. A single sub-lethal dose of irradiation has been shown to result in compensatory up-regulation of the myocardial connexin-43 (Cx43), activation of the protein kinase C (PKC) signaling along with the decline of microRNA (miR)-1 and an increase of miR-21 levels in the left ventricle (LV). We investigated whether drugs with antioxidant, anti-inflammatory or vasodilating properties, such as aspirin, atorvastatin, and sildenafil, may affect myocardial response in the LV and right ventricle (RV) following chest irradiation. Adult, male Wistar rats were subjected to a single sub-lethal dose of chest radiation at 25 Gy and treated with aspirin (3 mg/day), atorvastatin (0.25 mg/day), and sildenafil (0.3 mg/day) for six weeks. Cx43, PKCε and PKCδ proteins expression and levels of miR-1 as well as miR-21 were determined in the LV and RV. Results showed that the suppression of miR-1 was associated with an increase of total and phosphorylated forms of Cx43 as well as PKCε expression in the LV while having no effect in the RV post-irradiation as compared to the non-irradiated rats. Treatment with aspirin and atorvastatin prevented an increase in the expression of Cx43 and PKCε without change in the miR-1 levels. Furthermore, treatment with aspirin, atorvastatin, and sildenafil completely prevented an increase of miR-21 in the LV while having partial effect in the RV post irradiation. The increase in pro-apoptotic PKCδ was not affected by any of the used treatment. In conclusion, irradiation and drug-induced changes were less pronounced in the RV as compared to the LV. Treatment with aspirin and atorvastatin interfered with irradiation-induced compensatory changes in myocardial Cx43 protein and miR-21 by preventing their elevation, possibly via amelioration of oxidative stress and inflammation.

Keywords: irradiation; heart; connexin-43; miR-1; miR-21; atorvastatin; aspirin

---

1. Introduction

Cardiovascular injury due to radiation is the most common cause of adverse events among cancer survivors [1,2]. Key factors responsible for the establishment of cardiovascular injury, i.e., oxidative stress, inflammation, and epigenetic modifications, have been linked to potential treatments and been recently described [1,2]. Ionizing radiation induces oxidative stress and causes changes in the expression of several microRNAs (miRNA)s, including miR-1 and miR-21. An increase of miR-21 is involved in myocardial hypertrophy [3,4] and fibrosis [5]. An increase in miR-21 has also been associated with the up-regulation of the protein kinase C (PKC) δ [6], which is also implicated in tissue remodeling. Fibrosis and necrosis were reduced by the treatment with a free radical-scavenging component such as melatonin [7]. However, molecular mechanisms of the irradiation induced injury are unknown and there is currently a lack of treatment strategies.

Cardiac connexin-43 (Cx43) channels are essential for coordinated heart function because they ensure electrical coupling and direct intercellular communication. We and others [6,8] have shown that a single sub-lethal dose of irradiation results in up-regulation of Cx43, which has been associated with the protection of the heart against malignant arrhythmias [9] and infarction [10]. An increase in myocardial Cx43 expression and its active phosphorylated forms has been shown to be associated with the suppression of miR-1 (which regulates GJA1 gene transcription for Cx43) and the enhancement of PKCε (which phosphorylates Cx43) [6]. It appears that these early post-irradiation related myocardial alterations, including up-regulation of Cx43, are most likely compensatory responses of the heart to maintain its normal function [10–12]. Since irradiation induces inflammation and oxidative stress [12], we hypothesized that compounds exerting anti-inflammatory and antioxidant actions would interfere with irradiation-induced compensatory responses. To this context, we considered several drugs, which included acetylsalicylic acid (aspirin), a non-selective inhibitor of cyclooxygenase-1 and cyclooxygenase-2, which prevents formation of pro-inflammatory prostaglandins and thromboxanes. Antioxidant properties of acetylsalicylic acid are attributed to its ability of inhibiting lipid peroxidation and DNA damage [13]. Atorvastatin is widely used for treatment of human dislipidemia due to inhibition of the 3-hydroxy-3-methylglutaryl coenzyme A reductase. In addition, its pleiotropic effects are associated with anti-inflammatory and antioxidative actions [14] as well as promoting the availability of vascular nitric oxide [15]. Sildenafil, the inhibitor of phosphodiestherase 5, is used for its vasodilatation and activation of nitric oxide [16].

Our goal was to demonstrate whether treatment with the drugs targeting oxidative stress and inflammation might result in attenuation of irradiation induced myocardial compensatory responses previously reported [6,10]. In particular, we examined myocardial changes in Cx43, PKC, miR-1 and miR-21 in rats exposed to single chest irradiation.

2. Results

2.1. Main Characteristics of Experimental Rats

Comparing to non-irradiated rats, the body, heart, and left ventricular weight were significantly decreased in irradiated animals after six weeks. On the other hand, irradiation did not alter the right ventricular weight. Treatment with selected drugs also had no effect on these biometric parameters in any treated group, except for the heart weight in post-irradiated + sildenafil group. Data are summarized in the Table 1.

Table 1. Biometric parameters registered in control and irradiated Wistar rats.

GROUP	BW (g)	HW (g)	LVW (g)	RVW (g)
C	344.22 ± 28.40	0.89 ± 0.11	0.36 ± 0.07	0.09 ± 0.02
C-A	382.61 ± 32.19	0.92 ± 0.09	0.39 ± 0.04	0.12 ± 0.01
C-AT	371.01 ± 20.45	0.87 ± 0.07	0.37 ± 0.04	0.10 ± 0.02
C-S	363.63 ± 23.93	0.90 ± 0.10	0.39 ± 0.04	0.11 ± 0.02
I	252.24 ± 14.31 [a]	0.83 ± 0.05	0.25 ± 0.04 [a]	0.10 ± 0.04
I-A	227.41 ± 26.47 [c]	0.73 ± 0.09 [c]	0.24 ± 0.02 [c]	0.11 ± 0.03
I-AT	253.23 ± 31.82 [c]	0.77 ± 0.08	0.27 ± 0.03 [c]	0.13 ± 0.03
I-S	233.62 ± 14.50 [c]	0.67 ± 0.05 [b,c]	0.23 ± 0.02 [c]	0.12 ± 0.03

BW—body weight; HW—heart weight; LVW—left ventricular weight; RVW—right ventricular weight; C—control non-irradiated; C-A—control + aspirin; C-AT—control + atorvastatin; C-S—control + sildenafil; I—irradiated rats; I-A—irradiated + aspirin; I-AT—irradiated + atorvastatin; I-S—irradiated + sildenafil. Results are the mean ± SD of 6 hearts. [a] $p < 0.05$ vs. C (C vs. C-A, C-AT, C-S, I); [b] $p < 0.05$ vs. I (I vs. I-A, I-AT, I-S); [c] $p < 0.05$ treated C vs. treated I (C-A vs. I-A; C-AT vs. I-AT; C-S vs. I-S).

2.2. *Protein Expression of Myocardial Cx43 in Control and Irradiated Wistar Rats*

Western blot analysis showed that total Cx43 protein was increased in the LV ($p < 0.05$) and to a lesser extent in RV post-irradiation as compared to the non-irradiated group (Figure 1A,B,D,E). In parallel, the active phosphorylated forms of Cx43 were significantly increased in the LV and RV of irradiated rats versus the non-irradiated controls (Figure 1A,C,D,F). Treatment with aspirin and atorvastatin for six weeks (starting one day before irradiation) suppressed the elevation of the total as well as the phosphorylated forms of Cx43, significantly in the LV (Figure 1A–C) while having no effect in RV (Figure 1D–F) of post-irradiated animals. The administration of sildenafil had no significant effect on the irradiation-induced increase in myocardial Cx43, i.e., either on total levels or its phosphorylated forms after six weeks (Figure 1).

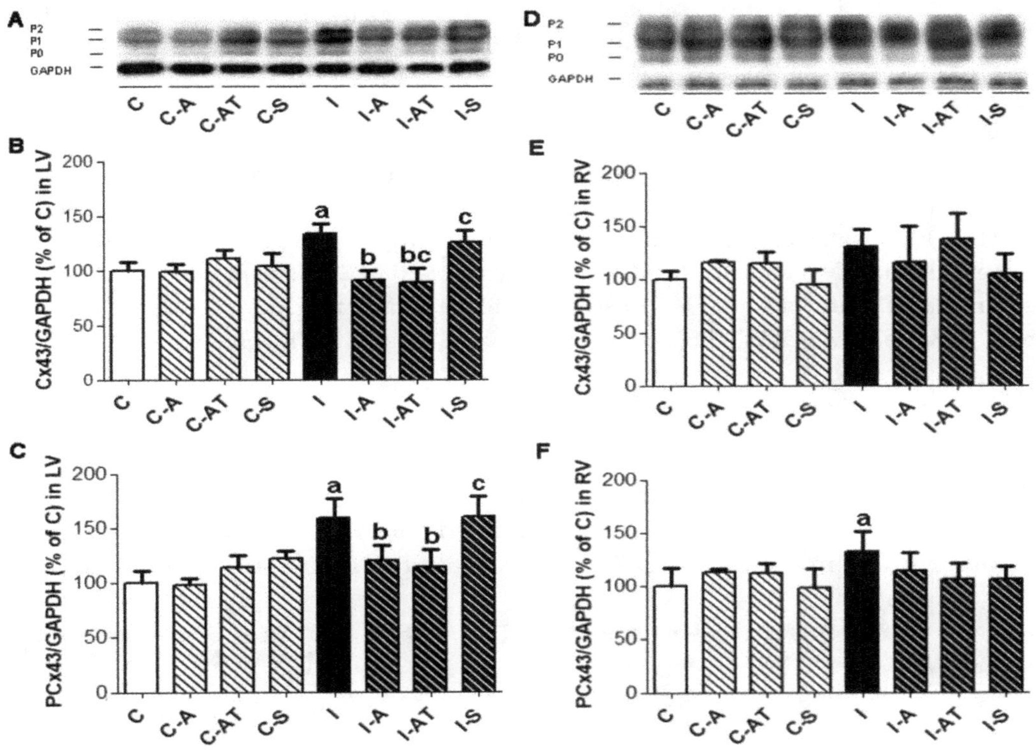

Figure 1. Representative immunoblots showing three forms of Cx43 (**A**,**D**) and densitometric quantification of total Cx43 expression (**B**,**E**), and its phosphorylated forms (**C**,**F**) normalized to GAPDH in the LV (left panel) and RV (right panel) of non-irradiated and post-irradiated Wistar rats with and without treatment. Abbreviations—P0: unphosphorylated form of Cx43; P1 and P2: phosphorylated forms of Cx43; GAPDH: housekeeper; C: control non-irradiated rats; C-A: control + aspirin; C-AT: control + atorvastatin; C-S: control + sildenafil; I: post-irradiated rats; I-A: post-irradiated + aspirin; I-AT: post-irradiated + atorvastatin; I-S: post-irradiated + sildenafil. Data are means ± SD of 6 hearts. [a] $p < 0.05$ vs. C (C vs. C-A, C-AT, C-S, I); [b] $p < 0.05$ vs. I (I vs. I-A, I-AT, I-S); [c] $p < 0.05$ treated C vs. treated I (C-A vs. I-A; C-AT vs. I-AT; C-S vs. I-S).

2.3. *Expression of Protein Kinase Cε in Control and Irradiated Wistar Rats*

PKCε was significantly increased in the LV (Figure 2A,B) but not in the RV (Figure 2C,D) of rats following irradiation when compared to the non-irradiated controls. Six weeks of treatment with aspirin and atorvastatin following irradiation normalized PKCε in the LV (Figure 2A,B) while having no effect in the RV (Figure 2C,D). Treatment with sildenafil had no effect on the PKCε expression of the irradiated rats. There was no change in the expression of PKCε in non-irradiated rats following treatment with drugs (Figure 2).

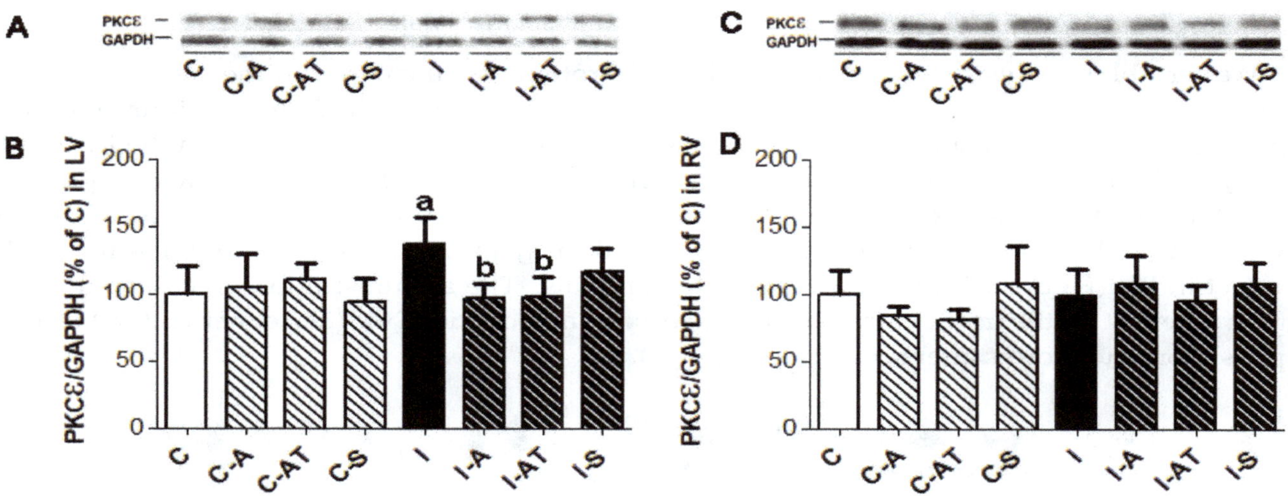

Figure 2. Representative immunoblots of PKCε expression (**A**,**C**) and its quantitative evaluation normalized to GAPDH in the LV ((**B**), left panel) and RV ((**D**), right panel) of non-irradiated and post-irradiated Wistar rats with and without treatment. Abbreviations—PKCε: protein kinase C epsilon; GAPDH: housekeeping protein; C: control non-irradiated rats; C-A: control + aspirin; C-AT: control + atorvastatin; C-S: control + sildenafil; I: post-irradiated rats; I-A: post-irradiated + aspirin; I-AT: post-irradiated + atorvastatin; I-S: post-irradiated + sildenafil. Data are means ± SD of 6 hearts. [a] $p < 0.05$ vs. C (C vs. C-A, C-AT, C-S, I); [b] $p < 0.05$ vs. I (I vs. I-A, I-AT, I-S).

2.4. *Expression of Protein Kinase C δ in Control and Irradiated Wistar Rats*

Similar to PKCε, the myocardial expression of PKCδ (Figure 3) was increased in response to irradiation. The increase was significant in the LV (Figure 3A,B) while no change was observed in the RV (Figure 3C,D) when compared to the to non-irradiated controls. Treatment with drugs had no effect on the expression of PKCδ in the LV or RV in the irradiated and non-irradiated groups (Figure 3).

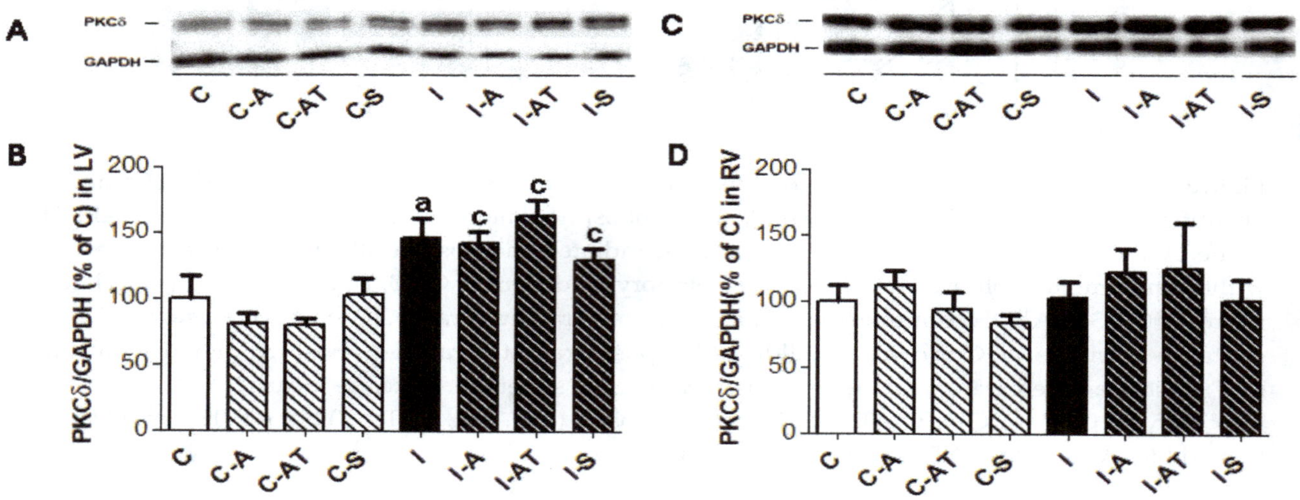

Figure 3. Representative immunoblots of PKCδ expression (**A**,**C**) and quantitative evaluation normalized to GAPDH in the LV ((**B**), left panel) and RV ((**D**), right panel) of non-irradiated and post-irradiated Wistar rats. Abbreviations—PKCδ: protein kinase C delta; GAPDH: housekeeping protein; C: control non-irradiated rats; C-A: control + aspirin; C-AT: control + atorvastatin; C-S: control + sildenafil; I: post-irradiated rats; I-A: post-irradiated + aspirin; I-AT: post-irradiated + atorvastatin; I-S: post-irradiated + sildenafil. Data are means ± SD of 6 hearts. [a] $p < 0.05$ vs. C (C vs. C-A, C-AT, C-S, I); [c] $p < 0.05$ treated C vs. treated I (C-A vs. I-A; C-AT vs. I-AT; C-S vs. I-S).

2.5. Myocardial Expression of miR-1 in Control and Irradiated Wistar Rats

miR-1 level decreased following six weeks after irradiation (Figure 4), which was signficant in the LV (Figure 4A) but not in the RV (Figure 4B). Treatment with the drugs had no significant effect on miR-1 level in post-irradiated as well as in non-irradiated groups (Figure 4).

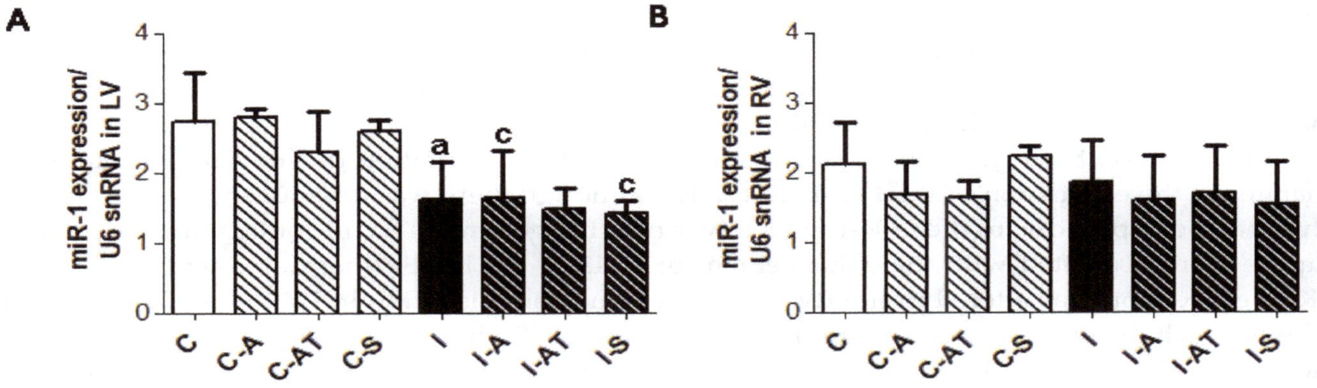

Figure 4. Myocardial expression of miR-1 in the LV ((**A**), left panel) and RV ((**B**), right panel) of non-irradiated and post-irradiated Wistar rats with and without treatment. Endogenous U6 small nuclear RNA (U6snRNA) was used to normalize miR-1. Abbreviations—C: control non-irradiated rats; C-A: control + aspirin; C-AT: control + atorvastatin; C-S: control + sildenafil; I: post-irradiated rats; I-A: post-irradiated + aspirin; I-AT: post-irradiated + atorvastatin; I-S: post-irradiated + sildenafil. Data are means ± SD of 5 hearts. [a] $p < 0.05$ vs. C (C vs. C-A, C-AT, C-S, I); [c] $p < 0.05$ treated C vs. treated I (C-A vs. I-A; C-AT vs. I-AT; C-S vs. I-S).

2.6. Expression of miR-21 in Control and Irradiated Wistar Rats

The expression of myocardial miR-21 was significantly increased in both the LV and RV of the post-irradiated rats compared to the non-irradiated controls (Figure 5). Six weeks of treatment with the selected drugs significantly suppressed miR-21 expression in the left (Figure 5A), although to a lesser extent in the RV (Figure 5B) following irradiation. There was no effect of drugs on miR-21 levels in the non-irradiated control groups (Figure 5).

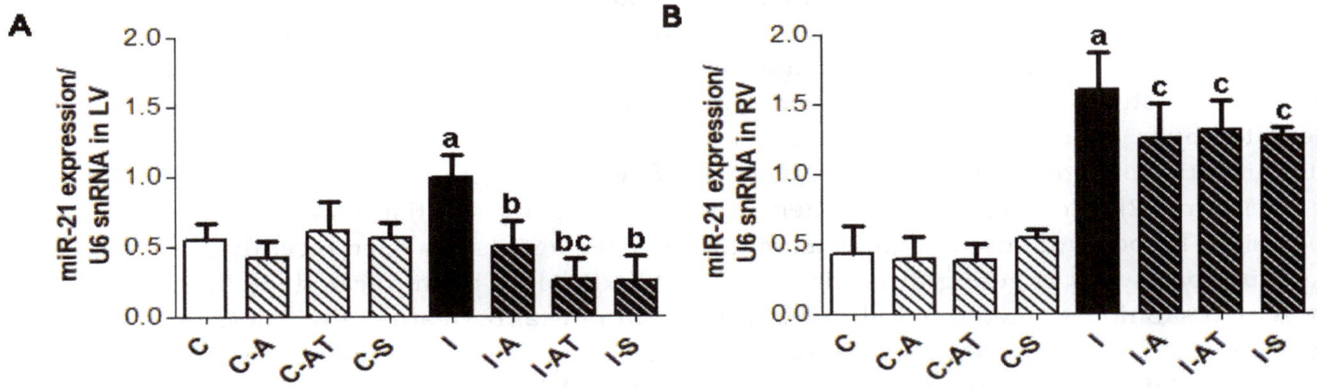

Figure 5. Myocardial expression of miR-21 in the LV (**A**) and RV (**B**) of non-irradiated and post-irradiated Wistar rats with and without treatment. Endogenous U6 small nuclear RNA (U6snRNA) was used to normalize miR-21. Abbreviations—C: control non-irradiated rats; C-A: control + aspirin; C-AT: control + atorvastatin; C-S: control + sildenafil; I: post-irradiated rats; I-A: post-irradiated + aspirin; I-AT: post-irradiated + atorvastatin; I-S: post-irradiated + sildenafil. Data are means ± SD of 5 hearts. [a] $p < 0.05$ vs. C (C vs. C-A, C-AT, C-S, I); [b] $p < 0.05$ vs. I (I vs. I-A, I-AT, I-S); [c] $p < 0.05$ treated C vs. treated I (C-A vs. I-A; C-AT vs. I-AT; C-S vs. I-S).

3. Discussion

In the present study, we showed that exposure of rats to a single dose of chest irradiation at 25 Gy caused up-regulation in the expression of Cx43, PKCε, and PKCδ in the LV following six weeks. In parallel, miR-1, which is known to repress GJA1 for Cx43 [3,6] was decreased. While miR-21, which is involved in myocardial remodeling and apoptosis [3,6], was increased following irradiation. These results are in accordance with our previous findings [6,10] and in line with the reported enhancement of myocardial Cx43 protein and mRNA expression found in the rabbit heart in response to heavy ion radiation [8,9]. Importantly, these alterations were associated with protection of the heart against arrhythmia and infarction [8,10].

In the present study, we have also demonstrated that irradiation did not induce significant changes in the expression of total Cx43 in the RV, although there was a trend towards an increase. This may be in part due to the miR-1, which was not changed in the RV in contrast to its significant suppression associated with the enhancement of Cx43 in the LV. Furthermore, neither PKCε nor PKCδ expression was altered in the RV unlike its significant elevation in LV following irradiation. Whether such distinct responses to irradiation in the LV and RV have any relationship with functional, metabolic, structural, and other differences of the heart chambers [17,18] needs to be investigated. Chamber related differences in Cx43 and PKC expression in response to altered thyroid status have been previously suggested [19]. A higher metabolic rate and mechanical load of the LV seems to be more prone to oxidative stress and injury. Nevertheless, our results suggest that cardiac response to chest irradiation is associated with the up-regulation of myocardial Cx43 connected with the suppression of miR-1 and enhanced PKCε and PKCδ signaling in the LV but not in the RV. On the other hand, the expression of miR-21 was significantly increased in both the LV and RV following irradiation. It is possible that the anti-apoptotic [20] and proliferation promoting effects of miR-21 [5] may be pro-survival to cardiac tissue during the early period in response to radiation-induced injury.

Our results also show that treatment of the irradiated rats with aspirin and atorvastatin prevented up-regulation of Cx43, i.e., its total and phosphorylated forms in the LV. Interestingly, none of the drugs reduced the level of miR-1 in the LV following irradiation. These data suggest that apart from the miR-1, other post-translational factors may modulate Cx43 levels in response to irradiation. Neither atorvastatin nor aspirin had any effect on the basal myocardial expression of Cx43 in the non-irradiated control rats.

The question arises, how aspirin or atorvastatin may affect changes in myocardial Cx43 protein levels induced by single chest irradiation? Considering that both compounds exert protection from oxidative stress and inflammation—the important culprits in irradiation-induced cardiac injury [1,2]—it is reasonable to speculate that these drugs may suppress these processes. If so, then cardiac stress would be attenuated and a subsequent compensatory response (most likely mediated by free radicals and pro-inflammatory molecules signaling) will be reduced. Indeed, the administration of antioxidants and/or scavengers of free radicals, such as hesperidin [21], melatonin [7] or selenium [22] prior to irradiation attenuated oxidative stress, inflammation, and cardiomyocyte necrosis. The potential use of statins as radioprotective agents has been recently reviewed, where signaling pathways targeting pro-inflammatory NF-κB might be implicated [1]. In support of this concept, it should be noted that unlike aspirin and atorvastatin, treatment with sildenafil (dominant vasculo-protective drug) did not affect the myocardial Cx43 levels in irradiated rats. Moreover, aspirin and atorvastatin but not sildenafil reduced expression of TNF-α in irradiated rats in our model, as reported previously [23].

In general, oxidative stress and/or inflammation contribute to the impairment of intercellular communication due to the acceleration of Cx43 and Cx43 interacting proteins that are in degradation and/or dysfunction [24]. Consequently, down-regulation of Cx43 due to chronic redox disorders and subclinical inflammation often accompanies cardiovascular disease [25,26]. On the other hand, acute heart injury (e.g., intermittent ischemia) triggers endogenous pro-survival molecular pathways, including up-regulation of Cx43, to protect heart function [27]. It appears that the heart may respond to stressors by compensatory/adaptive (such as up-regulation of Cx43) and by maladaptive/decompensatory changes (down-regulation of Cx43). Accordingly, enhanced Cx43 level observed in the compensatory hypertrophy was induced by pressure overload, while reduced Cx43 occurred in the decompensatory state [25].

Our results also show that the treatment of irradiated rats with aspirin and atorvastatin normalized the myocardial expression of PKCε, which is associated with the expression of phosphorylated forms of Cx43. These results suggest that oxidative stress and inflammation may modulate myocardial PKCε, signaling and its cardioprotective role as shown in various conditions [28]. Interestingly, treatment did not affect elevated myocardial PKCδ expression, i.e., its pro-hypertrophic signaling in irradiated rat heart. However, the expression of pro-fibrotic miR-21 was significantly decreased in the left heart ventricle by all tested drugs. Of note, miR-21 has been shown up-regulated in human fibroblast cells due to various stress-inducing conditions, including radiation [3,29]. Thus, more attention should be paid to elucidate the possible anti-fibrotic effects of atorvastatin, aspirin, and perhaps sildenafil. Importantly, microRNA-21 has been reported as a novel promising target in cancer radiation therapy [20] and atorvastatin was shown to suppress expansive remodeling by inhibition of macrophage infiltration [30].

Taken together, we assume that protection of the heart from oxidative stress and inflammation by appropriate drugs, including aspirin and atorvastatin or nonpharmacological compounds like melatonin [7], omega-PUFA [31] may counteract compensatory responses and attenuate adverse consequences of chest irradiation.

4. Materials and Methods

Animal experiments were approved by the Animal Research and Care Committee of the Institute for Heart Research, Slovak Academy of Sciences—Project 1873/11-221/3, approved on 30 September 2011 and in accordance with the rules issued by the State Veterinary Administration of the Slovak Republic, legislation No 289/2003. Rats were maintained on a 12:12 h's light/dark cycle with access to standard pellet and water *ad libitum*.

4.1. Experimental Model of Irradiation Induced Cardiac Injury

Three-month-old male Wistar rats were randomly divided into irradiated (n = 24) and non-irradiated (n = 24) groups. Rats were anesthetized with Narketan (115 mg/kg body weight) followed by myorelaxant Xylan (1 mg/kg body weight) and exposed to a single dose of 25 Gy of ionizing radiation given locally on mediastinum at the area of the heart using the electron linear accelerator UELR 5-1S (Producer NIIEFA St. Petersburg, RF, Russia), as described previously [6]. Control animals were shielded with lead plates. Non-irradiated controls (C) and irradiated (I) rats were treated one day before, the day of irradiation, and for the next six weeks with aspirin (A; 3 mg/day), atorvastatin (AT; 0.25 mg/day) or sildenafil (S; 0.3 mg/day) via a gastric tube. Doses of the drugs were calculated from the maximal therapeutic dose for humans in relation to the rat body weight.

At the end of the experiment, hearts were excised from the anesthetized animals (thiopental, 65 mg/kg body weight) followed by the registration of the whole heart as well as left (LV) and right ventricle (RV) weight. Frozen tissues from the heart ventricles were stored at −80 °C in freezer box and used for the analysis of Cx43, PKCε and PKCδ expression by the Western blot method and for miR-1 and miR-21 expression analysis by qRT-PCR.

4.2. Determination of Myocardial Cx43, PKCε and PKCδ Protein Expression

The western blot analysis was performed as previously described [6]. Briefly, the ventricular samples (n = 6 per group) were powdered and solubilized in SB20 (20% SDS, 10 mmol/L EDTA, 0.1 mol/L tris(hydroxymethyl) aminomethane (TRIS), pH 6.8 by sonicator UP 100H (Hielscher, Teltow, Germany). Total proteins (10–30 μg) from each sample were separated in 10% sodium dodecyl sulfate polyacrylamide gels, transferred onto a nitrocellulose membrane, and blocked with 5% non-fat dry milk in Tris-buffered saline. For the determination of Cx43, the membrane was incubated with a primary rabbit polyclonal antibody (diluted 1:4000; Anti-Connexin 43 C 6219; Sigma-Aldrich, St. Louis, MO, USA). For PKCε and PKCδ determination, the nitrocellulose membrane was incubated with primary rabbit polyclonal antibodies (PKCε Antibody, C-15: sc-214, Santa Cruz Biotechnology, Inc., PKCδ Antibody, C-17: sc-213, Santa Cruz Biotechnology, Inc., Santa Cruz, CA, USA) diluted 1:1000, overnight at 4 °C, followed by further incubation for 1 h at room temperature with a secondary donkey antibody (peroxidase-labeled anti-rabbit, 1:2000, Amersham Biosciences, Piscataway, NJ, USA). After ECL visualization, the densitometric analysis by Carestream Molecular Imaging Software (version 5.0, Carestream Health, New Haven, CT, USA.) was done using a KODAK In-Vivo Multispectral System FX. The measured values were normalized to the expression of GAPDH (glyceraldehyde-3-phosphate dehydrogenase) serving as a control [6].

4.3. *Estimation of Myocardial miR-1 and miR-21 Levels*

miR reverse transcription and TaqMan-based qRT-PCR analysis were performed as previously reported [6]. Total RNA including small RNA was isolated from the frozen ventricular tissue of the non-irradiated (n = 5 per group) and irradiated (n = 5 per group) Wistar rats using a miRNA mini kit according to the manufacturer's protocol (QIAGEN Sciences, Germantown, MD, USA). The concentration and purity of the isolated RNA was checked using a Nanodrop ND-1000 spectrophotometer (Agilent Technologies, Santa Clara, CA, USA). Briefly, 10 ng of total RNA were subjected for reverse transcription reaction with miRNA specific RT primers using microRNA reverse transcription kit (Applied Biosystems, Foster City, CA, USA) in accordance to the manufacturer's instructions. Real time PCR was performed using a Roche Light cycler 480 II (Roche Applied Science, Indianapolis, IN, USA). TaqMan miRNA assay probe (Applied Biosystems, Foster City, CA, USA) was applied to determine the expression level of miR-1 and miR-21. Endogenous U6 small nuclear RNA was used to normalize RNA content. Reverse transcription was performed using stem loop specific microRT primers under the following conditions: 16 °C for 30 min, 42 °C for 30 min, and 85 °C for 5 min. The obtained cDNA was diluted in 1:3 ratios and subjected to real-time PCR using a TaqMan amplicon specific assay probe under the following PCR cycle conditions: 95 °C for 10 min, 95 °C for 15 s, and 60 °C for 60 s [6].

4.4. *Statistical Analysis*

Data are expressed as means ± SD. One way two-tailed ANOVA and Tukey post hoc tests were used for statistical analysis. $p < 0.05$ was considered as statistically significant.

5. Conclusions

In conclusion, we have demonstrated that irradiation related changes are less pronounced in the RV as compared to the LV. Our results also suggest that treatment with aspirin and atorvastatin attenuate irradiation-induced up-regulation of myocardial Cx43 and PKCε signaling as well as miR-21 expression. Whether treatment related prevention or attenuation of irradiation-induced myocardial alterations at the early responsive period might help to prevent adverse late effects needs further investigations.

Acknowledgments: This study was supported by grants APVV-0241/11, APVV-15-0376 of Slovak Research and Development Agency and VEGA 2/0076/16, VEGA 2/0167/15 of Slovak Scientific Grant Agency and by EU Structural Fund ITMS 26230120006.

Author Contributions: Csilla Viczenczova: acquisition of data, data analysis/interpretation; Branislav Kura: acquisition of data, data analysis/interpretation; Tamara Egan Benova: acquisition of data, data analysis/interpretation; Chang Yin: acquisition of data, data analysis/interpretation; Rakesh C. Kukreja: formulation of the overall concept/design of experiments, editing of English language; Jan Slezak: formation of concept/design of experiment; Narcis Tribulova: formation of concept/design of experiment, critical revision of the manuscript, and approval of the article; Barbara Szeiffova Bacova: acquisition of data, data analysis/interpretation, approval of the article.

References

1. Cuomo, J.R.; Sharma, G.K.; Conger, P.D.; Weintraub, N.L. Novel concepts in radiation-induced cardiovascular disease. *World J. Cardiol.* **2016**, *8*, 504–519. [CrossRef] [PubMed]
2. Slezak, J.; Kura, B.; Ravingerova, T.; Tribulova, N.; Okruhlicova, L.; Barancik, M. Mechanisms of cardiac radiation injury and potential preventive approaches. *Can. J Physiol. Pharmacol.* **2015**, *27*, 1–17. [CrossRef] [PubMed]
3. Simone, N.L.; Soule, B.P.; Ly, D.; Saleh, A.D.; Savage, J.E.; Degraff, W.; Cook, J.; Harris, C.C.; Gius, D.; Mitchell, J.B. Ionizing radiation-induced oxidative stress alters miRNA expression. *PLoS ONE* **2009**, *4*, e6377. [CrossRef] [PubMed]
4. Kura, B.; Babal, P.; Slezak, J. Implication of microRNAs in the development and potential treatment of radiation—Induced heart disease. *Can. J. Physiol. Pharmacol.* **2017**, *95*, 1236–1244. [CrossRef] [PubMed]
5. Zhu, H.; Fan, G.C. Role of microRNAs in the reperfused myocardium towards post-infarct remodelling. *Cardiovasc. Res.* **2012**, *94*, 284–292. [CrossRef] [PubMed]
6. Viczenczova, C.; Szeiffova Bacova, B.; Egan Benova, T.; Kura, B.; Yin, C.; Weismann, P.; Kukreja, R.; Slezak, J.; Tribulova, N. Myocardial connexin-43 and PKC signalling are involved in adaptation of the heart to irradiation-induced injury: Implication of miR-1 and miR-21. *Gen. Physiol. Biophys.* **2016**, *35*, 215–222. [CrossRef] [PubMed]
7. Gürses, I.; Özeren, M.; Serin, M.; Yücel, N.; Erkal, H.S. Histopathological evaluation of melatonin as a protective agent in heart injury induced by radiation in a rat model. *Pathol. Res. Pract.* **2014**, *210*, 863–871. [CrossRef] [PubMed]
8. Amino, M.; Yoshioka, K.; Tanabe, T.; Tanaka, E.; Mori, H.; Furusawa, Y.; Zareba, W.; Yamazaki, M.; Nakagawa, H.; Honjo, H.; et al. Heavy ion radiation up-regulates connexin43 and ameliorates the arrhythmogenic substrates in rabbit hearts after myocardial infarction. *Cardiovasc. Res.* **2006**, *72*, 412–421. [CrossRef] [PubMed]
9. Amino, M.; Yoshioka, K.; Fujibayashi, D.; Hashida, T.; Furusawa, Y.; Zareba, W.; Ikari, Y.; Tanaka, E.; Mori, H.; Inokuchi, S.; et al. Year-long upregulation of connexin43 in rabbit hearts by heavy ion irradiation. *Am. J. Physiol. Heart Circ. Physiol.* **2010**, *298*, 1014–1021. [CrossRef] [PubMed]
10. Viczenczova, C.; Kura, B.; Chaudagar, K.K.; Szeiffova Bacova, B.; Egan Benova, T.; Barancik, M.; Knezl, V.; Ravingerova, T.; Tribulova, N.; Slezak, J. Myocardial connexin-43 is upregulated in response to acute cardiac injury in rats. *Can. J. Physiol. Pharmacol.* **2017**, *95*, 911–919. [CrossRef] [PubMed]
11. Song, J.; Yan, R.; Wu, Z.; Li, J.; Yan, M.; Hao, X.; Liu, J.; Li, S. ^{13}N-ammonia PET/CT detection of myocardial perfusion abnormalities in beagle dogs after local heart irradiation. *J. Nucl. Med.* **2017**, *58*, 605–610. [CrossRef] [PubMed]
12. Slezak, J.; Kura, B.; Babal, P.; Barancik, M.; Ferko, M.; Frimmel, K.; Kalocayova, B.; Kukreja, R.C.; Lazou, A.; Mezesova, L.; et al. Potential markers and metabolic processes involved in the mechanism of radiation-induced heart injury. *Can. J. Physiol. Pharmacol.* **2017**, *95*, 1190–1203. [CrossRef] [PubMed]
13. Shi, X.; Ding, M.; Dong, Z.; Chen, F.; Ye, J.; Wang, S.; Leonard, S.S.; Castranova, V.; Vallyathan, V. Antioxidant properties of aspirin: Characterization of the ability of aspirin to inhibit silica-induced lipid peroxidation, DNA damage, NF-kappaB activation, and TNF-alpha production. *Mol. Cell. Biochem.* **1999**, *199*, 93–102. [CrossRef] [PubMed]
14. Pignatelli, P.; Carnevale, R.; Pastori, D.; Cangemi, R.; Napoleone, L.; Bartimoccia, S.; Nocella, C.; Basili, S.; Violi, F. Immediate antioxidant and antiplatelet effect of atorvastatin via inhibition of Nox2. *Circulation* **2012**, *126*, 92–103. [CrossRef] [PubMed]
15. Lefer, A.M.; Scalia, R.; Lefer, D.J. Vascular effects of HMG CoA-reductase inhibitors (statins) unrelated to cholesterol lowering: New concepts for cardiovascular disease. *Cardiovasc. Res.* **2001**, *49*, 281–287. [CrossRef]
16. Webb, D.J.; Freestone, S.; Allen, M.J.; Muirhead, G.J. Sildenafil citrate and blood-pressure-lowering drugs: Results of drug interaction studies with an organic nitrate and a calcium antagonist. *Am. J. Cardiol.* **1999**, *83*, 21–28. [CrossRef]
17. Cihák, R.; Kolár, F.; Pelouch, V.; Procházka, J.; Ostádal, B.; Widimský, J. Functional changes in the right and left ventricle during development of cardiac hypertrophy and after its regression. *Cardiovasc. Res.* **1992**, *26*, 845–850. [CrossRef] [PubMed]

18. Noorman, M.; van Rijen, H.V.; van Veen, T.A.; de Bakker, J.M.; Stein, M. Differences in distribution of fibrosis in the ventricles underlie dominant arrhythmia vulnerability of the right ventricle in senescent mice. *Neth. Heart J.* **2008**, *16*, 356–358. [CrossRef] [PubMed]
19. Szeiffová Bačová, B.; Egan Beňová, T.; Viczenczová, C.; Soukup, T.; Rauchová, H.; Pavelka, S.; Knezl, V.; Barančík, M.; Tribulová, N. Cardiac connexin-43 and PKC signaling in rats with altered thyroid status without and with omega-3 fatty acids intake. *Physiol. Res.* **2016**, *65*, 77–90.
20. Liu, J.; Zhu, H.; Yang, X.; Ge, Y.; Zhang, C.; Qin, Q.; Lu, J.; Zhan, L.; Cheng, H.; Sun, X. MicroRNA-21 is a novel promising target in cancer radiation therapy. *Tumour Biol.* **2014**, *35*, 3975–3979. [CrossRef] [PubMed]
21. Rezaeyan, A.; Haddadi, G.H.; Hosseinzadeh, M.; Moradi, M.; Najafi, M. Radioprotective effects of hesperidin on oxidative damages and histopathological changes induced by X-irradiation in rats heart tissue. *J. Med. Phys.* **2016**, *41*, 182–191. [CrossRef] [PubMed]
22. Sieber, F.; Muir, S.A.; Cohen, E.P.; Fish, B.L.; Mäder, M.; Schock, A.M.; Althouse, B.J.; Moulder, J.E. Dietary selenium for the mitigation of radiation injury: Effects of selenium dose escalation and timing of supplementation. *Radiat. Res.* **2011**, *176*, 366–374. [CrossRef] [PubMed]
23. Kura, B.; Bagchi, A.S.; Akolkar, G.; Singal, P.K.; Slezak, J. Myocardial changes after mediastinal irradiation in rats: Molecular mechamisms and potential targets to minimize the adverse effects. In *Adaptation Biology and Medicine*; Kawai, Y., Hargens, A.R., Singal, P.K., Eds.; Narosa Publishing House Ltd.: New Delhi, India, 2017; pp. 93–122.
24. Smyth, J.W.; Hong, T.T.; Gao, D.; Vogan, J.M.; Jensen, B.C.; Fong, T.S.; Simpson, P.C.; Stainier, D.Y.; Chi, N.C.; Shaw, R.M. Limited forward trafficking of connexin 43 reduces cell-cell coupling in stressed human and mouse myocardium. *J. Clin. Investig.* **2010**, *120*, 266–279. [CrossRef] [PubMed]
25. Egan Benova, T.; Szeiffova Bacova, B.; Viczenczova, C.; Diez, E.; Barancik, M.; Tribulova, N. Protection of cardiac cell-to-cell coupling attenuate myocardial remodeling and proarrhythmia induced by hypertension. *Physiol. Res.* **2016**, *65*, 29–42.
26. Tribulova, N.; Szeiffova Bacova, B.; Benova, T.; Viczenczova, C. Can we protect from malignant arrhythmias by modulation of cardiac cell-to-cell coupling? *J. Electrocardiol.* **2015**, *48*, 434–440. [CrossRef] [PubMed]
27. Su, F.; Zhao, L.; Zhang, S.; Wang, J.; Chen, N.; Gong, Q.; Tang, J.; Wang, H.; Yao, J.; Wang, Q.; et al. Cardioprotection by PI3K-mediated signaling is required for anti-arrhythmia and myocardial repair in response to ischemic preconditioning in infarcted pig hearts. *Lab. Investig.* **2015**, *95*, 860–871. [CrossRef] [PubMed]
28. Jeyaraman, M.M.; Srisakuldee, W.; Nickel, B.E.; Kardami, E. Connexin43 phosphorylation and cytoprotection in the heart. *Biochim. Biophys. Acta* **2012**, *1818*, 2009–2013. [CrossRef] [PubMed]
29. Thum, T.; Gross, C.; Fiedler, J.; Fischer, T.; Kissler, S.; Bussen, M.; Galuppo, P.; Just, S.; Rottbauer, W.; Frantz, S.; et al. MicroRNA-21 contributes to myocardial disease by stimulating MAP kinase signalling in fibroblasts. *Nature* **2008**, *456*, 980–984. [CrossRef] [PubMed]
30. Qiang, B.; Toma, J.; Fujii, H.; Osherov, A.B.; Nili, N.; Sparkes, J.D.; Fefer, P.; Samuel, M.; Butany, J.; Leong-Poi, H.; et al. Statin therapy prevents expansive remodeling in venous bypass grafts. *Atherosclerosis* **2012**, *223*, 106–113. [CrossRef] [PubMed]
31. Fabian, C.J.; Kimler, B.F.; Hursting, S.D. Omega-3 fatty acids for breast cancer prevention and survivorship. *Breast Cancer Res.* **2015**, *17*, 62. [CrossRef] [PubMed]

6

Recent Advances in the Pathophysiology of Musculocontractural Ehlers-Danlos Syndrome

Tomoki Kosho [1,2,3,*], Shuji Mizumoto [4], Takafumi Watanabe [5], Takahiro Yoshizawa [6], Noriko Miyake [7] and Shuhei Yamada [4]

1 Department of Medical Genetics, Shinshu University School of Medicine, Matsumoto 390-8621, Japan
2 Center for Medical Genetics, Shinshu University Hospital, Matsumoto 390-8621, Japan
3 Research Center for Supports to Advanced Science, Matsumoto 390-8621, Japan
4 Department of Pathobiochemistry, Faculty of Pharmacy, Meijo University, Nagoya 468-8503, Japan; mizumoto@meijo-u.ac.jp (S.M.); shuheiy@meijo-u.ac.jp (S.Y.)
5 Laboratory of Anatomy, School of Veterinary Medicine, Rakuno Gakuen University, Ebetsu 069-8501, Japan; t-watanabe@rakuno.ac.jp
6 Division of Animal Research, Research Center for Supports to Advanced Science, Shinshu University, Matsumoto 390-8621, Japan; tyoshizawa@shinshu-u.ac.jp
7 Department of Human Genetics, Yokohama City University Graduate School of Medicine, Yokohama 236-0004, Japan; nmiyake@yokohama-cu.ac.jp
* Correspondence: ktomoki@shinshu-u.ac.jp

Abstract: Musculocontractural Ehlers–Danlos Syndome (mcEDS) is a type of EDS caused by biallelic pathogenic variants in the gene for carbohydrate sulfotransferase 14/dermatan 4-*O*-sulfotransferase 1 (*CHST14/D4ST1*, mcEDS-*CHST14*), or in the gene for dermatan sulfate epimerase (*DSE*, mcEDS-*DSE*). Thus far, 41 patients from 28 families with mcEDS-*CHST14* and five patients from four families with mcEDS-*DSE* have been described in the literature. Clinical features comprise multisystem congenital malformations and progressive connective tissue fragility-related manifestations. This review outlines recent advances in understanding the pathophysiology of mcEDS. Pathogenic variants in *CHST14* or *DSE* lead to reduced activities of relevant enzymes, resulting in a negligible amount of dermatan sulfate (DS) and an excessive amount of chondroitin sulfate. Connective tissue fragility is presumably attributable to a compositional change in the glycosaminoglycan chains of decorin, a major DS-proteoglycan in the skin that contributes to collagen fibril assembly. Collagen fibrils in affected skin are dispersed in the papillary to reticular dermis, whereas those in normal skin are regularly and tightly assembled. Glycosaminoglycan chains are linear in affected skin, stretching from the outer surface of collagen fibrils to adjacent fibrils; glycosaminoglycan chains are curved in normal skin, maintaining close contact with attached collagen fibrils. Homozygous (*Chst14*$^{-/-}$) mice have been shown perinatal lethality, shorter fetal length and vessel-related placental abnormalities. Milder phenotypes in mcEDS-*DSE* might be related to a smaller fraction of decorin DS, potentially through residual DSE activity or compensation by DSE2 activity. These findings suggest critical roles of DS and DS-proteoglycans in the multisystem development and maintenance of connective tissues, and provide fundamental evidence to support future etiology-based therapies.

Keywords: musculocontractural Ehlers–Danlos Syndome; carbohydrate sulfotransferase-14 (CHST14)/dermatan 4-*O*-sulfotransferase-1 (D4ST1); *CHST14*; dermatan sulfate epimerase (DSE); *DSE*; dermatan sulfate (DS); decorin; collagen

1. Introduction

Musculocontractural Ehlers–Danlos Syndome (mcEDS) is a type of EDS, caused by biallelic pathogenic variants in the gene for carbohydrate sulfotransferase 14/dermatan 4-*O*-sulfotransferase 1

(*CHST14*/*D4ST1*, mcEDS-*CHST14*) (MIM#601776), or in the gene for dermatan sulfate epimerase (*DSE*, mcEDS-*DSE*) (MIM#615539) [1–3]. mcEDS-*CHST14* was originally described as three independent conditions: A rare type of arthrogryposis syndrome "adducted thumb-clubfoot syndrome" [4]; a specific type of EDS "EDS, Kosho type" [5,6]; and a subset of kyphoscoliosis type without lysyl hydroxylase deficiency [7]. To date, 41 patients from 28 families have been reported to have mcEDS-*CHST14* [4–22]. mcEDS-*DSE* was identified in a patient with a phenotype similar to that of patients with mcEDS-*CHST14* [23], as well as in four additional patients from three families [18,24]. These disorders were defined as subtypes of EDS, based on the International Classification of the EDSs [3]. Clinical features are highly characteristic, comprising multisystem congenital malformations such as craniofacial features (e.g., large fontanelle, hypertelorism, short and downslanting palpebral fissures, blue sclerae, short nose with hypoplastic columella, low-set and rotated ears, high palate, long philtrum, thin upper lip vermilion, small mouth and micro-retrognathia), multiple congenital contractures (e.g., adduction–flexion contractures of thumbs and talipes equinovarus), and visceral and ocular malformations. Features also include progressive connective tissue fragility-related manifestations, such as skin hyperextensibility, bruisability, and fragility with atrophic scars; recurrent dislocations; progressive talipes or spinal deformities; pneumothorax or pneumohemothorax; large subcutaneous hematomas; and/or diverticular perforation (Figure 1) [1,2]. Major diagnostic criteria of the disorder are as follows: 1) congenital multiple contractures, characteristically adduction–flexion contractures and/or talipes equinovarus (clubfoot); 2) characteristic craniofacial features, which are evident at birth or in early infancy; 3) characteristic cutaneous features including hyperextensibility, bruisability and fragility with atrophic scars, as well as increased palmer wrinkles [3]. Minor criteria as follows: 1) recurrent/chronic dislocations, 2) pectus deformities (e.g., flat or excavated), 3) spinal deformities (e.g., scoliosis or kyphoscoliosis), 4) peculiar fingers (e.g., tapered, slender, or cylindrical), 5) progressive talipes deformities (e.g., valgus, planus, or cavum), 6) large subcutaneous hematomas, 7) chronic constipation, 8) colonic diverticula, 9) pneumothorax/pneumohemothorax, 10) nephrolithiasis/cystolithiasis, 11) hydronephrosis, 12) cryptorchidism in males, 13) strabismus, 14) refractive errors (e.g., myopia or astigmatism) and/or 15) glaucoma/elevated intraocular pressure [3].

In this review, we describe the comprehensive pathophysiological findings of mcEDS, as demonstrated in previous studies including our recent reports.

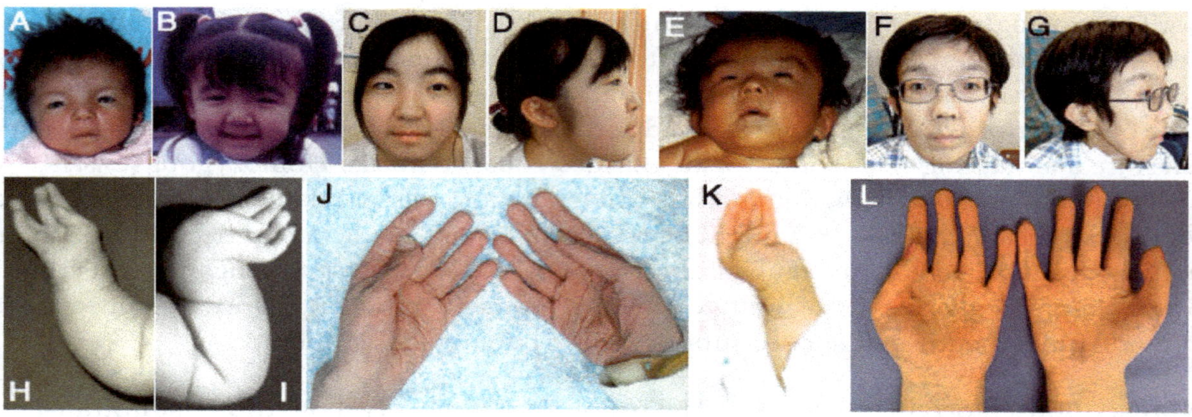

Figure 1. *Cont.*

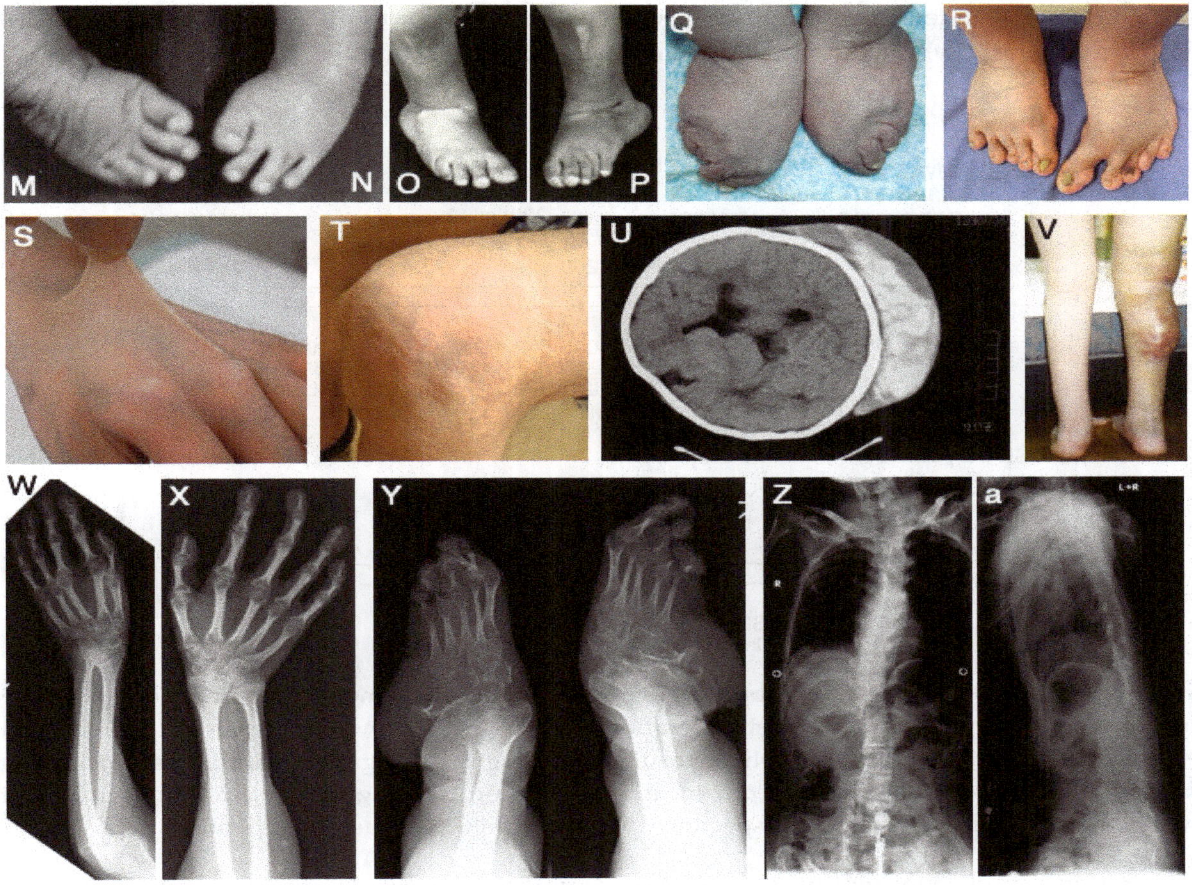

Figure 1. Clinical photographs and radiological images of patients with mcEDS-*CHST14*. Clinical photographs of a patient with heterozygous variants Pro281Leu/Try293Cys at age 23 days (**A**), 3 years (**B**), and 16 years (**C**,**D**); those of a patient with a homozygous variant Pro281Leu at age 2 months (**H**,**M**,**N**), 3 months (**I**), 6 years (**O**,**P**), and 28 years (**J**,**Q**); photographs of a patient with a homozygous variant "P281L" in the neonatal period (**E**) and at age 30 years (**F**,**G**,**T**); and photographs of a patient with heterozygous variants Pro281Leu /Cys289Ser at age 1 month (**K**), 16 years (**V**), and 19 years (**L**,**R**,**S**) [5]. Radiological image of a patient with heterozygous variants Pro281Leu /Try293Cys at age 6 years (**U**); images of a patient with a homozygous variant Pro281Leu at age 28 years (**W**–**Z**,**a**) [5,13]. (U, reproduced from Kosho et al. *Am. J. Med. Genet. Part A* **2005**, *138A*, 282–287, with permission from Wiley-Liss, Inc.; the other images, reproduced from Kosho et al. *Am. J. Med. Genet. Part A* **2010**, *152A*, 1333–1346, with permission from Wiley-Liss, Inc.).

2. Molecular Findings

Pathogenic variants have been detected throughout *CHST14* (NM_130468.4): 11 missense variants, five frameshift variants, and three nonsense variants in patients with mcEDS [4,6,7,14–19,22] (Figure 2). The p.(Pro281Leu) variant is most common (n = 10 families), followed by p.(Try293Cys) (n = 4), p.(Val49*) (n = 3), p.(Arg213Pro), and p.(Phe209Ser) (n = 2); p.(Arg29Glyfs*113), p.(Lys69*), p.(Gln113Argfs*14), p.(Arg135Gly), p.(Leu137Gln), p.(Cys152Leufs*10), p.(Arg218Ser), p.(Gly228Leufs*13), p.(Glu262Lys), p.(Tyr266*), p.(Arg274Pro), p.(Met280Leu), p.(Cys289Ser), p.(Trp327Cysfs*29), and p.(Glu334Glyfs*107) variants are particularly uncommon (n = 1 for all). Furthermore, p.(Gly19Trpfs*19) and p.(Lys26Alafs*16) variants have been detected in patients with features similar to those of mcEDS, among patients with hereditary connective tissue disorders and skeletal dysplasia, respectively (Figure 2A) [25,26]. Three missense variants have been detected in *DSE* (NM_013352.4): p.(Arg267Gly), p.(Ser268Leu), and p.(His588Arg); and one frameshift variant, p.(Pro384Trpfs*9), has also been detected (Figure 2B) [18,23,24]. Another frameshift variant, p.(Gly216Glufs*3), was detected in a patient with features similar to those of mcEDS, among patients with chondrodysplasia who exhibited multiple dislocations (Figure 2B) [27].

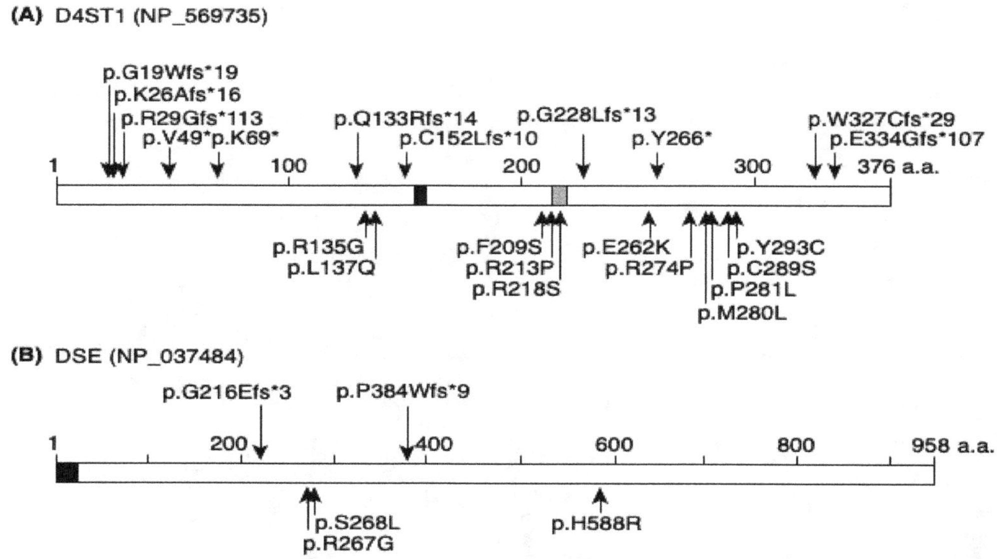

Figure 2. Published pathogenic protein changes of D4ST1 and DSE in mcEDS. (**A**) Previously published truncating and non-truncating protein alterations in D4ST1 are shown in upper and lower panels, respectively. Black box indicates 5′-phosphosulfate binding site and gray box indicates 3′-phosphate binding site. (**B**) Previously published truncating and non-truncating protein alterations in DSE are shown in upper and lower panels, respectively. Black box indicates the signal peptide.

No apparent genotype-phenotype correlations have been reported in patients with mcEDS-*CHST14*. Phenotypes of patients with mcEDS-*DSE* seem to be milder than those of patients with mcEDS-*CHST14* [18,24].

3. Glycobiological Findings

Normal, biosynthetic pathways of chondroitin sulfate (CS) and dermatan sulfate (DS) are shown in Figure 3A. Reduced activity of D4ST1 in fibroblast cultures of skin from a patient with mcEDS-*CHST14* caused by compound heterozygous p.(Pro281Leu)/(Tyr293Cys) substitutions in *CHST14*, as well as in fibroblasts from a patient with mcEDS-*CHST14* caused by a homozygous p.(Pro281Leu) substitution in *CHST14*, showed a marked reduction in D4ST1 activity (Figure 3B); this change in activity resulted in a negligible amount of DS and an excessive amount of CS (Figure 3C) [6].

Decorin, which consists of a core protein and a single glycosaminoglycan (GAG) chain, is a major DS-proteoglycan (PG) that plays an important role in the assembly of collagen fibrils in the skin [28]; it also plays roles in the pathophysiology of mcEDS-*CHST14* [1–4,6,7]. GAG chains of decorin-PG from skin fibroblasts of a patient with p.(Pro281Leu)/(Tyr293Cys) substitutions, as well as from skin fibroblasts of a patient with a homozygous p.(Pro281Leu) substitution, contained only CS and no DS; in contrast, GAG chains of decorin-PG from skin fibroblasts of healthy controls contained mainly DS (Figure 3D) [6,18]. 4-*O*-Sulfation in CS and DS chains functions as an inhibitor of DSE [29]. Thus, impaired 4-*O*-sulfation inhibition due to D4ST1 deficiency enables back-epimerization from L-iduronic acid (IdoUA) to D-glucuronic acid (GlcUA) (Figure 3E) [4,6,7]. In our laboratory, we have established a urinary disaccharide analysis of CS/DS chains through an anion-exchange chromatography after treatment with DS-specific degrading enzymes; this analysis method showed that no DS was present in the urine of eight patients with mcEDS-*CHST14* [30]. This result suggested a systemic depletion of DS in patients with mcEDS-*CHST14*; thus we presume that our urinary disaccharide analysis method can be implemented to allow a non-invasive screening for mcEDS-*CHST14* [30].

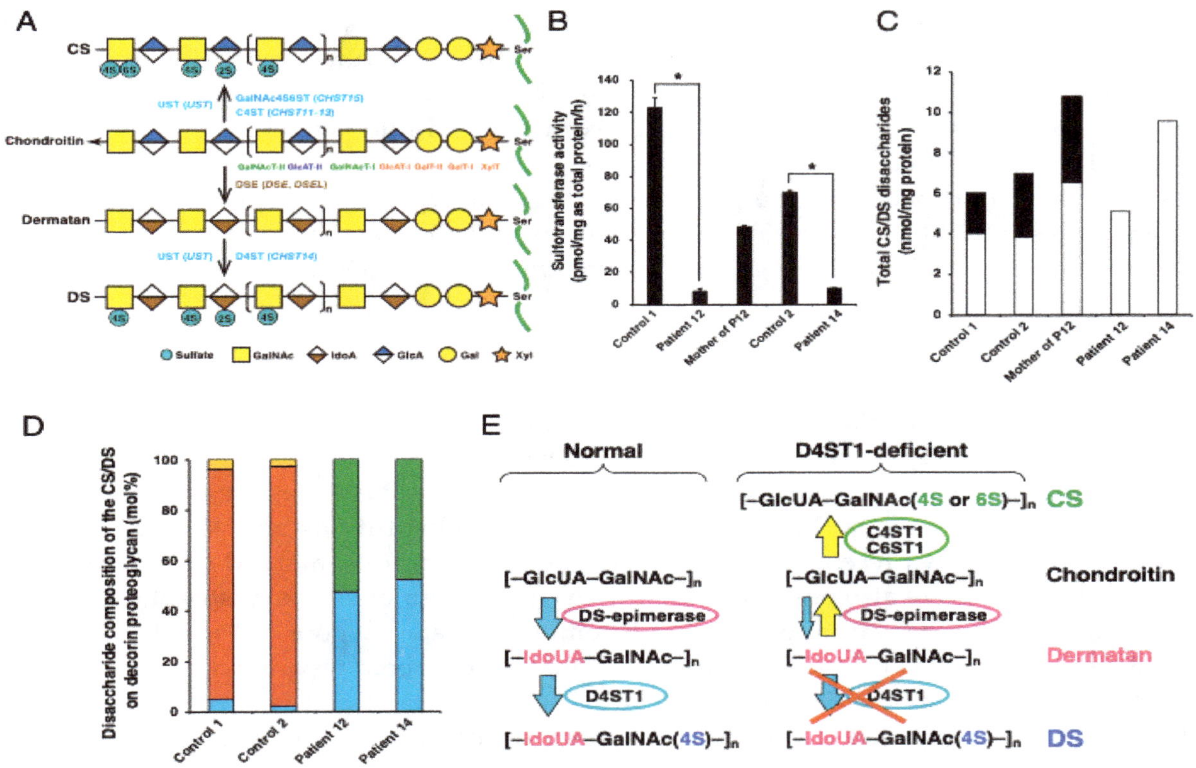

Figure 3. Biosynthesis of CS/DS and glycobiological analysis in mcEDS-*CHST14*. (**A**) Biosynthetic assembly of CS and DS chains by glycosyltransferases, epimerases, and sulfotransferases. It starts with the biosynthesis of a tetrasaccharide linker region, glucuronic acid-β1,3-galactose-β1,3-galactose-β1,4-xylose-β1-*O*-(GlcUA-Gal-Gal-Xyl-), onto serine residues of specific core proteins of PGs by β-xylosyltransferase (XylT), GalT-I, GalT-II and β1,3-glucuronosyltransferase-I (GlcAT-I), respectively. Subsequently, a repetitive disaccharide region [*N*-acetyl-D-galactosamine(GalNAc)-GlcUA)]$_n$ of chondroitin is elongated by the actions of *N*-acetyl-D-galactosaminyltransferase-I (GalNAcT-I), *N*-acetyl-D-galactosaminyltransferase-II (GalNAcT-II) and glucuronyltransferase-II (GlcAT-II), which are encoded by CS *N*-acetylgalactosaminyltransferase-1 and -2, chondroitin synthase-1, -2, and -3 and chondroitin polymerizing factor genes. Chondroitin chains are matured to CS through modifications by chondroitin 4-*O*-sulfotransferase (C4ST), chondroitin 6-*O*-sulfotransferase (C6ST) and uronyl 2-*O*-sulfotransferase (UST). A disaccharide-repeating region of dermatan is synthesized through epimerization of a carboxyl group at C5 from GlcUA to IdoUA by DSE. A mature DS chain is synthesized through modification with sulfation by D4ST1 and UST. (**B**) Sulfotransferase activity toward dermatan in fibroblast cultures of skin from two patients with mcEDS-*CHST14* (patient 12 with heterozygous variants Pro281Leu/Tyr293Cys; patient 14 with a homozygous variant Pro281Leu), the mother of patient 12, and a sex- and age-matched healthy volunteer [6]. * $p < 0.0001$ by two-tailed unpaired *t*-test. (**C**) Total amounts of CS and DS derived from fibroblast cultures of skin [6]. Total disaccharide contents of CS (white box) and DS (black box) were calculated based on the peak area in the chromatograms of the digests with chondroitinase AC and chondroitinase B, respectively. (**D**) Proportion of the disaccharide units in the CS-DS hybrid chain in decorin-PGs secreted by the fibroblasts [6]. Cyan, green, red and orange boxes are GlcUA-GalNAc(4S), GlcUA-GalNAc(6S), IdoUA-GalNAc(4S), and IdoUA(2S)-GalNAc(4S), respectively. Abbreviations of 2S, 4S and 6S indicate 2-*O*-, 4-*O*- and 6-*O*-sulfate, respectively. (**E**) Schematic diagram of the biochemical mechanism in the replacement of DS by CS in mcEDS-*CHST14*. Defect in D4ST1 enables a back-epimerization reaction that converts IdoUA back to GlcUA to form chondroitin by DSE, followed by the 4-*O*-sulfation and/or 6-*O*-sulfation of GalNAc residues in chondroitin by C4ST1 and C6ST1, respectively. (B–D, reproduced from Miyake et al. *Hum. Mutat.* **2010**, *31*, 1233–1239, with permission from Wiley-Liss, Inc.).

Regarding patients with mcEDS-*DSE*, reduced activity of DSE in fibroblast cultures of skin from a patient with a homozygous p.(Ser268Leu) substitution resulted in marked reduction of DS disaccharides, compared with healthy controls [23]. The total amount of CS in the cell fraction from affected skin fibroblasts was increased by approximately 1.5-fold, which might reflect increased synthesis and/or reduced conversion of CS chains [23]. A minor fraction of DS from decorin-PG was present in skin fibroblasts from a patient with a homozygous p.(Ser268Leu) substitution [23]; this suggested residual DSE activity or compensation by DSE2, which might be related to milder phenotypes in patients with mcEDS-*DSE* than in patients with mcEDS-*CHST14* [18].

4. Pathological Findings

The pathology of mcEDS-*CHST14*, as the simplest model for complete depletion of DS, has been extensively investigated using affected skin specimens. Light microscopy of skin specimens (hematoxylin and eosin staining) from patients with compound heterozygous p.(Pro281Leu)/(Cys289Ser) or p.(Pro281Leu)/(Tyr293Cys) substitutions showed that fine collagen fibers were predominantly present in the reticular to papillary dermis; marked reduction of normally thick collagen bundles were also observed (Figure 4A) [6]. Immunohistochemistry staining of decorin core protein in skin specimens from patients with compound heterozygous p.(Pro281Leu)/(CYs289Ser) or p.(Pro281Leu)/(Tyr293Cys) substitutions showed that decorin core protein was present on collagen fibers that were thin and filamentous without clear boundaries; in contrast, skin specimens from healthy controls showed decorin core protein on collagen fibers that were thick bundles with clear boundaries [31] (Figure 4B). Transmission electron microscopy of skin specimens from five patients with compound heterozygous p.(Pro281Leu)/(Cys289Ser), p.(Pro281Leu)/(Tyr293Cys), or p.(Phe209Ser)/(Pro281Leu) substitutions showed that collagen fibrils were dispersed in the papillary to reticular dermis, whereas skin specimens from healthy controls exhibited collagen fibrils that were regularly and tightly assembled (Figure 4C) [6,31]. Transmission electron microscopy-based cupromeronic blue staining to visualize GAG chains on affected skin samples showed that GAG chains were linear, stretching from the outer surface of collagen fibrils to adjacent fibrils, whereas skin samples from healthy controls exhibited curved GAG chains that maintained close contact with attached collagen fibrils (Figure 4D) [31]. This structural alteration of GAG chains of decorin is presumably related to the biochemical alteration from DS to CS: the structure of DS-GAG chains is flexible because L-IdoUA residues in DS can easily adopt any of the nearly equi-energetic $^1C_4$, $^2S_0$, and $^4C_1$ conformations, whereas the structure of CS-GAG chains is rigid because D-GlcUA in CS only adopts the $^4C_1$ conformation [6,32,33].

Furthermore, focused ion beam scanning electron microscopy using cupromeronic blue staining uncovered the structure of collagen fibrils in association with GAG chains (likely comprising decorin): GAG chains form a ring mesh-like structure with each ring surrounding a collagen fibril at its D band, fusing with adjacent rings to form a planar network [34]. Abnormally stretching CS-GAG chains of decorin in the affected skin would disrupt the ring-mesh structure of collagen fibrils (Figure 4E), which could result in substantial fragility.

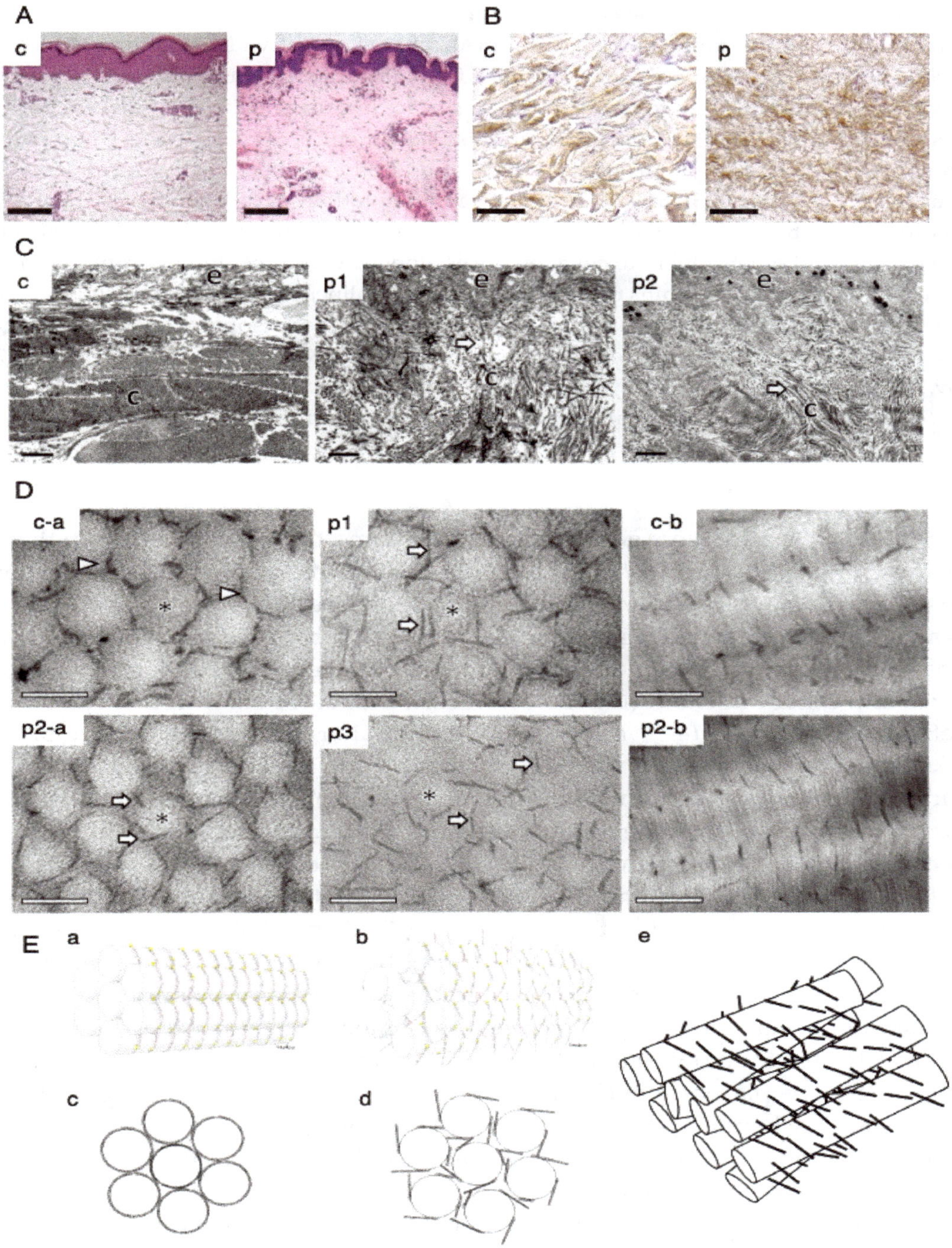

Figure 4. Skin pathology of mcEDS-*CHST14*. (**A**) Light microscopy (hematoxylin and eosin staining). In the skin specimen from a patient with heterozygous variants Pro281Leu/ Cys289Ser (panel p), fine collagen fibers are present predominantly in the reticular to papillary dermis with marked reduction of thick collagen bundles; thick collagen bundles are observed in a skin specimen from a healthy control volunteer (panel c) [6]. (**B**) Immunohistochemical staining for decorin core protein. Decorin core protein is present on collagen fibers in thick bundles in a skin specimen from a healthy control volunteer (panel c), but on thin and filamentous collagen fibers without clear boundaries in a skin specimen from a patient with heterozygous variants Pro281Leu/ Cys289Ser (panel p) [31] (**C**) Transmission electron microscopy. Collagen fibrils are regularly and tightly assembled in a skin specimen from a healthy control volunteer (panel c), but are dispersed in the papillary to reticular dermis in skin specimens from a patient with heterozygous variants Pro281Leu/ Tyr293Cys (panel p1)

and a patient with a novel homozygous variant (panel p2) [31]. (**D**) Transmission electron microscopy-based cupromeronic blue staining. GAG chains are curved and maintain close contact with attached collagen fibrils in the skin specimens from a healthy control volunteer (panels c-a, c-b); conversely, they are linear and stretch from the outer surface of collagen fibrils to adjacent fibrils in skin specimens from a patient with heterozygous variants Pro281Leu/ Tyr293Cys (panel p1), a patient with a novel homozygous variant (panels p2a and p2b) and another patient with heterozygous variants Pro281Leu/ Tyr293Cys (panel p3) [31]. (**E**) Schematic representations of collagen fibrils and GAG chains. Decorin core protein binds to D bands of collagen fibrils both in normal skin and in affected skin. GAG chains composed of DS adhere to collagen fibrils along D bands, beginning from the core protein (panels a and c), whereas GAG chains composed of CS extend linearly and perpendicularly to collagen fibrils from the core protein (panels b and d) [31]. Putative spatial disorganization of collagen fibril networks in the skin of patients (panel e) (A, reproduced from Miyake et al. *Hum. Mutat.* **2010**, *31*, 1233–1239, with permission from Wiley-Liss, Inc.; B–E, reproduced from Hirose et al. *Biochim. Biophys. Acta Gen. Subj.* **2019**, *1863*, 623–631, with permission from Elsevier, Inc.).

5. Animal Model-Based Findings

Knockout (*Chst14*$^{-/-}$) mice were generated through homologous recombination that targeted the only coding exon 1 (i.e., exon 1) of *Chst14* [35,36]. F2 mice showed reduced weight and/or length and reduced bone volume/thickness/density of their lumbar vertebrae [35]. *Chst14*$^{-/-}$ mice showed reduced neurogenesis and diminished proliferation of neural stem cells, accompanied by increased expression of glutamate aspartate transporter and epidermal growth factor, compared with findings in both wild-type (*Chst14*$^{+/+}$) mice and other knockout (*Chst11*$^{-/-}$) mice, a model for chondroitin 4-*O*-sulfotransferase 1 (C4ST1) deficiency [36]. *Chst14*$^{-/-}$ mice also had a smaller body mass (Figure 5A, B), reduced fertility, a kinked tail, and increased skin fragility compared with their wild-type (*Chst14*$^{+/+}$) littermates; however, brain weight and gross anatomy were not affected [36,37]. Schwann cells from *Chst14*$^{-/-}$ mice formed longer processes in vitro and exhibited greater proliferation than those from *Chst14*$^{+/+}$ mice. Functional recovery and axonal regrowth in *Chst14*$^{-/-}$ mice were initially accelerated after femoral nerve transection and suture; after 3 months, these characteristics were similar to those in *Chst14*$^{+/+}$ littermates. These findings suggested that DS, synthesized by Chst14/D4st1, might be of limited importance for neural development; moreover, it might contribute to the regeneration-restricting environment in the adult mammalian nervous system [38]. Only a few adult *Chst14*$^{-/-}$ mice were generated because of perinatal lethality in most of the homozygous mice; these adult *Chst14*$^{-/-}$ mice showed significantly shorter crown-rump length, compared with wild-type or heterozygous mice (Figure 5A–C) [37,38]. The placentas of *Chst14*$^{-/-}$ fetuses showed a reduced weight, alterations in the vascular structure and ischemic and/or necrotic-like changes (Figure 5D–G). Transmission electron microscopy of homozygous placentas demonstrated an abnormal capillary basement membrane structure in the placental villus, compared with wild-type or heterozygous placentas (Figure 5H–J). These findings showed that DS was essential for placental vascular development and perinatal fetal survival. In addition, DS was suggested to be related to the structure and/or function of capillary basement membranes, which constitutes an extracellular matrix [37].

C4st1, encoded by *Chst11*, transfers a sulfate group from 3′-phosphoadenosine 5′-phosphosulfates to the C4 position of GalNAc residues in chondroitin (Figure 3A). *Chst11*-mutant mice died within 6 hours of birth due to respiratory failure, severe dwarfism and chondrodysplasia (i.e., abnormalities in the cartilage growth plate and chondrocyte columns) [39]. Furthermore, marked reductions in the content and 4-*O*-sulfation of CS, as well as the downregulation of bone morphogenetic protein signaling and upregulation of transforming growth factor-β, have also been observed in *Chst11*-mutant mice. These findings suggest that Chst11/C4st1 and the 4-*O*-sulfation of CS chains are essential for early development and for bone morphogenetic protein and transforming growth factor-β in signaling pathways in cartilage. When considered in the context of *Chst14*$^{-/-}$ mouse phenotypes, the above findings suggest that 4-*O*-sulfation is required for the maturation of both CS and DS; moreover, CS and

DS exert distinct functions in the development of cartilage and skin, respectively. However, the DS content in *Chst11*-mutant mice remains to be elucidated [39].

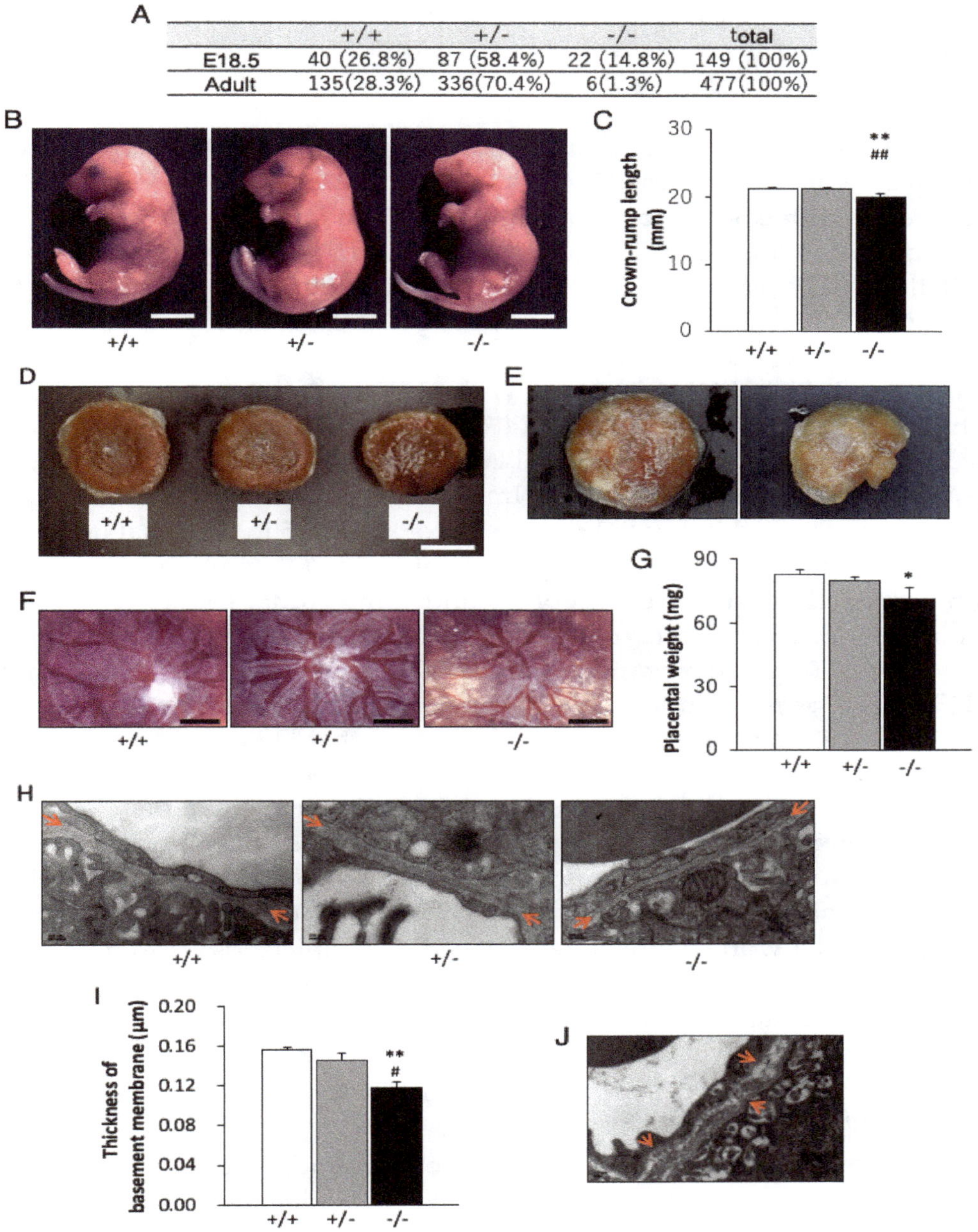

Figure 5. Mouse model for mcEDS-*CHST14*. (**A**) Numbers (percentages) of each type at embryonic (E18.5) and postnatal (adult) ages. Markedly greater numbers of homozygous fetuses are observed, compared with homozygous adults. (**B**) General appearances of wild-type (*Chst14*$^{+/+}$), heterozygous (*Chst14*$^{+/-}$) and homozygous (*Chst14*$^{-/-}$) fetuses [37]. (**C**) Crown-rump length of each type of fetus (bar: 5 mm). Homozygous mice demonstrate significantly shorter crown-rump length, compared with wild-type or heterozygous mice [37]. (**D**) Appearance of each type of placenta (bar: 5 mm) [37]. (**E**) Homozygous placentas exhibit appearances indicative of hypoxia (left) and necrosis (right) [37]. (**F**) Microphotographs of the chorionic plate side of the placentas (bar: 1 mm). Homozygous placentas demonstrate smaller vascular diameters, compared with wild-type or heterozygous placentas [37]. (**G**) Weight of each type of placenta (mean + standard error of the mean). (**H**) Transmission electron microscopy of capillary basement membrane in the labyrinth zone of each type of placenta (bar: 200 nm). Arrows indicate capillary basement membrane [37]. (**I**) Homozygous placentas show a significantly

thinner capillary basement membrane, compared with wild-type or heterozygous placentas [37]. (J) Homozygous placentas show structural abnormalities (arrows) in capillary basement membrane (bar: 0.2 μm) [37]. * $p < 0.05$, ** $p < 0.01$, compared with wild-type; # $p < 0.05$, ## $p < 0.01$, compared with heterozygous; one-way analysis of variance (ANOVA) followed by the Tukey–Kramer post hoc test. (A–J, reproduced from Yoshizawa et al. *Glycobiology* **2018**, *28*, 80–89, with permission from Oxford University Press, Inc.).

Biosynthesis of DS requires D4st1, dermatan sulfate epimerase 1 (DS-epi1) and dermatan sulfate epimerase 2 (DS-epi2), which are encoded by *Chst14*, *Dse* and *Dsel*, respectively [40–43]. Furthermore, D4ST1 interacts directly with DS-epi1, but not with DS-epi2, to form a hetero-complex that is required for the formation of IdoUA blocks in DS chains [44]. *DS-epi1*$^{-/-}$ mice showed greater skin fragility compared with wild-type littermates, due to altered collagen fibril morphology [45]; this phenotype was similar to that of *Chst14*$^{-/-}$ mice [38]. The numbers of IdoUA blocks were dramatically reduced in DS side chains of decorin-PG and biglycan-PG from the skin of *DS-epi1*$^{-/-}$ mice [45], which suggests that DS-epi1 mainly synthesizes IdoUA blocks in vivo. *DS-epi1*$^{-/-}$ embryos and newborn mice showed kinked tails, which is a common feature in *Chst14*$^{-/-}$ mice [38]; the *DS-epi1*$^{-/-}$ embryos and newborn mice also showed significantly thicker epidermal layers through histological staining, compared with heterozygous or wild-type littermates [45,46]. Immunohistochemical staining of epidermal layers in *DS-epi1*$^{-/-}$ newborns showed increased expression of keratin 5 in the basal layer and keratin 1 in the spinous layer [46]. Furthermore, a small portion of *DS-epi1*$^{-/-}$ embryos showed an abdominal wall defect with herniated intestines, exencephaly and spina bifida. Defective collagen structure in the dermis and imbalanced keratocyte maturation were presumed to cause developmental defects in *DS-epi1*$^{-/-}$ mice [46]. These observations indicate that *DS-epi1*$^{-/-}$ mice may constitute a useful model of mcEDS-*DSE*. *DS-epi2*$^{-/-}$ mice displayed no significant defects and DS-epi1 compensated for the absence of DS-epi2 in most tissue, which indicated that DS-epi1 is the major contributor of epimerase activity [47]. DS-epi2 exhibits higher expression than DS-epi1 in developing the mouse brain [48]. Although CS/DS chains in the brains of *DS-epi2*$^{-/-}$ newborn mice demonstrated a 38% reduction in IdoUA content, compared with wild-type littermates, the brains of adult knockout mice showed normal extracellular matrix features [47]. *DS-epi1*$^{-/-}$/*DS-epi2*$^{-/-}$ mice experienced perinatal death with variable phenotypes at late embryological stages and birth; these phenotypes included umbilical hernia, exencephaly, and a kinked tail, as well as complete loss of IdoUA residues in CS/DS chains [49]. However, a minority of embryos exhibited normal lung, bone, and cartilage features.

These findings indicate that DS, DS-PGs, DS-epi1 and/or DS-epi2 are important in early embryonic development and perinatal survival [49].

6. Ongoing Projects and Future Perspectives

Our group established a multicenter collaboration network to promote comprehensive basic research on mcEDS. In this network, genetic testing is provided as part of routine medical care covered by national health insurance, using a custom next generation sequencing-based panel that includes all EDS-related genes and genes for hereditary connective tissue disorders [50]. Whole exome sequencing is performed to identify other potential causative genes for mcEDS in patients with similar features who do not exhibit pathogenic variants in *CHST14* or *DSE*. Biochemical abnormalities of the extracellular matrix are investigated (e.g., various types of collagen and DS-PGs, including decorin and biglycan), using patient skin fibroblasts. Furthermore, mass spectrometry is performed to identify appropriate serum/plasma biomarker(s) that may be useful in the diagnosis or surveillance of disease progression. A subsequent pathological approach includes an elucidation of the structural alterations of collagen fibril networks and GAG chains of decorin in skin specimens from patients with mcEDS-*DSE*. Determination of the crystal structure of D4ST1 would be useful for understanding the effects of common missense variants (e.g., p.(Pro281Leu)) in *CHST14*. A technical breakthrough in the efficient generation of knockout mice for *Chst14* (e.g., CRISPR/cas9) is needed to continue mouse-based phenotypic and pathophysiological investigations. Considering the differences in the phenotypes between patients with mcEDS and *Chst14*$^{-/-}$ or *DS-epi1*$^{-/-}$ mice, experiments using other models that could reflect phenotypic and pathophysiological abnormalities in patients with mcEDS, such as induced pluripotent stem cells, would be particularly useful. All of these approaches will be valuable for further elucidating the critical roles of DS and DS-PGs, including decorin and biglycan, in the multisystem development and maintenance of connective tissues; in addition, they provide fundamental evidence for future etiology-based therapies, such as adeno-associated virus-based gene therapy.

Acknowledgments: We thank all the collaborators engaged in this project. We are also grateful to the patients and their families for participating in the studies described here. We thank Ryan Chastain-Gross, from Edanz Group (www.edanzediting.com/ac) for editing a draft of this manuscript. The drafting and revision of this review was supported by the Practical Research Project for Rare/Intractable Diseases #105 from the Japan Agency for Medical Research Development (AMED) (T.K., S.M., T.Y., N.M., and S.Y.); Grant-in-Aid for Young Scientists (B) (16K19396) (T.Y.); Grant-in-Aid for Scientific Research (C) from the Ministry of Education, Culture, Sports, Science and Technology of Japan (#16K08251, #19K07054) (S.M.) (#19K08745) (T.Y.); Grant-in-Aid for Scientific Research (B) from the Ministry of Education, Culture, Sports, Science and Technology of Japan (#19H03616) (T.K., S.M., T.W., T.Y., N.M., and S.Y.); Grant-in Aid for Research Center for Pathogenesis of Intractable Diseases from the Research Institute of Meijo University (S.M. and S.Y.).

References

1. Kosho, T. *CHST14/D4ST1* deficiency: New form of Ehlers-Danlos syndrome. *Pediatr. Int.* **2016**, *58*, 88–99. [CrossRef]
2. Brady, A.F.; Demirdas, S.; Fournel-Gigleux, S.; Ghali, N.; Giunta, C.; Kapferer-Seebacher, I.; Kosho, T.; Mendoza-Londono, R.; Pope, M.F.; Rohrbach, M.; et al. The Ehlers-Danlos syndromes, rare types. *Am. J. Med. Genet. C Semin. Med. Genet.* **2017**, *175*, 70–115. [CrossRef] [PubMed]
3. Malfait, F.; Francomano, C.; Byers, P.; Belmont, J.; Berglund, B.; Black, J.; Bloom, L.; Bowen, J.M.; Brady, A.F.; Burrows, N.P.; et al. The 2017 international classification of the Ehlers-Danlos syndromes. *Am. J. Med. Genet. C Semin. Med. Genet.* **2017**, *175*, 8–26. [CrossRef] [PubMed]
4. Dündar, M.; Müller, T.; Zhang, Q.; Pan, J.; Steinmann, B.; Vodopiutz, J.; Gruber, R.; Sonoda, T.; Krabichler, B.; Utermann, G.; et al. Loss of dermatan-4-sulfotransferase 1 function results in adducted thumb-clubfoot syndrome. *Am. J. Hum. Genet.* **2009**, *85*, 873–882. [CrossRef] [PubMed]
5. Kosho, T.; Miyake, N.; Hatamochi, A.; Takahashi, J.; Kato, H.; Miyahara, T.; Igawa, Y.; Yasui, H.; Ishida, T.; Ono, K.; et al. A new Ehlers-Danlos syndrome with craniofacial characteristics, multiple congenital contractures, progressive joint and skin laxity, and multisystem fragility-related manifestations. *Am. J. Med. Genet. Part A* **2010**, *152A*, 1333–1346. [CrossRef] [PubMed]
6. Miyake, N.; Kosho, T.; Mizumoto, S.; Furuichi, T.; Hatamochi, A.; Nagashima, Y.; Arai, E.; Takahashi, K.; Kawamura, R.; Wakui, K.; et al. Loss-of-function mutations of *CHST14* in a new type of Ehlers-Danlos syndrome. *Hum. Mutat.* **2010**, *31*, 966–974. [CrossRef] [PubMed]
7. Malfait, F.; Syx, D.; Vlummens, P.; Symoens, S.; Nampoothiri, S.; Hermanns-Lê, T.; Van Laer, L.; De Paepe, A. Musculocontractural Ehlers-Danlos syndrome (former EDS type VIB) and adducted thumb clubfoot syndrome (ATCS) represent a single clinical entity caused by mutations in the dermatan-4-sulfotransferase 1 encoding *CHST14* gene. *Hum. Mutat.* **2010**, *31*, 1233–1239. [CrossRef] [PubMed]
8. Dündar, M.; Demiryilmaz, F.; Demiryilmaz, I.; Kumandas, S.; Erkilic, K.; Kendirch, M.; Tuncel, M.; Ozyazgan, I.; Tolmie, J.L. An autosomal recessive adducted thumb-club foot syndrome observed in Turkish cousins. *Clin. Genet.* **1997**, *51*, 61–64. [CrossRef]
9. Sonoda, T.; Kouno, K. Two brothers with distal arthrogryposis, peculiar facial appearance, cleft palate, short stature, hydronephrosis, retentio testis, and normal intelligence: A new type of distal arthrogryposis? *Am. J. Med. Genet.* **2000**, *91*, 280–285. [CrossRef]
10. Dündar, M.; Kurtoglu, S.; Elmas, B.; Demiryilmaz, F.; Candemir, Z.; Ozkul, Y.; Durak, A.C. A case with adducted thumb and club foot syndrome. *Clin. Dysmorphol.* **2001**, *10*, 291–293. [CrossRef]
11. Janecke, A.R.; Unsinn, K.; Kreczy, A.; Baldissera, I.; Gassner, I.; Neu, N.; Utermann, G.; Müller, T. Adducted thumb-club foot syndrome in sibs of a consanguineous Austrian family. *J. Med. Genet.* **2001**, *38*, 265–269. [CrossRef] [PubMed]

12. Yasui, H.; Adachi, Y.; Minami, T.; Ishida, T.; Kato, Y.; Imai, K. Combination therapy of DDAVP and conjugated estrogens for a recurrent large subcutaneous hematoma in Ehlers-Danlos syndrome. *Am. J. Hematol.* **2003**, *72*, 71–72. [CrossRef] [PubMed]
13. Kosho, T.; Takahashi, J.; Ohashi, H.; Nishimura, G.; Kato, H.; Fukushima, Y. Ehlers-Danlos syndrome type VIB with characteristic facies, decreased curvatures of the spinal column, and joint contractures in two unrelated girls. *Am. J. Med. Genet. Part A* **2005**, *138A*, 282–287. [CrossRef] [PubMed]
14. Shimizu, K.; Okamoto, N.; Miyake, N.; Taira, K.; Sato, Y.; Matsuda, K.; Akimaru, N.; Ohashi, H.; Wakui, K.; Fukushima, Y.; et al. Delineation of dermatan 4-O-sulfotransferase 1 deficient Ehlers-Danlos syndrome: Observation of two additional patients and comprehensive review of 20 reported patients. *Am. J. Med. Genet. A* **2011**, *155A*, 1949–1958. [CrossRef]
15. Mendoza-Londono, R.; Chitayat, D.; Kahr, W.H.; Hinek, A.; Blaser, S.; Dupuis, L.; Goh, E.; Badilla-Porras, R.; Howard, A.; Mittaz, L.; et al. Extracellular matrix and platelet function in patients with musculocontractural Ehlers-Danlos syndrome caused by mutations in the *CHST14* gene. *Am. J. Med. Genet. A* **2012**, *158A*, 1344–1354. [CrossRef]
16. Voermans, N.C.; Kempers, M.; Lammens, M.; van Alfen, N.; Janssen, M.C.; Bönnemann, C.; van Engelen, B.G.; Hamel, B.C. Myopathy in a 20-year-old female patient with D4ST-1 deficient Ehlers-Danlos syndrome due to a homozygous *CHST14* mutation. *Am. J. Med. Genet. A* **2012**, *158A*, 850–855. [CrossRef]
17. Winters, K.A.; Jiang, Z.; Xu, W.; Li, S.; Ammous, Z.; Jayakar, P.; Wierenga, K.J. Re-assigned diagnosis of D4ST1-deficient Ehlers-Danlos syndrome (adducted thumb-clubfoot syndrome) after initial diagnosis of Marden-Walker syndrome. *Am. J. Med. Genet. A* **2012**, *158A*, 2935–2940. [CrossRef]
18. Syx, D.; Van Damme, T.; Symoens, S.; Maiburg, M.C.; van de Laar, I.; Morton, J.; Suri, M.; Del Campo, M.; Hausser, I.; Hermanns-Lê, T.; et al. Genetic heterogeneity and clinical variability in musculocontractural Ehlers-Danlos syndrome caused by impaired dermatan sulfate biosynthesis. *Hum. Mutat.* **2015**, *36*, 535–547. [CrossRef]
19. Janecke, A.R.; Li, B.; Boehm, M.; Krabichler, B.; Rohrbach, M.; Müller, T.; Fuchs, I.; Golas, G.; Katagiri, Y.; Ziegler, S.G.; et al. The phenotype of the musculocontractural type of Ehlers-Danlos syndrome due to *CHST14* mutations. *Am. J. Med. Genet. A* **2016**, *170A*, 103–115. [CrossRef]
20. Kono, M.; Hasegawa-Murakami, Y.; Sugiura, K.; Ono, M.; Toriyama, K.; Miyake, N.; Hatamochi, A.; Kamei, Y.; Kosho, T.; Akiyama, M. A 45-year-old woman with Ehlers-Danlos syndrome caused by dermatan 4-O-sulfotransferase-1 deficiency: Implications for early ageing. *Acta Derm. Venereol.* **2016**, *96*, 830–831. [CrossRef]
21. Mochida, K.; Amano, M.; Miyake, N.; Matsumoto, N.; Hatamochi, A.; Kosho, T. Dermatan 4-O-sulfotransferase 1-deficient Ehlers-Danlos syndrome complicated by a large subcutaneous hematoma on the back. *J. Dermatol.* **2016**, *43*, 832–833. [CrossRef] [PubMed]
22. Sandal, S.; Kaur, A.; Panigrahi, I. Novel mutation in the *CHST14* gene causing musculocontractural type of Ehlers-Danlos syndrome. *BMJ Case Rep.* **2018**, *pii*, bcr-2018-226165. [CrossRef] [PubMed]
23. Müller, T.; Mizumoto, S.; Suresh, I.; Komatsu, Y.; Vodopiutz, J.; Dundar, M.; Straub, V.; Lingenhel, A.; Melmer, A.; Lechner, S.; et al. Loss of dermatan sulfate epimerase (DSE) function results in musculocontractural Ehlers-Danlos syndrome. *Hum. Mol. Genet.* **2013**, *22*, 3761–3772. [CrossRef] [PubMed]
24. Schirwani, S.; Metcalfe, K.; Wagner, B.; Berry, I.; Sobey, G.; Jewell, R. DSE associated musculocontractural EDS, a milder phenotype or phenotypic variability. *Eur. J. Med. Genet.* **2019**. [CrossRef] [PubMed]
25. Alazami, A.M.; Al-Qattan, S.M.; Faqeih, E.; Alhashem, A.; Alshammari, M.; Alzahrani, F.; Al-Dosari, M.S.; Patel, N.; Alsagheir, A.; Binabbas, B.; et al. Expanding the clinical and genetic heterogeneity of hereditary disorders of connective tissue. *Hum. Genet.* **2016**, *135*, 525–540. [CrossRef] [PubMed]
26. Maddirevula, S.; Alsahli, S.; Alhabeeb, L.; Patel, N.; Alzahrani, F.; Shamseldin, H.E.; Anazi, S.; Ewida, N.; Alsaif, H.S.; Mohamed, J.Y.; et al. Expanding the phenome and variome of skeletal dysplasia. *Genet. Med.* **2018**, *20*, 1609–1616. [CrossRef]
27. Ranza, E.; Huber, C.; Levin, N.; Baujat, G.; Bole-Feysot, C.; Nitschke, P.; Masson, C.; Alanay, Y.; Al-Gazali, L.; Bitoun, P.; et al. Chondrodysplasia with multiple dislocations: Comprehensive study of a series of 30 cases. *Clin. Genet.* **2017**, *91*, 868–880. [CrossRef]
28. Nomura, Y. Structural change in decorin with skin aging. *Connect Tissue Res.* **2006**, *47*, 249–255. [CrossRef]

29. Malmström, A. Biosynthesis of dermatan sulfate. II. Substrate specificity of the C-5 uronosyl epimerase. *J. Biol. Chem.* **1984**, *259*, 161–165.
30. Mizumoto, S.; Kosho, T.; Hatamochi, A.; Honda, T.; Yamaguchi, T.; Okamoto, N.; Miyake, N.; Yamada, S.; Sugahara, K. Defect in dermatan sulfate in urine of patients with Ehlers-Danlos syndrome caused by a *CHST14/D4ST1* deficiency. *Clin. Biochem.* **2017**, *50*, 670–677. [CrossRef]
31. Hirose, T.; Takahashi, N.; Tangkawattana, P.; Minaguchi, J.; Mizumoto, S.; Yamada, S.; Miyake, N.; Hayashi, S.; Hatamochi, A.; Nakayama, J.; et al. Structural alteration of glycosaminoglycan side chains and spatial disorganization of collagen networks in the skin of patients with mcEDS-*CHST14*. *Biochim. Biophys. Acta Gen. Subj.* **2019**, *1863*, 623–631. [CrossRef] [PubMed]
32. Casu, B.; Petitou, M.; Provasoli, M.; Sinaÿ, P. Conformational flexibility: A new concept for explaining binding and biological properties of iduronic acid-containing glycosaminoglycans. *Trends Biochem. Sci.* **1988**, *13*, 221–225. [CrossRef]
33. Catlow, K.R.; Deakin, J.A.; Wei, Z.; Delehedde, M.; Femig, D.G.; Gherardi, E.; Gallagher, J.T.; Pavão, M.S.G.; Lyon, M. Interactions of hepatocyte growth factor/scatter factor with various glycosaminoglycans reveal an important interplay between the presence of iduronate and sulfate density. *J. Biol. Chem.* **2008**, *283*, 5235–5248. [CrossRef] [PubMed]
34. Watanabe, T.; Kametani, K.; Koyama, Y.I.; Suzuki, D.; Imamura, Y.; Takehana, K.; Hiramatsu, K. Ring-mesh model of proteoglycan glycosaminoglycan chains in tendon based on three-dimensional reconstruction by focused ion beam scanning electron microscopy. *J. Biol. Chem.* **2016**, *291*, 23704–23708. [CrossRef] [PubMed]
35. Tang, T.; Li, L.; Tang, J.; Li, Y.; Lin, W.Y.; Martin, F.; Grant, D.; Solloway, M.; Parker, L.; Ye, W.; et al. A mouse knockout library for secreted and transmembrane proteins. *Nat. Biotechnol.* **2010**, *28*, 749–755. [CrossRef] [PubMed]
36. Bian, S.; Akyüz, N.; Bernreuther, C.; Loers, G.; Laczynska, E.; Jakovcevski, I.; Schachner, M. Dermatan sulfotransferase Chst14/D4st1, but not chondroitin sulfotransferase Chst11/C4st1, regulates proliferation and neurogenesis of neural progenitor cells. *J. Cell Sci.* **2011**, *124*, 4051–4063. [CrossRef]
37. Yoshizawa, T.; Mizumoto, S.; Takahashi, Y.; Shimada, S.; Sugahara, K.; Nakayama, J.; Takeda, S.; Nomura, Y.; Nitahara-Kasahara, Y.; Okada, T.; et al. Vascular abnormalities in the placenta of *Chst14*$^{-/-}$ fetuses: Implications in the pathophysiology of perinatal lethality of the murine model and vascular lesions in human *CHST14/D4ST1* deficiency. *Glycobiology* **2018**, *28*, 80–89. [CrossRef]
38. Akyüz, N.; Rost, S.; Mehanna, A.; Bian, S.; Loers, G.; Oezen, I.; Mishra, B.; Hoffmann, K.; Guseva, D.; Laczynska, E.; et al. Dermatan 4-*O*-sulfotransferase1 ablation accelerates peripheral nerve regeneration. *Exp. Neurol.* **2013**, *247*, 517–530. [CrossRef]
39. Klüppel, M.; Wight, T.N.; Chan, C.; Hinek, A.; Wrana, J.L. Maintenance of chondroitin sulfation balance by chondroitin-4-sulfotransferase 1 is required for chondrocyte development and growth factor signaling during cartilage morphogenesis. *Development* **2005**, *132*, 3989–4003. [CrossRef]
40. Evers, M.R.; Xia, G.; Kang, H.G.; Schachner, M.; Baenziger, J.U. Molecular cloning and characterization of a dermatan-specific *N*-acetylgalactosamine 4-*O*-sulfotransferase. *J. Biol. Chem.* **2001**, *276*, 36344–36353. [CrossRef]
41. Mikami, T.; Mizumoto, S.; Kago, N.; Kitagawa, H.; Sugahara, K. Specificities of three distinct human chondroitin/dermatan *N*-acetylgalactosamine 4-*O*-sulfotransferases demonstrated using partially desulfated dermatan sulfate as an acceptor: Implication of differential roles in dermatan sulfate biosynthesis. *J. Biol. Chem.* **2003**, *278*, 36115–36127. [CrossRef] [PubMed]
42. Maccarana, M.; Olander, B.; Malmström, J.; Tiedemann, K.; Aebersold, R.; Lindahl, U.; Li, J.P.; Malmström, A. Biosynthesis of dermatan sulfate: Chondroitin-glucuronate C5-epimerase is identical to SART2. *J. Biol. Chem.* **2006**, *281*, 11560–11568. [CrossRef] [PubMed]
43. Pacheco, B.; Malmström, A.; Maccarana, M. Two dermatan sulfate epimerases form iduronic acid domains in dermatan sulfate. *J. Biol. Chem.* **2009**, *284*, 9788–9795. [CrossRef] [PubMed]
44. Tykesson, E.; Hassinen, A.; Zielinska, K.; Thelin, M.A.; Frati, G.; Ellervik, U.; Westergren-Thorsson, G.; Malmström, A.; Kellokumpu, S.; Maccarana, M. Dermatan sulfate epimerase 1 and dermatan 4-*O*-sulfotransferase 1 form complexes that generate long epimerized 4-*O*-sulfated blocks. *J. Biol. Chem.* **2018**, *293*, 13725–13735. [CrossRef]

45. Maccarana, M.; Kalamajski, S.; Kongsgaard, M.; Magnusson, S.P.; Oldberg, A.; Malmström, A. Dermatan sulfate epimerase 1-deficient mice have reduced content and changed distribution of iduronic acids in dermatan sulfate and an altered collagen structure in skin. *Mol. Cell Biol.* **2009**, *29*, 5517–5528. [CrossRef]
46. Gustafsson, R.; Stachtea, X.; Maccarana, M.; Grottling, E.; Eklund, E.; Malmström, A.; Oldberg, A. Dermatan sulfate epimerase 1 deficient mice as a model for human abdominal wall defects. *Birth Defects Res. A Clin. Mol. Teratol.* **2014**, *100*, 712–720. [CrossRef]
47. Bartolini, B.; Thelin, M.A.; Rauch, U.; Feinstein, R.; Oldberg, A.; Malmström, A.; Maccarana, M. Mouse development is not obviously affected by the absence of dermatan sulfate epimerase 2 in spite of a modified brain dermatan sulfate composition. *Glycobiology* **2012**, *22*, 1007–1016. [CrossRef]
48. Akatsu, C.; Mizumoto, S.; Kaneiwa, T.; Maccarana, M.; Malmström, A.; Yamada, S.; Sugahara, K. Dermatan sulfate epimerase 2 is the predominant isozyme in the formation of the chondroitin sulfate/dermatan sulfate hybrid structure in postnatal developing mouse brain. *Glycobiology* **2011**, *21*, 565–574. [CrossRef]
49. Stachtea, X.N.; Tykesson, E.; van Kuppevelt, T.H.; Feinstein, R.; Malmström, A.; Reijmers, R.M.; Maccarana, M. Dermatan sulfate-free mice display embryological defects and are neonatal lethal despite normal lymphoid and non-lymphoid organogenesis. *PLoS ONE* **2015**, *10*, e0140279. [CrossRef]
50. Koitabashi, N.; Yamaguchi, T.; Fukui, D.; Nakano, T.; Umeyama, A.; Toda, K.; Funada, R.; Ishikawa, M.; Kawamura, R.; Okada, K.; et al. Peripartum iliac arterial aneurysm and rupture in a patient with vascular Ehlers-Danlos syndrome diagnosed by next-generation sequencing. *Int. Heart J.* **2018**, *59*, 1180–1185. [CrossRef]

7

Connexins: Synthesis, Post-Translational Modifications and Trafficking in Health and Disease

Trond Aasen [1,*], Scott Johnstone [2,3,*], Laia Vidal-Brime [1], K. Sabrina Lynn [4] and Michael Koval [4,5,*]

1 Translational Molecular Pathology, Vall d'Hebron Institute of Research (VHIR), Autonomous University of Barcelona, CIBERONC, 08035 Barcelona, Spain; laia.vidal.b@gmail.com
2 Robert M. Berne Cardiovascular Research Center, University of Virginia School of Medicine, P.O. Box 801394, Charlottesville, VI 22908, USA
3 Institute of Cardiovascular and Medical Sciences, College of Medical, Veterinary and Life Sciences, University of Glasgow, Glasgow G12 8TT, UK
4 Division of Pulmonary, Allergy, Critical Care and Sleep Medicine, Department of Medicine, Emory University School of Medicine, Atlanta, GA 30322, USA; k.s.lynn@emory.edu
5 Department of Cell Biology, Emory University School of Medicine, Atlanta, GA 30322, USA
* Correspondence: trond.aasen@vhir.org (T.A.); srj6n@virginia.edu (S.J.); mhkoval@emory.edu (M.K.)

Abstract: Connexins are tetraspan transmembrane proteins that form gap junctions and facilitate direct intercellular communication, a critical feature for the development, function, and homeostasis of tissues and organs. In addition, a growing number of gap junction-independent functions are being ascribed to these proteins. The connexin gene family is under extensive regulation at the transcriptional and post-transcriptional level, and undergoes numerous modifications at the protein level, including phosphorylation, which ultimately affects their trafficking, stability, and function. Here, we summarize these key regulatory events, with emphasis on how these affect connexin multifunctionality in health and disease.

Keywords: connexins; gap junctions; transcription; translation; post-translational modifications; trafficking

1. Introduction

Since the cloning of the first connexins in the 1980s, steady progress towards elucidating their regulation and function as signaling hubs and mediators of direct intercellular communication has been made [1–3]. All connexins share a conserved four-transmembrane domain structure that assembles into hexameric pores known as connexons that can integrate into the cell membrane (Figure 1). Hundreds to thousands of these connexons typically dock with opposing connexons in an adjacent cell, creating intercellular channels forming a clustered gap junction plaque that permits direct flux of ions and small cytosolic signaling molecules between cells, commonly referred to as gap junctional intercellular communication (GJIC) (Figure 1). More recently, connexons have been shown to act as "hemichannels" to facilitate direct exchange of molecules between the cell cytosol and the extracellular milieu under specific conditions [4]. Additionally, numerous noncanonical channel-independent functions have been described, in particular for connexin 43 (Cx43), which are mediated through direct protein interactions and modulation of signaling pathways [5]. The complexity and isoform-specificity of the connexin gene family is reflected by their links to numerous human diseases, many of which are rare syndromes with unique genotype–phenotype associations [6,7]. This latter phenomenon is underscored by the observation that mutations in different connexins can cause the same disease, whereas varying mutations in one connexin gene can result in vastly divergent diseases and phenotypes. Dysregulation of connexins is also increasingly linked to many common and often morbid medical conditions—such as stroke, heart attack, and cancer—which have been linked to the discovery of an expanding number of new functional attributes through both gap junction-dependent and -independent mechanisms [2,3,6–9]. As such, exploring the clinical and therapeutic potential of connexins as drug targets is pertinent and ongoing [10–12]. Towards this, a deeper understanding of how these genes and proteins are regulated and function is essential. This review aims to summarize and underscore important and unique mechanisms that regulate connexin function in healthy and diseased states, which ultimately shed light on clinical observations and future therapeutic opportunities.

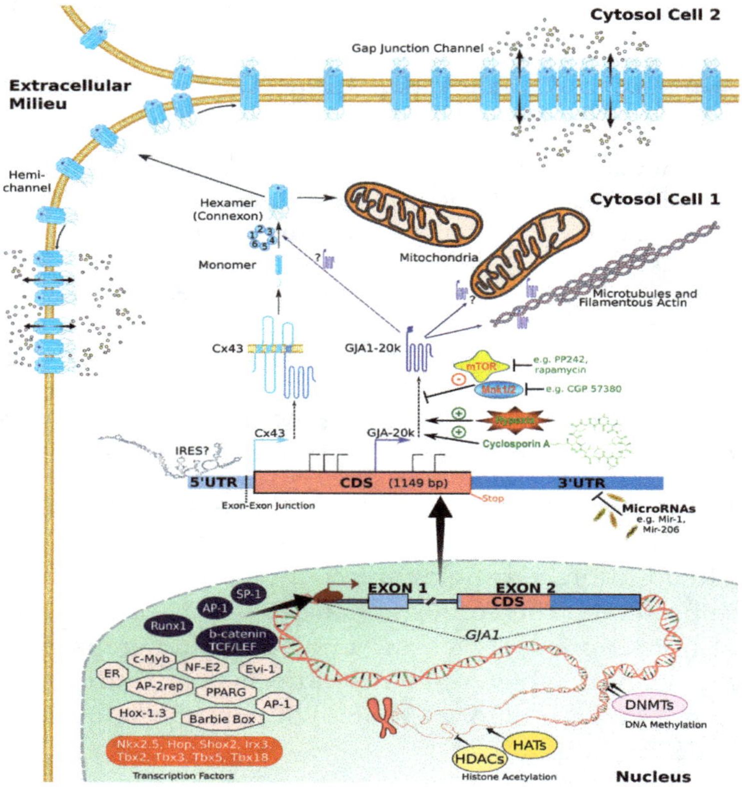

Figure 1. Connexins form hexameric connexons permeable to small molecules acting either as hemichannels or as intercellular channels. The human *GJA1* gene, encoding for connexin 43 (Cx43), contains two exons spanning a genomic region of 14,168 bp. Exon 1 contains 256 bp of the 5′ UTR (untranslated region), whereas exon 2 encompasses 16 bp of the 5′ UTR, the entire coding region (1149 bp), and the entire 3′ UTR region (1748 bp). Transcription of mRNA (3169 bp) is under regulation by numerous transcription factors as indicated in this figure and in the main text. Notably, Sp-1 and AP-1 are key regulators of Cx43 mRNA expression (grouped in blue). Multiple tissue-specific promoters are active, which has been well described in the heart (grouped in red). Additional transcription factors (grouped in light red) are derived from promoter analysis using the online Lasagna-Search tool (using a very strict cut-off of $p < 0.0001$ and Transfac transcription factor binding sites) [13]. Epigenetics regulate transcription, including through promoter hypermethylation by DNA methyltransferase enzymes (DNMTs). Acetylation by histone acetyltransferase enzymes (HATs) promote transcription, and the reverse reaction is mediated by histone deacetylases (HDACs). The transcript is also regulated by numerous microRNAs (see main text for details). In addition to full-length Cx43 (43 kilodalton (kDa)), the same mRNA can produce multiple truncated forms via internal translation initiation (indicated by arrows within the CDS (coding DNA sequence) of the mRNA, most notably the 20 kDa form named GJA1-20k). Truncated forms are also under translational regulation by a number of pathways such as mechanistic target of rapamycin (mTOR) and mitogen-activated protein kinase (MAPK)-interacting serine/threonine-protein kinase 1 (MNK1) and 2 (MNK2), and can be induced by inhibitors of these pathways as well as by other specific drugs such as cyclosporin A (the positive regulators are depicted in green). GJA1-20k is also induced by pathological states such as hypoxia. The function of GJA1-20k may include interaction with mitochondria and regulation of the actin cytoskeleton as well as regulation of Cx43 oligomerization and trafficking to the membrane. See main text for further details related to the figure.

2. Connexins: From Gene to Protein

2.1. Gene Structure and Splicing

Twenty-one human genes and 20 mouse genes encoding for connexin proteins have been identified, of which 19 are considered orthologous pairs [14,15]. The genes tend to have distinct chromosomal locations, although there are some regions of the genome containing clusters of connexin genes [14]. Most connexin genes share a common structure consisting of two exons separated by an intron of variable size. The majority of the 5′ UTR (untranslated region) is localized on exon 1, whereas the entire coding region and the 3′ UTR are found in exon 2. Some connexin genes contain more than two exons (for the 5′ UTR of the transcript), such as human *GJA5* (Cx40) [16], which contains three exons producing two distinct and tissue-specific transcripts, and *GJB6* (Cx30), described to contain six exons that allows for tissue-specific splicing [17]. Mouse connexin genes with three or more exons include *Gjb1* (Cx32) [18], *Gja1* (Cx43) [19], and *Gjc1* (Cx45) [20]. In a few cases, the coding region is also distributed over more than one exon [21–24]. A basal promoter (P1) is typically found within 300 bp upstream of the transcription initiation site of exon 1 [25]. However, splice isoforms have been reported due to alternate promoter usage, yielding different transcripts with the coding region being unaltered. As such, a deeper understanding of connexin gene structure, promoter usage, and splicing pattern is required for a full understanding of their impact in connexin-related diseases. For example, the human *GJB1* gene encoding Cx32 contains at least three exons (E1, E1B, and the coding exon E2) and produces two different alternatively spliced transcripts by using two tissue-specific promoters (P1 and P2) [26]. It is thus pertinent to include this region in mutational screening of dominant X-linked Charcot-Marie-Tooth (CMTX1) disease, a type of neuropathy that can be caused by mutations in Cx32 leading to defects in Schwann cell function, at least in cases where no mutations are found in the Cx32 coding region. Indeed, recent studies have identified mutations affecting *GJB1* splicing [27], and even deletion of the *GJB1* P2 promoter [28], as underlying causes of CMTX1. Others have shown that splicing mutations in *GJC2* encoding Cx47 can cause a severe form of Pelizaeus-Merzbacher-like disease [29]. Another splice-site mutation, in *GJB2* encoding Cx26, has been suggested to cause a mild postlingual onset form of hearing loss [30].

In addition to these more well-described biological phenomena, a few connexin pseudogenes (genes thought to originate from decay of genes that stems from duplication through evolution) have been identified in the human genome. The *GJA1* pseudogene (GJA1P) is located on human chromosome 5, whereas the regular *GJA1* gene encoding for Cx43 is located on chromosome 6. Although most pseudogenes are thought to be nonfunctional, GJA1P appears to be transcribed, possibly even translated, and may regulate tumor growth [31,32]. Mutations in GJA1P have also been associated with nonsyndromic deafness [33]. Functionally, GJA1P may influence *GJA1* expression levels by acting as a microRNA sponge [34]. In contrast, GJA6P seems to be a nonfunctional pseudogene, originated from the mouse *Gja6* connexin gene encoding Cx33, which has no human counterpart (Gene ID: 100126825). Another potential pseudogene has been inferred for *GJA4* (Gene ID: 100421028) encoding Cx37. The role of pseudogenes in disease is an emerging field, particularly among genes causing multiple different diseases or syndromic diseases, such as connexins.

2.2. Transcription Factors and Epigenetics

Connexins are expressed distinctively in almost all vertebrate cell types (excluding erythrocytes, mature sperm cells, and differentiated skeletal muscle cells) [35]. Some connexins (notably Cx43) are expressed in numerous cell types, whereas others show a more restricted expression profile (e.g., Cx50 that is mainly found in lens cells). Most tissues express multiple connexins. The epidermis of the skin, for example, is thought to express at least 10 different connexins whose expression partially overlap during keratinocyte stratification and differentiation [36–38]. Five of these connexins underlie 11 clinically different cutaneous disorders [37,39]. This spatiotemporal expression pattern is in large part controlled by transcription factors and epigenetic mechanisms. Several transcription factors acting as regulators of basal (ubiquitous) or cell-specific gene activity, and their upstream signal transduction pathways, have been implicated in the control of connexin expression (Figure 1). Notably, specificity protein 1 (Sp1), an important basal transcription factor that binds to GC box sequences in promoter regions, has been reported to favor transcriptional initiation of several connexin genes, including Cx26 [40], Cx32 [41,42], Cx40 [16,43–47], and Cx43 [45,48–53]. Examples of other important regulators that control connexin gene expression include: (i) Activator protein 1 (AP1) transcription factor, composed of proteins belonging to the c-Fos, c-Jun, activating transcription factor (ATF), and J domain containing protein(JDP) families that typically promote positive regulation. AP-1 sites have mainly been described in Cx43 [48,54,55], whereas putative sites have been identified in the Cx45 promoter [56]. (ii) The Wnt pathway: activation of this pathway leads to the formation of nuclear β catenin/TCF (T-cell factor) complexes that act as transcription factors by binding to specific TCF/LEF (lymphoid enhancer-binding factor) motifs present in the promoter of human *GJA1* and mouse *Gja1* encoding Cx43 [57]. From a physiological and disease point of view, this may also be relevant. For example, one study showed Wnt signaling could modulate Cx43-dependent GJIC in the heart, which ultimately may contribute to altered impulse propagation and arrhythmia in the myopathic heart [58]. The importance of GJIC in the heart is well documented and several cell-specific transcription factors have been shown to either activate or repress connexin gene expression in this setting (Figure 1 (red box), reviewed in [25,59]). These studies have revealed a role of: (i) homeobox proteins, transcription factors with a unique DNA-binding domain that target gene promoter sequences by self-complementarity (e.g., Nkx2.5, Hop, Shox2, Irx3); (ii) T-box (Tbx) proteins, transcription factors that possess a domain that recognizes a DNA binding element (e.g., Tbx2, Tbx3, Tbx5, Tbx18); and (iii) GATA proteins, important regulators of specific gene expression in different tissue (e.g., GATA-4) [25,59].

Besides the well-described transcriptional regulation of the cardiac connexins, other cases of tissue-specific regulation have been reported (for an overview, see [25]). Cx32 transcription has been found to be positively regulated by hepatocyte nuclear factor-1 (HNF-1) via Sp1 in liver cells [60], by the transcription factor Mist1 in secretory pancreatic acinar cells [61], and by the Sox10 in synergy with the early growth response-2 gene (Egr2) in Schwann cells [62]. This exemplifies how different transcription factors act in a tissue-dependent fashion. Complex transcriptional control thus allows for tissue-specific regulation of connexin expression. It also facilitates rapid response to environmental changes, for example, progesterone and estrogen act as positive and negative regulators, respectively, of Cx43 transcription in the myometrium during pregnancy and labor [63]. Transcription factors are also important during pathological states, such as in ischemia, where multiple connexins are emerging as important injury response mediators. Their roles in complex disease, such as cancer, are also being unraveled. In breast cancer, for example, Cx43 has been proposed to play a biphasic role acting both as a tumor promotor and a tumor suppressor depending on context such as cancer subtype and stage [3]. In this setting, the aforementioned role of progesterone and estrogen as regulators of Cx43 expression may be of importance. Recent evidence also suggests that the transcription factor FOXP3 directly binds to and inhibits RUNX1 in mammary epithelial cells, whereas in the absence of FOXP3 in breast tumors, RUNX1 downregulates Cx43 expression [64]. Understanding the role of transcription factors will provide further insight into loss and overexpression of connexins during tumor progression and other pathological states.

Connexin expression is also under significant epigenetic regulation (for recent extensive reviews see [25,65]). Two major epigenetic mechanisms have been described to regulate transcriptional control: DNA methylation and histone acetylation. Connexin gene inactivation due to hypermethylation of CpG islands in the promoter region has been described in various human carcinomas, including Cx26 in lung [66] and breast [67], Cx32 in a renal cell carcinoma cell line [68], and Cx43 in breast cancer [69]. In addition, a gradual decrease in Cx32 and Cx43 mRNA expression levels is associated with promoter hypermethylation in *Helicobacter pylori*-associated gastric tumorigenesis [70]. Transcriptional silencing via promoter hypermethylation is mediated by the enzyme DNA methyltransferase (DNMT). The use of demethylating drugs (DNMTs inhibitors), such as 5-aza-2-deoxycytidine and 5-azacytidine, has been proposed as a potential therapeutic solution in cancer, as an increase connexin expression and/or GJIC has been demonstrated in specific cases [68,71,72]. However, the correlation between hypermethylation and gene expression is not always direct and differs between connexin isoforms [72].

Histone acetylation and deacetylation—causing chromatin decondensation and condensation, respectively—constitute other important mechanisms of epigenetic regulation of connexin transcription [25,65]. While acetylation is catalyzed by histone acetyltransferase (HAT) enzymes and promotes transcription, the reverse reaction is mediated by histone deacetylase (HDAC) enzymes. Histone acetylation also affects connexin expression, and inhibitors of HDAC enzymes (HDACi)—such as trichostatin A, sodium butyrate, and 4-phenylbutarate—have been shown to enhance connexin and GJIC in a variety of cell populations, including in cancer cells [73], in which therapeutic and preventive roles for specific HDACi have been proposed. Histone deacetylase inhibition has also been shown to reduce Cx43 expression and gap junction communication in cardiac cells [74], which has implications with regards to potential side effects such as slow ventricular conduction or arrhythmias. Therefore, the action of HDACi seems to be connexin- and cell type-dependent. Curiously, Cx43 has been shown to influence histone acetylation of other genes; in a human pulmonary giant cell carcinoma cell line, the follistatin-like 1 (FSTL1) promoter was shown to be associated with acetylated histones H3 and H4 upon Cx43 transfection. Cx43 was proposed to act as a "histone deacetylase inhibitor" that modulates gene expression and inhibits tumor invasion [75].

The potential therapeutic role of epigenetic regulations has broad interest, particularly in complex diseases such as cancer, as exemplified above. However, the nonspecific nature of this gene regulatory mode complicates more direct and specific therapeutic targeting. Moreover, research is needed to determine if connexin levels are mainly mediated via HDACi histone modification [73,76], via non-histone protein modification of transcription factors, or via direct or indirect connexin protein modification such as Cx43 acetylation or phosphorylation [77–79].

2.3. *RNA Stability and MicroRNAs*

MicroRNAs (miRNAs) are short single-stranded noncoding RNAs that can regulate expression at a post-transcriptional level by base pairing to mRNA sequences (usually located at the 3′ UTR region), reducing protein expression levels via mRNA degradation, translational inhibition, or transient mRNA sequestration. Numerous microRNAs have been predicted to downregulate the expression of different connexin genes (for recent reviews see [65,80]). Cx43 is by far the best studied connexin, and a number of functional microRNAs targeting this gene have been identified, including miR-1, miR-23a, miR-186, miR-200a, miR-206, and miR-381 in human breast cancer [81], miR-20a in human prostate cancer [82], miR-221/222 in glioblastoma multiforme [83], and miR-206, miR-1, and miR-133 in cardiac myocytes and during skeletal myoblast differentiation [84–86].

Regulation of connexin expression by miRNAs has been described to be active in various disease states (for example, in cancer) by affecting hallmarks such as proliferation and invasion [82,83]. In therapeutic settings, options include targeting miRNAs that regulate connexins in order to reverse the malignant phenotype. This has been shown in several studies, including in human glioblastoma cells, where inhibition of miR-221/222 activity with antisense oligonucleotides led to the upregulation of Cx43 and restoration of GJIC [83].

As mentioned above, miR-1 acts in cardiac muscle and downregulates Cx43 expression. This has been related to several cardiopathologies in humans, including the regulation of cardiac arrhythmogenic potential [86]. In contrast, loss of miR-1, and thus increased Cx43 expression, has been linked to myotonic dystrophy [87]. Interestingly, a severe congenital heart defect, tetralogy of Fallot, is associated with downregulation of miR-1 and miR-206, which is thought to lead to an increase in Cx43 protein levels [88]. miR-1 downregulation of Cx43 in the bladder musculature has also been reported to have a role in overactive bladder syndrome [89].

Connexins are implicated in joint and bone disease [90]. Cx43 has an important role in osteoblast growth and differentiation, and various miRNAs (including miR-23a [91] and miR144-3p [92]) have been shown to target Cx43 in this setting. Cx43 can also influence the expression of miRNAs themselves, notably miR-21 in osteocytes, a pathway linked to osteocyte apoptosis and osteoclast formation/recruitment [93]. Moreover, direct transfer of miRNAs—through gap junctions—has been described, and is thought to play a role in bone development [94] as well as in aspects of tumor growth and tumor dormancy [3].

In addition to miRNAs, connexin transcript stability can be regulated by RNA-binding proteins (RBPs), such as human antigen R (HuR) that stabilizes the Cx43 mRNA by binding adenylate/uridine-rich elements (AREs) present in the Cx43 3′ UTR [95]. Other examples include S1516-binding protein elements, which may regulate Cx43 expression, particularly in Ras-transformed cancers [96]. For further insight into the epigenetic regulation of connexins, including by miRNAs, we refer to other more exhaustive recent reviews [65,80].

2.4. *Translational Regulation*

2.4.1. Internal Ribosome Entry Site (IRES)

Due to the key role of connexins in sustaining many cellular functions and tissue physiology, it has been suggested that connexin expression needs to be maintained at all times, even under conditions where the classical cap-dependent mRNA translation pathway is suppressed, such as during mitosis, apoptosis, differentiation, senescence, or cell stress [97,98]. Several internal ribosome entry site (IRESs) elements have been reported in the mRNA of connexins, notably in Cx43 [99] (Figure 1), Cx32 [100], and Cx26 [101]. An IRES is a nucleotide sequence, usually located within the 5′ UTR of the mRNA, which—in contrast with the canonical translation mechanism—allows for cap-independent translation initiation, a process regulated by specific RBPs also known as IRES trans-acting factors (ITAFs) [102,103]. However, numerous other translation initiation mechanisms are thought to exist [104] and whether true IRES-mediated translation occurs in the aforementioned connexins and other family members, is subject to caution, and additional specific molecular assays are warranted [105]. Additional work is also needed towards elucidating their functional relevance. One study suggests that IRES-mediated translation of Cx26 and Cx43 occurs in density-inhibited cancer cells (where cap-dependent translation is reduced), thus leading to the induction of GJIC and potentially reduced tumor growth [101]. Some data also points towards an important role of IRES-translation of connexins in human physiology. Notably, a specific mutation in the 5′ UTR IRES sequence of Cx32 is linked to neurodegenerative Charcot–Marie–Tooth disease [100].

2.4.2. Alternative Translation of Truncated Connexin Forms

Most IRES sequences are located in the 5′ UTR, yet a few examples exist (notably Notch2 [106]) where an IRES sequence is located within the coding region, allowing translation of truncated protein forms. A similar mechanism has been proposed for Cx55.5 in zebrafish, in which an 11 kilodalton (kDa) truncated C-terminal form is produced and localizes to the nucleus of outer retina cells [107,108].

In mammalian cells, the presence of truncated forms of Cx43 is often observed in immunoblots. In particular, a 20 kDa form (named GJA1-20k) is highly prevalent in cultured cells, which was described to arise from the Cx43 coding sequence and correspond to the C-terminal tail [109]. More recently, Smyth and Shaw described that GJA1-20k and several other less prevalent truncated forms can occur in normal tissue, and is due to internal translation initiation events [110]. Multiple groups have now confirmed this observation and further delineated key regulatory pathways, such as the mechanistic target of rapamycin (mTOR) [110,111] and the mitogen-activated protein kinase (MAPK)-interacting serine/threonine-protein kinase 1 (MNK1) and 2 (MNK2) [111] signaling cascades. Additionally, regulation occurs in response to important physiological conditions such as hypoxia [112] (Figure 1). Although an internal IRES element has been suggested [112], evidence suggests a highly unusual cap-dependent mechanism is critical for the efficient synthesis of these truncated forms [80,111].

The C-terminus of Cx43 has been extensively studied and is implicated in the regulation of a variety of biological events such as cell migration and proliferation, neuronal differentiation, and cytoskeletal changes (for a recent review see [5]). However, functional roles for specific internally truncated forms of Cx43 are currently being elucidated. Thus far, GJA1-20k has been shown to act as a potential chaperone for Cx43 [110,113] that facilitates microtubule-based mitochondrial transport and mitochondrial network integrity [114] (for details, see Section 4.3). Additionally, loss of GJA1-20k (but not full-length Cx43) has been reported in early-stage human breast cancers, followed by its re-expression in cell lines regulated by p53 activation via miR-125b [115]. Roles for these truncated forms of connexins in complex genetic disease is of future interest considering recent advancements in the potential for pharmacologic modulation of internal translation [80].

3. Post-Translational Regulation of Connexins

Post-translational modification of connexin proteins regulates many important aspects of their life-cycle, including synthesis, trafficking, channel gating, and protein–protein interactions. While highly conserved, variations occur throughout the connexin family in protein sequence, size of intracellular N-/C-terminus, and loop regions. Connexin extracellular loop regions contain disulfide bridges that form between cysteines to maintain membrane topology and facilitate docking with opposing connexons, allowing the formation of gap junctions [116]. Unlike many other membrane-bound proteins, connexins are not glycosylated, with membrane trafficking and protein folding being regulated through alternative pathways (for details, see Section 4). The relatively unstructured nature of intracellular connexin domains makes for an ideal environment for post-translational modification to induce conformational changes that regulate protein–protein interactions. The majority of connexins contain multiple consensus sites for modifications through phosphorylation, *S*-nitrosylation, SUMOylation, and others. There have been several recent and comprehensive reviews on connexin post-translational modifications [5,117–119]. Instead of recapitulating these articles, we will highlight some of the main aspects of post-translational modifications of connexins and discuss their relevance in human disease.

3.1. Phosphorylation

Phosphorylation is a key regulator of connexin proteins, hemichannels, and gap junction channels [120–122]. The addition of phosphate groups to specific amino acids—including serine (Ser, S), threonine (Thr, T), or tyrosine (Tyr, Y)—leads to changes in charge, hydrophobicity, and potential alterations in protein structure resulting from formation of hydrogen bond networks [123]. These can alter the way the connexin protein interacts with itself (e.g., channel regulation) or with other proteins (e.g., trafficking and protein–protein interactions).

Phosphorylation has been reported in a large number of connexins, e.g., Cx31 [124], Cx32 [125–127], Cx37, Cx40 and Cx45 [128,129], Cx43 [130,131], Cx46 and Cx50 [132–134], and Cx47 [135]. The majority of phosphorylation events are reported within the connexin C-terminus, with the exception of Cx26, which is not phosphorylated in its short 11 a.a. C-terminus [136,137]. However, mass spectrometry has demonstrated multiple potential Cx26 phosphorylation sites in the N-terminus, which are differentially regulated by hydroxylation, and further putative sites in the cytoplasmic loop, although the functions of these Cx26 phosphorylation sites are unknown [138,139]. There are some reports of intracellular loop phosphorylation—such as Cx56 [140] and Cx35 [141]—although this does not appear to be the case for Cx43 or other connexins [5,142,143]. There are no reports of N-terminus phosphorylation in other connexins, although Cx43–Ser5 is a potential candidate site [144]. The C-terminus of connexins are intrinsically disordered protein (IDP) regions with a high Ser/Thr/Tyr content, as described for Cx32, Cx40, Cx43, Cx45, and Cx50 [145–149]. Stable α-helical regions have been identified by nuclear magnetic resonance (NMR) and circular dichroism (CD) in the C-terminus of Cx43 [146,150] and other connexins, for example, Cx37, Cx45, and Cx50 [151–154]. However, stable alpha-helices are not a common feature of the connexin C-terminus. For instance, Cx40 only forms dynamic alpha-helices between Cys267–Gly285 [155]. Several lines of evidence—such as electrophoretic shifts on SDS-PAGE gels and NMR analysis—suggest that phosphorylation by enzymes, such as MAPK and Protein Kinase C (PKC), result in differential, transient increases in connexin C-terminal alpha-helical content [128,149,156–158].

The significance of the formation of alpha-helical domains is the potential for higher order secondary structures that regulate channel gating and protein partner binding. In Cx43, it has been demonstrated that the C-terminus interacts with the intercellular loop to regulate channel functions in a "ball-and-chain" type mechanism [159,160], although other factors relating to phosphorylation (e.g., charge and hydrophobicity) may also influence channel gating. Multisite phosphorylation of proteins is known to alter protein half-life, docking, and intracellular localization, which may also influence gap junction signaling [148,149,161]. Connexin 43, the most widely studied of the connexin family, has 30 putative phosphorylation sites which have been extensively demonstrated to be post-translationally modified, leading to alterations in gap junction signaling. For detailed reviews of these phosphorylation sites and their effects on channel regulation see [5,143,144,162–164]. The effects of post-translational modifications on connexins are also shown in Table 1.

Table 1. Connexin post-translational modifications (PTMs) and functional effects.

Connexin/Residue	PTM	GJIC	Expression	Refs.
Cx26 [m.s./a]:				
M1/K15/K102/K103/K105/K108/K112/K116	Acetylation	ND	ND	[138,139]
N14/N113/N170/N176	Hydroxylation	ND	ND	[138,139]
E42/E47/E114	carboxylation	ND	ND	[138,139]
K61/R75/K221/K223	Methylation	ND	ND	[138,139]
T123/T177/S183/T186/(Y233 or Y235 or Y240)	Phosphorylation	ND	ND	[138,139]
Cx31(m):				
263 [b]	CK1	No change	No change	[124]
266 [b]	CK1	No change	No change	[124]
Cx32:				
S229	PKC	Increase/Decrease	Increase/Decrease	[165]
S233	PKA/PKC	Increase/Decrease	Increase/Decrease	[120,138,165,166]
S240	ND	ND	ND	[138]
Y7/Y243	EGFR tyrosine kinase	ND	ND	[167]
Cx35/Cx36:				
S110	PKA/PKG	No change	Decrease	[141,168–170]
S276/293	PKA/PKG	No change	Decrease	[141,168–171]
S289	PKG (NO mediated)	ND	Decrease	[170]
Cx37:				
S275/S285/S302/S319/S321/S325/S329	PKC	Increased	Decrease	[128]

Table 1. *Cont.*

Connexin/Residue	PTM	GJIC	Expression	Refs.
Cx43:				
S5 [m.s.]	ND	ND	ND	[144]
K144	SUMO	Increase	Increase	[172]
K237	SUMO	Increase	Increase	[172]
S244 [m.s.]	CAMKII	ND	ND	[173]
Y247 [c]	Src	Decrease	Decrease [c]	[120,146,174–178]
S255 [m.s.]	CAMKII	ND	ND	[173]
	P34cdc2	Decrease	Decrease	[179,180]
	MAPK	No change/Decrease	No change	[120,131,148,181]
S257 [m.s.]	PKG/CAMKII	ND	ND	[173]
S262 [d]	P34cdc2	Decrease	Decrease	[179,180]
	MAPK	Decrease	Decrease/no change	[120,131,148,182,183]
	PKCε [a]	Decrease	Decrease	[131,181,182]
Y265 [c]	Src	Decrease	Decrease [c]	[120,146,174–178]
C271	Nitrosylation	Increase	No change	[184]
S279 [e]	MAPK	Decrease	Decrease/no change	[131,148,174]
	CDK5		Decrease	[185]
S282 [e]	MAPK	Decrease	Decrease/no change	[131,148,174]
	CDK5	Decrease	Decrease	[185]
S296 [m.s.]	CAMKII	ND	No change	[173,186]
S297 [m.s.]	CAMKII/PKCε	ND	No change	[173,186]
S306 [m.s.]	CAMKII	Decrease	Decrease associated with De-Phosph.	[173,186,187]
S314 [m.s.]	CAMKII	ND	ND	[173]
S325 [m.s.]	CAMKII	ND	ND	[173]
	CK1	Increase	Increase	[188]
S328 [m.s.]	CAMKII	ND	ND	[173]
	CK1	Increase	Increase	[188]
S330 [m.s.]	CAMKII	ND	ND	[173]
	CK1	Increase	Increase	[188]
S364 [m.s.]	CAMKII	ND	ND	[173]
	PKA	Increase	Increase	[120,189–191]
S365 [m.s.]	CAMKII	ND	ND	[173]
	PKA	Increase	Increase	
	PKC	Decrease	Decrease	[120,192–194]
S368 [f]	PKCα	Increase/Preserved/	Increase	[192–196]
	PKCε	Decrease [g]	Decrease	[120,193–199]
S369 [m.s.]	CAMKII	ND	ND	
	PKA	Increase	No change	[173]
	PKC	Increase	Increase	[5,120,192–194]
S372 [m.s.]	CAMKII	ND	ND	[173]
	PKC	Decrease	Decrease	[5,148,192,193,200,201]
S373 [g,m.s.]	Akt	Increase	Increase [e]	[200,201]
	CAMKII	ND	ND	[173]
	PKC	Decrease	Decrease	
	PKA	Increase	Increase	[120,148,192–194]

Table 1. *Cont.*

Connexin/Residue	PTM	GJIC	Expression	Refs.
Cx45:				
S326/Y337/ S381/S382/S384/ S385/S387/S393 m.s.	CAMKII	ND	ND	[129]
S326/S382/S384/ S387/S393 m.s.	CK1	ND	ND	[129]
Cx46 (Cx56 Chick homologue):				
S118	PKCε	ND	Decrease	[140,202]
Cx50:				
S363	CK1	Increase	Increase	[120,193]

Notes: [a] mass spec identified a number of potential phosphorylation sites in Cx26 but did not test functions, although mutations at many of these sites are associated with disease pathology [139]. [b] Direct phosphorylation not shown, S263 and S266 on Cx31 contain consensus sequence for Ck1 which, when deleted, alters functions. [c] Src may not alter function of formed gap junctions. [d] Currently debated as to whether Cx43-S262 is a CDK1/CDC2/PKC/MAPK site, and several lines of evidence indicate that this is most likely an ERK-regulated site [148]. [e] Functions of S279/S282 typically shown by single phosphorylation antibodies or multiple site directed mutagenesis including both residues. Decrease GJIC as a result of reduced open probability. [f] Phosphorylation of S368 by phorbyl esters, e.g., TPA, are associated with PKCε phosphorylation and reduced communication. In ischemia, treatment by peptides, e.g., rotagaptide, increase S368 phosphorylation by PKCα, leading to increases in GJIC. [g] While initial phosphorylation at S373 is associated with a temporal increase in GJ size, it is thought to be the start in the process that leads to internalization. Abbreviations: ND, not demonstrated; (m), mouse; m.s., mass spectrometry-based identification approach. GJIC, gap junction intercellular communication; EGFR, epidermal growth factor receptor; PKA/PKC, Protein kinase A/ Protein kinase C; NO, nitric oxide; SUMO, small ubiquitin-like modifier.

Phosphorylation is a key regulator of physiological states in tissues, and changes in the phosphorylation status has been observed in several disease states. Within the vasculature, heterocellular endothelial cell–smooth muscle cell contacts, called the myoendothelial junctions (MEJs), express Cx37, Cx40, and Cx43, allowing for the direct exchange of intercellular signaling ions and molecules such as Ca^{2+} and IP_3 [203,204]. At the MEJ, Cx43 and Cx37 are regulated by post-translational modifications, including phosphorylation and *S*-nitrosylation (for details, see Section 3.2). In vitro and ex vivo data demonstrate that gap junctions at MEJs allow for the movement of Ca^{2+} and IP_3 between endothelial and vascular smooth muscle cells, which is in part regulated via Cx43-Ser368 [205].

In the healthy heart, Cx43 is primarily localized to the intercalated disc region of cardiomyocytes. Opening of Cx43-containing channels and signal conduction is facilitated by phosphorylation at residues including Ser365, 325, 328, and 330 [206–208]. Phosphorylation acts as a molecular switch, regulating gap junction opening. In ventricular arrhythmias following myocardial infarction, raised intracellular Ca^{2+} concentration leads to de-phosphorylation of Cx43-Ser365, which acts as the gatekeeper to phosphorylation of Cx43-Ser368. This resulting increase in Cx43-Ser368 reduces GJIC and promotes a redistribution of Cx43 to lateral regions of the cardiac myocytes, disrupting signaling in the heart [208–210].

Formation of large cardiac gap junction plaques at the intercalated disc is modulated through Cx43 interactions with zonula occludens 1 (ZO-1) [211–214]. In turn, this protein–protein interaction is regulated by PKC phosphorylation of Cx43 at Ser368, which inhibits ZO-1-mediated disassembly of gap junctions [215]. In ischemic heart disease, Cx43 is lost at the intercalated disc, but Cx43-Ser368 phosphorylation can act to indirectly stabilize the protein [196]. Multiple studies have investigated the effects of targeting the C-terminus of Cx43 in ischemia/reperfusion injuries, reducing infarct size, and other diseases [11,216]. A peptide that mimics the terminal region of the Cx43 known as ACT1 can disrupt Cx43/ZO-1 interaction [214,217]. This peptide promotes phosphorylation of Cx43-Ser368 via upregulation of PKCε activity, inhibits Cx43-ZO-1 binding, and improves cardiac function following ischemic insult in mice [215]. Similar results have been found for other connexin mimetic peptides targeting the Cx43 C-terminus (e.g., antiarrhythmic peptide 10 (AAP10) and rotigaptide (ZP123)), causing increases in Cx43-Ser368 phosphorylation through PKCα (reported to stabilize protein expression and increase GJIC) associated with improved cardiac functions in experimental animal models and early tests demonstrating no adverse effects in humans [192,218–222]. However, it should be noted that a similar peptide, danegaptide (a stabilized form of rotigaptide), failed to change clinical outcomes in ischemic reperfusion injuries in human Phase II testing (NCT01977755, completed 2016) [223].

In vascular disease, phosphorylation-mediated connexin–protein interactions and GJIC have been found to regulate disease state. Oxidized phospholipids found within atherosclerotic plaques increase MAPK and PKC phosphorylation of Cx43 and are associated with increased inflammation and cellular proliferation [130,224–227]. In response to the release of growth factors in disease, Cx43 is phosphorylated at MAPK residues (Cx43-Ser255, -Ser262, -Ser279, -Ser282), promoting direct interactions with the cyclin E/CDK2 complex and enhancing smooth muscle cell proliferation [131]. Conversely, PKC phosphorylation of Cx37 alters GJIC, which is linked with growth suppressive effects (e.g., reducing vasculogenesis and angiogenesis) [228–233]. Mutation of all seven Cx37 Ser > Ala essentially closes Cx37 GJs and hemichannels and inhibits both proliferation and cell death, whereas mutation of only three (Cx37-Ser275, -Ser302 and -Ser328) partially inhibits channel opening and decreases cellular death in rat insulinoma cells [128].

Phosphorylation also plays an important role in altered localization and function of connexins in cancer [3]. Several oncogenes and proto-oncogenes robustly inhibit GJIC, including HRAS [234], c-Src [235], and v-Src [178]. Curiously, the tyrosine-protein kinase c-Src has a reciprocal relationship with Cx43 that regulates its activity, where Cx43 is shown to bind with phosphatases (e.g., PTEN and Csk) reducing c-Src activity [236]. Conversely, Src phosphorylation of tyrosine residues on Cx43 (Cx43-Tyr243/-Tyr265) mediates interactions with endosomal machinery, leading to internalization of Cx43 and reduced expression [118,237]. Numerous tumor promoters, such as phorbol esters, also rapidly inhibit Cx43-mediated GJIC [238–240] through PKC- and ERK-mediated phosphorylation events [181,241]. On the contrary, loss of phosphorylation can also negatively affect GJIC. One recent study showed that the levels of total Cx43 protein and Cx43 phosphorylated at Ser368 and Ser279/282 were high in normal tissue but low to absent in malignant pancreatic tissue [79]. Altered Cx43-phosphorylation can be indicative of prognosis in some tumors, such as gliomas [242]. Phosphorylation of other connexins can also affect GJIC and the cancer phenotype, notably PKC-mediated phosphorylation of Cx37 [128]. Targeting dysregulated phosphorylation events of connexins in cancer may be one therapeutic angle towards restoring connexin function or GJIC. Indeed, the chemotherapeutic drug gefitinib has been suggested to upregulate GJIC by inhibiting Src and PKC-modulated Cx43 phosphorylation [243]. However, resistance to cisplatin-based chemotherapy has been suggested to be due to Src-induced Cx43 phosphorylation and loss of GJIC [244].

During wound healing, phosphorylation may also play a role in coordinating GJIC and connexin redistribution [245–247]. Initial responses to wounding include a generalized loss in Cx43, which may be modulated by increases in cyclic adenosine monophosphate (cAMP). In wound models, 8-bromo-cAMP-treated embryonic stem cells promote enhanced wound repair associated with reduced membrane bound Cx43, disruption in Cx43-ZO-1 interactions, and reduced GJIC [248]. However, the mechanisms regulating this are unclear, since cAMP-associated kinases have been previously described to increase PKA-mediated Cx43 synthesis, phosphorylation (Cx43-Ser364), GJ assembly, and GJIC in other model systems [189,249]. Phosphorylation is extremely dynamic within the wound and appears to be coordinated with the stage of repair. Initial increases in Cx43-Ser373, driven by AKT, can be seen between 1 and 30 min after wounding occurs, disrupting interactions with ZO-1, initially stabilizing Cx43 at the membrane, but is followed by rapid internalization of Cx43 [200]. Following wounding, transient increases (24–72 h) in PKC-mediated Cx43-Ser368 phosphorylation in regions proximal to the injured sited are associated with a loss of GJIC [250,251]. These data and others suggest that a combination of phosphorylation events sequentially regulate connexin signaling during wound repair [252].

In disease states such as diabetes, nonhealing wounds lead to complications, including ulcerations in skin tissues. In streptozotocin-induced diabetic mice, Cx43 dynamics are different from normal skin tissues, with increased expression of dermal Cx43 associated with reduction in keratinocyte migration [253]. Similar observations have been made in human diabetic ulcers, with Cx43 found to remain at elevated levels as compared to normal skin wounds [254]. In vitro and ex vivo evidence suggests that peptides aimed at disrupting gap junction and hemichannel communication (e.g., Gap27) can improve wound healing, which is associated with increased Cx43-Ser368 phosphorylation [251]. Recent studies have also shown that increases in Cx43-Ser368 phosphorylation following topical application of the ACT1 peptide is associated with clinically significant improvements in scar reduction and wound closure rates [255].

3.2. S-Nitrosylation

S-Nitrosylation occurs through covalent binding of nitric oxide (NO) to reactive cysteine(s) and can result in structural alterations of proteins leading to functional changes [256]. Protein *S*-nitrosylation is highly dependent on the cysteine oxidation state and surrounding amino acids, meaning that not all cysteines in a protein can be *S*-nitrosylated. While there are cysteine residues on the extracellular loops of all connexins, these have not been demonstrated to be *S*-nitrosylation targets [257]. Within the C-terminus of Cx43, there are three cysteines (Cx43-Cys260, -Cys271, and -Cys298), but only Cx43-Cys271 has been demonstrated to be *S*-nitrosylated, leading to an increase in GJ permeability in endothelial cells and at the MEJ [184]. Direct *S*-nitrosylation of other connexins has not been demonstrated, although there are multiple lines of evidence demonstrating that nitric oxide (NO) activation leads to regulation of gap junction and hemichannel signaling [258]. Within the vasculature, NO plays an important role in vasodilation. Figueroa et al. found that vascular connexins channels formed by Cx37, Cx40, and Cx43 are activated by and directly permeable to NO, and have suggested that this is an alternative method to NO transfer across plasma membranes [259]. Cx37 is enriched at the MEJ of resistance arteries and is reported to be important in the regulation of NO-mediated Ca^{2+} regulation via reducing Cx37-mediated gap junctional coupling between endothelial cells and smooth muscle cells [260]. However, unlike Cx43, the effects of NO on Cx37 gap junction channels are thought to be indirect, with no known cysteine modification occurring. Rather, the phosphorylated tyrosine residue (Cx37-Tyr332) is protected from de-phosphorylation by Src homology region 2 (Shp2) phosphatase, which is inhibited in the presence of NO, reducing MEJ transfer of Ca^{2+} signaling through Cx37 GJ [261]. Thus, *S*-nitrosylation appears to have diverse effects, depending on GJ composition particularly at the MEJ [261].

3.3. Other Post-Translational Modifications: SUMOylation, Ubiquitination, and Acetylation

A number of post-translational modifications are associated with regulation of connexin protein turnover, for example, ubiquitination, SUMOylation, and acetylation. Small ubiquitin-like modifier proteins (e.g., SUMO-1/-2/-3) interact with lysine residues on proteins, altering protein targeting and turnover [262]. So far, there is only evidence for direct Cx43 SUMOylation at lysine residues (Cx43-Lys144, -Lys237) within its intracellular loop and C-terminus [172]. Overexpression of all three SUMO proteins in HeLa cells increases Cx43 expression, promotes gap junction formation, and increases signaling. However, the exact mechanism by which SUMOylation regulates protein expression is not known. The amino acids sequences surrounding Cx43-Lys144 and Cx43-Lys237 are not common motifs associated with SUMOylation, although the same motifs of a conserved Lys144 followed by an upstream large hydrophobic amino acid (valine) are found in at least six other connexins, suggesting a common regulatory pathway [172].

Once at the plasma membrane, the majority of connexins are rapidly turned over with half-lives estimated between 1.5 and 5 h for Cx43 and Cx26 and up to 24 h for other isoforms such as Cx46 [124,263–266]. While connexins use a multitude of pathways for internalization and degradation, the process typically involves formation of an endosome (termed connexosome [267]), where older gap junctions are internalized to be targeted to the lysosome for degradation, although there is also evidence for endosomal recycling back to the membrane [214,268,269]. Endosomal formation is driven by multiple proteins in complex, including interactions with ZO-1, tubulin, and others. In the case of Cx43, this interaction (with ZO-1) is regulated via Cx43-Ser373 and Cx43-Ser368 phosphorylation [200,214,270,271]. Monoubiquitinylation typically acts as a signal for internalization of proteins via endosomes to lysosomes, leading to degradation [272,273]. Multiple covalently linked ubiquitin molecules bind lysine residues within the target protein, which are then recognized by receptors and targeted for degradation by the 26S proteasome [274–276] and by autophagy [277–279]. Recent evidence has demonstrated a complementary role for Cx43 in regulating autophagy, in that Cx43 at the plasma membrane interacts with several pre-autophagosomal proteins, including Atg16, but not other autophagosome proteins, such as LC3 [280]. When the cells are under stress, such as nutrient depletion, Cx43 becomes ubiquitinylated and internalized, causing recruitment of other factors (Atg5, Atg12, and LC3) to form fully functional autophagosomes. While regulated autophagy can have a protective effect in stressed cells, there is also evidence linking aberrant autophagy and Cx43 degradation from intercalated discs to heart failure [281], suggesting the potential for a novel pharmacologic approach to treat cardiac failure.

Proteasomal–ubiquitin pathways have been proposed to indirectly regulate Cx43 through interaction with the ZO-1 protein, thus disrupting part of the process that is critical for Cx43 membrane organization [214,282]. Multiple studies suggest that other connexin proteins (e.g., Cx50, Cx43, and Cx31.1) are regulated by ubiquitination [283]. Several studies show that ubiquitin regulates internalization of Cx43 via clathrin-mediated endocytosis, by both tyrosine (Y)-dependent sorting signal (YXXΦ, where X is any amino acid and Φ is an amino acid with a bulky hydrophobic side chain) and tyrosine-independent, EPS15-dependent pathways [284,285]. However, the route through which ubiquitin regulates the connexins has not been fully delineated, with studies in Cx43 demonstrating that the C-terminal lysines are dispensable for protein turnover [286]. Despite this, there is increasing evidence that Cx43 is modified in response to ubiquitin, and corresponding ligases are controlled in part by phosphorylation events, such as MAPK and PKC phosphorylation [287,288]. A number of ubiquitin-binding proteins (e.g., EPS15, p62, Hrs, and TSG101) are rec ruited to Cx43 to facilitate its internalization and sorting to the lysosome [289,290]. In addition, TSG101 has been found to interact with Cx30.2, Cx31, Cx36, and Cx45 [290]. While classic lysine-based motifs may not be responsible for direct ubiquitin binding, more recent studies have shown that proline-rich regions of the Cx43 C-terminus (xPPxY) bind to ubiquitin ligase. A number of ubiquitin ligases have also been associated with direct binding, internalization, and degradation of Cx43 (e.g., Trim21 [291], WWP1 [292], SMURF2 [293], and NEDD4 [287–289,294]). NEDD4 also has been directly associated with loss of Cx43 at the plasma membrane in experimental models [287].

The process of degradation may be further regulated by connexin N-terminal acetylation, which can act to regulate protein stability in the membrane. In mouse cardiac myocytes, N-terminal acetylation through binding of P300/CBP-associated factor with Cx43 leads to a loss of Cx43 at the intercalated disc, a lateral reorganization of the protein, reduced gap junction formation in cardiac myocytes, and internalization in NIH-3T3 (mouse embryo) fibroblasts [77]. These patterns of disorganization of Cx43 are similar to those seen in mouse models of Duchenne cardiomyopathies, where NO and oxidative stress lead to an imbalance in acetylation/deacetylation and alterations in cardiac conduction. Similarly in dogs, cardiac pacing leads to increased Cx43 acetylation, suggesting that this mechanism is important in regulating signaling in physiology and pathology of the cardiac system [77,295,296].

4. Connexin Trafficking

Formation of gap junctions by connexins is regulated by the delivery of newly synthesized channels to the plasma membrane and is balanced by the removal of channels via endocytosis [263,297,298]. As mentioned above, since connexin turnover is generally quite rapid and influenced by post-translational modifications, the dynamic regulation of connexins by secretion and turnover provides a means to control gap junction formation, composition, and, thus, GJIC.

4.1. Control of Oligomerization

Secretion of newly synthesized connexins from the endoplasmic reticulum (ER) through the Golgi apparatus is coordinately regulated with oligomerization into hexameric hemichannels [299]. Based on structural homology, connexins can be separated into two distinct oligomerization groups. *GJB1–GJB7* (so-called β connexins, including Cx26 and Cx32) follow a more traditional pathway, where full oligomerization into hexamers is required prior to transport from the ER to the cis-Golgi apparatus [300–302]. By contrast, other connexins are stabilized by a connexin-specific quality control apparatus as monomers that are subsequently transported to the trans-Golgi network (TGN) where they then have the capacity to oligomerize [301,303]. The best-studied connexin known to oligomerize in the TGN is Cx43, although there is also experimental evidence for Cx40 and Cx46 oligomerization late in the secretory pathway [304,305]. By homology, it is likely that most non-beta connexins will also follow the late oligomerization pathway that has been demonstrated for Cx43 [299].

Several lines of evidence suggest that the transition from monomeric to hexameric Cx43 requires a conformational change, largely centered on the third transmembrane domain (TM3) where it is stabilized in a monomeric conformation by motifs containing charged amino acids on both ends of the TM domain (Figure 2) [300,305]. At the cytoplasmic interface of the Cx43 TM3 domain is an LR motif containing a highly charged arginine residue, and at the extracellular interface is a glutamine-containing motif with a QYFLYGF amino acid consensus sequence. The extracellular loop domain of Cx43 also interacts with a chaperone protein, ERp29, that is required to stabilize monomeric Cx43 [300].

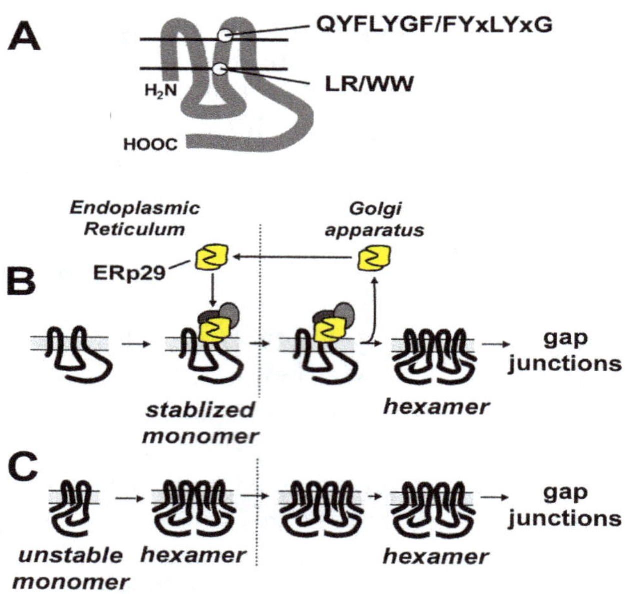

Figure 2. Differential connexin oligomerization. (**A**) Line diagram showing two key connexin motifs adjacent to the third transmembrane domain. Connexins (such as Cx43), which oligomerize in the Golgi apparatus (**B**), have a cytosolic LR and extracellular QYFLYGF motif that interacts with ERp29 (yellow) and other putative chaperones (grey ovals) that stabilize monomeric connexins until they transition from the endoplasmic reticulum (ER) to the Golgi apparatus (delineated by the dashed lines). In the Golgi apparatus, ERp29 dissociates from monomeric connexins and then recycles back to the ER, enabling connexins to oligomerize into hexameric hemichannels. By contrast, connexins (such as Cx32) that have a WW and a FYxLYxG motif cannot interact with ERp29—they are inserted into the ER membrane as unstable monomers and thus immediately oligomerize (**C**).

By contrast, beta connexins lack charged residues adjacent to the TM3 domain. They instead have a di-tryptophan (WW) motif that is less stringently localized to the membrane/cytosol interface, and they lack the ability to interact with ERp29. Thus, beta connexins are not stable as monomers and instead oligomerize in the ER (Figure 2) [300–302]. Since motifs associated with the TM3 domain also have been implicated in regulating connexin hetero-oligomerization [299,306], this implicates a role for spatial separation of connexin oligomerization in regulating the extent and stoichiometry of heteromeric channel formation.

4.2. Connexin Quality Control

The differences in quality control for Cx26 and Cx43 were directly observed for native connexins in human airway epithelial cells derived from a cystic fibrosis (CF) patient expressing the CF transmembrane conductance regulator (CFTR) protein harboring the Fdel508 mutation [307]. In these cells, Cx43 trafficking and function is impaired, yet Cx26 transport and assembly into gap junction channels is normal. Interestingly, CFTR also interacts with ERp29 [308], and Cx43-mediated GJIC by Fdel508-CFTR-expressing cells is restored by treatment with 4-phenylbutyrate, a drug that upregulates ERp29 expression [307,308]. In addition, 4-phenylbutyrate has been shown to upregulate GJIC in several other contexts [309–314], further underscoring a role for ERp29 and other 4-phenylbutyrate-sensitive factors in connexin quality control.

Aberrant accumulation of connexins in the ER clearly decreases the pool of connexins available to produce gap junction channels at the cell surface. However, ER accumulation of connexins has also been found to induce an unfolded protein response (UPR) that, in turn, has the capacity to impair cell function and lead to human disease. UPR induced by mutant connexins has been directly demonstrated for Cx50 mutations associated with cataract [315–317] and Cx31 mutations that cause the skin disease erythrokeratoderma variabilis (EKV) [318] or hearing impairment [319]. The association of UPR with human diseases related to misfolded connexins suggests the possibility that treatments alleviating ER stress, such as 4-phenylbutyrate, may have therapeutic value by promoting proper protein folding and trafficking as well as increasing GJIC. Also, as mentioned above, the ability of 4-phenylbutyrate to enhance GJIC also may contribute to its potential as an anticancer therapeutic, and may be related to increased ERp29 activity [320].

4.3. Connexin Cytoplasmic Domains and the Cytoskeleton

In addition to motifs adjacent to the TM3 domain, there are several lines of evidence in support of connexin C-terminal domains in regulating connexin trafficking. As described above, in addition to containing several motifs that can be post-translationally modified, the semi-structured nature of the C-terminus [153,155,321] enables it to be conformationally labile and to interact with several different classes of cytosolic scaffold proteins and the cytoskeleton that can influence connexin targeting (reviewed in [5] for Cx43). For instance, several truncated connexins lack the ability to be efficiently trafficked to the plasma membrane or be endocytosed [322,323]. The connexin C-terminal domains also have the capacity to homo- and hetero-dimerize [153,155,159,324] as well as interact with other connexin domains, including the cytoplasmic loop [155,325,326] that can influence connexin targeting, oligomerization, and function.

Interestingly, it was determined that there is reciprocal regulation of Cx43 and Cx46 in the lens, where conditions such as activation of PKC caused an increase in Cx46 transcription and expression that was associated with a concomitant decrease in Cx43, via ubiquitination and proteasomal degradation [327]. In fact, transfecting cells with Cx46 was sufficient to induce Cx43 degradation and this effect required the C-terminus of Cx46, since a Cx46 tail truncation mutant had no effect on Cx43 expression. Increased Cx50 also had no effect on Cx43. However, transfecting cells with a soluble Cx46 tail construct had the ability to decrease Cx43 expression. Since the decrease in Cx43 was induced by an intracellular pool of Cx46, this raises the possibility that crosstalk between Cx46 and Cx43 may be related to differential oligomerization [304]. However, this remains to be determined.

As another instance where the C-terminus plays a key role in regulating Cx43 trafficking, it has been shown that amino N-terminal truncated forms of Cx43 are also expressed by cells, through alternative internal translation via one of six different AUG initiation sites (see Section 2.4.2) [328]. The most prominent of these is GJA1-20k, which consists of a portion of the TM4 domain as well as the entire C-terminus [110] (Figure 1). GJA1-20k expression promotes formation of Cx43 gap junction channels, resulting in an increase in intercellular communication [110,113]. As discussed in Section 2.4.2, alternative translation of Cx43, including production of GJA1-20k, is inhibited by mTOR [110,111] and Mnk1/2 kinases [111], suggesting that metabolic stress regulates gap junctional coupling through mTOR- and Mnk1/2-mediated pathways as a means to protect cells both by enabling scarce metabolites to be distributed via intercellular communication as well as limiting damage by restricting generation of reactive oxygen species [329].

How GJA1-20k regulates channel formation by Cx43 is still under investigation. One intriguing possibility is that GJA1-20k acts as a chaperone protein that promotes Cx43 oligomerization, as was recently demonstrated to regulate the decrease in gap junction formation and function that can occur in the epithelial to mesenchyme transition [330] (Figure 1).

Another likely role for GJA1-20k relates to cytoskeletal control of Cx43 trafficking, since it has been shown that the C-terminus of Cx43 and, therefore, GJA-20k as well, interacts with both microtubules and filamentous actin [331–333]. Microtubules and actin perform complementary functions in regulating connexin trafficking, where microtubules help facilitate rapid transport of Cx43-containing vesicles to sites of junction formation [332], whereas actin has a more subtle role in regulating connexin trafficking, since quantitative live cell-imaging shows that transport of Cx43-containing vesicles temporarily pauses when they interact with actin filaments, perhaps as a means to enhance sorting or to remodel vesicle composition [331]. Also, transfecting HeLa cells with GJA1-20k nucleates the formation of actin filaments [113], suggesting a role for GJA1-20k in altering the itinerary of Cx43 trafficking in the cell. Reverse regulation is also suggested by studies where gap junction inhibitors resulted in misalignment of actin filaments across the monolayer and reduced calcium signaling in rat astrocytes [334]. Furthermore, treatment of astrocytes with an actin polymerization inhibitor cytochalasin D or anti-actin antibodies reduced GJIC, as visualized by a reduction in the spread of microinjected neurobiotin between cells [335].

4.4. Regulation of Gap Junction Plaque Morphology

Actin has also been implicated in regulating gap junction plaque morphology. Double knockout of the actin capping protein tropomodulin 1 and intermediate filament protein CP49 in lens fiber cells led to a significant decrease in Cx46 plaque volume and increase in plaque number, affecting gap junction coupling and function in the lens tissue [336]. Regulation of plaque size by actin is likely to be coordinated by interactions involving the C-terminus of connexins and zonula occludens 1 (ZO-1). For example, enhanced green fluorescent protein (EGFP)-tagged Cx43 incapable of interacting with ZO-1 produces plaques that are not size regulated [337]. By contrast, the perimeter of gap junction plaques (the perinexus) is ringed by Cx43/ZO-1 complexes, whereas the center of plaques is largely devoid of ZO-1 [338]. Inhibition of Cx43/ZO-1 interactions cause an increase in gap junction plaque size. Consistent with this possibility, Cx43 phosphorylation inhibits ZO-1 binding and facilitates connexin channel endocytosis [339]. Additional roles for ZO-1, connexin phosphorylation, and ubiquitinylation in regulating connexin endocytosis and degradation are described in Sections 3.2 and 3.3, above.

Although the precise mechanism whereby ZO-1 limits plaque formation is still under investigation, it seems plausible that it may be analogous to the role of ZO-1 in regulating tight junctions, where claudin/ZO-1/actin interactions have a junction-stabilizing influence on the apical junctional complex, whereas, in the absence of ZO-1, there is increased access of myosin that increases tight junction dynamics and tension [340,341]. Consistent with this possibility, myosin VI has also been found to have a specific role in increasing gap junction plaque size, analogous to treatments inhibiting Cx43/ZO-1 interactions [342].

Whether regulation of plaque assembly strictly follows the perinexus model has recently been challenged by observations of Cx36 plaque formation [343]. Pulse-chase experiments with Cx36 indicated addition of Cx36 to both the ends and the middle of preexisting gap junction plaques, with diffusion of Cx36 throughout the plaque. When the experiments were repeated with Cx43, there appeared to be less diffusion of newly added Cx43 in preexisting plaques [343]. Targeted delivery of connexins has only recently been observed. Through interactions with plus-end binding protein EB1 and the dynein/dynactin complex, microtubule plus-ends are tethered to adherens junctions at the plasma membrane, leading to the targeted deposition of connexin hemichannels and gap junction plaque formation [332]. These two models begin to bring to light the vast complexity of connexin trafficking and gap junction formation, suggesting a network of cytoskeleton and protein-binding partners tailored to specific connexins that was previously unrealized.

A less understood but intriguing role for the cytoskeleton in gap junction biology is the creation of unique junctional subregions involved in gap junction dynamics. Using an EGFP-tagged Cx32 construct, particularly dynamic regions at the edges of gap junction plaques were observed as invaginated tubular structures, where plaque fragments pinched off into the cytoplasm [344]. These tubulovesicular extensions of gap junction plaques were recently observed with Cx36 and termed filadendrites [345]. Filadendrites at the edges of gap junction plaques appeared to be the same thickness as the plaque, suggesting that the filadendrites were a continuation of the gap junction plaques themselves. Filadendrites were also observed in interior regions of the gap junction plaques, but appeared to be much thinner than the gap junction plaques. From pulse-chase labeling of Cx36, it was observed that filadendrites exhibited some of the same dynamic properties as the earlier observed Cx32 invaginations, constantly pinching off and fusing with the gap junction plaque. Labeling of actin filaments showed colocalization with Cx36 filadendrites, suggesting that the actin cytoskeleton could be one of the drivers behind the formation of these dynamic structures. Treatment with the actin polymerization inhibitor Latrunculin A or actin depolymerization inducer cytochalasin D reduced the presence of filadendrites, indicating that the driving force behind the dynamic gap junction plaques requires actin polymerization [345].

Similar structures have been noted at other junctions. Primary human keratinocytes treated with pemphigus vulgaris (PV) IgG containing antibodies targeted to the adherens junction protein desmoglein 3 (Dsg3) exhibited reorganized Dsg3 at the membrane into projections perpendicular to the membrane plane. These projections, termed linear arrays, are similar to the filadendrites in that they are sites of disassembly of junction components and active endocytosis at the junctions. Linear arrays also colocalized with actin filaments oriented perpendicular to the plasma membrane, similar to those observed in filadendrites. Furthermore, linear arrays were associated with decreased cell adhesion, suggesting a functional effect of these junctional subregions [346,347]. A comparable structure formed by tight junction proteins, termed tight junction spikes, have been observed to correlate with treatments that enhance junction disassembly and paracellular leak, including oxidative stress induced by chronic alcohol exposure, transforming growth factor (TGF)-β1 treatment, and inhibition of NF-κB [348–350]. In alveolar epithelial cells, actin filaments colocalized with the tight junction protein claudin-18 in tight junction spikes. Spikes were also found to be sites of budding and fusion of vesicles carrying tight junction proteins, both indicators of active tight junction remodeling. Treatment of lung alveolar epithelial cells with granulocyte-macrophage colony-stimulating factor (GM-CSF) reduced actin filament colocalization with claudin-18 containing tight junction spikes, whereas keratinocyte growth factor treatment inhibited spike formation and instead promoted formation of cortical actin as opposed to actin stress fibers [350,351]. Taken together, these findings indicate that these similar junctional subregions observed universally across several different classes of intercellular junctions, including gap junctions, could represent a common mechanism of junction protein turnover, where the junctions partition themselves into unique filamentous structures. Whether these structures serve to restrict turnover of junction proteins to specific subdomains or whether they nucleate the formation of signaling complexes that recruit specialized subsets of cytosolic binding partners remains to be determined.

5. Conclusions and Future Perspectives

In order to fully understand the complex role of connexins in health and disease, it is essential to elucidate their regulation at all steps, from gene transcription, protein synthesis, post-translational modifications, and trafficking to their regulation at the cell membrane. This review is intended to highlight some of the progress made in these areas in relation to health and disease, giving examples of how this knowledge is pertinent for future therapeutic applications. Going forward, understanding how modulation of connexins occurs at any of these stages will require additional work and insight, which over time may lead to more fruitful and safer strategies to alleviate patient suffering. For example, the danegaptide trials that were based on strong preclinical data suggested that alterations to the trafficking and increased Cx43 signaling in the heart would have a profound effect in reducing ischemic reperfusion injury and reduce cardiac tissue damage. However, Phase II clinical trials in humans failed to show an effect, highlighting the complex nature of targeting gap junctions as a treatment modality including differences in how connexins are regulated in model systems as opposed to human disease. Additional caution is also needed for therapeutic approaches in cancer, where it is now clear that connexins have distinct roles that both promote and inhibit cell growth and metastasis.

Despite substantial progress, it is important to acknowledge the complexity of gap junctions that serve as a conduit that enables cells to share thousands of different signaling molecules. Additionally, the complex connexin protein interactome underscores the non-junctional functions of connexins, including their ability to act as a signaling platform. In particular, it is critical to identify connexin-specific functions that are unique and targetable. This is best approached by understanding how connexins are regulated at multiple levels by multiple mechanisms, from gene transcription and translation to post-translational modification, and as a specifically localized multiprotein complex.

Acknowledgments: Trond Aasen acknowledges support from Instituto de Salud Carlos III grants PI13/00763, PI16/00772 and CPII16/00042, co-financed by the European Regional Development Fund (ERDF). Supported by NIH R01-AA025854 and R01-HL137112 (Michael Koval) and F31-HL139109 (K. Sabrina Lynn).

References

1. Goodenough, D.A.; Paul, D.L. Gap junctions. *Cold Spring Harb. Perspect. Biol.* **2009**, *1*, a002576. [CrossRef] [PubMed]
2. Esseltine, J.L.; Laird, D.W. Next-generation connexin and pannexin cell biology. *Trends Cell Biol.* **2016**, *26*, 944–955. [CrossRef] [PubMed]
3. Aasen, T.; Mesnil, M.; Naus, C.C.; Lampe, P.D.; Laird, D.W. Gap junctions and cancer: Communicating for 50 years. *Nat. Rev. Cancer* **2016**, *16*, 775–788. [CrossRef] [PubMed]
4. Saez, J.C.; Leybaert, L. Hunting for connexin hemichannels. *FEBS Lett.* **2014**, *588*, 1205–1211. [CrossRef] [PubMed]
5. Leithe, E.; Mesnil, M.; Aasen, T. The connexin 43 C-terminus: A tail of many tales. *Biochim. Biophys. Acta* **2018**, *1860*, 48–64. [CrossRef] [PubMed]
6. Delmar, M.; Laird, D.W.; Naus, C.C.; Nielsen, M.S.; Verselis, V.K.; White, T.W. Connexins and disease. *Cold Spring Harb. Perspect. Biol.* **2017**. [CrossRef] [PubMed]
7. Srinivas, M.; Verselis, V.K.; White, T.W. Human diseases associated with connexin mutations. *Biochim. Biophys. Acta* **2018**, *1860*, 192–201. [CrossRef] [PubMed]
8. Kelly, J.J.; Simek, J.; Laird, D.W. Mechanisms linking connexin mutations to human diseases. *Cell Tissue Res.* **2015**, *360*, 701–721. [CrossRef] [PubMed]
9. Aasen, T. Connexins: Junctional and non-junctional modulators of proliferation. *Cell Tissue Res.* **2015**, *360*, 685–699. [CrossRef] [PubMed]
10. Leybaert, L.; Lampe, P.D.; Dhein, S.; Kwak, B.R.; Ferdinandy, P.; Beyer, E.C.; Laird, D.W.; Naus, C.C.; Green, C.R.; Schulz, R. Connexins in cardiovascular and neurovascular health and disease: Pharmacological implications. *Pharmacol. Rev.* **2017**, *69*, 396–478. [CrossRef] [PubMed]
11. Becker, D.L.; Phillips, A.R.; Duft, B.J.; Kim, Y.; Green, C.R. Translating connexin biology into therapeutics. *Semin. Cell Dev. Biol.* **2016**, *50*, 49–58. [CrossRef] [PubMed]

12. Grek, C.L.; Rhett, J.M.; Ghatnekar, G.S. Cardiac to cancer: Connecting connexins to clinical opportunity. *FEBS Lett.* **2014**, *588*, 1349–1364. [CrossRef] [PubMed]
13. Lee, C.; Huang, C.H. Lasagna-search: An integrated web tool for transcription factor binding site search and visualization. *BioTechniques* **2013**, *54*, 141–153. [CrossRef] [PubMed]
14. Söhl, G.; Willecke, K. An update on connexin genes and their nomenclature in mouse and man. *Cell Commun. Adhes.* **2003**, *10*, 173–180. [CrossRef] [PubMed]
15. Beyer, E.C.; Berthoud, V.M. Gap junction gene and protein families: Connexins, innexins, and pannexins. *Biochim. Biophys. Acta* **2018**, *1860*, 5–8. [CrossRef] [PubMed]
16. Dupays, L.; Mazurais, D.; Rücker-Martin, C.; Calmels, T.; Bernot, D.; Cronier, L.; Malassiné, A.; Gros, D.; Théveniau-Ruissy, M. Genomic organization and alternative transcripts of the human connexin40 gene. *Gene* **2003**, *305*, 79–90. [CrossRef]
17. Essenfelder, G.M.; Larderet, G.; Waksman, G.; Lamartine, J. Gene structure and promoter analysis of the human gjb6 gene encoding connexin30. *Gene* **2005**, *350*, 33–40. [CrossRef] [PubMed]
18. Sohl, G.; Theis, M.; Hallas, G.; Brambach, S.; Dahl, E.; Kidder, G.; Willecke, K. A new alternatively spliced transcript of the mouse connexin32 gene is expressed in embryonic stem cells, oocytes, and liver. *Exp. Cell Res.* **2001**, *266*, 177–186. [CrossRef] [PubMed]
19. Pfeifer, I.; Anderson, C.; Werner, R.; Oltra, E. Redefining the structure of the mouse connexin43 gene: Selective promoter usage and alternative splicing mechanisms yield transcripts with different translational efficiencies. *Nucleic Acids Res.* **2004**, *32*, 4550–4562. [CrossRef] [PubMed]
20. Anderson, C.L.; Zundel, M.A.; Werner, R. Variable promoter usage and alternative splicing in five mouse connexin genes. *Genomics* **2005**, *85*, 238–244. [CrossRef] [PubMed]
21. Cicirata, F.; Parenti, R.; Spinella, F.; Giglio, S.; Tuorto, F.; Zuffardi, O.; Gulisano, M. Genomic organization and chromosomal localization of the mouse connexin36 (*mCx36*) gene. *Gene* **2000**, *251*, 123–130. [CrossRef]
22. Von Maltzahn, J.; Euwens, C.; Willecke, K.; Söhl, G. The novel mouse connexin39 gene is expressed in developing striated muscle fibers. *J. Cell Sci.* **2004**, *117*, 5381–5392. [CrossRef] [PubMed]
23. Hombach, S.; Janssen-Bienhold, U.; Sohl, G.; Schubert, T.; Bussow, H.; Ott, T.; Weiler, R.; Willecke, K. Functional expression of connexin57 in horizontal cells of the mouse retina. *Eur. J. Neurosci.* **2004**, *19*, 2633–2640. [CrossRef] [PubMed]
24. Söhl, G.; Joussen, A.; Kociok, N.; Willecke, K. Expression of connexin genes in the human retina. *BMC Ophthalmol.* **2010**, *10*, 27. [CrossRef] [PubMed]
25. Oyamada, M.; Takebe, K.; Oyamada, Y. Regulation of connexin expression by transcription factors and epigenetic mechanisms. *Biochim. Biophys. Acta Biomembr.* **2013**, *1828*, 118–133. [CrossRef] [PubMed]
26. Neuhaus, I.M.; Bone, L.; Wang, S.; Ionasescu, V.; Werner, R. The human connexin32 gene is transcribed from two tissue-specific promoters. *Biosci. Rep.* **1996**, *16*, 239–248. [CrossRef] [PubMed]
27. Murphy, S.M.; Polke, J.; Manji, H.; Blake, J.; Reiniger, L.; Sweeney, M.; Houlden, H.; Brandner, S.; Reilly, M.M. A novel mutation in the nerve-specific 5′ UTR of the GJB1 gene causes X-linked charcot-marie-tooth disease. *J. Peripher. Nerv. Syst. JPNS* **2011**, *16*, 65–70. [CrossRef] [PubMed]
28. Kulshrestha, R.; Burton-Jones, S.; Antoniadi, T.; Rogers, M.; Jaunmuktane, Z.; Brandner, S.; Kiely, N.; Manuel, R.; Willis, T. Deletion of p2 promoter of *GJB1* gene a cause of charcot-marie-tooth disease. *Neuromuscul. Disord. NMD* **2017**, *27*, 766–770. [CrossRef] [PubMed]
29. Al-Yahyaee, S.A.; Al-Kindi, M.; Jonghe, P.D.; Al-Asmi, A.; Al-Futaisi, A.; Vriendt, E.D.; Deconinck, T.; Chand, P. Pelizaeus-merzbacher-like disease in a family with variable phenotype and a novel splicing *GJC2* mutation. *J. Child Neurol.* **2013**, *28*, 1467–1473. [CrossRef] [PubMed]
30. Gandia, M.; Del Castillo, F.J.; Rodriguez-Alvarez, F.J.; Garrido, G.; Villamar, M.; Calderon, M.; Moreno-Pelayo, M.A.; Moreno, F.; del Castillo, I. A novel splice-site mutation in the *GJB2* gene causing mild postlingual hearing impairment. *PLoS ONE* **2013**, *8*, e73566. [CrossRef] [PubMed]
31. Kandouz, M.; Bier, A.; Carystinos, G.D.; Alaoui-Jamali, M.A.; Batist, G. Connexin43 pseudogene is expressed in tumor cells and inhibits growth. *Oncogene* **2004**, *23*, 4763–4770. [CrossRef] [PubMed]
32. Bier, A.; Oviedo-Landaverde, I.; Zhao, J.; Mamane, Y.; Kandouz, M.; Batist, G. Connexin43 pseudogene in breast cancer cells offers a novel therapeutic target. *Mol. Cancer Ther.* **2009**, *8*, 786–793. [CrossRef] [PubMed]
33. Hong, H.M.; Yang, J.J.; Shieh, J.C.; Lin, M.L.; Li, S.Y. Novel mutations in the connexin43 (*GJA1*) and *GJA1* pseudogene may contribute to nonsyndromic hearing loss. *Hum. Genet.* **2010**, *127*, 545–551. [CrossRef] [PubMed]

34. Poliseno, L.; Salmena, L.; Zhang, J.; Carver, B.; Haveman, W.J.; Pandolfi, P.P. A coding-independent function of gene and pseudogene mRNAs regulates tumour biology. *Nature* **2010**, *465*, 1033–1038. [CrossRef] [PubMed]
35. Rackauskas, M.; Neverauskas, V.; Skeberdis, V.A. Diversity and properties of connexin gap junction channels (review). *Medicina (Kaunas Lithuania)* **2010**, *46*, 1–12. [PubMed]
36. Di, W.L.; Rugg, E.L.; Leigh, I.M.; Kelsell, D.P. Multiple epidermal connexins are expressed in different keratinocyte subpopulations including connexin 31. *J. Investig. Dermatol.* **2001**, *117*, 958–964. [CrossRef] [PubMed]
37. Scott, C.A.; Tattersall, D.; O'Toole, E.A.; Kelsell, D.P. Connexins in epidermal homeostasis and skin disease. *Biochim. Biophys. Acta* **2012**, *1818*, 1952–1961. [CrossRef] [PubMed]
38. Faniku, C.; Wright, C.S.; Martin, P.E. Connexins and pannexins in the integumentary system: The skin and appendages. *Cell. Mol. Life Sci. CMLS* **2015**, *72*, 2937–2947. [CrossRef] [PubMed]
39. Lilly, E.; Sellitto, C.; Milstone, L.M.; White, T.W. Connexin channels in congenital skin disorders. *Semin. Cell Dev. Biol.* **2016**, *50*, 4–12. [CrossRef] [PubMed]
40. Tu, Z.J.; Kiang, D.T. Mapping and characterization of the basal promoter of the human connexin26 gene. *Biochim. Biophys. Acta* **1998**, *1443*, 169–181. [CrossRef]
41. Bai, S.; Spray, D.C.; Burk, R.D. Identification of proximal and distal regulatory elements of the rat connexin32 gene. *BBA Gene Struct. Expr.* **1993**, *1216*, 197–204. [CrossRef]
42. Field, J.M.L.; Tate, L.A.; Chipman, J.K.; Minchin, S.D. Identification of functional regulatory regions of the connexin32 gene promoter. *Biochim. Biophys. Acta Gene Struct. Expr.* **2003**, *1628*, 22–29. [CrossRef]
43. Seul, K.H.; Tadros, P.N.; Beyer, E.C. Mouse connexin40: Gene structure and promoter analysis. *Genomics* **1997**, *46*, 120–126. [CrossRef] [PubMed]
44. Bierhuizen, M.F.A.; Van Amersfoorth, S.C.M.; Groenewegen, W.A.; Vliex, S.; Jongsma, H.J. Characterization of the rat connexin40 promoter: Two Sp1/Sp3 binding sites contribute to transcriptional activation. *Cardiovasc. Res.* **2000**, *46*, 511–522. [CrossRef]
45. Echetebu, C.O.; Ali, M.; Izban, M.G.; MacKay, L.; Garfield, R.E. Localization of regulatory protein binding sites in the proximal region of human myometrial connexin 43 gene. *Mol. Hum. Reprod.* **1999**, *5*, 757–766. [CrossRef] [PubMed]
46. Teunissen, B.E.J.; van Amersfoorth, S.C.M.; Opthof, T.; Jongsma, H.J.; Bierhuizen, M.F.A. Sp1 and Sp3 activate the rat connexin40 proximal promoter. *Biochem. Biophys. Res. Commun.* **2002**, *292*, 71–78. [CrossRef] [PubMed]
47. Linhares, V.L.F.; Almeida, N.A.S.; Menezes, D.C.; Elliott, D.A.; Lai, D.; Beyer, E.C.; Campos De Carvalho, A.C.; Costa, M.W. Transcriptional regulation of the murine connexin40 promoter by cardiac factors nkx2-5, gata4 and tbx5. *Cardiovasc. Res.* **2004**, *64*, 402–411. [CrossRef] [PubMed]
48. Geimonen, E.; Boylston, E.; Royek, A.; Andersen, J. Elevated connexin-43 expression in term human myometrium correlates with elevated C-jun expression and is independent of myometrial estrogen receptors. *J. Clin. Endocrinol. Metab.* **1998**, *83*, 1177–1185. [CrossRef] [PubMed]
49. Fernandez-Cobo, M.; Stewart, D.; Drujan, D.; De Maio, A. Promoter activity of the rat connexin 43 gene in nrk cells. *J. Cell. Biochem.* **2001**, *81*, 514–522. [CrossRef]
50. Teunissen, B.E.J.; Jansen, A.T.; Van Amersfoorth, S.C.M.; O'Brien, T.X.; Jongsma, H.J.; Bierhuizen, M.F.A. Analysis of the rat connexin 43 proximal promoter in neonatal cardiomyocytes. *Gene* **2003**, *322*, 123–136. [CrossRef] [PubMed]
51. Vine, A.L.; Leung, Y.M.; Bertram, J.S. Transcriptional regulation of connexin 43 expression by retinoids and carotenoids: Similarities and differences. *Mol. Carcinog.* **2005**, *43*, 75–85. [CrossRef] [PubMed]
52. Hernandez, M.; Shao, Q.; Yang, X.J.; Luh, S.P.; Kandouz, M.; Batist, G.; Laird, D.W.; Alaoui-Jamali, M.A. A histone deacetylation-dependent mechanism for transcriptional repression of the gap junction gene *cx43* in prostate cancer cells. *Prostate* **2006**, *66*, 1151–1161. [CrossRef] [PubMed]
53. Villares, G.J.; Dobroff, A.S.; Wang, H.; Zigler, M.; Melnikova, V.O.; Huang, L.; Bar-Eli, M. Overexpression of protease-activated receptor-1 contributes to melanoma metastasis via regulation of connexin 43. *Cancer Res.* **2009**, *69*, 6730–6737. [CrossRef] [PubMed]
54. Geimonen, E.; Jiang, W.; Ali, M.; Fishman, G.I.; Garfield, R.E.; Andersen, J. Activation of protein kinase c in human uterine smooth muscle induces connexin-43 gene transcription through an AP-1 site in the promoter sequence. *J. Biol. Chem.* **1996**, *271*, 23667–23674. [CrossRef] [PubMed]

55. Ghouili, F.; Martin, L.J. Cooperative regulation of GJA1 expression by members of the AP-1 family cjun and cfos in TM3 leydig and TM4 sertoli cells. *Gene* **2017**, *635*, 24–32. [CrossRef] [PubMed]
56. Baldridge, D.; Lecanda, F.; Shin, C.S.; Stains, J.; Civitelli, R. Sequence and structure of the mouse connexin45 gene. *Biosci. Rep.* **2001**, *21*, 683–689. [CrossRef] [PubMed]
57. Van der Heyden, M.A.; Rook, M.B.; Hermans, M.M.; Rijksen, G.; Boonstra, J.; Defize, L.H.; Destree, O.H. Identification of connexin43 as a functional target for Wnt signalling. *J. Cell Sci.* **1998**, *111 Pt 12*, 1741–1749. [PubMed]
58. Ai, Z.; Fischer, A.; Spray, D.C.; Brown, A.M.; Fishman, G.I. Wnt-1 regulation of connexin43 in cardiac myocytes. *J. Clin. Investig.* **2000**, *105*, 161–171. [CrossRef] [PubMed]
59. Teunissen, B.E.; Bierhuizen, M.F. Transcriptional control of myocardial connexins. *Cardiovasc. Res.* **2004**, *62*, 246–255. [CrossRef] [PubMed]
60. Koffler, L.D.; Fernstrom, M.J.; Akiyama, T.E.; Gonzalez, F.J.; Ruch, R.J. Positive regulation of connexin32 transcription by hepatocyte nuclear factor-1α. *Arch. Biochem. Biophys.* **2002**, *407*, 160–167. [CrossRef]
61. Rukstalis, J.M.; Kowalik, A.; Zhu, L.; Lidington, D.; Pin, C.L.; Konieczny, S.F. Exocrine specific expression of connexin32 is dependent on the basic helix-loop-helix transcription factor mist1. *J. Cell Sci.* **2003**, *116*, 3315–3325. [CrossRef] [PubMed]
62. Bondurand, N.; Girard, M.; Pingault, V.; Lemort, N.; Dubourg, O.; Goossens, M. Human connexin 32, a gap junction protein altered in the X-linked form of charcot-marie-tooth disease, is directly regulated by the transcription factor SOX10. *Hum. Mol. Genet.* **2001**, *10*, 2783–2795. [CrossRef] [PubMed]
63. Petrocelli, T.; Lye, S.J. Regulation of transcripts encoding the myometrial gap junction protein, connexin-43, by estrogen and progesterone. *Endocrinology* **1993**, *133*, 284–290. [CrossRef] [PubMed]
64. Recouvreux, M.S.; Grasso, E.N.; Echeverria, P.C.; Rocha-Viegas, L.; Castilla, L.H.; Schere-Levy, C.; Tocci, J.M.; Kordon, E.C.; Rubinstein, N. RUNX1 and FOXP3 interplay regulates expression of breast cancer related genes. *Oncotarget* **2016**, *7*, 6552–6565. [CrossRef] [PubMed]
65. Vinken, M. Regulation of connexin signaling by the epigenetic machinery. *Biochim. Biophys. Acta* **2015**, *1859*, 262–268. [CrossRef] [PubMed]
66. Chen, Y.; Huhn, D.; Knosel, T.; Pacyna-Gengelbach, M.; Deutschmann, N.; Petersen, I. Downregulation of connexin 26 in human lung cancer is related to promoter methylation. *Int. J. Cancer* **2005**, *113*, 14–21. [CrossRef] [PubMed]
67. Tan, L.W.; Bianco, T.; Dobrovic, A. Variable promoter region cpg island methylation of the putative tumor suppressor gene connexin 26 in breast cancer. *Carcinogenesis* **2002**, *23*, 231–236. [CrossRef] [PubMed]
68. Hirai, A.; Yano, T.; Nishikawa, K.; Suzuki, K.; Asano, R.; Satoh, H.; Hagiwara, K.; Yamasaki, H. Down-regulation of connexin 32 gene expression through DNA methylation in a human renal cell carcinoma cell. *Am. J. Nephrol.* **2003**, *23*, 172–177. [CrossRef] [PubMed]
69. Chen, J.T.; Cheng, Y.W.; Chou, M.C.; Sen-Lin, T.; Lai, W.W.; Ho, W.L.; Lee, H. The correlation between aberrant connexin 43 mRNA expression induced by promoter methylation and nodal micrometastasis in non-small cell lung cancer. *Clin. Cancer Res.* **2003**, *9*, 4200–4204. [PubMed]
70. Wang, Y.; Huang, L.H.; Xu, C.X.; Xiao, J.; Zhou, L.; Cao, D.; Liu, X.M.; Qi, Y. Connexin 32 and 43 promoter methylation in helicobacter pylori-associated gastric tumorigenesis. *World J. Gastroenterol. WJG* **2014**, *20*, 11770–11779. [CrossRef] [PubMed]
71. Yi, Z.C.; Wang, H.; Zhang, G.Y.; Xia, B. Downregulation of connexin 43 in nasopharyngeal carcinoma cells is related to promoter methylation. *Oral Oncol.* **2007**, *43*, 898–904. [CrossRef] [PubMed]
72. Sirnes, S.; Honne, H.; Ahmed, D.; Danielsen, S.A.; Rognum, T.O.; Meling, G.I.; Leithe, E.; Rivedal, E.; Lothe, R.A.; Lind, G.E. DNA methylation analyses of the connexin gene family reveal silencing of *GJC1* (connexin45) by promoter hypermethylation in colorectal cancer. *Epigenetics* **2011**, *6*, 602–609. [CrossRef] [PubMed]
73. Ogawa, T.; Hayashi, T.; Tokunou, M.; Nakachi, K.; Trosko, J.E.; Chang, C.C.; Yorioka, N. Suberoylanilide hydroxamic acid enhances gap junctional intercellular communication via acetylation of histone containing connexin 43 gene locus. *Cancer Res.* **2005**, *65*, 9771–9778. [CrossRef] [PubMed]
74. Xu, Q.; Lin, X.; Andrews, L.; Patel, D.; Lampe, P.D.; Veenstra, R.D. Histone deacetylase inhibition reduces cardiac connexin43 expression and gap junction communication. *Front. Pharmacol.* **2013**, *4*, 44. [CrossRef] [PubMed]

75. Zhao, W.; Han, H.B.; Zhang, Z.Q. Suppression of lung cancer cell invasion and metastasis by connexin43 involves the secretion of follistatin-like 1 mediated via histone acetylation. *Int. J. Biochem. Cell Biol.* **2011**, *43*, 1459–1468. [CrossRef] [PubMed]
76. Hohl, M.; Thiel, G. Cell type-specific regulation of RE-1 silencing transcription factor (REST) target genes. *Eur. J. Neurosci.* **2005**, *22*, 2216–2230. [CrossRef] [PubMed]
77. Colussi, C.; Rosati, J.; Straino, S.; Spallotta, F.; Berni, R.; Stilli, D.; Rossi, S.; Musso, E.; Macchi, E.; Mai, A.; et al. Nepsilon-lysine acetylation determines dissociation from gap junctions and lateralization of connexin 43 in normal and dystrophic heart. *Proc. Natl. Acad. Sci. USA* **2011**, *108*, 2795–2800. [CrossRef] [PubMed]
78. Colussi, C.; Berni, R.; Rosati, J.; Straino, S.; Vitale, S.; Spallotta, F.; Baruffi, S.; Bocchi, L.; Delucchi, F.; Rossi, S.; et al. The histone deacetylase inhibitor suberoylanilide hydroxamic acid reduces cardiac arrhythmias in dystrophic mice. *Cardiovasc. Res.* **2010**, *87*, 73–82. [CrossRef] [PubMed]
79. Forster, T.; Rausch, V.; Zhang, Y.; Isayev, O.; Heilmann, K.; Schoensiegel, F.; Liu, L.; Nessling, M.; Richter, K.; Labsch, S.; et al. Sulforaphane counteracts aggressiveness of pancreatic cancer driven by dysregulated CX43-mediated gap junctional intercellular communication. *Oncotarget* **2014**, *5*, 1621–1634. [CrossRef] [PubMed]
80. Salat-Canela, C.; Munoz, M.J.; Sese, M.; Ramon y Cajal, S.; Aasen, T. Post-transcriptional regulation of connexins. *Biochem. Soc. Trans.* **2015**, *43*, 465–470. [CrossRef] [PubMed]
81. Ming, J.; Zhou, Y.; Du, J.; Fan, S.; Pan, B.; Wang, Y.; Fan, L.; Jiang, J. Identification of miR-200a as a novel suppressor of connexin 43 in breast cancer cells. *Biosci. Rep.* **2015**, *35*. [CrossRef] [PubMed]
82. Li, X.; Pan, J.H.; Song, B.; Xiong, E.Q.; Chen, Z.W.; Zhou, Z.S.; Su, Y.P. Suppression of CX43 expression by miR-20a in the progression of human prostate cancer. *Cancer Biol. Ther.* **2012**, *13*, 890–898. [CrossRef] [PubMed]
83. Hao, J.; Zhang, C.; Zhang, A.; Wang, K.; Jia, Z.; Wang, G.; Han, L.; Kang, C.; Pu, P. MiR-221/222 is the regulator of CX43 expression in human glioblastoma cells. *Oncol. Rep.* **2012**, *27*, 1504–1510. [CrossRef] [PubMed]
84. Anderson, C.; Catoe, H.; Werner, R. MiR-206 regulates connexin43 expression during skeletal muscle development. *Nucleic Acids Res.* **2006**, *34*, 5863–5871. [CrossRef] [PubMed]
85. Hak, K.K.; Yong, S.L.; Sivaprasad, U.; Malhotra, A.; Dutta, A. Muscle-specific microRNA miR-206 promotes muscle differentiation. *J. Cell Biol.* **2006**, *174*, 677–687. [CrossRef]
86. Yang, B.; Lin, H.; Xiao, J.; Lu, Y.; Luo, X.; Li, B.; Zhang, Y.; Xu, C.; Bai, Y.; Wang, H.; et al. The muscle-specific microRNA miR-1 regulates cardiac arrhythmogenic potential by targeting *GJA1* and *KCNJ2*. *Nat. Med.* **2007**, *13*, 486–491. [CrossRef] [PubMed]
87. Rau, F.; Freyermuth, F.; Fugier, C.; Villemin, J.P.; Fischer, M.C.; Jost, B.; Dembele, D.; Gourdon, G.; Nicole, A.; Duboc, D.; et al. Misregulation of miR-1 processing is associated with heart defects in myotonic dystrophy. *Nat. Struct. Mol. Biol.* **2011**, *18*, 840–845. [CrossRef] [PubMed]
88. Wu, Y.; Ma, X.J.; Wang, H.J.; Li, W.C.; Chen, L.; Ma, D.; Huang, G.Y. Expression of CX43-related microRNAs in patients with tetralogy of fallot. *World J. Pediatr. WJP* **2014**, *10*, 138–144. [CrossRef] [PubMed]
89. Imamura, M.; Sugino, Y.; Long, X.; Slivano, O.J.; Nishikawa, N.; Yoshimura, N.; Miano, J.M. Myocardin and microRNA-1 modulate bladder activity through connexin 43 expression during post-natal development. *J. Cell. Physiol.* **2013**, *228*, 1819–1826. [CrossRef] [PubMed]
90. Donahue, H.J.; Qu, R.W.; Genetos, D.C. Joint diseases: From connexins to gap junctions. *Nat. Rev. Rheumatol.* **2017**, *14*, 42–51. [CrossRef] [PubMed]
91. Gindin, Y.; Jiang, Y.; Francis, P.; Walker, R.L.; Abaan, O.D.; Zhu, Y.J.; Meltzer, P.S. MiR-23a impairs bone differentiation in osteosarcoma via down-regulation of *GJA1*. *Front. Genet.* **2015**, *6*, 233. [CrossRef] [PubMed]
92. Sun, Y.X.; Zhang, J.F.; Xu, J.; Xu, L.L.; Wu, T.Y.; Wang, B.; Pan, X.H.; Li, G. MicroRNA-144-3p inhibits bone formation in distraction osteogenesis through targeting connexin 43. *Oncotarget* **2017**, *8*, 89913–89922. [CrossRef] [PubMed]
93. Davis, H.M.; Pacheco-Costa, R.; Atkinson, E.G.; Brun, L.R.; Gortazar, A.R.; Harris, J.; Hiasa, M.; Bolarinwa, S.A.; Yoneda, T.; Ivan, M.; et al. Disruption of the CX43/miR21 pathway leads to osteocyte apoptosis and increased osteoclastogenesis with aging. *Aging Cell* **2017**, *16*, 551–563. [CrossRef] [PubMed]
94. Plotkin, L.I.; Pacheco-Costa, R.; Davis, H.M. MicroRNAs and connexins in bone: Interaction and mechanisms of delivery. *Curr. Mol. Biol. Rep.* **2017**, *3*, 63–70. [CrossRef] [PubMed]

95. Ale-Agha, N.; Galban, S.; Sobieroy, C.; Abdelmohsen, K.; Gorospe, M.; Sies, H.; Klotz, L.O. Hur regulates gap junctional intercellular communication by controlling β-catenin levels and adherens junction integrity. *Hepatology* **2009**, *50*, 1567–1576. [CrossRef] [PubMed]
96. Lee, K.W.; Chun, K.S.; Lee, J.S.; Kang, K.S.; Surh, Y.J.; Lee, H.J. Inhibition of cyclooxygenase-2 expression and restoration of gap junction intercellular communication in h-ras-transformed rat liver epithelial cells by caffeic acid phenethyl ester. *Ann. N. Y. Acad. Sci.* **2004**, *1030*, 501–507. [CrossRef] [PubMed]
97. Ul-Hussain, M.; Dermietzel, R.; Zoidl, G. Connexins and cap-independent translation: Role of internal ribosome entry sites. *Brain Res.* **2012**, *1487*, 99–106. [CrossRef] [PubMed]
98. Werner, R. IRES elements in connexin genes: A hypothesis explaining the need for connexins to be regulated at the translational level. *IUBMB Life* **2000**, *50*, 173–176. [CrossRef] [PubMed]
99. Schiavi, A.; Hudder, A.; Werner, R. Connexin43 mRNA contains a functional internal ribosome entry site. *FEBS Lett.* **1999**, *464*, 118–122. [CrossRef]
100. Hudder, A.; Werner, R. Analysis of a charcot-marie-tooth disease mutation reveals an essential internal ribosome entry site element in the connexin-32 gene. *J. Biol. Chem.* **2000**, *275*, 34586–34591. [CrossRef] [PubMed]
101. Lahlou, H.; Fanjul, M.; Pradayrol, L.; Susini, C.; Pyronnet, S. Restoration of functional gap junctions through internal ribosome entry site-dependent synthesis of endogenous connexins in density-inhibited cancer cells. *Mol. Cell. Biol.* **2005**, *25*, 4034–4045. [CrossRef] [PubMed]
102. Martinez-Salas, E.; Lozano, G.; Fernandez-Chamorro, J.; Francisco-Velilla, R.; Galan, A.; Diaz, R. RNA-binding proteins impacting on internal initiation of translation. *Int. J. Mol. Sci.* **2013**, *14*, 21705–21726. [CrossRef] [PubMed]
103. Faye, M.D.; Holcik, M. The role of IRES trans-acting factors in carcinogenesis. *Biochim. Biophys. Acta* **2015**, *1849*, 887–897. [CrossRef] [PubMed]
104. Komar, A.A.; Mazumder, B.; Merrick, W.C. A new framework for understanding IRES-mediated translation. *Gene* **2012**, *502*, 75–86. [CrossRef] [PubMed]
105. Thompson, S.R. So you want to know if your message has an IRES? *Wiley Interdiscip. Rev. RNA* **2012**, *3*, 697–705. [CrossRef] [PubMed]
106. Lauring, A.S.; Overbaugh, J. Evidence that an IRES within the Notch2 coding region can direct expression of a nuclear form of the protein. *Mol. Cell* **2000**, *6*, 939–945. [CrossRef]
107. Ul-Hussain, M.; Zoidl, G.; Klooster, J.; Kamermans, M.; Dermietzel, R. IRES-mediated translation of the carboxy-terminal domain of the horizontal cell specific connexin CX55.5 in vivo and in vitro. *BMC Mol. Biol.* **2008**, *9*, 52. [CrossRef] [PubMed]
108. Ul-Hussain, M.; Dermietzel, R.; Zoidl, G. Characterization of the internal IRES element of the zebrafish connexin55.5 reveals functional implication of the polypyrimidine tract binding protein. *BMC Mol. Biol.* **2008**, *9*, 92. [CrossRef] [PubMed]
109. Joshi-Mukherjee, R.; Coombs, W.; Burrer, C.; de Mora, I.A.; Delmar, M.; Taffet, S.M. Evidence for the presence of a free C-terminal fragment of cx43 in cultured cells. *Cell Commun. Adhes.* **2007**, *14*, 75–84. [CrossRef] [PubMed]
110. Smyth, J.W.; Shaw, R.M. Autoregulation of connexin43 gap junction formation by internally translated isoforms. *Cell Rep.* **2013**, *5*, 611–618. [CrossRef] [PubMed]
111. Salat-Canela, C.; Sese, M.; Peula, C.; Ramon y Cajal, S.; Aasen, T. Internal translation of the connexin 43 transcript. *Cell Commun. Signal.* **2014**, *12*, 31. [CrossRef] [PubMed]
112. Ul-Hussain, M.; Olk, S.; Schoenebeck, B.; Wasielewski, B.; Meier, C.; Prochnow, N.; May, C.; Galozzi, S.; Marcus, K.; Zoidl, G.; et al. Internal ribosomal entry site (IRES) activity generates endogenous carboxyl-terminal domains of CX43 and is responsive to hypoxic conditions. *J. Biol. Chem.* **2014**, *289*, 20979–20990. [CrossRef] [PubMed]
113. Basheer, W.A.; Xiao, S.; Epifantseva, I.; Fu, Y.; Kleber, A.G.; Hong, T.; Shaw, R.M. GJA1-20k arranges actin to guide CX43 delivery to cardiac intercalated discs. *Circ. Res.* **2017**, *121*, 1069–1080. [CrossRef] [PubMed]
114. Fu, Y.; Zhang, S.S.; Xiao, S.; Basheer, W.A.; Baum, R.; Epifantseva, I.; Hong, T.; Shaw, R.M. Cx43 isoform GJA1-20k promotes microtubule dependent mitochondrial transport. *Front. Physiol.* **2017**, *8*, 905. [CrossRef] [PubMed]
115. Maqbool, R.; Rashid, R.; Ismail, R.; Niaz, S.; Chowdri, N.A.; Hussain, M.U. The carboxy-terminal domain of connexin 43 (CT-CX43) modulates the expression of p53 by altering miR-125b expression in low-grade human breast cancers. *Cell. Oncol.* **2015**, *38*, 443–451. [CrossRef] [PubMed]

116. Foote, C.I.; Zhou, L.; Zhu, X.; Nicholson, B.J. The pattern of disulfide linkages in the extracellular loop regions of connexin 32 suggests a model for the docking interface of gap junctions. *J. Cell Biol.* **1998**, *140*, 1187–1197. [CrossRef] [PubMed]
117. Johnstone, S.R.; Billaud, M.; Lohman, A.W.; Taddeo, E.P.; Isakson, B.E. Posttranslational modifications in connexins and pannexins. *J. Membr. Biol.* **2012**, *245*, 319–332. [CrossRef] [PubMed]
118. Solan, J.L.; Lampe, P.D. Specific Cx43 phosphorylation events regulate gap junction turnover in vivo. *FEBS Lett.* **2014**, *588*, 1423–1429. [CrossRef] [PubMed]
119. Pogoda, K.; Kameritsch, P.; Retamal, M.A.; Vega, J.L. Regulation of gap junction channels and hemichannels by phosphorylation and redox changes: A revision. *BMC Cell Biol.* **2016**, *17* (Suppl. 1), 11. [CrossRef] [PubMed]
120. Lampe, P.D.; Lau, A.F. The effects of connexin phosphorylation on gap junctional communication. *Int. J. Biochem. Cell Biol.* **2004**, *36*, 1171–1186. [CrossRef]
121. Solan, J.L.; Lampe, P.D. Connexin phosphorylation as a regulatory event linked to gap junction channel assembly. *Biochim. Biophys. Acta* **2005**, *1711*, 154–163. [CrossRef] [PubMed]
122. Saez, J.C.; Martinez, A.D.; Branes, M.C.; Gonzalez, H.E. Regulation of gap junctions by protein phosphorylation. *Braz. J. Med. Biol. Res.* **1998**, *31*, 593–600. [CrossRef] [PubMed]
123. Stultz, C.M.; Levin, A.D.; Edelman, E.R. Phosphorylation-induced conformational changes in a mitogen-activated protein kinase substrate. Implications for tyrosine hydroxylase activation. *J. Biol. Chem.* **2002**, *277*, 47653–47661. [CrossRef] [PubMed]
124. Diestel, S.; Eckert, R.; Hülser, D.; Traub, O. Exchange of serine residues 263 and 266 reduces the function of mouse gap junction protein connexin31 and exhibits a dominant-negative effect on the wild-type protein in hela cells. *Exp. Cell Res.* **2004**, *294*, 446–457. [CrossRef] [PubMed]
125. Qin, J.; Chang, M.; Wang, S.; Liu, Z.; Zhu, W.; Wang, Y.; Yan, F.; Li, J.; Zhang, B.; Dou, G.; et al. Connexin 32-mediated cell-cell communication is essential for hepatic differentiation from human embryonic stem cells. *Sci. Rep.* **2016**, *6*, 37388. [CrossRef] [PubMed]
126. Ghosh, P.; Ghosh, S.; Das, S. Self-regulation of rat liver gap junction by phosphorylation. *Biochim. Biophys. Acta* **2002**, *1564*, 500–504. [CrossRef]
127. Ghosh, P. Self-phosphorylation modulates the gating of rat liver gap junction channels: A nonstationary noise analysis. *Biophys. Chem.* **2007**, *127*, 97–102. [CrossRef] [PubMed]
128. Jacobsen, N.L.; Pontifex, T.K.; Li, H.; Solan, J.L.; Lampe, P.D.; Sorgen, P.L.; Burt, J.M. Regulation of cx37 channel and growth-suppressive properties by phosphorylation. *J. Cell Sci.* **2017**, *130*, 3308–3321. [CrossRef] [PubMed]
129. Bao, M.; Kanter, E.M.; Huang, R.Y.; Maxeiner, S.; Frank, M.; Zhang, Y.; Schuessler, R.B.; Smith, T.W.; Townsend, R.R.; Rohrs, H.W.; et al. Residual Cx45 and its relationship to Cx43 in murine ventricular myocardium. *Channels (Austin)* **2011**, *5*, 489–499. [CrossRef] [PubMed]
130. Johnstone, S.R.; Ross, J.; Rizzo, M.J.; Straub, A.C.; Lampe, P.D.; Leitinger, N.; Isakson, B.E. Oxidized phospholipid species promote in vivo differential Cx43 phosphorylation and vascular smooth muscle cell proliferation. *Am. J. Pathol.* **2009**, *175*, 916–924. [CrossRef] [PubMed]
131. Johnstone, S.R.; Kroncke, B.M.; Straub, A.C.; Best, A.K.; Dunn, C.A.; Mitchell, L.A.; Peskova, Y.; Nakamoto, R.K.; Koval, M.; Lo, C.W.; et al. Mapk phosphorylation of connexin 43 promotes binding of cyclin e and smooth muscle cell proliferation. *Circ. Res.* **2012**, *111*, 201–211. [CrossRef] [PubMed]
132. Pelletier, R.M.; Akpovi, C.D.; Chen, L.; Kumar, N.M.; Vitale, M.L. Complementary expression and phosphorylation of Cx46 and Cx50 during development and following gene deletion in mouse and in normal and orchitic mink testes. *Am. J. Physiol. Regul. Integr. Comp. Physiol.* **2015**, *309*, R255–R276. [CrossRef] [PubMed]
133. Walter, W.J.; Zeilinger, C.; Bintig, W.; Kolb, H.A.; Ngezahayo, A. Phosphorylation in the C-terminus of the rat connexin46 (rCx46) and regulation of the conducting activity of the formed connexons. *J. Bioenergy Biomembr.* **2008**, *40*, 397–405. [CrossRef] [PubMed]
134. Liu, J.; Ek Vitorin, J.F.; Weintraub, S.T.; Gu, S.; Shi, Q.; Burt, J.M.; Jiang, J.X. Phosphorylation of connexin 50 by protein kinase a enhances gap junction and hemichannel function. *J. Biol. Chem.* **2011**, *286*, 16914–16928. [CrossRef] [PubMed]
135. May, D.; Tress, O.; Seifert, G.; Willecke, K. Connexin47 protein phosphorylation and stability in oligodendrocytes depend on expression of connexin43 protein in astrocytes. *J. Neurosci.* **2013**, *33*, 7985–7996. [CrossRef] [PubMed]

136. Traub, O.; Look, J.; Dermietzel, R.; Brummer, F.; Hulser, D.; Willecke, K. Comparative characterization of the 21-kD and 26-kD gap junction proteins in murine liver and cultured hepatocytes. *J. Cell Biol.* **1989**, *108*, 1039–1051. [CrossRef] [PubMed]
137. Elvira, M.; Díez, J.A.; Wang, K.K.; Villalobo, A. Phosphorylation of connexin-32 by protein kinase C prevents its proteolysis by mu-calpain and m-calpain. *J. Biol. Chem.* **1993**, *268*, 14294–14300. [PubMed]
138. Locke, D.; Koreen, I.V.; Harris, A.L. Isoelectric points and post-translational modifications of connexin26 and connexin32. *FASEB J.* **2006**, *20*, 1221–1223. [CrossRef] [PubMed]
139. Locke, D.; Bian, S.; Li, H.; Harris, A.L. Post-translational modifications of connexin26 revealed by mass spectrometry. *Biochem. J.* **2009**, *424*, 385–398. [CrossRef] [PubMed]
140. Berthoud, V.M.; Beyer, E.C.; Kurata, W.E.; Lau, A.F.; Lampe, P.D. The gap-junction protein connexin 56 is phosphorylated in the intracellular loop and the carboxy-terminal region. *Eur. J. Biochem.* **1997**, *244*, 89–97. [CrossRef] [PubMed]
141. Ouyang, X.; Winbow, V.M.; Patel, L.S.; Burr, G.S.; Mitchell, C.K.; O'Brien, J. Protein kinase a mediates regulation of gap junctions containing connexin35 through a complex pathway. *Brain Res. Mol. Brain Res.* **2005**, *135*, 1–11. [CrossRef] [PubMed]
142. Johnstone, S.; Isakson, B.; Locke, D. Biological and biophysical properties of vascular connexin channels. *Int. Rev. Cell Mol. Biol.* **2009**, *278*, 69–118. [CrossRef] [PubMed]
143. Solan, J.L.; Lampe, P.D. Connexin43 phosphorylation: Structural changes and biological effects. *Biochem. J.* **2009**, *419*, 261–272. [CrossRef] [PubMed]
144. Chen, V.C.; Gouw, J.W.; Naus, C.C.; Foster, L.J. Connexin multi-site phosphorylation: Mass spectrometry-based proteomics fills the gap. *Biochim. Biophys. Acta* **2013**, *1828*, 23–34. [CrossRef] [PubMed]
145. Sorgen, P.L.; Duffy, H.S.; Spray, D.C.; Delmar, M. Ph-dependent dimerization of the carboxyl terminal domain of cx43. *Biophys. J.* **2004**, *87*, 574–581. [CrossRef] [PubMed]
146. Sorgen, P.L.; Duffy, H.S.; Sahoo, P.; Coombs, W.; Delmar, M.; Spray, D.C. Structural changes in the carboxyl terminus of the gap junction protein connexin43 indicates signaling between binding domains for c-Src and zonula occludens-1. *J. Biol. Chem.* **2004**, *279*, 54695–54701. [CrossRef] [PubMed]
147. Bouvier, D.; Kieken, F.; Kellezi, A.; Sorgen, P.L. Structural changes in the carboxyl terminus of the gap junction protein connexin 40 caused by the interaction with c-Src and zonula occludens-1. *Cell Commun. Adhes.* **2008**, *15*, 107–118. [CrossRef] [PubMed]
148. Solan, J.L.; Lampe, P.D. Spatio-temporal regulation of connexin43 phosphorylation and gap junction dynamics. *Biochim. Biophys. Acta* **2018**, *1860*, 83–90. [CrossRef] [PubMed]
149. Grosely, R.; Kopanic, J.L.; Nabors, S.; Kieken, F.; Spagnol, G.; Al-Mugotir, M.; Zach, S.; Sorgen, P.L. Effects of phosphorylation on the structure and backbone dynamics of the intrinsically disordered connexin43 C-terminal domain. *J. Biol. Chem.* **2013**, *288*, 24857–24870. [CrossRef] [PubMed]
150. Sorgen, P.L.; Duffy, H.S.; Cahill, S.M.; Coombs, W.; Spray, D.C.; Delmar, M.; Girvin, M.E. Sequence-specific resonance assignment of the carboxyl terminal domain of connexin43. *J. Biomol. NMR* **2002**, *23*, 245–246. [CrossRef] [PubMed]
151. Shi, Q.; Banks, E.A.; Yu, X.S.; Gu, S.; Lauer, J.; Fields, G.B.; Jiang, J.X. Amino acid residue val362 plays a critical role in maintaining the structure of C terminus of connexin 50 and in lens epithelial-fiber differentiation. *J. Biol. Chem.* **2010**, *285*, 18415–18422. [CrossRef] [PubMed]
152. Kopanic, J.L.; Sorgen, P.L. Chemical shift assignments of the connexin45 carboxyl terminal domain: Monomer and dimer conformations. *Biomol. NMR Assign.* **2013**, *7*, 293–297. [CrossRef] [PubMed]
153. Kopanic, J.L.; Al-mugotir, M.H.; Kieken, F.; Zach, S.; Trease, A.J.; Sorgen, P.L. Characterization of the connexin45 carboxyl-terminal domain structure and interactions with molecular partners. *Biophys. J.* **2014**, *106*, 2184–2195. [CrossRef] [PubMed]
154. Kyle, J.W.; Berthoud, V.M.; Kurutz, J.; Minogue, P.J.; Greenspan, M.; Hanck, D.A.; Beyer, E.C. The n terminus of connexin37 contains an α-helix that is required for channel function. *J. Biol. Chem.* **2009**, *284*, 20418–20427. [CrossRef] [PubMed]
155. Bouvier, D.; Spagnol, G.; Chenavas, S.; Kieken, F.; Vitrac, H.; Brownell, S.; Kellezi, A.; Forge, V.; Sorgen, P.L. Characterization of the structure and intermolecular interactions between the connexin40 and connexin43 carboxyl-terminal and cytoplasmic loop domains. *J. Biol. Chem.* **2009**, *284*, 34257–34271. [CrossRef] [PubMed]

156. Grosely, R.; Kieken, F.; Sorgen, P.L. ^{1}h, ^{13}c, and ^{15}n backbone resonance assignments of the connexin43 carboxyl terminal domain attached to the 4th transmembrane domain in detergent micelles. *Biomol. NMR Assign.* **2013**, *7*, 299–303. [CrossRef] [PubMed]
157. Sosinsky, G.E.; Solan, J.L.; Gaietta, G.M.; Ngan, L.; Lee, G.J.; Mackey, M.R.; Lampe, P.D. The C-terminus of connexin43 adopts different conformations in the golgi and gap junction as detected with structure-specific antibodies. *Biochem. J.* **2007**, *408*, 375–385. [CrossRef] [PubMed]
158. Grosely, R.; Kieken, F.; Sorgen, P.L. Optimizing the solution conditions to solve the structure of the connexin43 carboxyl terminus attached to the 4(th) transmembrane domain in detergent micelles. *Cell Commun. Adhes.* **2010**, *17*, 23–33. [CrossRef] [PubMed]
159. Hirst-Jensen, B.J.; Sahoo, P.; Kieken, F.; Delmar, M.; Sorgen, P.L. Characterization of the PH-dependent interaction between the gap junction protein connexin43 carboxyl terminus and cytoplasmic loop domains. *J. Biol. Chem.* **2007**, *282*, 5801–5813. [CrossRef] [PubMed]
160. Duffy, H.S.; Sorgen, P.L.; Girvin, M.E.; O'Donnell, P.; Coombs, W.; Taffet, S.M.; Delmar, M.; Spray, D.C. Ph-dependent intramolecular binding and structure involving Cx43 cytoplasmic domains. *J. Biol. Chem.* **2002**, *277*, 36706–36714. [CrossRef] [PubMed]
161. Cohen, P. The regulation of protein function by multisite phosphorylation—A 25 year update. *Trends Biochem. Sci.* **2000**, *25*, 596–601. [CrossRef]
162. Axelsen, L.N.; Calloe, K.; Holstein-Rathlou, N.H.; Nielsen, M.S. Managing the complexity of communication: Regulation of gap junctions by post-translational modification. *Front. Pharmacol.* **2013**, *4*, 130. [CrossRef] [PubMed]
163. Ek-Vitorin, J.F.; Burt, J.M. Structural basis for the selective permeability of channels made of communicating junction proteins. *Biochim. Biophys. Acta* **2013**, *1828*, 51–68. [CrossRef] [PubMed]
164. Moreno, A.P. Connexin phosphorylation as a regulatory event linked to channel gating. *Biochim. Biophys. Acta* **2005**, *1711*, 164–171. [CrossRef] [PubMed]
165. Saez, J.C.; Nairn, A.C.; Czernik, A.J.; Spray, D.C.; Hertzberg, E.L.; Greengard, P.; Bennett, M.V. Phosphorylation of connexin 32, a hepatocyte gap-junction protein, by cAMP-dependent protein kinase, protein kinase C and Ca^{2+}/calmodulin-dependent protein kinase II. *Eur. J. Biochem.* **1990**, *192*, 263–273. [CrossRef] [PubMed]
166. Takeda, A.; Saheki, S.; Shimazu, T.; Takeuchi, N. Phosphorylation of the 27-kDa gap junction protein by protein kinase c in vitro and in rat hepatocytes. *J. Biochem.* **1989**, *106*, 723–727. [CrossRef] [PubMed]
167. Diez, J.A.; Elvira, M.; Villalobo, A. The epidermal growth factor receptor tyrosine kinase phosphorylates connexin32. *Mol. Cell. Biochem.* **1998**, *187*, 201–210. [CrossRef] [PubMed]
168. Kothmann, W.W.; Li, X.; Burr, G.S.; O'Brien, J. Connexin 35/36 is phosphorylated at regulatory sites in the retina. *Vis. Neurosci.* **2007**, *24*, 363–375. [CrossRef] [PubMed]
169. Li, H.; Chuang, A.Z.; O'Brien, J. Photoreceptor coupling is controlled by connexin 35 phosphorylation in zebrafish retina. *J. Neurosci.* **2009**, *29*, 15178–15186. [CrossRef] [PubMed]
170. Patel, L.S.; Mitchell, C.K.; Dubinsky, W.P.; O'Brien, J. Regulation of gap junction coupling through the neuronal connexin Cx35 by nitric oxide and cGMP. *Cell Commun. Adhes.* **2006**, *13*, 41–54. [CrossRef] [PubMed]
171. Li, H.; Chuang, A.Z.; O'Brien, J. Regulation of photoreceptor gap junction phosphorylation by adenosine in zebrafish retina. *Vis. Neurosci.* **2014**, *31*, 237–243. [CrossRef] [PubMed]
172. Kjenseth, A.; Fykerud, T.A.; Sirnes, S.; Bruun, J.; Yohannes, Z.; Kolberg, M.; Omori, Y.; Rivedal, E.; Leithe, E. The gap junction channel protein connexin 43 is covalently modified and regulated by sumoylation. *J. Biol. Chem.* **2012**, *287*, 15851–15861. [CrossRef] [PubMed]
173. Huang, R.Y.; Laing, J.G.; Kanter, E.M.; Berthoud, V.M.; Bao, M.; Rohrs, H.W.; Townsend, R.R.; Yamada, K.A. Identification of CaMKII phosphorylation sites in connexin43 by high-resolution mass spectrometry. *J. Proteome Res.* **2011**, *10*, 1098–1109. [CrossRef] [PubMed]
174. Cottrell, G.T.; Lin, R.; Warn-Cramer, B.J.; Lau, A.F.; Burt, J.M. Mechanism of v-Src- and mitogen-activated protein kinase-induced reduction of gap junction communication. *Am. J. Physiol. Cell Physiol.* **2003**, *284*, C511–C520. [CrossRef] [PubMed]
175. Lin, R.; Warn-Cramer, B.J.; Kurata, W.E.; Lau, A.F. v-Src phosphorylation of connexin 43 on Tyr247 and Tyr265 disrupts gap junctional communication. *J. Cell Biol.* **2001**, *154*, 815–827. [CrossRef] [PubMed]

176. Giepmans, B.N.; Hengeveld, T.; Postma, F.R.; Moolenaar, W.H. Interaction of c-Src with gap junction protein connexin-43. Role in the regulation of cell-cell communication. *J. Biol. Chem.* **2001**, *276*, 8544–8549. [CrossRef] [PubMed]
177. Zhou, L.; Kasperek, E.M.; Nicholson, B.J. Dissection of the molecular basis of pp60(v-Src) induced gating of connexin 43 gap junction channels. *J. Cell Biol.* **1999**, *144*, 1033–1045. [CrossRef] [PubMed]
178. Swenson, K.I.; Piwnica-Worms, H.; McNamee, H.; Paul, D.L. Tyrosine phosphorylation of the gap junction protein connexin43 is required for the pp60v-Src-induced inhibition of communication. *Cell Regul.* **1990**, *1*, 989–1002. [CrossRef] [PubMed]
179. Lampe, P.D.; Kurata, W.E.; Warn-Cramer, B.J.; Lau, A.F. Formation of a distinct connexin43 phosphoisoform in mitotic cells is dependent upon p34cdc2 kinase. *J. Cell Sci.* **1998**, *111 Pt 6*, 833–841. [PubMed]
180. Kanemitsu, M.Y.; Jiang, W.; Eckhart, W. Cdc2-mediated phosphorylation of the gap junction protein, connexin43, during mitosis. *Cell Growth Differ.* **1998**, *9*, 13–21. [PubMed]
181. Sirnes, S.; Kjenseth, A.; Leithe, E.; Rivedal, E. Interplay between pkc and the map kinase pathway in connexin43 phosphorylation and inhibition of gap junction intercellular communication. *Biochem. Biophys. Res. Commun.* **2009**, *382*, 41–45. [CrossRef] [PubMed]
182. Doble, B.W.; Dang, X.; Ping, P.; Fandrich, R.R.; Nickel, B.E.; Jin, Y.; Cattini, P.A.; Kardami, E. Phosphorylation of serine 262 in the gap junction protein connexin-43 regulates DNA synthesis in cell-cell contact forming cardiomyocytes. *J. Cell Sci.* **2004**, *117*, 507–514. [CrossRef] [PubMed]
183. Srisakuldee, W.; Jeyaraman, M.M.; Nickel, B.E.; Tanguy, S.; Jiang, Z.S.; Kardami, E. Phosphorylation of connexin-43 at serine 262 promotes a cardiac injury-resistant state. *Cardiovasc. Res.* **2009**, *83*, 672–681. [CrossRef] [PubMed]
184. Straub, A.C.; Billaud, M.; Johnstone, S.R.; Best, A.K.; Yemen, S.; Dwyer, S.T.; Looft-Wilson, R.; Lysiak, J.J.; Gaston, B.; Palmer, L.; et al. Compartmentalized connexin 43 *S*-nitrosylation/denitrosylation regulates heterocellular communication in the vessel wall. *Arterioscler. Thromb. Vasc. Biol.* **2011**, *31*, 399–407. [CrossRef] [PubMed]
185. Qi, G.J.; Chen, Q.; Chen, L.J.; Shu, Y.; Bu, L.L.; Shao, X.Y.; Zhang, P.; Jiao, F.J.; Shi, J.; Tian, B. Phosphorylation of connexin 43 by cdk5 modulates neuronal migration during embryonic brain development. *Mol. Neurobiol.* **2016**, *53*, 2969–2982. [CrossRef] [PubMed]
186. Procida, K.; Jorgensen, L.; Schmitt, N.; Delmar, M.; Taffet, S.M.; Holstein-Rathlou, N.H.; Nielsen, M.S.; Braunstein, T.H. Phosphorylation of connexin43 on serine 306 regulates electrical coupling. *Heart Rhythm* **2009**, *6*, 1632–1638. [CrossRef] [PubMed]
187. Hund, T.J.; Decker, K.F.; Kanter, E.; Mohler, P.J.; Boyden, P.A.; Schuessler, R.B.; Yamada, K.A.; Rudy, Y. Role of activated CaMKII in abnormal calcium homeostasis and i(na) remodeling after myocardial infarction: Insights from mathematical modeling. *J. Mol. Cell. Cardiol.* **2008**, *45*, 420–428. [CrossRef] [PubMed]
188. Cooper, C.D.; Lampe, P.D. Casein kinase 1 regulates connexin-43 gap junction assembly. *J. Biol. Chem.* **2002**, *277*, 44962–44968. [CrossRef] [PubMed]
189. Paulson, A.F.; Lampe, P.D.; Meyer, R.A.; TenBroek, E.; Atkinson, M.M.; Walseth, T.F.; Johnson, R.G. Cyclic AMP and LDL trigger a rapid enhancement in gap junction assembly through a stimulation of connexin trafficking. *J. Cell Sci.* **2000**, *113 Pt 17*, 3037–3049. [PubMed]
190. Darrow, B.J.; Fast, V.G.; Kleber, A.G.; Beyer, E.C.; Saffitz, J.E. Functional and structural assessment of intercellular communication. Increased conduction velocity and enhanced connexin expression in dibutyryl camp-treated cultured cardiac myocytes. *Circ. Res.* **1996**, *79*, 174–183. [CrossRef] [PubMed]
191. TenBroek, E.M.; Lampe, P.D.; Solan, J.L.; Reynhout, J.K.; Johnson, R.G. Ser364 of connexin43 and the upregulation of gap junction assembly by camp. *J. Cell Biol.* **2001**, *155*, 1307–1318. [CrossRef] [PubMed]
192. Axelsen, L.N.; Stahlhut, M.; Mohammed, S.; Larsen, B.D.; Nielsen, M.S.; Holstein-Rathlou, N.H.; Andersen, S.; Jensen, O.N.; Hennan, J.K.; Kjolbye, A.L. Identification of ischemia-regulated phosphorylation sites in connexin43: A possible target for the antiarrhythmic peptide analogue rotigaptide (ZP123). *J. Mol. Cell. Cardiol.* **2006**, *40*, 790–798. [CrossRef] [PubMed]
193. Shah, M.M.; Martinez, A.M.; Fletcher, W.H. The connexin43 gap junction protein is phosphorylated by protein kinase a and protein kinase c: In vivo and in vitro studies. *Mol. Cell. Biochem.* **2002**, *238*, 57–68. [CrossRef] [PubMed]
194. Yogo, K.; Ogawa, T.; Akiyama, M.; Ishida, N.; Takeya, T. Identification and functional analysis of novel phosphorylation sites in Cx43 in rat primary granulosa cells. *FEBS Lett.* **2002**, *531*, 132–136. [CrossRef]

195. Zou, J.; Yue, X.Y.; Zheng, S.C.; Zhang, G.; Chang, H.; Liao, Y.C.; Zhang, Y.; Xue, M.Q.; Qi, Z. Cholesterol modulates function of connexin 43 gap junction channel via PKC pathway in H9c2 cells. *Biochim. Biophys. Acta* **2014**, *1838*, 2019–2025. [CrossRef] [PubMed]
196. Ek-Vitorin, J.F.; King, T.J.; Heyman, N.S.; Lampe, P.D.; Burt, J.M. Selectivity of connexin 43 channels is regulated through protein kinase C-dependent phosphorylation. *Circ. Res.* **2006**, *98*, 1498–1505. [CrossRef] [PubMed]
197. Xie, Y.; Liu, S.; Hu, S.; Wei, Y. Cardiomyopathy-associated gene 1-sensitive PKC-dependent connexin 43 expression and phosphorylation in left ventricular noncompaction cardiomyopathy. *Cell. Physiol. Biochem.* **2017**, *44*, 828–842. [CrossRef] [PubMed]
198. Bao, X.; Altenberg, G.A.; Reuss, L. Mechanism of regulation of the gap junction protein connexin 43 by protein kinase C-mediated phosphorylation. *Am. J. Physiol. Cell Physiol.* **2004**, *286*, C647–C654. [CrossRef] [PubMed]
199. Liao, C.K.; Cheng, H.H.; Wang, S.D.; Yeih, D.F.; Wang, S.M. Pkcvarepsilon mediates serine phosphorylation of connexin43 induced by lysophosphatidylcholine in neonatal rat cardiomyocytes. *Toxicology* **2013**, *314*, 11–21. [CrossRef] [PubMed]
200. Dunn, C.A.; Lampe, P.D. Injury-triggered akt phosphorylation of Cx43: A ZO-1-driven molecular switch that regulates gap junction size. *J. Cell Sci.* **2014**, *127*, 455–464. [CrossRef] [PubMed]
201. Park, D.J.; Wallick, C.J.; Martyn, K.D.; Lau, A.F.; Jin, C.; Warn-Cramer, B.J. Akt phosphorylates connexin43 on ser373, a "mode-1" binding site for 14-3-3. *Cell Commun. Adhes.* **2007**, *14*, 211–226. [CrossRef] [PubMed]
202. Berthoud, V.M.; Westphale, E.M.; Grigoryeva, A.; Beyer, E.C. Pkc isoenzymes in the chicken lens and TPA-induced effects on intercellular communication. *Investig. Ophthalmol. Vis. Sci.* **2000**, *41*, 850–858.
203. Isakson, B.E. Localized expression of an Ins(1,4,5)P3 receptor at the myoendothelial junction selectively regulates heterocellular Ca2+ communication. *J. Cell Sci.* **2008**, *121*, 3664–3673. [CrossRef] [PubMed]
204. Isakson, B.E.; Ramos, S.I.; Duling, B.R. Ca2+ and inositol 1,4,5-trisphosphate-mediated signaling across the myoendothelial junction. *Circ. Res.* **2007**, *100*, 246–254. [CrossRef] [PubMed]
205. Straub, A.C.; Johnstone, S.R.; Heberlein, K.R.; Rizzo, M.J.; Best, A.K.; Boitano, S.; Isakson, B.E. Site-specific connexin phosphorylation is associated with reduced heterocellular communication between smooth muscle and endothelium. *J. Vasc. Res.* **2010**, *47*, 277–286. [CrossRef] [PubMed]
206. Revel, J.P.; Karnovsky, M.J. Hexagonal array of subunits in intercellular junctions of the mouse heart and liver. *J. Cell Biol.* **1967**, *33*, C7–C12. [CrossRef] [PubMed]
207. Solan, J.L.; Marquez-Rosado, L.; Sorgen, P.L.; Thornton, P.J.; Gafken, P.R.; Lampe, P.D. Phosphorylation at s365 is a gatekeeper event that changes the structure of Cx43 and prevents down-regulation by PKC. *J. Cell Biol.* **2007**, *179*, 1301–1309. [CrossRef] [PubMed]
208. Lampe, P.D.; Cooper, C.D.; King, T.J.; Burt, J.M. Analysis of connexin43 phosphorylated at s325, s328 and s330 in normoxic and ischemic heart. *J. Cell Sci.* **2006**, *119*, 3435–3442. [CrossRef] [PubMed]
209. Jabr, R.I.; Hatch, F.S.; Salvage, S.C.; Orlowski, A.; Lampe, P.D.; Fry, C.H. Regulation of gap junction conductance by calcineurin through Cx43 phosphorylation: Implications for action potential conduction. *Pflugers Arch.* **2016**, *468*, 1945–1955. [CrossRef] [PubMed]
210. Schulz, R.; Gres, P.; Skyschally, A.; Duschin, A.; Belosjorow, S.; Konietzka, I.; Heusch, G. Ischemic preconditioning preserves connexin 43 phosphorylation during sustained ischemia in pig hearts in vivo. *FASEB J.* **2003**, *17*, 1355–1357. [CrossRef] [PubMed]
211. Rhett, J.M.; Gourdie, R.G. The perinexus: A new feature of Cx43 gap junction organization. *Heart Rhythm* **2012**, *9*, 619–623. [CrossRef] [PubMed]
212. Palatinus, J.A.; O'Quinn, M.P.; Barker, R.J.; Harris, B.S.; Jourdan, J.; Gourdie, R.G. ZO-1 determines adherens and gap junction localization at intercalated disks. *Am. J. Physiol. Heart Circ. Physiol.* **2011**, *300*, H583–H594. [CrossRef] [PubMed]
213. Zhu, C.; Barker, R.J.; Hunter, A.W.; Zhang, Y.; Jourdan, J.; Gourdie, R.G. Quantitative analysis of ZO-1 colocalization with Cx43 gap junction plaques in cultures of rat neonatal cardiomyocytes. *Microsc. Microanal.* **2005**, *11*, 244–248. [CrossRef] [PubMed]
214. Hunter, A.W.; Barker, R.J.; Zhu, C.; Gourdie, R.G. Zonula occludens-1 alters connexin43 gap junction size and organization by influencing channel accretion. *Mol. Biol. Cell* **2005**, *16*, 5686–5698. [CrossRef] [PubMed]

215. O'Quinn, M.P.; Palatinus, J.A.; Harris, B.S.; Hewett, K.W.; Gourdie, R.G. A peptide mimetic of the connexin43 carboxyl terminus reduces gap junction remodeling and induced arrhythmia following ventricular injury. *Circ. Res.* **2011**, *108*, 704–715. [CrossRef] [PubMed]
216. Schulz, R.; Görge, P.M.; Görbe, A.; Ferdinandy, P.; Lampe, P.D.; Leybaert, L. Connexin 43 is an emerging therapeutic target in ischemia/reperfusion injury, cardioprotection and neuroprotection. *Pharmacol. Ther.* **2015**, *153*, 90–106. [CrossRef] [PubMed]
217. Soder, B.L.; Propst, J.T.; Brooks, T.M.; Goodwin, R.L.; Friedman, H.I.; Yost, M.J.; Gourdie, R.G. The connexin43 carboxyl-terminal peptide act1 modulates the biological response to silicone implants. *Plast. Reconstr. Surg.* **2009**, *123*, 1440–1451. [CrossRef] [PubMed]
218. Su, G.Y.; Wang, J.; Xu, Z.X.; Qiao, X.J.; Zhong, J.Q.; Zhang, Y. Effects of rotigaptide (ZP123) on connexin43 remodeling in canine ventricular fibrillation. *Mol. Med. Rep.* **2015**, *12*, 5746–5752. [CrossRef] [PubMed]
219. Stahlhut, M.; Petersen, J.S.; Hennan, J.K.; Ramirez, M.T. The antiarrhythmic peptide rotigaptide (ZP123) increases connexin 43 protein expression in neonatal rat ventricular cardiomyocytes. *Cell Commun. Adhes.* **2006**, *13*, 21–27. [CrossRef] [PubMed]
220. Dhein, S.; Larsen, B.D.; Petersen, J.S.; Mohr, F.W. Effects of the new antiarrhythmic peptide ZP123 on epicardial activation and repolarization pattern. *Cell Commun. Adhes.* **2003**, *10*, 371–378. [CrossRef] [PubMed]
221. Xing, D.; Kjolbye, A.L.; Nielsen, M.S.; Petersen, J.S.; Harlow, K.W.; Holstein-Rathlou, N.H.; Martins, J.B. ZP123 increases gap junctional conductance and prevents reentrant ventricular tachycardia during myocardial ischemia in open chest dogs. *J. Cardiovasc. Electrophysiol.* **2003**, *14*, 510–520. [CrossRef] [PubMed]
222. Kjølbye, A.L.; Haugan, K.; Hennan, J.K.; Petersen, J.S. Pharmacological modulation of gap junction function with the novel compound rotigaptide: A promising new principle for prevention of arrhythmias. *Basic Clin. Pharmacol. Toxicol.* **2007**, *101*, 215–230. [CrossRef] [PubMed]
223. Skyschally, A.; Walter, B.; Schultz Hansen, R.; Heusch, G. The antiarrhythmic dipeptide ZP1609 (danegaptide) when given at reperfusion reduces myocardial infarct size in pigs. *Naunyn-Schmiedeberg's Arch. Pharmacol.* **2013**, *386*, 383–391. [CrossRef] [PubMed]
224. Cherepanova, O.A.; Pidkovka, N.A.; Sarmento, O.F.; Yoshida, T.; Gan, Q.; Adiguzel, E.; Bendeck, M.P.; Berliner, J.; Leitinger, N.; Owens, G.K. Oxidized phospholipids induce type viii collagen expression and vascular smooth muscle cell migration. *Circ. Res.* **2009**, *104*, 609–618. [CrossRef] [PubMed]
225. Kadl, A.; Meher, A.K.; Sharma, P.R.; Lee, M.Y.; Doran, A.C.; Johnstone, S.R.; Elliott, M.R.; Gruber, F.; Han, J.; Chen, W.S.; et al. Identification of a novel macrophage phenotype that develops in response to atherogenic phospholipids via nrf2. *Circ. Res.* **2010**, *107*, 737–746. [CrossRef] [PubMed]
226. Leitinger, N. Oxidized phospholipids as triggers of inflammation in atherosclerosis. *Mol. Nutr. Food Res.* **2005**, *49*, 1063–1071. [CrossRef] [PubMed]
227. Chatterjee, S.; Berliner, J.A.; Subbanagounder, G.G.; Bhunia, A.K.; Koh, S. Identification of a biologically active component in minimally oxidized low density lipoprotein (MM-LDL) responsible for aortic smooth muscle cell proliferation. *Glycoconj. J.* **2004**, *20*, 331–338. [CrossRef] [PubMed]
228. Good, M.E.; Nelson, T.K.; Simon, A.M.; Burt, J.M. A functional channel is necessary for growth suppression by Cx37. *J. Cell Sci.* **2011**, *124*, 2448–2456. [CrossRef] [PubMed]
229. Good, M.E.; Ek-Vitorín, J.F.; Burt, J.M. Extracellular loop cysteine mutant of Cx37 fails to suppress proliferation of rat insulinoma cells. *J. Membr. Biol.* **2012**, *245*, 369–380. [CrossRef] [PubMed]
230. Good, M.E.; Ek-Vitorin, J.F.; Burt, J.M. Structural determinants and proliferative consequences of connexin 37 hemichannel function in insulinoma cells. *J. Biol. Chem.* **2014**, *289*, 30379–30386. [CrossRef] [PubMed]
231. Traub, O.; Hertlein, B.; Kasper, M.; Eckert, R.; Krisciukaitis, A.; Hülser, D.; Willecke, K. Characterization of the gap junction protein connexin37 in murine endothelium, respiratory epithelium, and after transfection in human hela cells. *Eur. J. Cell Biol.* **1998**, *77*, 313–322. [CrossRef]
232. Morel, S.; Burnier, L.; Roatti, A.; Chassot, A.; Roth, I.; Sutter, E.; Galan, K.; Pfenniger, A.; Chanson, M.; Kwak, B.R. Unexpected role for the human Cx37 C1019T polymorphism in tumour cell proliferation. *Carcinogenesis* **2010**, *31*, 1922–1931. [CrossRef] [PubMed]
233. Larson, D.M.; Seul, K.H.; Berthoud, V.M.; Lau, A.F.; Sagar, G.D.; Beyer, E.C. Functional expression and biochemical characterization of an epitope-tagged connexin37. *Mol. Cell. Biol. Res. Commun.* **2000**, *3*, 115–121. [CrossRef] [PubMed]

234. Vanhamme, L.; Rolin, S.; Szpirer, C. Inhibition of gap-junctional intercellular communication between epithelial cells transformed by the activated h-ras-1 oncogene. *Exp. Cell Res.* **1989**, *180*, 297–301. [CrossRef]
235. Azarnia, R.; Reddy, S.; Kmiecik, T.E.; Shalloway, D.; Loewenstein, W.R. The cellular *SRC* gene product regulates junctional cell-to-cell communication. *Science* **1988**, *239*, 398–401. [CrossRef] [PubMed]
236. Gonzalez-Sanchez, A.; Jaraiz-Rodriguez, M.; Dominguez-Prieto, M.; Herrero-Gonzalez, S.; Medina, J.M.; Tabernero, A. Connexin43 recruits PTEN and Csk to inhibit c-Src activity in glioma cells and astrocytes. *Oncotarget* **2016**, *7*, 49819–49833. [CrossRef] [PubMed]
237. Johnson, K.E.; Mitra, S.; Katoch, P.; Kelsey, L.S.; Johnson, K.R.; Mehta, P.P. Phosphorylation on ser-279 and ser-282 of connexin43 regulates endocytosis and gap junction assembly in pancreatic cancer cells. *Mol. Biol. Cell* **2013**, *24*, 715–733. [CrossRef] [PubMed]
238. Brissette, J.L.; Kumar, N.M.; Gilula, N.B.; Dotto, G.P. The tumor promoter 12-O-tetradecanoylphorbol-13-acetate and the ras oncogene modulate expression and phosphorylation of gap junction proteins. *Mol. Cell. Biol.* **1991**, *11*, 5364–5371. [CrossRef] [PubMed]
239. Oh, S.Y.; Grupen, C.G.; Murray, A.W. Phorbol ester induces phosphorylation and down-regulation of connexin 43 in wb cells. *Biochim. Biophys. Acta* **1991**, *1094*, 243–245. [CrossRef]
240. Asamoto, M.; Oyamada, M.; el Aoumari, A.; Gros, D.; Yamasaki, H. Molecular mechanisms of TPA-mediated inhibition of gap-junctional intercellular communication: Evidence for action on the assembly or function but not the expression of connexin 43 in rat liver epithelial cells. *Mol. Carcinog.* **1991**, *4*, 322–327. [CrossRef] [PubMed]
241. Ruch, R.J.; Trosko, J.E.; Madhukar, B.V. Inhibition of connexin43 gap junctional intercellular communication by tpa requires erk activation. *J. Cell. Biochem.* **2001**, *83*, 163–169. [CrossRef] [PubMed]
242. Ye, X.Y.; Jiang, Q.H.; Hong, T.; Zhang, Z.Y.; Yang, R.J.; Huang, J.Q.; Hu, K.; Peng, Y.P. Altered expression of connexin43 and phosphorylation connexin43 in glioma tumors. *Int. J. Clin. Exp. Pathol.* **2015**, *8*, 4296–4306. [PubMed]
243. Wu, J.F.; Ji, J.; Dong, S.Y.; Li, B.B.; Yu, M.L.; Wu, D.D.; Tao, L.; Tong, X.H. Gefitinib enhances oxaliplatin-induced apoptosis mediated by Src and PKC-modulated gap junction function. *Oncol. Rep.* **2016**, *36*, 3251–3258. [CrossRef] [PubMed]
244. Peterson-Roth, E.; Brdlik, C.M.; Glazer, P.M. Src-induced cisplatin resistance mediated by cell-to-cell communication. *Cancer Res.* **2009**, *69*, 3619–3624. [CrossRef] [PubMed]
245. Wong, P.; Tan, T.; Chan, C.; Laxton, V.; Chan, Y.W.; Liu, T.; Wong, W.T.; Tse, G. The role of connexins in wound healing and repair: Novel therapeutic approaches. *Front. Physiol.* **2016**, *7*, 596. [CrossRef] [PubMed]
246. Becker, D.L.; Thrasivoulou, C.; Phillips, A.R. Connexins in wound healing; perspectives in diabetic patients. *Biochim. Biophys. Acta* **2012**, *1818*, 2068–2075. [CrossRef] [PubMed]
247. Cogliati, B.; Vinken, M.; Silva, T.C.; Araújo, C.M.M.; Aloia, T.P.A.; Chaible, L.M.; Mori, C.M.C.; Dagli, M.L.Z. Connexin 43 deficiency accelerates skin wound healing and extracellular matrix remodeling in mice. *J. Dermatol. Sci.* **2015**, *79*, 50–56. [CrossRef] [PubMed]
248. Kim, M.O.; Ryu, J.M.; Suh, H.N.; Park, S.H.; Oh, Y.M.; Lee, S.H.; Han, H.J. Camp promotes cell migration through cell junctional complex dynamics and actin cytoskeleton remodeling: Implications in skin wound healing. *Stem Cells Dev.* **2015**, *24*, 2513–2524. [CrossRef] [PubMed]
249. Mehta, P.P.; Yamamoto, M.; Rose, B. Transcription of the gene for the gap junctional protein connexin43 and expression of functional cell-to-cell channels are regulated by camp. *Mol. Biol. Cell* **1992**, *3*, 839–850. [CrossRef] [PubMed]
250. Richards, T.S.; Dunn, C.A.; Carter, W.G.; Usui, M.L.; Olerud, J.E.; Lampe, P.D. Protein kinase C spatially and temporally regulates gap junctional communication during human wound repair via phosphorylation of connexin43 on serine368. *J. Cell Biol.* **2004**, *167*, 555–562. [CrossRef] [PubMed]
251. Pollok, S.; Pfeiffer, A.C.; Lobmann, R.; Wright, C.S.; Moll, I.; Martin, P.E.; Brandner, J.M. Connexin 43 mimetic peptide gap27 reveals potential differences in the role of Cx43 in wound repair between diabetic and non-diabetic cells. *J. Cell. Mol. Med.* **2011**, *15*, 861–873. [CrossRef] [PubMed]
252. Solan, J.L.; Lampe, P.D. Kinase programs spatiotemporally regulate gap junction assembly and disassembly: Effects on wound repair. *Semin. Cell Dev. Biol.* **2016**, *50*, 40–48. [CrossRef] [PubMed]
253. Wang, C.M.; Lincoln, J.; Cook, J.E.; Becker, D.L. Abnormal connexin expression underlies delayed wound healing in diabetic skin. *Diabetes* **2007**, *56*, 2809–2817. [CrossRef] [PubMed]

254. Brandner, J.M.; Houdek, P.; Hüsing, B.; Kaiser, C.; Moll, I. Connexins 26, 30, and 43: Differences among spontaneous, chronic, and accelerated human wound healing. *J. Investig. Dermatol.* **2004**, *122*, 1310–1320. [CrossRef] [PubMed]
255. Grek, C.L.; Montgomery, J.; Sharma, M.; Ravi, A.; Rajkumar, J.S.; Moyer, K.E.; Gourdie, R.G.; Ghatnekar, G.S. A multicenter randomized controlled trial evaluating a Cx43-mimetic peptide in cutaneous scarring. *J. Investig. Dermatol.* **2017**, *137*, 620–630. [CrossRef] [PubMed]
256. Stamler, J.S.; Simon, D.I.; Osborne, J.A.; Mullins, M.E.; Jaraki, O.; Michel, T.; Singel, D.J.; Loscalzo, J. S-nitrosylation of proteins with nitric oxide: Synthesis and characterization of biologically active compounds. *Proc. Natl. Acad. Sci. USA* **1992**, *89*, 444–448. [CrossRef] [PubMed]
257. Retamal, M.A.; García, I.E.; Pinto, B.I.; Pupo, A.; Báez, D.; Stehberg, J.; Del Rio, R.; González, C. Extracellular cysteine in connexins: Role as redox sensors. *Front. Physiol.* **2016**, *7*, 1. [CrossRef] [PubMed]
258. Contreras, J.E.; Sánchez, H.A.; Eugenin, E.A.; Speidel, D.; Theis, M.; Willecke, K.; Bukauskas, F.F.; Bennett, M.V.; Sáez, J.C. Metabolic inhibition induces opening of unapposed connexin 43 gap junction hemichannels and reduces gap junctional communication in cortical astrocytes in culture. *Proc. Natl. Acad. Sci. USA* **2002**, *99*, 495–500. [CrossRef] [PubMed]
259. Figueroa, X.F.; Lillo, M.A.; Gaete, P.S.; Riquelme, M.A.; Sáez, J.C. Diffusion of nitric oxide across cell membranes of the vascular wall requires specific connexin-based channels. *Neuropharmacology* **2013**, *75*, 471–478. [CrossRef] [PubMed]
260. Pogoda, K.; Füller, M.; Pohl, U.; Kameritsch, P. No, via its target Cx37, modulates calcium signal propagation selectively at myoendothelial gap junctions. *Cell Commun. Signal. CCS* **2014**, *12*, 33. [CrossRef] [PubMed]
261. Pogoda, K.; Mannell, H.; Blodow, S.; Schneider, H.; Schubert, K.M.; Qiu, J.; Schmidt, A.; Imhof, A.; Beck, H.; Tanase, L.I.; et al. No augments endothelial reactivity by reducing myoendothelial calcium signal spreading: A novel role for Cx37 (connexin 37) and the protein tyrosine phosphatase SHP-2. *Arterioscler. Thromb. Vasc. Biol.* **2017**, *37*, 2280–2290. [CrossRef] [PubMed]
262. Gareau, J.R.; Lima, C.D. The sumo pathway: Emerging mechanisms that shape specificity, conjugation and recognition. *Nat. Rev. Mol. Cell Biol.* **2010**, *11*, 861–871. [CrossRef] [PubMed]
263. Laird, D.W. Life cycle of connexins in health and disease. *Biochem. J.* **2006**, *394*, 527–543. [CrossRef] [PubMed]
264. Jiang, J.X.; Paul, D.L.; Goodenough, D.A. Posttranslational phosphorylation of lens fiber connexin46: A slow occurrence. *Investig. Ophthalmol. Vis. Sci.* **1993**, *34*, 3558–3565.
265. Beardslee, M.A.; Laing, J.G.; Beyer, E.C.; Saffitz, J.E. Rapid turnover of connexin43 in the adult rat heart. *Circ. Res.* **1998**, *83*, 629–635. [CrossRef] [PubMed]
266. Fallon, R.F.; Goodenough, D.A. Five-hour half-life of mouse liver gap-junction protein. *J. Cell Biol.* **1981**, *90*, 521–526. [CrossRef] [PubMed]
267. Norris, R.P.; Baena, V.; Terasaki, M. Localization of phosphorylated connexin 43 using serial section immunogold electron microscopy. *J. Cell Sci.* **2017**, *130*, 1333–1340. [CrossRef] [PubMed]
268. Boassa, D.; Solan, J.L.; Papas, A.; Thornton, P.; Lampe, P.D.; Sosinsky, G.E. Trafficking and recycling of the connexin43 gap junction protein during mitosis. *Traffic* **2010**, *11*, 1471–1486. [CrossRef] [PubMed]
269. Piehl, M.; Lehmann, C.; Gumpert, A.; Denizot, J.P.; Segretain, D.; Falk, M.M. Internalization of large double-membrane intercellular vesicles by a clathrin-dependent endocytic process. *Mol. Biol. Cell* **2007**, *18*, 337–347. [CrossRef] [PubMed]
270. Hunter, A.W.; Gourdie, R.G. The second pdz domain of zonula occludens-1 is dispensable for targeting to connexin 43 gap junctions. *Cell Commun. Adhes.* **2008**, *15*, 55–63. [CrossRef] [PubMed]
271. Chen, C.H.; Mayo, J.N.; Gourdie, R.G.; Johnstone, S.R.; Isakson, B.E.; Bearden, S.E. The connexin 43/ZO-1 complex regulates cerebral endothelial f-actin architecture and migration. *Am. J. Physiol. Cell Physiol.* **2015**, *309*, C600–C607. [CrossRef] [PubMed]
272. Leithe, E.; Sirnes, S.; Fykerud, T.; Kjenseth, A.; Rivedal, E. Endocytosis and post-endocytic sorting of connexins. *Biochim. Biophys. Acta* **2012**, *1818*, 1870–1879. [CrossRef] [PubMed]
273. Falk, M.M.; Fong, J.T.; Kells, R.M.; O'Laughlin, M.C.; Kowal, T.J.; Thevenin, A.F. Degradation of endocytosed gap junctions by autophagosomal and endo-/lysosomal pathways: A perspective. *J. Membr. Biol.* **2012**, *245*, 465–476. [CrossRef] [PubMed]
274. Leithe, E.; Rivedal, E. Ubiquitination of gap junction proteins. *J. Membr. Biol.* **2007**, *217*, 43–51. [CrossRef] [PubMed]

275. Willis, M.S.; Townley-Tilson, W.H.; Kang, E.Y.; Homeister, J.W.; Patterson, C. Sent to destroy: The ubiquitin proteasome system regulates cell signaling and protein quality control in cardiovascular development and disease. *Circ. Res.* **2010**, *106*, 463–478. [CrossRef] [PubMed]
276. Voges, D.; Zwickl, P.; Baumeister, W. The 26s proteasome: A molecular machine designed for controlled proteolysis. *Annu. Rev. Biochem.* **1999**, *68*, 1015–1068. [CrossRef] [PubMed]
277. Bejarano, E.; Girao, H.; Yuste, A.; Patel, B.; Marques, C.; Spray, D.C.; Pereira, P.; Cuervo, A.M. Autophagy modulates dynamics of connexins at the plasma membrane in a ubiquitin-dependent manner. *Mol. Biol. Cell* **2012**, *23*, 2156–2169. [CrossRef] [PubMed]
278. Fong, J.T.; Kells, R.M.; Gumpert, A.M.; Marzillier, J.Y.; Davidson, M.W.; Falk, M.M. Internalized gap junctions are degraded by autophagy. *Autophagy* **2012**, *8*, 794–811. [CrossRef] [PubMed]
279. Lichtenstein, A.; Minogue, P.J.; Beyer, E.C.; Berthoud, V.M. Autophagy: A pathway that contributes to connexin degradation. *J. Cell Sci.* **2011**, *124*, 910–920. [CrossRef] [PubMed]
280. Bejarano, E.; Yuste, A.; Patel, B.; Stout, R.F., Jr.; Spray, D.C.; Cuervo, A.M. Connexins modulate autophagosome biogenesis. *Nat. Cell Biol.* **2014**, *16*, 401–414. [CrossRef] [PubMed]
281. Hesketh, G.G.; Shah, M.H.; Halperin, V.L.; Cooke, C.A.; Akar, F.G.; Yen, T.E.; Kass, D.A.; Machamer, C.E.; Van Eyk, J.E.; Tomaselli, G.F. Ultrastructure and regulation of lateralized connexin43 in the failing heart. *Circ. Res.* **2010**, *106*, 1153–1163. [CrossRef] [PubMed]
282. Leithe, E.; Rivedal, E. Ubiquitination and down-regulation of gap junction protein connexin-43 in response to 12-O-tetradecanoylphorbol 13-acetate treatment. *J. Biol. Chem.* **2004**, *279*, 50089–50096. [CrossRef] [PubMed]
283. Zhu, X.; Ruan, Z.; Yang, X.; Chu, K.; Wu, H.; Li, Y.; Huang, Y. Connexin 31.1 degradation requires the clathrin-mediated autophagy in NSCLC cell h1299. *J. Cell. Mol. Med.* **2015**, *19*, 257–264. [CrossRef] [PubMed]
284. Catarino, S.; Ramalho, J.S.; Marques, C.; Pereira, P.; Girao, H. Ubiquitin-mediated internalization of connexin43 is independent of the canonical endocytic tyrosine-sorting signal. *Biochem. J.* **2011**, *437*, 255–267. [CrossRef] [PubMed]
285. Girao, H.; Pereira, P. The proteasome regulates the interaction between Cx43 and ZO-1. *J. Cell. Biochem.* **2007**, *102*, 719–728. [CrossRef] [PubMed]
286. Dunn, C.A.; Su, V.; Lau, A.F.; Lampe, P.D. Activation of AKT, not connexin 43 protein ubiquitination, regulates gap junction stability. *J. Biol. Chem.* **2012**, *287*, 2600–2607. [CrossRef] [PubMed]
287. Totland, M.Z.; Bergsland, C.H.; Fykerud, T.A.; Knudsen, L.M.; Rasmussen, N.L.; Eide, P.W.; Yohannes, Z.; Sorensen, V.; Brech, A.; Lothe, R.A.; et al. The E3 ubiquitin ligase nedd4 induces endocytosis and lysosomal sorting of connexin 43 to promote loss of gap junctions. *J. Cell Sci.* **2017**, *130*, 2867–2882. [CrossRef] [PubMed]
288. Spagnol, G.; Kieken, F.; Kopanic, J.L.; Li, H.; Zach, S.; Stauch, K.L.; Grosely, R.; Sorgen, P.L. Structural studies of the NEDD4 WW domains and their selectivity for the connexin43 (Cx43) carboxyl terminus. *J. Biol. Chem.* **2016**, *291*, 7637–7650. [CrossRef] [PubMed]
289. Girao, H.; Catarino, S.; Pereira, P. Eps15 interacts with ubiquitinated Cx43 and mediates its internalization. *Exp. Cell Res.* **2009**, *315*, 3587–3597. [CrossRef] [PubMed]
290. Auth, T.; Schluter, S.; Urschel, S.; Kussmann, P.; Sonntag, S.; Hoher, T.; Kreuzberg, M.M.; Dobrowolski, R.; Willecke, K. The TSG101 protein binds to connexins and is involved in connexin degradation. *Exp. Cell Res.* **2009**, *315*, 1053–1062. [CrossRef] [PubMed]
291. Chen, V.C.; Kristensen, A.R.; Foster, L.J.; Naus, C.C. Association of connexin43 with E3 ubiquitin ligase TRIM21 reveals a mechanism for gap junction phosphodegron control. *J. Proteome Res.* **2012**, *11*, 6134–6146. [CrossRef] [PubMed]
292. Basheer, W.A.; Harris, B.S.; Mentrup, H.L.; Abreha, M.; Thames, E.L.; Lea, J.B.; Swing, D.A.; Copeland, N.G.; Jenkins, N.A.; Price, R.L.; et al. Cardiomyocyte-specific overexpression of the ubiquitin ligase WWP1 contributes to reduction in connexin 43 and arrhythmogenesis. *J. Mol. Cell. Cardiol.* **2015**, *88*, 1–13. [CrossRef] [PubMed]
293. Fykerud, T.A.; Kjenseth, A.; Schink, K.O.; Sirnes, S.; Bruun, J.; Omori, Y.; Brech, A.; Rivedal, E.; Leithe, E. Smad ubiquitination regulatory factor-2 controls gap junction intercellular communication by modulating endocytosis and degradation of connexin43. *J. Cell Sci.* **2012**, *125*, 3966–3976. [CrossRef] [PubMed]
294. Fang, W.L.; Lai, S.Y.; Lai, W.A.; Lee, M.T.; Liao, C.F.; Ke, F.C.; Hwang, J.J. CRTC2 and NEDD4 ligase involvement in FSH and TGFβ1 upregulation of connexin43 gap junction. *J. Mol. Endocrinol.* **2015**, *55*, 263–275. [CrossRef] [PubMed]

295. Colussi, C.; Gurtner, A.; Rosati, J.; Illi, B.; Ragone, G.; Piaggio, G.; Moggio, M.; Lamperti, C.; D'Angelo, G.; Clementi, E.; et al. Nitric oxide deficiency determines global chromatin changes in duchenne muscular dystrophy. *FASEB J.* **2009**, *23*, 2131–2141. [CrossRef] [PubMed]
296. Meraviglia, V.; Azzimato, V.; Colussi, C.; Florio, M.C.; Binda, A.; Panariti, A.; Qanud, K.; Suffredini, S.; Gennaccaro, L.; Miragoli, M.; et al. Acetylation mediates Cx43 reduction caused by electrical stimulation. *J. Mol. Cell. Cardiol.* **2015**, *87*, 54–64. [CrossRef] [PubMed]
297. Carette, D.; Gilleron, J.; Denizot, J.P.; Grant, K.; Pointis, G.; Segretain, D. New cellular mechanisms of gap junction degradation and recycling. *Biol. Cell Auspices Eur. Cell Biol. Org.* **2015**, *107*, 218–231. [CrossRef] [PubMed]
298. Koval, M. Pathways and control of connexin oligomerization. *Trends Cell Biol.* **2006**, *16*, 159–166. [CrossRef] [PubMed]
299. Koval, M.; Molina, S.A.; Burt, J.M. Mix and match: Investigating heteromeric and heterotypic gap junction channels in model systems and native tissues. *FEBS Lett.* **2014**, *588*, 1193–1204. [CrossRef] [PubMed]
300. Das, S.; Smith, T.D.; Sarma, J.D.; Ritzenthaler, J.D.; Maza, J.; Kaplan, B.E.; Cunningham, L.A.; Suaud, L.; Hubbard, M.J.; Rubenstein, R.C.; et al. ERP29 restricts connexin43 oligomerization in the endoplasmic reticulum. *Mol. Biol. Cell* **2009**, *20*, 2593–2604. [CrossRef] [PubMed]
301. Maza, J.; Das Sarma, J.; Koval, M. Defining a minimal motif required to prevent connexin oligomerization in the endoplasmic reticulum. *J. Biol. Chem.* **2005**, *280*, 21115–21121. [CrossRef] [PubMed]
302. Jara, O.; Acuna, R.; Garcia, I.E.; Maripillan, J.; Figueroa, V.; Saez, J.C.; Araya-Secchi, R.; Lagos, C.F.; Perez-Acle, T.; Berthoud, V.M.; et al. Critical role of the first transmembrane domain of Cx26 in regulating oligomerization and function. *Mol. Biol. Cell* **2012**, *23*, 3299–3311. [CrossRef] [PubMed]
303. Musil, L.S.; Goodenough, D.A. Multisubunit assembly of an integral plasma membrane channel protein, gap junction connexin43, occurs after exit from the ER. *Cell* **1993**, *74*, 1065–1077. [CrossRef]
304. Koval, M.; Harley, J.E.; Hick, E.; Steinberg, T.H. Connexin46 is retained as monomers in a trans-golgi compartment of osteoblastic cells. *J. Cell Biol.* **1997**, *137*, 847–857. [CrossRef] [PubMed]
305. Smith, T.D.; Mohankumar, A.; Minogue, P.J.; Beyer, E.C.; Berthoud, V.M.; Koval, M. Cytoplasmic amino acids within the membrane interface region influence connexin oligomerization. *J. Membr. Biol.* **2012**, *245*, 221–230. [CrossRef] [PubMed]
306. Lagree, V.; Brunschwig, K.; Lopez, P.; Gilula, N.B.; Richard, G.; Falk, M.M. Specific amino-acid residues in the N-terminus and TM3 implicated in channel function and oligomerization compatibility of connexin43. *J. Cell Sci.* **2003**, *116*, 3189–3201. [CrossRef] [PubMed]
307. Molina, S.A.; Stauffer, B.; Moriarty, H.K.; Kim, A.H.; McCarty, N.A.; Koval, M. Junctional abnormalities in human airway epithelial cells expressing F508DEL CFTR. *Am. J. Physiol. Lung Cell. Mol. Physiol.* **2015**, *309*, L475–L487. [CrossRef] [PubMed]
308. Suaud, L.; Miller, K.; Alvey, L.; Yan, W.; Robay, A.; Kebler, C.; Kreindler, J.L.; Guttentag, S.; Hubbard, M.J.; Rubenstein, R.C. Erp29 regulates deltaf508 and wild-type cystic fibrosis transmembrane conductance regulator (CFTR) trafficking to the plasma membrane in cystic fibrosis (CF) and non-CF epithelial cells. *J. Biol. Chem.* **2011**, *286*, 21239–21253. [CrossRef] [PubMed]
309. Das Sarma, J.; Kaplan, B.E.; Willemsen, D.; Koval, M. Identification of Rab20 as a potential regulator of connexin43 trafficking. *Cell Commun. Adhes.* **2008**, *15*, 65–74. [CrossRef] [PubMed]
310. Asklund, T.; Appelskog, I.B.; Ammerpohl, O.; Ekstrom, T.J.; Almqvist, P.M. Histone deacetylase inhibitor 4-phenylbutyrate modulates glial fibrillary acidic protein and connexin 43 expression, and enhances gap-junction communication, in human glioblastoma cells. *Eur. J Cancer* **2004**, *40*, 1073–1081. [CrossRef] [PubMed]
311. Hattori, Y.; Fukushima, M.; Maitani, Y. Non-viral delivery of the connexin 43 gene with histone deacetylase inhibitor to human nasopharyngeal tumor cells enhances gene expression and inhibits in vivo tumor growth. *Int. J. Oncol.* **2007**, *30*, 1427–1439. [CrossRef] [PubMed]
312. Khan, Z.; Akhtar, M.; Asklund, T.; Juliusson, B.; Almqvist, P.M.; Ekstrom, T.J. Hdac inhibition amplifies gap junction communication in neural progenitors: Potential for cell-mediated enzyme prodrug therapy. *Exp. Cell Res.* **2007**, *313*, 2958–2967. [CrossRef] [PubMed]
313. Berthoud, V.M.; Minogue, P.J.; Guo, J.; Williamson, E.K.; Xu, X.; Ebihara, L.; Beyer, E.C. Loss of function and impaired degradation of a cataract-associated mutant connexin50. *Eur. J. Cell Biol.* **2003**, *82*, 209–221. [CrossRef] [PubMed]

314. Kaufman, J.; Gordon, C.; Bergamaschi, R.; Wang, H.Z.; Cohen, I.S.; Valiunas, V.; Brink, P.R. The effects of the histone deacetylase inhibitor 4-phenylbutyrate on gap junction conductance and permeability. *Front. Pharmacol.* **2013**, *4*, 111. [CrossRef] [PubMed]
315. Berthoud, V.M.; Minogue, P.J.; Lambert, P.A.; Snabb, J.I.; Beyer, E.C. The cataract-linked mutant connexin50D47A causes endoplasmic reticulum stress in mouse lenses. *J. Biol. Chem.* **2016**, *291*, 17569–17578. [CrossRef] [PubMed]
316. Lichtenstein, A.; Gaietta, G.M.; Deerinck, T.J.; Crum, J.; Sosinsky, G.E.; Beyer, E.C.; Berthoud, V.M. The cytoplasmic accumulations of the cataract-associated mutant, connexin50P88S, are long-lived and form in the endoplasmic reticulum. *Exp. Eye Res.* **2009**, *88*, 600–609. [CrossRef] [PubMed]
317. Alapure, B.V.; Stull, J.K.; Firtina, Z.; Duncan, M.K. The unfolded protein response is activated in connexin 50 mutant mouse lenses. *Exp. Eye Res.* **2012**, *102*, 28–37. [CrossRef] [PubMed]
318. Tattersall, D.; Scott, C.A.; Gray, C.; Zicha, D.; Kelsell, D.P. Ekv mutant connexin 31 associated cell death is mediated by er stress. *Hum. Mol. Genet.* **2009**, *18*, 4734–4745. [CrossRef] [PubMed]
319. Xia, K.; Ma, H.; Xiong, H.; Pan, Q.; Huang, L.; Wang, D.; Zhang, Z. Trafficking abnormality and ER stress underlie functional deficiency of hearing impairment-associated connexin-31 mutants. *Protein Cell* **2010**, *1*, 935–943. [CrossRef] [PubMed]
320. Chen, S.; Zhang, D. Friend or foe: Endoplasmic reticulum protein 29 (ERP29) in epithelial cancer. *FEBS Open Biol.* **2015**, *5*, 91–98. [CrossRef] [PubMed]
321. Li, H.; Spagnol, G.; Pontifex, T.K.; Burt, J.M.; Sorgen, P.L. Chemical shift assignments of the connexin37 carboxyl terminal domain. *Biomol. NMR Assign.* **2017**, *11*, 137–141. [CrossRef] [PubMed]
322. Schlingmann, B.; Schadzek, P.; Hemmerling, F.; Schaarschmidt, F.; Heisterkamp, A.; Ngezahayo, A. The role of the C-terminus in functional expression and internalization of rat connexin46 (rcx46). *J. Bioenergy Biomembr.* **2013**, *45*, 59–70. [CrossRef] [PubMed]
323. Laing, J.G.; Koval, M.; Steinberg, T.H. Association with ZO-1 correlates with plasma membrane partitioning in truncated connexin45 mutants. *J. Membr. Biol.* **2005**, *207*, 45–53. [CrossRef] [PubMed]
324. Trease, A.J.; Capuccino, J.M.V.; Contreras, J.; Harris, A.L.; Sorgen, P.L. Intramolecular signaling in a cardiac connexin: Role of cytoplasmic domain dimerization. *J. Mol. Cell. Cardiol.* **2017**, *111*, 69–80. [CrossRef] [PubMed]
325. Calero, G.; Kanemitsu, M.; Taffet, S.M.; Lau, A.F.; Delmar, M. A 17MER peptide interferes with acidification-induced uncoupling of connexin43. *Circ. Res.* **1998**, *82*, 929–935. [CrossRef] [PubMed]
326. Stergiopoulos, K.; Alvarado, J.L.; Mastroianni, M.; Ek-Vitorin, J.F.; Taffet, S.M.; Delmar, M. Hetero-domain interactions as a mechanism for the regulation of connexin channels. *Circ. Res.* **1999**, *84*, 1144–1155. [CrossRef] [PubMed]
327. Banerjee, D.; Das, S.; Molina, S.A.; Madgwick, D.; Katz, M.R.; Jena, S.; Bossmann, L.K.; Pal, D.; Takemoto, D.J. Investigation of the reciprocal relationship between the expression of two gap junction connexin proteins, connexin46 and connexin43. *J. Biol. Chem.* **2011**, *286*, 24519–24533. [CrossRef] [PubMed]
328. Basheer, W.; Shaw, R. The "tail" of connexin43: An unexpected journey from alternative translation to trafficking. *Biochim. Biophys. Acta* **2016**, *1863*, 1848–1856. [CrossRef] [PubMed]
329. Wellen, K.E.; Thompson, C.B. Cellular metabolic stress: Considering how cells respond to nutrient excess. *Mol. Cell* **2010**, *40*, 323–332. [CrossRef] [PubMed]
330. James, C.C.; Zeitz, M.J.; Calhoun, P.J.; Lamouille, S.; Smyth, J.W. Altered translation initiation of GJA1 limits gap junction formation during epithelial-mesenchymal transition. *Mol. Biol. Cell* **2018**, *29*, 797–808. [CrossRef]
331. Smyth, J.W.; Vogan, J.M.; Buch, P.J.; Zhang, S.S.; Fong, T.S.; Hong, T.T.; Shaw, R.M. Actin cytoskeleton rest stops regulate anterograde traffic of connexin 43 vesicles to the plasma membrane. *Circ. Res.* **2012**, *110*, 978–989. [CrossRef] [PubMed]
332. Shaw, R.M.; Fay, A.J.; Puthenveedu, M.A.; von Zastrow, M.; Jan, Y.N.; Jan, L.Y. Microtubule plus-end-tracking proteins target gap junctions directly from the cell interior to adherens junctions. *Cell* **2007**, *128*, 547–560. [CrossRef] [PubMed]
333. Giepmans, B.N.; Verlaan, I.; Hengeveld, T.; Janssen, H.; Calafat, J.; Falk, M.M.; Moolenaar, W.H. Gap junction protein connexin-43 interacts directly with microtubules. *Curr. Biol.* **2001**, *11*, 1364–1368. [CrossRef]
334. Yamane, Y.; Shiga, H.; Asou, H.; Ito, E. Gap junctional channel inhibition alters actin organization and calcium propagation in rat cultured astrocytes. *Neuroscience* **2002**, *112*, 593–603. [CrossRef]

335. Theiss, C.; Meller, K. Microinjected anti-actin antibodies decrease gap junctional intercellular commmunication in cultured astrocytes. *Exp. Cell Res.* **2002**, *281*, 197–204. [CrossRef] [PubMed]
336. Cheng, C.; Nowak, R.B.; Gao, J.; Sun, X.; Biswas, S.K.; Lo, W.K.; Mathias, R.T.; Fowler, V.M. Lens ion homeostasis relies on the assembly and/or stability of large connexin 46 gap junction plaques on the broad sides of differentiating fiber cells. *Am. J. Physiol. Cell Physiol.* **2015**, *308*, C835–C847. [CrossRef] [PubMed]
337. Lauf, U.; Giepmans, B.N.; Lopez, P.; Braconnot, S.; Chen, S.C.; Falk, M.M. Dynamic trafficking and delivery of connexons to the plasma membrane and accretion to gap junctions in living cells. *Proc. Natl. Acad. Sci. USA* **2002**, *99*, 10446–10451. [CrossRef] [PubMed]
338. Rhett, J.M.; Jourdan, J.; Gourdie, R.G. Connexin 43 connexon to gap junction transition is regulated by zonula occludens-1. *Mol. Biol. Cell* **2011**, *22*, 1516–1528. [CrossRef] [PubMed]
339. Thevenin, A.F.; Margraf, R.A.; Fisher, C.G.; Kells-Andrews, R.M.; Falk, M.M. Phosphorylation regulates connexin43/zo-1 binding and release, an important step in gap junction turnover. *Mol. Biol. Cell* **2017**, *28*, 3595–3608. [CrossRef] [PubMed]
340. Van Itallie, C.M.; Fanning, A.S.; Bridges, A.; Anderson, J.M. Zo-1 stabilizes the tight junction solute barrier through coupling to the perijunctional cytoskeleton. *Mol. Biol. Cell* **2009**, *20*, 3930–3940. [CrossRef] [PubMed]
341. Fanning, A.S.; Van Itallie, C.M.; Anderson, J.M. Zonula occludens-1 and -2 regulate apical cell structure and the zonula adherens cytoskeleton in polarized epithelia. *Mol. Biol. Cell* **2012**, *23*, 577–590. [CrossRef] [PubMed]
342. Waxse, B.J.; Sengupta, P.; Hesketh, G.G.; Lippincott-Schwartz, J.; Buss, F. Myosin vi facilitates connexin 43 gap junction accretion. *J. Cell Sci.* **2017**, *130*, 827–840. [CrossRef] [PubMed]
343. Wang, H.Y.; Lin, Y.P.; Mitchell, C.K.; Ram, S.; O'Brien, J. Two-color fluorescent analysis of connexin 36 turnover: Relationship to functional plasticity. *J. Cell Sci.* **2015**, *128*, 3888–3897. [CrossRef] [PubMed]
344. Windoffer, R.; Beile, B.; Leibold, A.; Thomas, S.; Wilhelm, U.; Leube, R.E. Visualization of gap junction mobility in living cells. *Cell Tissue Res.* **2000**, *299*, 347–362. [CrossRef] [PubMed]
345. Wang, Y. Two-Color Fluorescent Analysis of Connexin 36 Turnover—Relationship to Functional plasticity. Ph.D. Dissertation, University of Texas, Houston, UT, USA, May 2015. GSBS Dissertations and Theses (Open Access).
346. Stahley, S.N.; Saito, M.; Faundez, V.; Koval, M.; Mattheyses, A.L.; Kowalczyk, A.P. Desmosome assembly and disassembly are membrane raft-dependent. *PLoS ONE* **2014**, *9*, e87809. [CrossRef] [PubMed]
347. Jennings, J.M.; Tucker, D.K.; Kottke, M.D.; Saito, M.; Delva, E.; Hanakawa, Y.; Amagai, M.; Kowalczyk, A.P. Desmosome disassembly in response to pemphigus vulgaris igg occurs in distinct phases and can be reversed by expression of exogenous DSG3. *J. Investig. Dermatol.* **2011**, *131*, 706–718. [CrossRef] [PubMed]
348. Schlingmann, B.; Overgaard, C.E.; Molina, S.A.; Lynn, K.S.; Mitchell, L.A.; Dorsainvil White, S.; Mattheyses, A.L.; Guidot, D.M.; Capaldo, C.T.; Koval, M. Regulation of claudin/zonula occludens-1 complexes by hetero-claudin interactions. *Nat. Commun.* **2016**, *7*, 12276. [CrossRef] [PubMed]
349. Ward, C.; Schlingmann, B.; Stecenko, A.A.; Guidot, D.M.; Koval, M. Nf-kb inhibitors impair lung epithelial tight junctions in the absence of inflammation. *Tissue Barriers* **2015**, *3*, e982424. [CrossRef] [PubMed]
350. Overgaard, C.E.; Schlingmann, B.; Dorsainvil White, S.; Ward, C.; Fan, X.; Swarnakar, S.; Brown, L.A.; Guidot, D.M.; Koval, M. The relative balance of GM-CSF and tgfbeta1 regulates lung epithelial barrier function. *Am. J. Physiol. Lung Cell. Mol. Physiol.* **2015**, *308*, L1212–L1223. [CrossRef] [PubMed]
351. Lafemina, M.J.; Rokkam, D.; Chandrasena, A.; Pan, J.; Bajaj, A.; Johnson, M.; Frank, J.A. Keratinocyte growth factor enhances barrier function without altering claudin expression in primary alveolar epithelial cells. *Am. J. Physiol. Lung Cell. Mol. Physiol.* **2010**, *299*, L724–L734. [CrossRef] [PubMed]

8

Connexins and Pannexins: Important Players in Tumorigenesis, Metastasis and Potential Therapeutics

Sheila V. Graham [1,†], Jean X. Jiang [2,†] and Marc Mesnil [3,*]

1 Centre for Virus Research, Institute of Infection Immunity and Inflammation, College of Medical Veterinary and Life Sciences, Room 254 Jarrett Building, Garscube Estate, University of Glasgow, Glasgow G61 1QH, UK; Sheila.Graham@gla.ac.uk

2 Department of Biochemistry and Structural Biology, University of Texas, Health Science Center, 7703 Floyd Curl Drive, San Antonio, TX 78229, USA; jiangj@uthscsa.edu

3 STIM Laboratory, ERL 7003CNRS/Building B36, University of Poitiers, 1 rue Georges BonnetTSA 51 106, 86073 Poitiers, CEDEX 09, France

* Correspondence: marc.mesnil@univ-poitiers.fr

† These authors contributed equally to this work.

Abstract: Since their characterization more than five decades ago, gap junctions and their structural proteins—the connexins—have been associated with cancer cell growth. During that period, the accumulation of data and molecular knowledge about this association revealed an apparent contradictory relationship between them and cancer. It appeared that if gap junctions or connexins can down regulate cancer cell growth they can be also implied in the migration, invasion and metastatic dissemination of cancer cells. Interestingly, in all these situations, connexins seem to be involved through various mechanisms in which they can act either as gap-junctional intercellular communication mediators, modulators of signalling pathways through their interactome, or as hemichannels, which mediate autocrine/paracrine communication. This complex involvement of connexins in cancer progression is even more complicated by the fact that their hemichannel function may overlap with other gap junction-related proteins, the pannexins. Despite this complexity, the possible involvements of connexins and pannexins in cancer progression and the elucidation of the mechanisms they control may lead to use them as new targets to control cancer progression. In this review, the involvements of connexins and pannexins in these different topics (cancer cell growth, invasion/metastasis process, possible cancer therapeutic targets) are discussed.

Keywords: cancer; connexin; growth control; invasion; metastasis; pannexin; therapeutics

---

1. Introduction

The majority of cancers in adults are solid tumours [1]. Whatever their tissue origin, those tumours are characterized by two fundamental properties, which are, first, an uncontrolled cell proliferation forming the tumour itself and then an acquired invasion capacity leading to the dissemination of cancer cells in the organism. Fifty years of investigation have shown involvement of gap junctions (GJs) or their molecular components, the connexins (Cxs), in these two fundamental characteristics of cancer progression [2–4]. More recently, it appeared that the involvement of Cxs could be complicated by the fact that they can act independently from the establishment of gap-junctional intercellular communication (GJIC). For instance, Cxs may be involved in these mechanisms through their interactome to modulate signalling pathways [5] or by acting as hemichannels (Hcs) mediating autocrine/paracrine communication [6]. This last activity may overlap with pannexins (Panxs) which are Cx-related proteins (Figure 1) [7].

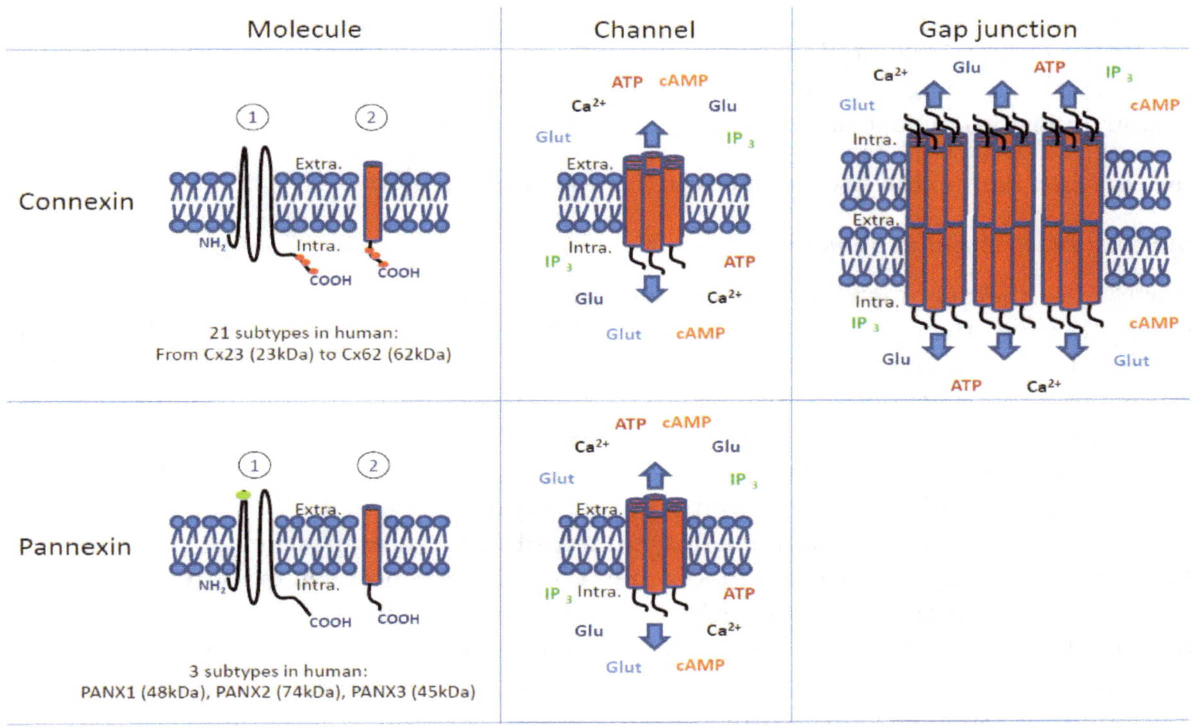

Figure 1. Connexin and pannexin molecules and channels formed by these molecules. As molecules, connexins (Cx) and pannexins (Panx) have similar topology with four transmembrane and intracellular (Intra.) NH_2 and COOH domains. In the left panels, both kinds of molecules are shown in a "spread" way to distinguish their topology (1) and in a "condensed" way (2) to better represent as transmembrane subunits of channels (centre panels) and gap junctions (right panel). In humans, 21 subtypes of connexins have been characterized, which are differentially expressed in tissues [8]. They are named according to their expected molecular weight (kDa) from the smallest connexin (Cx23: 23 kDa) to the largest one (Cx62: 62 kDa). The best-known member of the connexin family is the connexin43 (Cx43) which is the most common in the organism. Only 3 pannexin subtypes are known in human (PANX1, PANX2, PANX3) [9,10]. Except for Cx26, connexins can be phosphorylated mostly at their intracellular COOH tail (red spots) [11]. The level of phosphorylation potentially modifies channel gating, interaction with intracellular or other membrane proteins (connexin interactome) and thus their function and life cycle [11,12]. So far, pannexins do not appear to be regulated by phosphorylation as connexins are but they are more characterized as potentially N-glycosylated (green spots) molecules at their extracellular (Extra.) domain. Both connexins and pannexins can aggregate to form hexameric transmembrane channels permitting the passive passage of ions (e.g., Ca^{2+}) and small (<1–1.5 kDa) hydrophilic molecules such as nutrients (e.g., glucose: Glu), amino acids (e.g., glutamate: Glut), nucleotides (e.g., ATP) and second messengers (e.g., cAMP and IP_3). Theoretically, connexin-made channels (connexons also called hemichannels) and pannexin-made channels (pannexons) are permeable to the same type of ions and molecules even if pannexons permeability has been mostly studied for ATP, Ca^{2+} and glutamate (Glut). Moreover, connexons from one cell can dock with connexons of juxtaposed cells forming intercellular channels aggregated in gap junctions which permit the direct intercellular transfer from cytosol to cytosol (gap-junctional intercellular communication, GJIC) of same ions and molecules as isolated connexons. So far, no pannexon-made gap junctions have been described in physiological/pathological conditions. The term connexon is mostly used to define the transmembrane unit of gap junctions. When isolated in the plasma membrane, connexons are usually called hemichannels and can open with various stimuli such as, for example, hypoxia. For clarity in the figure, putative phosphorylation sites (red spots) and N-glycosylated sites (green spots) are not shown in channels and gap junctions.

Possible involvements of Cxs and Panxs in cancer progression and the elucidation of the mechanisms they control lead to their use as new possible targets to control cancer progression [13,14]. Here, we will review the involvement of Cxs and Panxs in these different topics, which are cancer cell proliferation, invasion/metastasis process and as possible targets for cancer control.

2. Connexins and Pannexins Involvement in Tumour Cell Growth

2.1. Connexins Involvement in Tumour Cell Growth

Shortly after their characterization, GJs were thought to be involved in growth regulation [15]. This assumption was the consequence of the possibility to estimate GJ functions through electrical coupling or diffusion of small hydrophilic fluorescent tracers [16,17]. By using such approaches, it rapidly appeared that cells derived from solid tumours (hepatoma, thyroid tumours, etc.) were not able to communicate through GJs [18,19]. These seminal studies introduced the notion that lack of GJ coupling could be a fundamental process in cancer leading to the formation of solid tumours by uncontrolled cell growth [15]. In other terms, growth regulation was the very first physiological role attributed to GJs and their mediation of a direct intercellular communication.

During the following decades, the involvement of GJIC in cancer cell growth regulation has been supported by a wide range of data. An early observation was about tumour promoter agents acting as inhibitors of GJIC [20,21]. This was observed in several models and reinforced the parallel between decreased GJIC and increased cell growth [22,23]. This parallel was extended to all kinds of phenomena able to inhibit GJIC such as cancer-causing viruses [24]. And such a phenomenon was so widely observed that it has been proposed that any GJIC inhibitor could be a potential tumour promoter [25]. If the tumour promoting effects of these chemicals were mostly known from in vitro studies, in some cases, GJIC inhibition effect could also be observed in vivo with transgenic mice exhibiting higher tumour susceptibility when defective for specific Cxs [26,27]. One of these best examples is liver since Cx32 gene knockout (KO) mice were shown to be more susceptible than wild-type mice to liver carcinogenesis after chemical treatments or even spontaneously [26]. This example was relevant to rodent and human situations for which liver tumours were correlated with lack of GJIC either by loss of expression or aberrant cytoplasmic localization of Cx32, respectively [28,29].

Conversely, strategies permitting the recovery of GJIC, by increasing Cx expression from non-communicating cancer cells, were expected to decrease cell growth. And indeed, globally this was the case as shown by approaches using chemical treatments or cDNA transfection. Chemicals known to be putative chemopreventing agents (flavonoids, carotenoids, retinoic acids, etc.) appeared to act on transformed cell lines by inducing GJIC and decreasing cell growth [30,31]. Cx cDNA transfection in GJIC-defective cancer cell lines brought similar conclusions that Cx expression is accompanied by decreased cell growth. This was observed in a variety of cancer cells (hepatoma, glioma, breast, etc.) in vitro and in vivo [32]. However, the type of transfected Cx was important since such an effect was mostly observed when the Cx of the normal tissue (before transformation or cancer progression) was re-expressed [33,34]. These results suggested that a recovery of GJIC is not sufficient by itself to have tumour suppressive effects but should be specifically controlled by the Cx subtype depending probably on the permeability capacity of the GJ it forms.

Thus, significant data accumulated over 50 years supported a similar conclusion. Whatever the models or the approaches (in situ detection of Cxs in tumours, cancer cell lines, chemical treatments, transgenic mice, cDNA transfection, etc.), the global conclusion is that Cx expression/GJIC is inversely correlated to cell growth. All these data have been analysed and synthesized in many reviews during past decades [2–4,32]. By considering all these observations, two kinds of molecular mechanisms can explain the involvement of Cxs in tumour cell growth regulation. The first one is to describe how Cxs, when present, can control cell growth. The second kind of molecular mechanisms, which are also needed for explaining the link between Cxs and cell growth, has to elucidate the origin of the lack of

Cx expression or function which is observed in tumour cells. These are the two kinds of mechanisms that will be reviewed below.

2.1.1. How Can the Presence of Connexins Regulate Cell Growth?

Most data attempting to elucidate how Cxs control cell growth came from Cx cDNA transfection in cancer cell lines. And from such approaches, whatever the cell types which were used (osteosarcoma, liver or lung carcinoma cells, etc.), a constant observation was that the increased expression of the original Cxs was followed by a longer G1 cell cycle phase slowing down the cell proliferation rate (Figure 2). A global analysis of these results suggests that this effect was the consequence of p27 accumulation [35,36]. From this common fact, diverse observations were made such as inhibition of enzymatic activity of Cyclin-dependent kinases (CDK) [36] and decreased amount of Cyclin D1 [37] and S-phase kinase-associated protein 2 (Skp2) [36,38,39]. To our knowledge, so far, no direct molecular link between Cx presence and the regulation of cell cycle has been demonstrated. Besides such an effect of Cxs on nuclear regulation of the cell cycle, it has been shown that Cxs can also act on the level of expression of growth factors. For instance, Cx43 re-expression but not Cx32, in C6 glioma cells is related to a decreased amount of milk fat globule-EGF factor 8 (MFG-E8) mRNA through an unknown mechanism (Figure 2) [40]. Therefore, Cx expression is mostly related to change of expression of growth factors or/and cell cycle regulators (p27, Cyclin D1, etc.). The most obvious scenarios for explaining how Cxs, when localized at the plasma membrane, can control gene expression might be through two major pathways. A first one would be through the Cx interactome by controlling growth transduction signalling and the second would be by diffusing growth regulators through GJs. Interestingly, as reported in the literature, both mechanisms have been observed and can explain the specificity of cell growth control induced by Cxs.

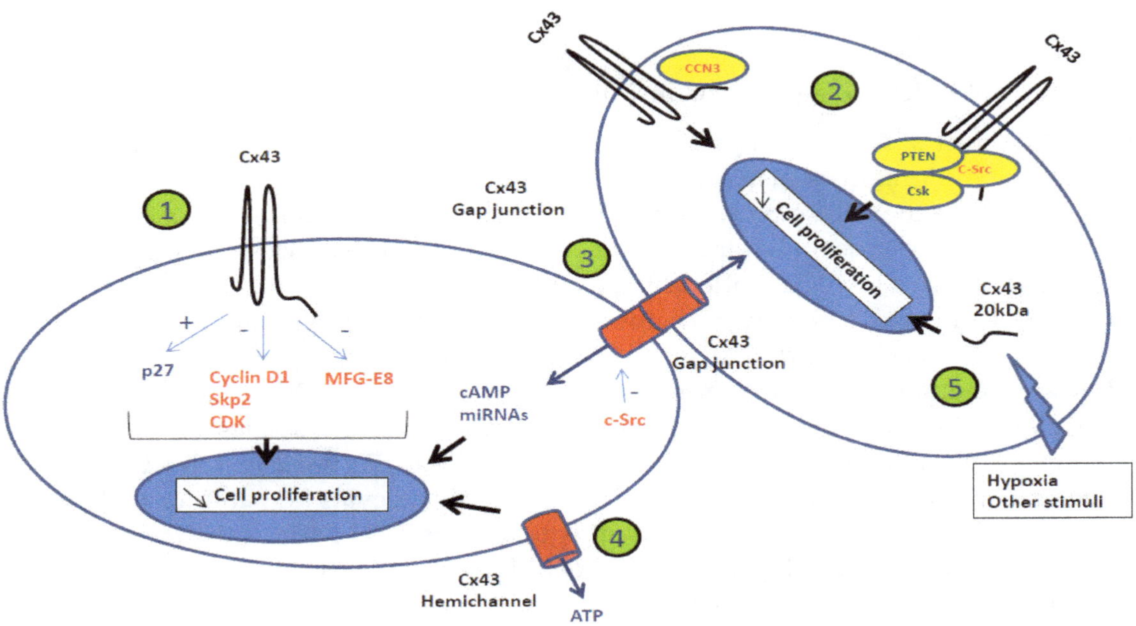

Figure 2. Connexin-mediated negative control of cell proliferation. Cx43 negatively regulates cell growth by acting differently on activators (red) and inhibitors (blue) of cell proliferation. This regulation is mediated through various mechanisms in which Cx43 acts by itself (1), as a sequestrator (2) of growth regulators (e.g., CCN3, PTEN, Csk, c-Src), as a mediator of GJIC (3), through hemichannel activity (4) or its 20 kDa carboxyl tail (CT)-domain (5). These various mechanisms act on the nucleus (thick black arrows) to decrease cell proliferation. Some of these mechanisms are mediated by hemichannel or gap-junction permeability (thick blue arrows). Positive (+)/negative (−) effects of Cx43 on cell cycle regulators (p27, Cyclin D1, etc.) and c-Src effect on Cx43 are also shown (thin blue arrows).

Gap-Junctional Intercellular Communication and Cell Growth Control

As mentioned above, the effect of Cx43 and Cx32 on cell growth has been extensively studied through various experimental models (cDNA transfection, transgenic mice, etc.) and appears to be specific. This specificity can be explained by their differential permeability which is illustrated by adenosine whose permeability is shifted from Cx32 to Cx43 channels by adding phosphate residues [41]. From such an observation, Cx channels appear as putative filters of intercellular signals that can be the consequence of the channel itself (diameter, amino-acid composition) or the configuration of the carboxyl tail (CT) which is sensitive to phosphorylation such as Cx43 channels closed by Src activation [42]. To our knowledge, a direct link between GJIC and growth regulation can be found in three situations. The first one is about the osteoblastic model in which extracellular growth stimulation induces the synthesis of second messengers that transit through GJs to activate extracellular signal-regulated kinase (ERK) and phosphatidylinositol-4,5-bisphosphate 3-kinase (PI3)/Akt serine/threonine kinase 1 (Akt) pathways. The translocation of ERK into the nucleus activates transcription factors that recognize a Cx-response element (CxRE) and induce osteocalcin and collagen I-1 expression [43]. Another example finally could explain the specific tumour suppressor effect of Cx26 on HeLa cells that was described two decades ago [33]. This effect seems to be the consequence of the maintenance of Cx26-mediated GJIC during the G2/M phase which permits intercellular cyclic 3′,5′-adenosine monophosphate (cAMP) redistribution able to delay the cell cycle progression (Figure 2) [44]. And more recently, it was shown that not only metabolites like cAMP could act as growth regulators passing through GJIC but also microRNAs (miRNAs) (Figure 2). As an example, the transmission of anti-proliferative effects from miR-124-3p-transfected to non-transfected glioma cells was mediated by GJIC [45]. Similarly, GJIC was shown to inhibit cancer cell growth by transferring miRNAs from endothelial cells in vitro [46]. And interestingly, it was observed that miRNA transfer can occur also by delivering from exosomes in which Cx43 facilitates the release of content into target cells [47].

Cell Growth Control Independent from Gap-Junctional Intercellular Communication

The specific effect of Cxs in cell growth control can come also from their cytoplasmic domains (internal loop and CT domain) which are unique in length and amino-acid sequences [8]. It has been known for a long time that these parts and in particular the CT domain, can interact directly with cytosolic/membrane proteins. Such interactomes have been mostly described for Cx43 for which about 40 different proteins have been identified as interacting ones [12,48]. From such observations, it became clear that the interactome may participate both to cell growth regulation by controlling channel permeability (i.e., channel closure due to Src-induced tyrosine phosphorylation of the Cx43 CT domain) or by modulating signalling pathways from the plasma membrane to the nucleus. For this last case, it has been postulated that the CT domain of Cxs could control, through sequestration, the translocation of putative transcription factors from the cytosol to the nucleus (Figure 2). Such a behaviour has been described for Cx32 with Discs large homolog 1 (hDlg1) in hepatocytes [49] and for Cx43 with CCN3 in rat C6 glioma cells [50,51]. In this last case, down regulation of Cx43 permits the translocation of CCN3 to the nucleus which activates cell growth (Figure 2) [50]. Such a situation can explain why glioma cell growth is higher when Cx43 expression is repressed and vice-versa. A similar situation has been shown for the transcription factor ZO-1–associated nucleic acid–binding protein (ZONAB) [52]. More recently, the tumour suppressive effect of Cx43 expression could be explained by the region 266–283 in the CT domain of Cx43 which is able to recruit PTEN and C-Terminal src kinase (Csk) to inhibit the oncogenic activity of c-Src (Figure 2) [53]. It is also possible that such a phenomenon could still happen when Cx43 is localized in the cytoplasm. Even if it has not been described yet, it would explain the down regulation of growth which was observed in human glioblastoma cells after transfection of Cx43 which was mainly localized in the cytoplasm [54].

In this last example, Cx43 signal was also detected in the nucleus of the cells [54]. The anti-proliferative effect associated with a nuclear signal of Cx43 is more intriguing. This effect could be due to the Cx43 CT domain since the transfection of that part only was followed by decreased growth in several cell types (HeLa, Neuro2a and HEK293 cells) [55–57]. It has been suggested that the Cx43 CT domain would then act as a transcription factor but this hypothesis has not been proven yet (Figure 2). However, a 20 kDa isoform which corresponds to the Cx43 CT domain is known to be translated in some cell types under certain conditions activated in cancer cells and hypoxia [58]. Its function is not known yet even if it has been shown to act as a chaperone protein for trafficking of Cx43 to the cell membrane [59] and for microtubule dependent mitochondrial transport [60].

Finally, to be complete, Cxs are known to form Hcs in the plasma membrane (Figure 1) [61]. Study of those Hcs has been growing this last decade, especially for Cx43 but their link with cell proliferation is still not obvious even if adenosine triphosphate (ATP) release and modulation of Ca^{2+} concentrations were correlated with decreased cell proliferation in several cell types [62]. In osteocytes, they have been found to be involved in suppression of breast cancer cell growth and bone metastasis using transgenic mouse models expressing dominant-negative mutants inhibiting either GJIC and/or Hcs [63]. With recent development of new research tools, such as Cx-interacting peptides, antibodies and dominant-negative mutants, the distinctive mechanisms of GJs versus Hcs, although still limited start to be elucidated. However, the action of Cx Hcs can still be confounded with Panx channels (Figure 1).

2.1.2. What Does Prevent Connexin Expression or Function during Tumour Progression?

The expression of Cxs is often decreased in tumours whatever their origin [32]. Such a decreased expression may then participate to increase tumour growth by preventing the molecular mechanisms controlled by the presence of Cxs that were reviewed in the previous section. The molecular events leading to the disappearance of Cxs are not known precisely but could come from two mechanisms acting either at the transcriptional or at the post-transcriptional levels of Cx expression.

At the transcriptional level, similar to other genes which are shut down during tumour progression, Cx genes could be the target of epigenetic control. However, data about such a transcriptional control of Cx expression are not abundant in the cancer context even if it was suggested two decades ago [64]. In HeLa cells, silencing of the Cx43 gene was thought to be controlled by DNA methylation [65]. Loss of Cx32 function through hypermethylation is necessary for the development of renal cell carcinoma at the early carcinogenic process [66,67]. The CpG island hypermethylation level was associated with heavy smoking, poorly-differentiated tumour and low expression of Cx43 in non-small cell lung cancer [68]. More recently, hypermethylation of the Cx45 gene has been linked to its reduced expression in colon cancer [69]. This field of research is probably under investigated and would reveal if pursued that epigenetic phenomena are more involved than expected in the control of Cx expression.

At the post transcriptional level, Cx function can be regulated by ubiquitination, glycosylation, S-nitrosylation and in particular, phosphorylation of the CT domain. This has been mostly studied for Cx43 whose phosphorylation regulates GJIC through different mechanisms such as Cx trafficking, connexon assembly, channel gating and GJ degradation [11]. And indeed, in the cancer context, many oncogenes encode for kinases (i.e., c-Src) or proteins activating kinases (growth factor receptors) that are known to phosphorylate Cx43 and modulate its function [70]. As an example among others, epidermal growth factor (EGF) inhibits GJIC by inducing mitogen-activated protein kinase (MAPK)-mediated phosphorylation of Cx43 [71,72]. A similar effect has been observed for platelet-derived growth factor (PDGF) which activates MAPK and protein kinase C (PKC) pathways [73]. Interestingly, such a phosphorylation of the Cx43 CT domain establishes a direct link between growth stimulation and GJIC inhibition, which appears to be either the consequence of channel gating or Cx degradation [74].

Still at the post transcriptional level, an emerging field is about repression of Cx expression by miRNAs. For instance, mi-R-221/222 complex and miR-125b have been shown to downregulate Cx43 expression in glioma [75,76] or miR-20a in prostate cancer [77]. This field is still emerging and no doubt that it will be more involved in Cx gene regulation in future years.

Finally, the lack of expression or function of Cxs could be also theoretically the consequence of mutations affecting either the coding region of the Cx genes or their promoters. However, contrary to classical tumour suppressors (p53, Rb, etc.), such mutations have been rarely reported in the cancer context [32]. The most convincing result revealed a mutation affecting the Cx43 CT domain in human colon adenocarcinomas, which resulted in a restricted expression in invasive parts of the tumours [78]. To our knowledge, such an observation has not been confirmed. The fact that Cx mutations are not involved in human cancer is intriguing when considering their involvement in several human hereditary diseases [79]. So far, none of these diseases are known to be associated with a particular cancer susceptibility except for Cx26 mutations in the case of keratitis ichthyosis deafness (KID) syndrome which are associated with squamous cell carcinomas in 15% of patients [79]. The apparent general lack of association with cancer is probably the consequence of a lack of follow up of such patients.

2.2. *Pannexins Involvement in Tumour Cell Growth*

Originally, Panxs (3 members in mammals: Panxs1, 2 and 3) were identified as GJ proteins exhibiting homology with the invertebrate GJ proteins, the innexins [9]. Present in chordates, contrary to Cxs and despite a similar topology, they are not able to form functional GJs but form single membrane channels releasing autocrine and paracrine signals similar to Cx Hcs [10].

Data about a possible relationship between Panx expression and cancer progression or cancer cell growth are not so developed as they are for Cxs. In general, it seems that Panxs exhibit a so-called tumour suppressive effect similar to what is observed with Cxs. Such an analogy started during the last decade with the analysis of the brain cancer gene expression database REMBRANDT which revealed that the expression level of PANX2 and also PANX1 is positively correlated to post diagnosis survival of glioma patients [80]. To some extent, these observations were confirmed by the tumour suppressive effect induced both by Panx1 and Panx2 overexpression in rat C6 glioma cells in vitro and in vivo conditions [81,82]. In those cells, Panx1 expression had a wide range of anti-tumour activity by reducing in vitro cell proliferation, cell motility, anchorage-independent growth and tumour growth in nude mice. Interestingly, these effects, which are globally similar (except cell motility) with those observed after Cx43 transfection, were accompanied by an increased GJIC [81].

Similar observations have been obtained from skin where PANX1 and PANX3 levels are reduced both in human keratinocyte-derived basal cell carcinomas and squamous cell carcinomas [83]. This is in line with studies showing that those Panxs reduce growth of rat epidermal keratinocytes when overexpressed [84]. Such a growth inhibition was also observed for Panx3 in chondrocytes and osteoprogenitor cells by inhibiting the WNT pathway and via calcium-mediated regulation of p21 [85,86]. Recently, Panx3 was shown to inhibit the odontoblast proliferation through AMP-activated protein kinase (AMPK)/p21 signalling pathway and promote cell differentiation by bone morphogenetic protein (BMP)/Smad signalling pathway [87].

However, the situation is not so clear and probably depends on the cell type by considering melanocytes in which Panx1 expression is low whereas increased expression is correlated with melanoma aggressiveness [88]. More data are necessary before understanding the real involvement of Panxs in cancer cell growth control.

3. Connexins and Pannexins: Involvement in Tumour Metastasis and Microenvironment

3.1. *The Process of Metastasis*

In order to become metastatic, a clone of cancer cells must acquire aggressive growth properties and/or stem cell-like properties and the tumour microenvironment can drive acquisition of migratory and invasive properties through epithelial to mesenchymal transition (EMT). In the majority of tumours, which are epithelial in origin, cells must be able to breach the basement membrane, invade into the stroma and into blood vessels (intravasation) that infiltrate the tumour site. In the vasculature, they will adhere to blood vessel walls and be transported to distant sites where they emerge from the circulation (extravasation) to initiated new tumours. Finally, establishment of metastatic tumours requires survival and growth in the new tissue microenvironment. During all of these processes metastatic cells must evade the anti-tumoral immune response (Figure 3).

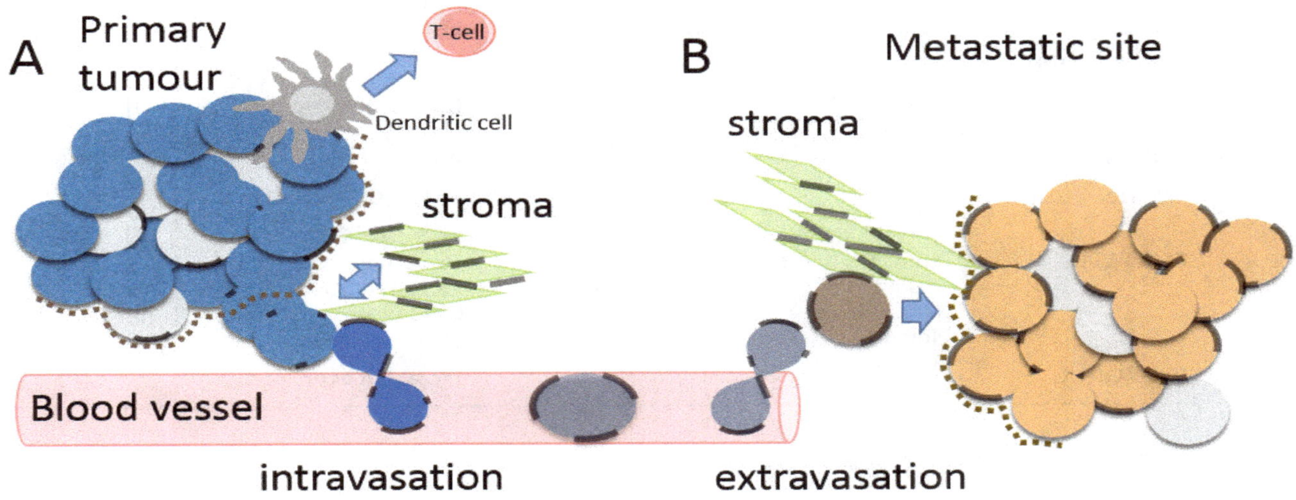

Figure 3. Gap-junctional intercellular communication in the tumour microenvironment and upon metastasis. (**A**) The tumour microenvironment consists of tumour cells (blue cells), non-tumour cells (light grey cells), immune cells including dendritic cells (dark grey cell) and CD8$^+$ T-cells (pink cell), the basement membrane (brown dotted line) and the stroma (green cells). Tumour cells often display reduced gap junctions (transparent black lines) but can form heterotypic gap junctions with dendritic cells. Once they invade through to the stroma they can also form junctions with stromal cells. Upon intravasation into blood vessels tumour cells create gap junctions with endothelial cells lining the blood vessels; (**B**) Upon extravasation into a metastatic site, metastatic cells (orange cells) initiate gap-junctional intercellular communication with stromal cells and with other cells in the metastatic tumour microenvironment (light grey cells) and this may facilitate establishment of metastases. Depending on the site of metastasis, tumour cells may interact with cells of the immune system.

3.2. Connexin Involvement in Tumour Metastasis and Microenvironment

3.2.1. The Role of Connexins in Cancer Progression

Cxs can change expression levels, be re-localized [89–92] and/or exhibit altered phosphorylation upon progression to invasive tumour (Table 1) [93]. The resulting loss of functional GJs could alter tumour cell interaction with its microenvironment and promote EMT and migration from the primary tumour. Conversely, Cx expression can facilitate intravasation and adhesion to endothelial cells, enabling increased survival in the circulation. There is also evidence that Cx expression promotes exit from blood vessels into the metastatic site, where GJIC may be reinitiated [94] (Figure 3). However, Cxs may both promote tumour cell dormancy and cell survival, at metastatic sites. These effects may be reliant on tumour/stromal interactions and cooperation between invasive/metastatic cells and GJ formation in the tumour microenvironment and are likely to be Cx type, tumour type and cancer-stage-specific.

Table 1. Selected representative examples of changes in connexins during tumour progression and metastasis.

TISSUE	ORGANISM	CONNEXIN	REGULATION	REFERENCE
PRECANCERS AND PRIMARY TUMOURS				
PANCREATIC DUCTAL ADENOCARCINOMA	Mouse	Cx43	Increased levels Changes in phosphorylation	[89]
CERVICAL CANCER	Human	Cx26, Cx30, Cx43	Loss of connexin expression	[95–97]
BREAST CANCER	Human	Cx26, Cx43	Loss of Cx43 gap junctions	[98–101]
PROSTATE CANCER	Human	Cx32, Cx43	Decreased expression	[102]
COLON CANCER	Human	Cx32, Cx43	Gradual loss of expression	[92]
MELANOMA	Human	Cx26, Cx30	Increased expression	[103]
PRIMARY TUMOUR TO METASTASIS				
BREAST CANCER	Human	Cx26, Cx43		[101,104–108]
BRAIN	Human, rat Human	Cx30 Cx43	Reduced expression	[109] [110,111]
PROSTATE	Human cell lines	Cx43	Increased Cx43 associated with increased invasion	[112]
LIVER	Rat cell lines Human	Cx43 Cx26	Cx43 overexpression High expression	[113] [114]
MELANOMA	Human Human cell lines	Cx26	Increased expression	[103,115] [116]

3.2.2. Invasion and the Local Microenvironment

E-cadherin is required for invasion in EMT and its loss is a marker of tumour progression. During invasion, cells display decreased GJIC, modification of cell-matrix interactions and acquisition of proteolytic properties to degrade the basal laminal proteins. Following this, altered stromal cells and microenvironment facilitate the motility of invasive cells through the extracellular matrix. All of these processes could be potentially altered by changes in Cx expression. For example, transfection of poorly coupled mouse epidermal cells with an E-cadherin expression construct increased GJIC [117]. Conversely, in prostate cancer cells, Cx43 levels correlated with levels of the transcription factor Snail-1 that inhibits expression of E-cadherin to promote EMT [118]. High levels of Cx43 and Snail-1 resulted in increased tumour cell invasion and Cx43 was downregulated upon Snail-1 silencing and vice versa. In keeping with these findings of a Cx43-Snail-1 axis controlling tumour cell behaviour, Cx43 expression could reverse A549 lung tumour cell resistance to the chemotherapeutic drug cisplatin by downregulating E-cadherin and EMT, while siRNA depletion of Cx43 initiated EMT [119]. Melanoma, breast, prostate and gastric cancers all display upregulated Cx43 and Cx26 in invasive lesions and metastases (Table 1) [101,103,104,112,115].

3.2.3. Promoting Metastasis: Connexins and Cell Motility

Early studies revealed that HeLa cervical cancer cells overexpressing Cx43 gained invasive properties in a chicken heart spheroid assay [120]. In a mouse melanoma model of metastasis following subcutaneous injection, clone F10 was less metastatic than the high Cx26-expressing clone BL6 but became as metastatic as BL6 upon Cx26 overexpression and BL6 cells expressing dominant negative Cx26 showed reduced metastatic potential [116]. γ-irradiation of C6 glioma cells induced Cx43 expression and increased ERK signalling and cell migration and a high Cx43 expressing clone displayed increased motility and invasion [121]. Conversely, knocking down Cx43 abrogated p38 MAPK activation and radiation-induced C6 cell migration [122]. Although GJIC was decreased upon Cx43 small interfering RNA (siRNA) depletion in the high Cx43 expressing C6 cells, GJ inhibitors did not alter motility indicating that Cx43 itself was responsible for the pro-metastatic effects [121]. Similarly, in a six-cell model of hepatocellular carcinoma, following injection into the tail vein of mice, only those lines with high metastatic potential formed foci in the lungs of the animals and this was reversible by depletion of Cx43 expression [113]. Another study found that blocking GJIC in GL15 glioblastoma cells increased motility in an in vitro 3D culture model [123]. However, blocking heterologous GJIC in ex vivo brain tissue by carbenoxolone reduced cell migration [123].

Cxs can facilitate adhesion of migrating cells to the endothelial layer of blood vessels and/or to specific distal sites (Figure 3). For instance, metastatic lung cancer cells could adhere to endothelial cells through GJs [124] as could metastasis-enabled melanoma cells ectopically expressing Cx26 in in vitro cultured vein segments [116]. In the case of colon cancer cells, conditioned medium from primary tumour cells enhanced phosphorylation of Cx43 and GJ formation between tumour and endothelial cells via the molecular chaperone heat shock protein 27 (HSP27), while metastatic colon cancer cells induced expression of Cx32 through action of the chemokine receptor CXCR2 [125]. Breast cancer cells that formed functional Cx43 GJs with endothelial cells facilitated migration out of the endothelial layer in in vitro culture [126] implicating Cx43 in the extravasation phase of metastasis. In zebrafish and chick embryo models, breast cancer and melanoma cell metastasis was dependent upon Cx43 and Cx26 to initiate brain metastatic lesions in association with the vasculature. Inhibition of Cx43-mediated GJIC inhibited extravasation, as did knock down of the EMT transcription factor twist [127].

3.2.4. Involvement of Gap Junctions and Hemichannels in Metastasis

Apparently contradictory effects of Cx43 in metastasis have been observed in different studies. When a functional null mutant Cx43 mouse line (G60S: that also has dominant negative effects on endogenous Cx43 activity) was crossed with erythroblastic leukemia viral oncogene homologue (ErbB) overexpressing mice [128], there was delayed onset and fewer and smaller primary breast tumours than in wild type mice but increased metastases to the lung [128]. In contrast, Cx43 overexpression in highly metastatic lung cancer cells reversed the metastatic tumour phenotype [129] but decreased Cx43 gene expression yielded breast cancer cells with increased metastatic potential [130,131]. In a two-cell model of prostate cancer, overexpressed Cx43 was present only in the cytoplasm and repressed proliferation, adhesion and invasion of normally invasive PC-3 cells. In contrast, overexpression of Cx43 in poorly metastatic LNCaP cells, re-established GJIC and increased bone metastasis in mice [132]. Stable overexpression of Cx43 in the MDA-MB-435 breast cancer cell line did not alter GJIC, invasion or migration in vitro. However, when injected into mice, the cells exhibited a reduced growth rate and fewer lung metastases [106]. This phenomenon was found to be GJIC-independent and it was suggested that it could be related to reduced N-cadherin expression, which would inhibit EMT. In another study, GJIC was restored in the same metastatic breast cancer cell line upon ectopic expression of the breast cancer metastasis suppressor gene BRMS1 [130]. The BRMS1-expressing cells showed increased levels of Cx43 but reduced Cx32, leading to loss of GJIC between breast cancer cells and between them and breast epithelial cells [130]. An in vivo murine study revealed that metastatic breast cancer cells in the bone formed more active GJs with osteoblasts than with themselves and BRMS1 expression increased homotypic GJIC. The breast cancer cells with increased heterotypic, relative to homotypic, GJ channels with osteoblasts were more metastatic than those that did not [105]. This suggests that the relative percentage of homo- and heterotypic GJ channels in tumour cells can influence metastasis. Moreover, it suggests that heterotypic GJs could be an important survival mechanism of tumour cells in the metastatic tumour microenvironment. It can be concluded that the precise timing of elevated or reduced Cx expression could be key to any effects during tumour progression.

Compared to GJs changes in Hc activity can produce different effects in metastasizing tumour cells. In a bone metastatic clone of MDA-MB-231 breast cancer cells, decreased Cx26 and Cx43 levels correlated with metastatic potential partly through alterations in Hc activity [107]. Similarly, a recent study reported suppression of breast cancer cell metastasis to the bone through osteocytic Cx43 Hcs [63]. Drug or mechanically-induced opening of Cx43 Hcs to release ATP from osteocytes led to inhibition of invasion and migration of the cancer cells. Analysis of a dominant negative Cx43 mutant that blocks GJs but not Hcs, revealed that Cx43 Hcs protected against tumour progression and metastasis [63]. The precise role of Cxs in tumour progression and metastasis might depend on the nature of the tumour, the properties of the cancer cell itself, the site of metastasis and the possibility of forming functional GJs at that site. It is clear that the tumour microenvironment drives cancer metastasis and Cx43 seems to stimulate growth of brain metastases after extravasation and tumour vasculature remodelling [133]. Protocadherin 7, a brain-specific cadherin, promoted Cx43-GJ assembly between breast and lung tumour cells and astrocytes. These GJs allowed cyclic guanosine monophosphate (cGAMP) to activate the stimulator of interferon genes (STING) pathway in astrocytes to induce an interferon response. The resulting changes in cell signalling could enhance growth of metastatic cells [133].

3.2.5. The Tumour Microenvironment

The tumour microenvironment, whether at the primary or secondary sites, is key to tumour cell survival and tumour progression [134]. In agreement with the hypothesis that Cxs control the microenvironment, Cx43-transfected glioma cells, which formed GJs with astrocytes in the striata of rats, were able to disseminate throughout the brain parenchyma. Cx43 itself, unlinked to GJIC, was shown to induce adhesive properties in the malignant glioma cells, which formed aggregates and were more invasive [135]. Also in rats, formation of GJIC with fibroblasts in co-culture stimulated prostate cancer cell migration [136,137]. However, Cx32 expression in metastatic renal cancer cells caused abrogation of invasive capacity via inactivation of c-Src signalling [138]. Tumour-associated immune cells are components of the tumour microenvironment. Heterotypic Cx43-GJs between tumour cells and dendritic cells can transmit melanoma antigenic peptides leading to activation of cytotoxic T-cells in vitro [139]. In vivo demonstration of Cx43-GJ transmission of antigenic peptides between antigen presenting cells has also been demonstrated [140]. GJ transmission of miRNAs between immune cells in the microenvironment and tumour cells is also expected to be a major regulator of metastasis because of the key role of many miRNAs in tumour suppression, while others can promote tumour progression [141].

3.3. *Pannexins and Metastasis*

The potential role of Panxs in metastasis is relatively unexplored. However, high levels of PANX1 mRNA were associated with metastatic spread in a two-cell model of hepatocellular carcinoma [142]. A key advance in understanding the role of Panxs in metastasis came from a study of the isogenic melanoma cell lines, F10 and BL6, mentioned previously. PANX1 levels were greatest in the most metastatic BL6 line [88]. PANX1 knock down reverted BL6 cells to a more normal melanocyte phenotype and these cells had reduced levels of vimentin and β-catenin, both markers of melanoma progression [88]. Importantly, in vivo data in a chick embryo xenograft model showed that reducing PANX1 expression reduced tumour growth and metastasis to the liver. A recent RNASeq analysis of breast cancer cells with different metastatic capacities revealed that cell lines with high metastatic potential had significantly enriched mutant mRNA encoding a N-terminal truncated PANX1 channel [143]. Truncated PANX-1, in association with wild type PANX1, seemed to confer a gain-of-function to channel activity and was found to promote metastatic cell survival. This appeared to be due to protection of tumour cells exiting the microvasculature via restrictive spaces between endothelial cells by enhancing ATP release from the Panx channels stimulated by mechanical deformation and abrogation of cell death [143]. In melanomas, P2X7/PANX1 channel activity has been linked to regulation of the NLRP3 inflammasome, which can result in release of pro-inflammatory, tumour promoting cytokines. Downstream effects on the tumour microenvironment could stimulate tumour growth and invasion. Of course, like Cxs, Panxs might also be found in future to repress tumour progression and metastasis.

4. Connexin and Pannexin Channels in Potential Cancer Therapeutics

4.1. Connexin Channels in Potential Cancer Therapeutics

The usefulness of Cxs and GJs as potential therapeutic targets for treating cancer has been studied for over four decades [4,144,145]. In recent years, several approaches have been developed in animal models to determine treatment modality by manipulating Cx channels. Although preclinical studies targeting connexin channels are still in their infancy, they hold great promise as de novo targets for cancer treatment.

4.1.1. Chemical Compounds in Modulating Connexins and Potential Cancer Therapy

Major attempts have focused on enhancement of GJIC function due to its impairment in primary cancer cells. Multiple chemical compounds have been used (e.g., retinoids, vitamin D, carotenoids, cAMP and lovastatin), which can fully or partially reverse the deficiency of GJIC in tumorigenic cells [146]. Lypopene, a carotenoid stimulates GJIC and Cx43 expression and inhibits the growth of the breast cancer MCF-7 cell line [147]. Extracts from the zooxanthellate jellyfish that show antioxidant activity exhibit higher levels of GJIC and cytotoxicity in MCF-7 cells than human epidermal keratinocytes [148].

An experimental approach was developed that killed tumorigenic cells based on GJIC selectively formed between them. In this study, tumorigenic BALB/c 3T3 and rat liver cells were loaded with Lucifer yellow (LY) and co-cultured with non-tumorigenic cells. By irradiation with blue light, only tumorigenic cells containing LY died but not the surrounding non-tumorigenic cells without LY [149]. This study further showed that when dibutyryl cAMP, retinoic acid, fluocinolone acetonide or dexamethasone were used during cell transformation, there was a reduction of transformed BALB/c 3T3 cell foci. These chemicals also increased and established GJIC between tumour cells and surrounding non-tumour cells, suggesting that the effects of chemicals on reversing the phenotypes of transformed cells rely on the establishment or enhancement of GJIC between tumour and normal cells.

Several cholesterol-lowering statin drugs (lovastatin, simvastatin, etc.) are suggested as anticancer reagents and high levels of mevalonate production are documented in various types of malignancies. Therefore, inhibition of the mevalonate producer, β-Hydroxy β-methylglutaryl-CoA (HMG-CoA) reductase, by statins offers a great potential for cancer treatment [150]. An earlier study shows that lovastatin increases GJIC in transformed E9 mouse lung carcinoma cells through the inhibition of PKC, although Cx43 expression and phosphorylation are not affected [151]. Moreover, apigenin, a flavonoid and lovastatin that is known to increase GJIC enhances bystander effect of the herpes simplex virus thymidine kinase/ganciclovir with reduction of cancer cell recovery on MCA38 adenocarcinoma cells, while neither chemical alone has such effect [152]. In vivo injection of both chemicals achieves 60–70% complete remission of tumour implanted in mice [152]. Simvastatin induced up-regulation of GJIC in Leydig tumour cells and this upregulation sensitized tumour cells to etoposide, a chemotherapeutic drug [153]. Simvastatin inhibited Cx43 phosphorylation by PKC and enhanced Cx43 membrane localization to promote formation of GJs (Ser368 phosphorylation promotes Cx43 internalization). However, a follow up study by the same group reported a protective function of simvastatin against toxicity by cisplatin on normal Sertoli cells [154]. This effect occurs at high cell density where GJIC forms and decreased GJIC by inhibitors or knocking down Cx43 by siRNA attenuates cell protective role of simvastatin. These two studies elucidate differential roles of GJIC by statins in chemotherapy by sensitizing drug effect on cancer cells and ameliorating toxicity in normal cells.

For Cx43 Hcs in cancer development, carbon monoxide (CO), a promising molecule to treat several diseases including cancer has been shown to inhibit their function [155]. CO donors inhibit Hc uptake in tumour cell lines (MCF-7 and HeLa cells) expressing exogenous Cx43 or Cx46 [156]. However, in general, scarce information is currently available describing the involvement of Cx Hcs in cancer cells.

Cxs can directly mediate the effect of chemotherapeutic drugs on cytotoxicity and apoptosis of cancer cells. Upregulation of Cx43 by cisplatin improves its resistance in a mesothelioma cell line (H28) [157]. GJIC inhibition fails to abrogate this effect but it is Cx43-dependent through the suppression of c-Src activation. Cx43 is increased in H28 cells by sunitinib treatment, which promotes apoptosis via the inhibition of receptor tyrosine kinase (RTK) signalling. This effect is likely to be mediated through direct interaction of Cx43 with an apoptotic related protein, Bax [158]. The Cx43 enhanced apoptotic effect of sunitinib was via enhancement of activation of Bax localized at the mitochondrial membrane and the phosphorylation of c-Jun N-terminal kinase (JNK) [159]. Several studies focus on the strategy of enhancing Cx expression in cancer cells. *Ganoderma lucidum*, an herbal mushroom known to inhibit tumour growth can increase Cx43 expression as well as vascular endothelial growth factor (VEGF) and inhibit growth of human ovarian cancer cells [160]. Such effect was abrogated by knocking down Cx43 expression. The bioactive substance sulforaphane inhibits cancer stem cells in aggressive pancreatic ductal adenocarcinoma through increased Cx43 and E-cadherin expression [161]. This treatment also inhibits the cancer stem cell markers c-Met and CD133, alters activation of several kinases and substrates, Glycogen synthase kinase 3 (GSK3), JNK and PKC and enhances GJ channels. Therefore, chemicals that can enhance GJs and Cx expression exhibit a high potency in suppressing cancer cell proliferation and tumour growth.

4.1.2. Connexin-Targeting Strategies in Potential Cancer Therapy

In recent years, several Cx mimetic peptides that reproduced portions of Cx sequences have been widely used in basic research as well as preclinical and therapeutic development [145]. Cx43-GJIC is decreased in breast cancer cells and efforts have been made to restore GJIC in these cells. αCT1, a mimetic peptide that targets CT domain of Cx43 can sustain and enhance GJIC function and has shown a great promise in promoting wound healing in skin by reducing scar formation [162]. A recent study shows that this peptide enhances Cx43 GJIC and reduces proliferation or survival of MCF7 and MDA-MB231 breast cancer cells but has no effect on MCF10A non-transformed cells [163]. A combination of αCT1 with tamoxifen or lapatinib augmented their effects on oestrogen receptor-positive MCF7 or Her2-positive BT474 breast cancer cells. Furthermore, treatment with αCT1 peptide sensitized human O-6-methylguanine-DNA methyltransferase (MGMT)-deficient and chemotherapeutic agent temozolomide (TMZ)-resistant glioblastoma (GBM) cells and combined treatment with the peptide and TMZ further incur autophagy and apoptosis of TMZ-resistance GMB cells [164]. A recent study shows that a cell-penetrating Cx mimetic peptide, TAT-Cx43(266-283) inhibits c-Src and focal adhesion kinase (FAK), upregulates phosphatase and tensin homology and reduces the growth, migration and survival of glioma stem cells (GSCs) from patients [165]. A Cx43 mimetic peptide juxtamembrane 2 (JM2) that is based on the Cx43 microtubule-binding domain inhibits Cx43 trafficking to the cell surface by promoting microtubule polymerization and reduces Hc numbers in the membrane for proinflammatory function. The authors imply that this peptide may have therapeutic value in treating proliferative diseases and cancer [166]. However, it is important to note that the recovery of GJIC does not consistently entail normalization of the tumour cells.

There are several reports concerning use of antibodies against Cxs. When a labelled monoclonal antibody against the second Cx43 extracellular loop domain was intravenously injected into rats with intracranial C6 glioma, antibody signals were detected in reactive, glial fibrillar acidic protein (GFAP)-positive astrocytes [167]. PEGylated immunoliposomes carrying monoclonal antibodies against GFAP and the above-described Cx43 monoclonal antibody were detected at the periphery of the glioma using either fluorescent or a paramagnetic probe [168]. These studies imply that these antibodies could potentially be used for targeted delivery of drugs to the zone of high-grade gliomas. Furthermore, magnetic resonance imaging data show that weekly administration of this Cx43 antibody at a dose of 5 mg/kg significantly reduces low-differentiated glioma volume and increases lifespan with a full recovery without delayed relapses in 19% animals [169]. Both Cx43 and brain-specific anion transporter (BSAT1) are preferably expressed in the brain tumour and peritumoral areas. Cisplatin-loaded nanogel conjugated with monoclonal Cx43 antibody [170] and BSAT1 was used to treat rats bearing tumours and the median survival was greater than control groups [171]. Vector nanogels seemed to reduce systemic toxicity of cisplatin [170]. Intriguingly, a combination of this Cx43 antibody with TMZ completely abolishes the antitumor effect of this antibody while combination treatment with γ-irradiation greatly inhibits tumour development and prolongs survival median to 60 days versus 38 days [172]. Recently, a magnetic resonance imaging (MRI) study further shows that uptake of Gd-based contrast agent with the same monoclonal Cx43 antibody is more than 4 times higher than nonspecific IgG-contrast agent and this Cx43 antibody conjugated agent markedly enhances visualization of glioma in vivo [173]. Although the specific molecular mechanism of this antibody is unknown, this Cx43-targeting monoclonal antibody could be developed as a potential drug and/or diagnostic agent for glioma therapies.

Finally, recombinant lentiviruses carrying siRNA were used to knockdown Cx37 expression in subcutaneous gastric tumours in mice [174]. Reduced levels of Cx37 are associated with higher apoptotic index of tumour cells in vivo. Cx46 is also detected in GBM cancer stem cells, while Cx43 is predominantly expressed in non-stem cells [175]. Besides Cx43, Cx46 is shown to express in GBM cancer stem cells (CSCs) that forms GJIC, while Cx43 is present in non-CSCs. During cancer differentiation, Cx46 is reduced associated with an increase of Cx43 and knocking down Cx46 by short hairpin RNA (shRNA) reduces stem cell maintenance.

Drug resistance is a major challenge for cancer treatment. Cisplatin is a commonly used chemotherapeutic agent for advanced non-small cell lung cancer but prolonged treatment leads to resistance due to development of EMT [119]. Overexpression of Cx43 reverses EMT and cisplatin resistance while Cx43 deletion initiates EMT and drug resistance in human lung cancer cell line A549. Patients with GBM, an aggressive adult primary brain tumour with poor prognosis, develop resistance to TMZ chemotherapy. In contrast to the situation in lung cancer, Cx43 is increased with the formation of GJIC in the resistant tumour cells and this increase is induced by epidermal growth factor receptor (EGFR) activated JNK-ERK1/2-AP-1 signalling [176]. Moreover, Cx43 expression in human glioma cells enhances resistance to TMZ via a mitochondrial apoptosis pathway by the reduction in Bax/Bcl-2 ratio and the release of cytochrome C [177]. Consistently, a recent study [178] showed that TMZ-resistant subline of U251 human GBM cells exhibited elevated Cx43 level compared to parental U251 cells, which was companied with increased EMT markers including vimentin, N-cadherin and β-catenin and decreased cell migration, monocyte adhesion and levels of vascular cell adhesion molecule (VCAM)-1. These studies suggest that depending upon cancer types, Cx43 expression and GJIC could be involved in either promoting or inhibiting sensitization of resistant cells to the chemotherapy. However, the underlying mechanisms remain elusive.

Recently, a new paradigm was proposed based on the data obtained in chronic inflammatory disorders and trauma in the eye that protecting cancer vasculature leads to reduced tumour hypoxia and promote survival of normal cells [179]. Given that Cx43 Hcs are involved in vascular leakage and endothelial cell death [180], modulation of these channels may provide an alternative for cancer treatment. Together, with advanced understanding of the mechanism of Cx channels in various types and stages of cancer development and metastasis, new lines of drugs that target them in cancer therapy are moving closer to reality.

4.2. Pannexin Channels in Potential Cancer Therapeutics

A great progress has been made in recent years for our understanding of Panx biology and physiology. However, compared to that of Cxs, the potential therapeutic application of Panxs in cancer is still limited.

4.2.1. Pannexin Channel Activation and Potential Cancer Therapy

Panx channels mediate ATP release and anti-tumour immune responses are associated with such a release from apoptotic cancer cells to engage P2 purinergic receptor signalling in leukocytes. A study shows that apoptotic reagents activate Panx1 channels via caspase-3 cleavage, which leads to ATP release in Jurkat T cell acute lymphocytes in chemotherapeutic drug-induced apoptosis [181,182]. Panx1 level is much higher in leukemic T lymphocytes than untransformed T lymphoblasts. Interestingly, chemotherapeutic drugs also cause ATP release with inhibition of caspase activation, which implies a Panx-independent mechanism. This study suggests that Panx1 channels and ATP release may mediate paracrine interaction between dying tumour cells and leukocytes in anti-tumour responses. A follow up study by the same group shows that activation of Panx1 channels by ATP is determined by expression level of particular ectonnucleotidases in tumour cell variants in Jurkat cell lines with and without the Fas-associated death domain (FADD) or receptor-interacting protein kinase 1 (RIP1) cell death regulatory proteins [183]. They noticed that robust levels of extracellular ATP/AMP were accumulated in apoptosis-deficient cells, not in apoptotic cells with the activation of Panx1 channels in response to chemotherapeutic drugs. Panx1 channel assists in accumulating immune-stimulatory ATP versus immunosuppressive adenosine within the tumour microenvironment. In support of the role of ATP and Panx1 channels in mediating immune response, a very recent study shows that ATP increases migration of dendritic cells through the activation of Panx1 channel and P2X7 receptor (P2X7R) [183]. In this study, they show that ATP actives P2X7R, which leads to opening of Panx1 channels and consequently results in more ATP release, re-organization of the actin cytoskeleton and faster migration of dendritic cells. Additionally, in vivo data show that Panx1 channels are required for the homing of dendritic cells to lymph nodes but not for maturation. Therefore, given that ATP acts as danger signal that recruits phagocytes including dendritic cells to cancer sites, activation of Panx channels through therapeutic drugs could hinder tumour growth and metastasis. Moreover, an US Food and Drug Administration (FDA)-approved anti-parasitic drug, Ivermectin allosterically regulates P2X4 receptors in breast cancer cells through opening of the P2X4/P2X7-gated Panx1 channels, which is associated with ATP release and consequently, cancer cell death [184]. Additionally, Ivermectin induces activation of autophagy and enrichment of inflammation mediators, ATP and high-mobility-group B (HMGB), suggesting that modulation of purinergic receptor signalling could be used as a platform for cancer immunotherapy [185].

4.2.2. Pannexin in Potential Cancer Diagnosis

A clinical report shows high relative expression of Panx3 in a patient with primary cutaneous sweat gland carcinomas with histologic features of a high-grade osteosarcoma [186]. By using quantitative trait loci (QTL) analysis, sequence comparison between strains and gene network analysis, this report links both body mass index (BMI) and tumorigenesis with Panx3 as a candidate gene in a genetically heterogeneous mouse model with carcinogen-induced cancer. A mutation encoding a truncated Panx1 (1–89) was identified which was enriched in highly metastatic breast cancer cells [143]. This truncated form of Panx1 further enhanced ATP release. In contrast to general belief of Panx channels in promoting cancer cell death, this paper suggests that ATP release by Panx1 suppresses deformation-induced apoptosis through P2Y receptor signalling and inhibition of Panx1 channels could reduce the efficiency of breast cancer metastasis. This could be partially explained by excess release of ATP by mutated Panx1 channels. Panx1 is present in skin melanocytes and is upregulated during melanoma tumour progression and tumorigenesis [88]. Knockdown of Panx1 in tumour cells decreases tumour cell growth, which indicates Panx1 as a potential target for treating melanoma. More studies are required to assess the expression levels of Panx subtypes in various types and stages of cancer.

4.2.3. Pannexin Channels in Pain Management Related to Cancer Treatment

Repeated treatment with the chemotherapeutic drug oxaliplatin is limited due to the development of a neuropathic pain in cancer patients. Functional recruitment of Panx1 mediates the increase of P2X7Rs in cerebrocortical nerve terminal in oxaliplatin-treated rats. Moreover, P2X7R antagonists and Panx1 inhibitors, Erioglaucine and ^{10}Panx peptide reverts neuropathic pain caused by oxaliplatin, while Panx1 inhibitors do not interfere the cytotoxic effect of oxaliplatin on human colon cancer cells HT-29 [187]. Consistently, a recent study shows that Panx1 expressed in immune cells plays a critical role for pain-like effects after nerve injury and this response is abrogated in Panx1 gene deficient mice [188]. These studies suggest that therapeutic modulation of Panx1 could be useful for treating neuropathic pain associated with cancer and cancer treatment.

5. Discussion and Conclusions

The involvement in cancer of GJs and their structural proteins, the Cxs, is a long story [4]. It rose just after the discovery of these particular intercellular junctions, which appeared to be absent in cancer cells. These very first observations suggested that the lack of GJIC could contribute to the lack of cell growth control which characterizes tumorigenesis [18]. Therefore, cell growth control was assumed to be one of the fundamental roles played by GJs. However, if this implication was assumed fifty years ago, the precise molecular mechanisms controlling cell growth came very late and are still unclear. There is a kind of paradox between the amount of observations accumulated for decades confirming a possible role of GJs as guardians of cellular homeostasis and replication and the lack of sufficient evidence explaining such a phenomenon.

Indeed, despite few exceptions, all kinds of observations were suggesting that the lack of GJs or Cxs is correlated to the lack of cell growth control and vice versa This consensus was supported by observations collected from a tremendous variety of models (cancer cell lines, primary cultures of tumour cells, in situ from biopsies, Cx-cDNA transfected cells, Cx-KO mice, chemical treatments decreasing or upregulating GJIC, etc.) whatever the species origins [32]. However, despite this consensus of observations, the assumption that GJs and Cxs were so-called tumour suppressors was not fully supported by several facts. First, GJs and Cxs did not behave as classical tumour suppressors since Cx gene mutations never appeared in tumours as commonly shown as for p53, Rb and so forth [32]. Second, no clear molecular mechanisms underlying the growth control that GJs and Cxs could exert has been established contrary to what was observed with classical tumour suppressors. These two aspects probably restricted GJs and Cxs to be considered as a real hallmark of cancer despite all the consensus studies we mentioned above [189]. The few molecular mechanisms that could explain the cell growth control exerted by GJs and Cxs seems to be "diffuse" and not so straightforward as growth signalling pathways described for oncogenes and tumour suppressors. Indeed, the involvement of Cxs in cell growth control is not clear at the molecular level and appears to be either GJIC-dependent or not. When this involvement was found to depend on GJIC, Cxs permit the intercellular diffusion of metabolites acting on cell growth control (i.e., Cx26 and the diffusion of cAMP, all along the cell cycle phases in HeLa cells) [44]. When this growth control is GJIC-independent, Cxs seem to act through their CT domain as a sequestrator preventing the nuclear translocation of cell growth regulators [53]. By comparing to our knowledge about cell growth control, Cxs seems to be a "helper" instead of a master regulator of cell growth control. Hopefully, future studies will bring more clear-cut information about the real involvement of GJs and Cxs in cancer cell growth [190].

In addition, we have also to consider that exceptions were observed in the consensus supporting the parallel between GJIC and cell growth control. These exceptions, supported by experimental observations, led to the hypothesis that Cxs could be protumoral actors when expressed at late stage of cancer progression. Indeed, from about twenty years ago, it appeared that Cxs could favour migration and invasion of cancer cells and participate to their dissemination [2,94]. A new wave of data then confirmed this new assumption that Cxs are actively involved in the late stages of carcinogenesis and participate to the aggressiveness of solid tumours. Very interestingly, from this more recent domain of investigation, Cxs were shown to play a role not only on migration and invasion of cancer cells but also on metastasis development by acting on intravasation, extravasation and dormancy of the metastatic cells. Within a few years, the Cx cancer statute has been changed then from tumour suppressor to tumour enhancer. Contrary to what appears at a first glance, this is not contradictory since an inverted correlation is often observed between cell proliferation and invasion capacity [191].

As for cell growth control, the molecular mechanisms underlying the involvement of Cxs in cell migration are not very clear. Once again, Cxs seem to control cell migration either through channel-dependent or –independent mechanisms. In the first case, the establishment of heterologous GJIC between cancer cells and cells of the tumour microenvironment may increase motility (such as glioma cells communicating with astrocytes) and further, helps to intravasation and extravasation [124–127,192]. When isolated in extracellular matrix, Cxs act on motility through GJIC-independent mechanisms by its CT domain. This has been particularly studied for Cx43 and even if the precise molecular events are not elucidated yet, it seems that the CT domain is involved by interacting with the actin cytoskeleton and helps to manage directional migration of the cancer cells [193]. Interestingly, such a phenomenon would not be pathological by itself since this process is present in migrations occurring in normal situations such as embryogenesis (neuron precursors migrating to the cortex) and leucocyte migration [194–196]. Other data also suggest that Cxs could be involved in formation of invadopodia and secretion of proteases during invasion process and also in metastasis targeting [132]. The molecular processes of all these phenomena are far from being to be elucidated. More data are needed to explain at the molecular level how Cxs can control cancer cell invasion and metastasis. These data are necessary for targeting Cxs to prevent eventually cancer invasion. This is of fundamental importance when considering that the majority of cancer deaths are the consequence of metastasis [1].

To conclude, there are globally sufficient data showing that Cxs are involved in carcinogenesis, especially in the progression of solid tumours. However, despite these data, the molecular mechanisms of the Cx involvement in carcinogenesis are not sufficiently elucidated yet. This lack of knowledge limits to use them as general therapeutical targets for cancer control. Moreover, the multifunctional sides of Cxs able to act as mediator of GJIC, through their interactome or even as Hcs make difficult to define their real implication in cancer. In addition, the similarity of Panxs with Cx Hcs adds another complexity to this area of research since this family of proteins seems to share functions with Cxs both in cell proliferation control and invasion. Facing this complexity, the only way to decipher the real impact of Cxs or Panxs in the cancer cell behaviour is to consider their involvement specifically in particular types of tumours but not globally [190]. One strategy could be by increasing in situ observations in order to localize precisely Cx/Panx expressions in the complex heterogeneity of specific human tumours and reveal the possible links of Cx/Panx localizations with the tumour behaviour. In particular, it could prove definitively the apparently opposed roles of Cxs in cell growth control and in cancer cell invasion through their differential expression either in the core of the tumour or in its invasive edges [111]. Therefore, due to uniqueness of the action of subtypes of Cxs and Cx channels on various types and stages of cancers, therapeutic approaches ought to be developed based on precise mechanism elucidated with more targeting approaches. This aligns with the current trend of drug development in treating cancer with precision medicine.

Acknowledgments: J.X.J. was supported by US National Institutes of Health grant CA196214, US Department of Defence (DoD) grant BC161273 and Welch Foundation grant AQ-1507; M.M. was supported by Ligue contre le Cancer (Comités de la Charente, Charente-Maritime, Deux-Sèvres, Morbihan et Vienne); S.V.G. was supported by Worldwide Cancer Research grant 08-0159 and acknowledges funding from the Medical Research Council as core funding for the MRC University of Glasgow Centre for Virus Research.

References

1. Forman, D.; Ferlay, J. The global and regional burden of cancer. In *World Cancer Report*; Stewart, B.W., Wild, C.P., Eds.; International Agency for Research on Cancer: Lyon, France, 2014; pp. 16–53, ISBN 978-92-832-0429-9.
2. Cronier, L.; Crespin, S.; Strale, P.O.; Defamie, N.; Mesnil, M. Gap junctions and cancer: New functions for an old story. *Antioxid. Redox Signal.* **2009**, *11*, 323–338. [CrossRef] [PubMed]

3. Naus, C.C.; Laird, D.W. Implications and challenges of connexin connections to cancer. *Nat. Rev. Cancer* **2010**, *10*, 435–441. [CrossRef] [PubMed]
4. Aasen, T.; Mesnil, M.; Naus, C.C.; Lampe, P.D.; Laird, D.W. Gap junctions and cancer: Communicating for 50 years. *Nat. Rev. Cancer* **2016**, *16*, 775–788. [CrossRef] [PubMed]
5. Hervé, J.C.; Bourmeyster, N.; Sarrouilhe, D.; Duffy, H.S. Gap junctional complexes: From partners to functions. *Prog. Biophys. Mol. Biol.* **2007**, *94*, 29–65. [CrossRef] [PubMed]
6. Aasen, T. Connexins: Junctional and non-junctional modulators of proliferation. *Cell Tissue Res.* **2015**, *360*, 685–699. [CrossRef] [PubMed]
7. Schalper, K.A.; Carvajal-Hausdorf, D.; Oyarzo, M.P. Possible role of hemichannels in cancer. *Front. Physiol.* **2014**, *5*, 237. [CrossRef] [PubMed]
8. Willecke, K.; Eiberger, J.; Degen, J.; Eckardt, D.; Romualdi, A.; Güldenagel, M.; Deutsch, U.; Söhl, G. Structural and functional diversity of connexin genes in the mouse and human genome. *Biol. Chem.* **2002**, *383*, 725–737. [CrossRef] [PubMed]
9. Panchin, Y.; Kelmanson, I.; Matz, M.; Lukyanov, K.; Usman, N.; Lukyanov, S. A ubiquitous family of putative gap junction molecules. *Curr. Biol.* **2000**, *10*, R473–474. [CrossRef]
10. Bond, S.R.; Naus, C.C. The pannexins: Past and present. *Front. Physiol.* **2014**, *5*, 58. [CrossRef] [PubMed]
11. Solan, J.L.; Lampe, P.D. Spatio-temporal regulation of connexin43 phosphorylation and gap junction dynamics. *Biochim. Biophys. Acta* **2018**, *1860*, 83–90. [CrossRef] [PubMed]
12. Hervé, J.C.; Derangeon, M.; Sarrouilhe, D.; Giepmans, B.N.; Bourmeyster, N. Gap junctional channels are parts of multiprotein complexes. *Biochim. Biophys. Acta* **2012**, *1818*, 1844–1865. [CrossRef] [PubMed]
13. Naus, C.C.; Giaume, C. Bridging the gap to therapeutic strategies based on connexin/pannexin biology. *J. Transl. Med.* **2016**, *14*, 330. [CrossRef] [PubMed]
14. Kandouz, M.; Batist, G. Gap junctions and connexins as therapeutic targets in cancer. *Expert Opin. Ther. Targets* **2010**, *14*, 681–692. [CrossRef] [PubMed]
15. Loewenstein, W.R. Junctional intercellular communication and the control of growth. *Biochim. Biophys. Acta* **1979**, *560*, 1–65. [CrossRef]
16. Loewenstein, W.R.; Socolar, S.J.; Higashino, S.; Kanno, Y.; Davidson, N. Intercellular Communication: Renal, Urinary Bladder, Sensory, and Salivary Gland Cells. *Science* **1965**, *149*, 295–298. [CrossRef] [PubMed]
17. Kanno, Y.; Loewenstein, W.R. Cell-to-cell passage of large molecules. *Nature* **1966**, *212*, 629–630. [CrossRef] [PubMed]
18. Loewenstein, W.R.; Kanno, Y. Intercellular communication and the control of tissue growth: Lack of communication between cancer cells. *Nature* **1966**, *209*, 1248–1249. [CrossRef] [PubMed]
19. Loewenstein, W.R.; Kanno, Y. Intercellular communication and tissue growth. I. Cancerous growth. *J. Cell Biol.* **1967**, *33*, 225–234. [CrossRef] [PubMed]
20. Yotti, L.P.; Chang, C.C.; Trosko, J.E. Elimination of metabolic cooperation in Chinese hamster cells by a tumor promoter. *Science* **1979**, *206*, 1089–1091. [CrossRef] [PubMed]
21. Murray, A.W.; Fitzgerald, D.J. Tumor promoters inhibit metabolic cooperation in cocultures of epidermal and 3T3 cells. *Biochem. Biophys. Res. Commun.* **1979**, *91*, 395–401. [CrossRef]
22. Yamasaki, H. Cell-cell interaction and carcinogenesis. *Toxicol. Pathol.* **1986**, *14*, 363–369. [CrossRef] [PubMed]
23. Trosko, J.E.; Jone, C.; Chang, C.C. Oncogenes, inhibited intercellular communication and tumor promotion. *Princess Takamatsu Symp.* **1983**, *14*, 101–113. [PubMed]
24. Atkinson, M.M.; Anderson, S.K.; Sheridan, J.D. Modification of gap junctions in cells transformed by a temperature-sensitive mutant of Rous sarcoma virus. *J. Membr. Biol.* **1986**, *91*, 53–64. [CrossRef] [PubMed]
25. Barrett, J.C.; Kakunaga, T.; Kuroki, T.; Neubert, D.; Trosko, J.E.; Vasiliev, J.M.; Williams, G.M.; Yamasaki, H. Short-term assays to predict carcinogenicity. In-vitro assays that may be predictive of tumour-promoting agents. *IARC Sci. Publ.* **1986**, 287–302.
26. Temme, A.; Buchmann, A.; Gabriel, H.D.; Nelles, E.; Schwarz, M.; Willecke, K. High incidence of spontaneous and chemically induced liver tumors in mice deficient for connexin32. *Curr. Biol.* **1997**, *7*, 713–716. [CrossRef]
27. Avanzo, J.L.; Mesnil, M.; Hernandez-Blazquez, F.J.; Mackowiak, I.I.; Mori, C.M.; da Silva, T.C.; Oloris, S.C.; Gárate, A.P.; Massironi, S.M.; Yamasaki, H.; et al. Increased susceptibility to urethane-induced lung tumors in mice with decreased expression of connexin43. *Carcinogenesis* **2004**, *25*, 1973–1982. [CrossRef] [PubMed]

28. Fitzgerald, D.J.; Mesnil, M.; Oyamada, M.; Tsuda, H.; Ito, N.; Yamasaki, H. Changes in gap junction protein (connexin 32) gene expression during rat liver carcinogenesis. *J. Cell Biochem.* **1989**, *41*, 97–102. [CrossRef] [PubMed]
29. Krutovskikh, V.; Mazzoleni, G.; Mironov, N.; Omori, Y.; Aguelon, A.M.; Mesnil, M.; Berger, F.; Partensky, C.; Yamasaki, H. Altered homologous and heterologous gap-junctional intercellular communication in primary human liver tumors associated with aberrant protein localization but not gene mutation of connexin 32. *Int. J. Cancer* **1994**, *56*, 87–94. [CrossRef] [PubMed]
30. Hossain, M.Z.; Wilkens, L.R.; Mehta, P.P.; Loewenstein, W.; Bertram, J.S. Enhancement of gap junctional communication by retinoids correlates with their ability to inhibit neoplastic transformation. *Carcinogenesis* **1989**, *10*, 1743–1748. [CrossRef] [PubMed]
31. Vine, A.L.; Bertram, J.S. Cancer chemoprevention by connexins. *Cancer Metastasis Rev.* **2002**, *21*, 199–216. [CrossRef] [PubMed]
32. Mesnil, M.; Crespin, S.; Avanzo, J.L.; Zaidan-Dagli, M.L. Defective gap junctional intercellular communication in the carcinogenic process. *Biochim. Biophys. Acta* **2005**, *1719*, 125–145. [CrossRef] [PubMed]
33. Mesnil, M.; Krutovskikh, V.; Piccoli, C.; Elfgang, C.; Traub, O.; Willecke, K.; Yamasaki, H. Negative growth control of HeLa cells by connexin genes: Connexin species specificity. *Cancer Res.* **1995**, *55*, 629–639. [PubMed]
34. Mesnil, M. Connexins and cancer. *Biol. Cell* **2002**, *94*, 493–500. [CrossRef]
35. Chen, S.C.; Pelletier, D.B.; Ao, P.; Boynton, A.L. Connexin43 reverses the phenotype of transformed cells and alters their expression of cyclin/cyclin-dependent kinases. *Cell Growth Differ.* **1995**, *6*, 681–690. [PubMed]
36. Zhang, Y.W.; Morita, I.; Ikeda, M.; Ma, K.W.; Murota, S. Connexin43 suppresses proliferation of osteosarcoma U2OS cells through post-transcriptional regulation of p27. *Oncogene* **2001**, *20*, 4138–4149. [CrossRef] [PubMed]
37. Koffler, L.; Roshong, S.; Kyu Park, I.; Cesen-Cummings, K.; Thompson, D.C.; Dwyer-Nield, L.D.; Rice, P.; Mamay, C.; Malkinson, A.M.; Ruch, R.J. Growth inhibition in G(1) and altered expression of cyclin D1 and p27(kip-1) after forced connexin expression in lung and liver carcinoma cells. *J. Cell Biochem.* **2000**, *79*, 347–354. [CrossRef]
38. Zhang, Y.W.; Kaneda, M.; Morita, I. The gap junction-independent tumor-suppressing effect of connexin 43. *J. Biol. Chem.* **2003**, *278*, 44852–44856. [CrossRef] [PubMed]
39. Zhang, Y.W.; Nakayama, K.; Nakayama, K.; Morita, I. A novel route for connexin 43 to inhibit cell proliferation: Negative regulation of S-phase kinase-associated protein (Skp2). *Cancer Res.* **2003**, *63*, 1623–1630. [PubMed]
40. Goldberg, G.S.; Bechberger, J.F.; Tajima, Y.; Merritt, M.; Omori, Y.; Gawinowicz, M.A.; Narayanan, R.; Tan, Y.; Sanai, Y.; Yamasaki, H.; et al. Connexin43 suppresses MFG-E8 while inducing contact growth inhibition of glioma cells. *Cancer Res.* **2000**, *60*, 6018–6026. [PubMed]
41. Goldberg, G.S.; Moreno, A.P.; Lampe, P.D. Gap junctions between cells expressing connexin 43 or 32 show inverse permselectivity to adenosine and ATP. *J. Biol. Chem.* **2002**, *277*, 36725–36730. [CrossRef] [PubMed]
42. Swenson, K.I.; Piwnica-Worms, H.; McNamee, H.; Paul, D.L. Tyrosine phosphorylation of the gap junction protein connexin43 is required for the pp60v-src-induced inhibition of communication. *Cell Regul.* **1990**, *1*, 989–1002. [CrossRef] [PubMed]
43. Stains, J.P.; Civitelli, R. Cell-to-cell interactions in bone. *Biochem. Biophys. Res. Commun.* **2005**, *328*, 721–727. [CrossRef] [PubMed]
44. Chandrasekhar, A.; Kalmykov, E.A.; Polusani, S.R.; Mathis, S.A.; Zucker, S.N.; Nicholson, B.J. Intercellular redistribution of cAMP underlies selective suppression of cancer cell growth by connexin26. *PLoS ONE* **2013**, *8*, e82335. [CrossRef] [PubMed]
45. Suzhi, Z.; Liang, T.; Yuexia, P.; Lucy, L.; Xiaoting, H.; Yuan, Z.; Qin, W. Gap Junctions Enhance the Antiproliferative Effect of MicroRNA-124–3p in Glioblastoma Cells. *J. Cell Physiol.* **2015**, *230*, 2476–2488. [CrossRef] [PubMed]
46. Thuringer, D.; Jego, G.; Berthenet, K.; Hammann, A.; Solary, E.; Garrido, C. Gap junction-mediated transfer of miR-145–5p from microvascular endothelial cells to colon cancer cells inhibits angiogenesis. *Oncotarget* **2016**, *7*, 28160–28168. [CrossRef] [PubMed]
47. Soares, A.R.; Martins-Marques, T.; Ribeiro-Rodrigues, T.; Ferreira, J.V.; Catarino, S.; Pinho, M.J.; Zuzarte, M.; Isabel Anjo, S.; Manadas, B.P.G.; Sluijter, J.; et al. Gap junctional protein Cx43 is involved in the communication between extracellular vesicles and mammalian cells. *Sci. Rep.* **2015**, *5*, 13243. [CrossRef] [PubMed]

48. Laird, D.W. The gap junction proteome and its relationship to disease. *Trends Cell Biol.* **2010**, *20*, 92–101. [CrossRef] [PubMed]
49. Duffy, H.S.; Iacobas, I.; Hotchkiss, K.; Hirst-Jensen, B.J.; Bosco, A.; Dandachi, N.; Dermietzel, R.; Sorgen, P.L.; Spray, D.C. The gap junction protein connexin32 interacts with the Src homology3/hook domain of discs large homolog 1. *J. Biol. Chem.* **2007**, *282*, 9789–9796. [CrossRef] [PubMed]
50. Fu, C.T.; Bechberger, J.F.; Ozog, M.A.; Perbal, B.; Naus, C.C. CCN3 (NOV) interacts with connexin43 in C6 glioma cells: Possible mechanism of connexin-mediated growth suppression. *J. Biol. Chem.* **2004**, *279*, 36943–36950. [CrossRef] [PubMed]
51. Gellhaus, A.; Dong, X.; Propson, S.; Maass, K.; Klein-Hitpass, L.; Kibschull, M.; Traub, O.; Willecke, K.; Perbal, B.; Lye, S.J.; et al. Connexin43 interacts with NOV: A possible mechanism for negative regulation of cell growth in choriocarcinoma cells. *J. Biol. Chem.* **2004**, *279*, 36931–36942. [CrossRef] [PubMed]
52. Penes, M.C.; Li, X.; Nagy, J.I. Expression of zonula occludens-1 (ZO-1) and the transcription factor ZO-1-associated nucleic acid-binding protein (ZONAB)-MsY3 in glial cells and colocalization at oligodendrocyte and astrocyte gap junctions in mouse brain. *Eur. J. Neurosci.* **2005**, *22*, 404–418. [CrossRef] [PubMed]
53. González-Sánchez, A.; Jaraíz-Rodríguez, M.; Domínguez-Prieto, M.; Herrero-González, S.; Medina, J.M.; Tabernero, A. Connexin43 recruits PTEN and Csk to inhibit c-Src activity in glioma cells and astrocytes. *Oncotarget* **2016**, *7*, 49819–49833. [CrossRef] [PubMed]
54. Huang, R.P.; Fan, Y.; Hossain, M.Z.; Peng, A.; Zeng, Z.L.; Boynton, A.L. Reversion of the neoplastic phenotype of human glioblastoma cells by connexin 43 (cx43). *Cancer Res.* **1998**, *58*, 5089–5096. [PubMed]
55. Dang, X.; Doble, B.W.; Kardami, E. The carboxy-tail of connexin-43 localizes to the nucleus and inhibits cell growth. *Mol. Cell Biochem.* **2003**, *242*, 35–38. [CrossRef] [PubMed]
56. Moorby, C.; Patel, M. Dual functions for connexins: Cx43 regulates growth independently of gap junction formation. *Exp. Cell Res.* **2001**, *271*, 238–248. [CrossRef] [PubMed]
57. Dang, X.; Jeyaraman, M.; Kardami, E. Regulation of connexin-43-mediated growth inhibition by a phosphorylatable amino-acid is independent of gap junction-forming ability. *Mol. Cell. Biochem.* **2006**, *289*, 201–217. [CrossRef] [PubMed]
58. Ul-Hussain, M.; Olk, S.; Schoenebeck, B.; Wasielewski, B.; Meier, C.; Prochnow, N.; May, C.; Galozzi, S.; Marcus, K.; Zoidl, G.; et al. Internal ribosomal entry site (IRES) activity generates endogenous carboxyl-terminal domains of Cx43 and is responsive to hypoxic conditions. *J. Biol. Chem.* **2014**, *289*, 20979–20990. [CrossRef] [PubMed]
59. Smyth, J.W.; Shaw, R.M. Autoregulation of connexin43 gap junction formation by internally translated isoforms. *Cell Rep.* **2013**, *5*, 611–618. [CrossRef] [PubMed]
60. Fu, Y.; Zhang, S.S.; Xiao, S.; Basheer, W.A.; Baum, R.; Epifantseva, I.; Hong, T.; Shaw, R.M. Cx43 Isoform GJA1–20k Promotes Microtubule Dependent Mitochondrial Transport. *Front. Physiol.* **2017**, *8*, 905. [CrossRef] [PubMed]
61. Bruzzone, S.; Guida, L.; Zocchi, E.; Franco, L.; De Flora, A. Connexin 43 hemi channels mediate Ca^{2+}-regulated transmembrane NAD+ fluxes in intact cells. *FASEB J.* **2001**, *15*, 10–12. [CrossRef] [PubMed]
62. Song, D.; Liu, X.; Liu, R.; Yang, L.; Zuo, J.; Liu, W. Connexin 43 hemichannel regulates H9c2 cell proliferation by modulating intracellular ATP and (Ca^{2+}). *Acta Biochim. Biophys. Sin.* **2010**, *42*, 472–482. [CrossRef] [PubMed]
63. Zhou, J.Z.; Riquelme, M.A.; Gu, S.; Kar, R.; Gao, X.; Sun, L.; Jiang, J.X. Osteocytic connexin hemichannels suppress breast cancer growth and bone metastasis. *Oncogene* **2016**, *35*, 5597–5607. [CrossRef] [PubMed]
64. Yamasaki, H.; Omori, Y.; Zaidan-Dagli, M.L.; Mironov, N.; Mesnil, M.; Krutovskikh, V. Genetic and epigenetic changes of intercellular communication genes during multistage carcinogenesis. *Cancer Detect Prev.* **1999**, *23*, 273–279. [CrossRef] [PubMed]
65. King, T.J.; Fukushima, L.H.; Donlon, T.A.; Hieber, A.D.; Shimabukuro, K.A.; Bertram, J.S. Correlation between growth control, neoplastic potential and endogenous connexin43 expression in HeLa cell lines: Implications for tumor progression. *Carcinogenesis* **2000**, *21*, 311–315. [CrossRef] [PubMed]
66. Yano, T.; Ito, F.; Yamasaki, H.; Hagiwara, K.; Ozasa, H.; Nakazawa, H.; Toma, H. Epigenetic inactivation of connexin 32 in renal cell carcinoma from hemodialytic patients. *Kidney Int.* **2004**, *65*, 1519. [CrossRef] [PubMed]

67. Sumiko, S.; Hiromi, H.; Hiromi, S.; Keiko, F.; Shigeto, K.; Taiichiro, S.; Toyohiko, A.; Kiyokazu, H.; Hiroshi, Y.; Tomohiro, Y. Prevention of renal cell carcinoma from hemodialysis patients by regulating epigenetic factors. *Kidney Int.* **2005**, *67*, 2506–2507. [CrossRef] [PubMed]
68. Jinn, Y.; Inase, N. Connexin 43, E-cadherin, beta-catenin and ZO-1 expression, and aberrant methylation of the connexin 43 gene in NSCLC. *Anticancer Res.* **2010**, *30*, 2271–2278. [PubMed]
69. Sirnes, S.; Honne, H.; Ahmed, D.; Danielsen, S.A.; Rognum, T.O.; Meling, G.I.; Leithe, E.; Rivedal, E.; Lothe, R.A.; Lind, G.E. DNA methylation analyses of the connexin gene family reveal silencing of GJC1 (Connexin45) by promoter hypermethylation in colorectal cancer. *Epigenetics* **2011**, *6*, 602–609. [CrossRef] [PubMed]
70. Warn-Cramer, B.J.; Lau, A.F. Regulation of gap junctions by tyrosine protein kinases. *Biochim. Biophys. Acta* **2004**, *1662*, 81–95. [CrossRef] [PubMed]
71. Warn-Cramer, B.J.; Cottrell, G.T.; Burt, J.M.; Lau, A.F. Regulation of connexin-43 gap junctional intercellular communication by mitogen-activated protein kinase. *J. Biol. Chem.* **1998**, *273*, 9188–9196. [CrossRef] [PubMed]
72. Lau, A.F.; Kanemitsu, M.Y.; Kurata, W.E.; Danesh, S.; Boynton, A.L. Epidermal growth factor disrupts gap-junctional communication and induces phosphorylation of connexin43 on serine. *Mol. Biol. Cell* **1992**, *3*, 865–874. [CrossRef] [PubMed]
73. Hossain, M.Z.; Ao, P.; Boynton, A.L. Platelet-derived growth factor-induced disruption of gap junctional communication and phosphorylation of connexin43 involves protein kinase C and mitogen-activated protein kinase. *J. Cell Physiol.* **1998**, *176*, 332–341. [CrossRef]
74. Leithe, E.; Mesnil, M.; Aasen, T. The connexin43 C-terminus: A tail of many tales. *Biochim. Biophys. Acta* **2018**, *1860*, 48–64. [CrossRef] [PubMed]
75. Hao, J.; Zhang, C.; Zhang, A.; Wang, K.; Jia, Z.; Wang, G.; Han, L.; Kang, C.; Pu, P. miR-221/222 is the regulator of Cx43 expression in human glioblastoma cells. *Oncol. Rep.* **2012**, *27*, 1504–1510. [PubMed]
76. Jin, Z.; Xu, S.; Yu, H.; Yang, B.; Zhao, H.; Zhao, G. miR-125b inhibits Connexin43 and promotes glioma growth. *Cell Mol. Neurobiol.* **2013**, *33*, 1143–1148. [CrossRef] [PubMed]
77. Li, X.; Pan, J.H.; Song, B.; Xiong, E.Q.; Chen, Z.W.; Zhou, Z.S.; Su, Y.P. Suppression of CX43 expression by miR-20a in the progression of human prostate cancer. *Cancer Biol. Ther.* **2012**, *13*, 890–898. [CrossRef] [PubMed]
78. Dubina, M.V.; Iatckii, N.A.; Popov, D.E.; Vasiliev, S.V.; Krutovskikh, V.A. Connexin 43, but not connexin 32, is mutated at advanced stages of human sporadic colon cancer. *Oncogene* **2002**, *21*, 4992–4996. [CrossRef] [PubMed]
79. Srinivas, M.; Verselis, V.K.; White, T.W. Human diseases associated with connexin mutations. *Biochim. Biophys. Acta* **2018**, *1860*, 192–201. [CrossRef] [PubMed]
80. Litvin, O.; Tiunova, A.; Connell-Alberts, Y.; Panchin, Y.; Baranova, A. What is hidden in the pannexin treasure trove: The sneak peek and the guesswork. *J. Cell Mol. Med.* **2006**, *10*, 613–634. [CrossRef] [PubMed]
81. Lai, C.P.; Bechberger, J.F.; Thompson, R.J.; MacVicar, B.A.; Bruzzone, R.; Naus, C.C. Tumor-suppressive effects of pannexin 1 in C6 glioma cells. *Cancer Res.* **2007**, *67*, 1545–1554. [CrossRef] [PubMed]
82. Lai, C.P.; Bechberger, J.F.; Naus, C.C. Pannexin2 as a novel growth regulator in C6 glioma cells. *Oncogene* **2009**, *28*, 4402–4408. [CrossRef] [PubMed]
83. Cowan, K.N.; Langlois, S.; Penuela, S.; Cowan, B.J.; Laird, D.W. Pannexin1 and Pannexin3 exhibit distinct localization patterns in human skin appendages and are regulated during keratinocyte differentiation and carcinogenesis. *Cell Commun. Adhes.* **2012**, *19*, 45–53. [CrossRef] [PubMed]
84. Celetti, S.J.; Cowan, K.N.; Penuela, S.; Shao, Q.; Churko, J.; Laird, D.W. Implications of pannexin 1 and pannexin 3 for keratinocyte differentiation. *J. Cell Sci.* **2010**, *123*, 1363–1372. [CrossRef] [PubMed]
85. Iwamoto, T.; Nakamura, T.; Doyle, A.; Ishikawa, M.; de Vega, S.; Fukumoto, S.; Yamada, Y. Pannexin 3 regulates intracellular ATP/cAMP levels and promotes chondrocyte differentiation. *J. Biol. Chem.* **2010**, *285*, 18948–18958. [CrossRef] [PubMed]
86. Ishikawa, M.; Iwamoto, T.; Fukumoto, S.; Yamada, Y. Pannexin 3 inhibits proliferation of osteoprogenitor cells by regulating Wnt and p21 signaling. *J. Biol. Chem.* **2014**, *289*, 2839–2851. [CrossRef] [PubMed]
87. Iwamoto, T.; Nakamura, T.; Ishikawa, M.; Yoshizaki, K.; Sugimoto, A.; Ida-Yonemochi, H.; Ohshima, H.; Saito, M.; Yamada, Y.; Fukumoto, S. Pannexin 3 regulates proliferation and differentiation of odontoblasts via its hemichannel activities. *PLoS ONE* **2017**, *12*, e0177557. [CrossRef] [PubMed]

88. Penuela, S.; Gyenis, L.; Ablack, A.; Churko, J.M.; Berger, A.C.; Litchfield, D.W.; Lewis, J.D.; Laird, D.W. Loss of pannexin 1 attenuates melanoma progression by reversion to a melanocytic phenotype. *J. Biol. Chem.* **2012**, *287*, 29184–29193. [CrossRef] [PubMed]
89. Solan, J.L.; Hingorani, S.R.; Lampe, P.D. Changes in Connexin43 Expression and Localization during Pancreatic Cancer Progression. *J. Membr. Biol.* **2012**, *245*, 255–262. [CrossRef] [PubMed]
90. Aasen, T.; Hodgins, M.B.; Edward, M.; Graham, S.V. The relationship between connexins, gap junctions, tissue architecture and tumour invasion, as studied in a novel in vitro model of HPV-16-associated cervical cancer progression. *Oncogene* **2003**, *22*, 7969–7980. [CrossRef] [PubMed]
91. Kanczuga-Koda, L.; Sulkowski, S.; Lenczewski, A.; Koda, M.; Wincewicz, A.; Baltaziak, M.; Sulkowska, M. Increased expression of connexins 26 and 43 in lymph node metastases of breast cancer. *J. Clin. Pathol.* **2006**, *59*, 429–433. [CrossRef] [PubMed]
92. Kanczuga-Koda, L.; Koda, M.; Sulkowski, S.; Wincewicz, A.; Zalewski, B.; Sulkowska, M. Gradual loss of functional gap junction within progression of colorectal cancer—A shift from membranous Cx32 and Cx43 expression to cytoplasmic pattern during colorectal carcinogenesis. *In Vivo* **2010**, *24*, 101–107. [PubMed]
93. Lowenstein, W.R. Junctional intercellular communication by phosphorylation. *Biochem. Soc. Symp.* **1985**, *50*, 43–58. [PubMed]
94. Defamie, N.; Chepied, A.; Mesnil, M. Connexins, gap junctions and tissue invasion. *FEBS Lett.* **2014**, *588*, 1331–1338. [CrossRef] [PubMed]
95. McNutt, N.; Hershberg, R.; Weinstein, R. Further observations on the occurrence of nexuses in benign and malignant human cervical epithelium. *J. Cell Biol.* **1971**, *51*, 805–825. [CrossRef] [PubMed]
96. King, T.; Fukushima, L.; Hieber, A.; Shimabukuro, A.; Sakr, W.; Bertram, J. Reduced levels of connexin 43 in cervical dysplasia: Inducible expression in a cervical carcinoma line decreases neoplastic potential with implications for tumour progression. *Carcinogenesis* **2000**, *21*, 1097–1109. [CrossRef] [PubMed]
97. Aasen, T.; Graham, S.V.; Edward, M.; Hodgins, M.B. Reduced expression of multiple gap junction proteins is a feature of cervical dysplasia. *Mol. Cancer* **2005**, *4*, 1–5. [CrossRef] [PubMed]
98. Jamieson, S.; Going, J.J.; D'Arcy, R.; George, W.D. Expression of gap junction proteins connexin 26 and connexin 43 in normal human breast and in breast tumours. *J. Pathol.* **1998**, *184*, 37–43. [CrossRef]
99. Laird, D.W.; Fistouris, P.; Batist, G.; Alpert, L.; Huynh, H.T.; Carysrinos, G.; Alaoui-Jamali, M.A. Deficiency of connexin43 gap junctions is an independent marker for breast tumors. *Cancer Res.* **1999**, *59*, 4104–4110. [PubMed]
100. Singal, R.; Tu, Z.; Vanwert, J.; Ginder, G.; Kiang, D. Modulation of the connexin26 tumour suppressor gene expression through methylation in human mammary epithelial cell lines. *Anticancer Res.* **2000**, *20*, 59–64. [PubMed]
101. Naoi, Y.; Miyoshi, Y.; Taguchi, T.; Kim, S.J.; Arai, T.; Tamaki, Y.; Noguchi, S. Connexin26 expression is associated with lymphatic vessel invasion and poor prognosis in human breast cancer. *Breast Cancer Res. Treat.* **2007**, *106*, 11–17. [CrossRef] [PubMed]
102. Habermann, H.; Ray, V.; Habermann, W.; Prins, G.S. Alterations in gap junction protein expression in human benign prostatic hyperplasia and prostate cancer. *J. Urol.* **2002**, *167*, 655–660. [CrossRef]
103. Haass, N.K.; Ripperger, D.; Wladykowski, E.; Dawson, P.; Gimotty, P.A.; Blome, C.; Fischer, F.; Schmage, P.; Moll, I.; Brandner, J.M. Melanoma progression exhibits a significant impact on connexin expression patterns in the epidermal tumor microenvironment. *Histochem. Cell Biol.* **2009**, *133*, 113–124. [CrossRef] [PubMed]
104. Elzarrad, M.K.; Haroon, A.; Willecke, K.; Dobrowolski, R.; Gillespie, M.N.; Al-Mehdi, A.-B. Connexin-43 upregulation in micrometastases and tumor vasculature and its role in tumor cell attachment to pulmonary endothelium. *BMC Med.* **2008**, *6*, 20. [CrossRef] [PubMed]
105. Kapoor, P.; Saunders, M.M.; Li, Z.; Zhou, Z.; Sheaffer, N.; Kunze, E.L.; Samant, R.S.; Welch, D.R.; Donahue, H.J. Breast cancer metastatic potential: Correlation with increased heterotypic gap junctional intercellular communication between breast cancer cells and osteoblastic cells. *Int. J. Cancer* **2004**, *111*, 693–697. [CrossRef] [PubMed]
106. Li, Z.; Zhou, Z.; Donahue, H.J. Alterations in Cx43 and OB-cadherin affect breast cancer cell metastatic potential. *Clin. Exp. Metastasis* **2008**, *25*, 265–272. [CrossRef] [PubMed]
107. Li, Z.; Zhou, Z.; Welch, D.R.; Donahue, H.J. Expressing connexin 43 in breast cancer cells reduces their metastasis to lungs. *Clin. Exp. Metastasis* **2008**, *25*, 893–901. [CrossRef] [PubMed]

108. Chao, Y.; Wu, Q.; Acquafondata, M.; Dhir, R.; Wells, A. Partial Mesenchymal to Epithelial Reverting Transition in Breast and Prostate Cancer Metastases. *Cancer Microenviron.* **2012**, *5*, 19–28. [CrossRef] [PubMed]
109. Arun, S.; Ravisankar, S.; Vanisree, A.J. Implication of connexin30 on the stemness of glioma: Connexin30 reverses the malignant phenotype of glioma by modulating IGF-1R, CD133 and cMyc. *J. Neuro-Oncol.* **2017**, *135*, 473–485. [CrossRef] [PubMed]
110. Dong, H.; Zhou, X.; Wang, X.; Yang, Y.; Luo, J.; Liu, Y.; Mao, Q. Complex role of connexin 43 in astrocytic tumors and possible promotion of gliom-associated epileptic discharge. *Mol. Med. Rep.* **2017**, *16*, 7890–7900. [CrossRef] [PubMed]
111. Crespin, S.; Fromont, G.; Wager, M.; Levillain, P.; Cronier, L.; Monvoisin, A.; Defamie, N.; Mesnil, M. Expression of a gap junction protein, connexin43, in a large panel of human gliomas: New insights. *Cancer Med.* **2016**, *5*, 1742–1752. [CrossRef] [PubMed]
112. Zhang, A.; Hitomi, M.; Bar-Shain, N.; Dalimov, Z.; Ellis, L.; Velpula, K.K.; Fraizer, G.C.; Gourdie, R.G.; Lathia, J.D. Connexin 43 expression is associated with increased malignancy in prostate cancer cell lines and functions to promote migration. *Oncotarget* **2015**, *6*, 11640–11651. [CrossRef] [PubMed]
113. Ogawa, K.; Pitchakarn, P.; Suzuki, S.; Chewonarin, T.; Tang, M.; Takahashi, S.; Naiki-Ito, A.; Sato, S.; Takahashi, S.; Asamoto, M.; et al. Silencing of connexin 43 suppresses invasion, migration and lung metastasis of rat hepatocellular carcinoma cells. *Cancer Sci.* **2012**, *103*, 860–867. [CrossRef] [PubMed]
114. Ezumi, K.; Yamamoto, H.; Murata, K.; Higashiyama, M.; Damdinsuren, B.; Nakamura, Y.; Kyo, N.; Okami, J.; Ngan, C.Y.; Takemasa, I.; et al. Aberrant Expression of Connexin 26 Is Associated with Lung Metastasis of Colorectal Cancer. *Clin. Cancer Res.* **2008**, *14*, 677–684. [CrossRef] [PubMed]
115. Saito-Katsuragi, M.; Asada, H.; Niizeki, H.; Katoh, F.; Masuzawa, M.; Tsutsumi, M.; Kuniyasu, H.; Ito, A.; Nojima, H.; Miyagawa, S. Role for connexin 26 in metastasis of human malignant melanoma. *Cancer* **2007**, *110*, 1162–1172. [CrossRef] [PubMed]
116. Ito, A.; Katoh, F.; Kataoka, T.R.; Okada, M.; Tsubota, N.; Asada, H.; Yoshikawa, K.; Maeda, S.; Kitamura, Y.; Yamasaki, H.; et al. A role for heterologous gap junctions between melanoma and endothelial cells in metastasis. *J. Clin. Investig.* **2000**, *105*, 1189–1197. [CrossRef] [PubMed]
117. Jongen, W.M.; Fitzgerald, D.J.; Asamoto, M.; Piccoli, C.; Slaga, T.J.; Gros, D.; Takeichi, M.; Yamasaki, H. Regulation of connexin 43-mediated gap junctional intercellular communication by Ca^{2+} in mouse epidermal cells is controlled by E-cadherin. *J. Cell Biol.* **1991**, *114*, 545–555. [CrossRef] [PubMed]
118. Ryszawy, D.; Sarna, M.; Rak, M.; Szpak, K.; Kędracka-Krok, S.; Michalik, M.; Siedlar, M.; Zuba-Surma, E.; Burda, K.; Korohoda, W.; et al. Functional links between Snail-1 and Cx43 account for the recruitment of Cx43-positive cells into the invasive front of prostate cancer. *Carcinogenesis* **2014**, *35*, 1920–1930. [CrossRef] [PubMed]
119. Yu, M.; Zhang, C.; Li, L.; Dong, S.; Zhang, N.; Tong, X. Cx43 reverses the resistance of A549 lung adenocarcinoma cells to cisplatin by inhibiting EMT. *Oncol. Rep.* **2014**, *31*, 2751–2758. [CrossRef] [PubMed]
120. Graeber, S.H.M.; Hülser, D.F. Connexin Transfection Induces Invasive Properties in HeLa Cells. *Exp. Cell Res.* **1998**, *243*, 142–149. [CrossRef] [PubMed]
121. Bates, D.C.; Sin, W.C.; Aftab, Q.; Naus, C.C. Connexin43 enhances glioma invasion by a mechanism involving the carboxy terminus. *Glia* **2007**, *55*, 1554–1564. [CrossRef] [PubMed]
122. Ghosh, S.; Kumar, A.; Tripathi, R.P.; Chandna, S. Connexin-43 regulates p38-mediated cell migration and invasion induced selectively in tumour cells by low doses of γ-radiation in an ERK-1/2-independent manner. *Carcinogenesis* **2014**, *35*, 383–395. [CrossRef] [PubMed]
123. Oliveira, R.; Christov, C.; Guillamo, J.S.; de Boüard, S.; Palfi, S.; Venance, L.; Tardy, M.; Peschanski, M. Contribution of gap junctional communication between tumor cells and astroglia to the invasion of the brain parenchyma by human glioblastomas. *BMC Cell Biol.* **2005**, *6*, 7. [CrossRef] [PubMed]
124. El-Sabban, M.E.; Pauli, B.U. Adhesion-mediated gap junctional communication between lung metastatic cancer cells and endothelium. *Invasion Metastasis* **1994**, *14*, 164–176. [PubMed]
125. Thuringer, D.; Berthenet, K.; Cronier, L.; Solary, E.; Garrido, C. Primary tumor- and metastasis-derived colon cancer cells differently modulate connexin expression and function in human capillary endothelial cells. *Oncotarget* **2015**, *6*, 28800–28815. [CrossRef] [PubMed]
126. Pollmann, M.-A.; Shao, Q.; Laird, D.W.; Sandig, M. Connexin 43 mediated gap junctional communication enhances breast tumor cell diapedesis in culture. *Breast Cancer Res.* **2005**, *7*, R522–R534. [CrossRef] [PubMed]

127. Stoletov, K.; Strnadel, J.; Zardouzian, E.; Momiyama, M.; Park, F.D.; Kelber, J.A.; Pizzo, D.P.; Hoffman, R.; VandenBerg, S.R.; Klemke, R.L. Role of connexins in metastatic breast cancer and melanoma brain colonization. *J. Cell Sci.* **2013**, *126*, 904–913. [CrossRef] [PubMed]
128. Plante, I.; Stewart, M.K.G.; Barr, K.; Allan, A.L.; Laird, D.W. Cx43 suppresses mammary tumor metastasis to the lung in a Cx43 mutant mouse model of human disease. *Oncogene* **2011**, *30*, 1681–1692. [CrossRef] [PubMed]
129. Zhang, Z.Q.; Zhang, W.; Wang, N.Q.; Bani-Yaqhoub, M.; Lin, Z.X.; Naus, C.C. Suppression of tumorigenicity of human lung carcinoma cells after transfection with connexin 43. *Carcinogenesis* **1998**, *19*, 1889–1894. [CrossRef] [PubMed]
130. Saunders, M.M.; Seraj, M.J.; Li, Z.; Zhou, Z.; Winter, C.R.; Welch, D.R.; Donahue, H.J. Breast Cancer Metastatic Potential Correlates with a Breakdown in Homospecific and Heterospecific Gap Junctional Intercellular Communication. *Cancer Res.* **2001**, *61*, 1765–1767. [PubMed]
131. Shao, Q.; Wang, H.; McLachlan, E.; Veitch, G.I.L.; Laird, D.W. Down-regulation of Cx43 by Retroviral Delivery of Small Interfering RNA Promotes an Aggressive Breast Cancer Cell Phenotype. *Cancer Res.* **2005**, *65*, 2705–2711. [CrossRef] [PubMed]
132. Lamiche, C.; Clarhaut, J.; Strale, P.-O.; Crespin, S.; Pedretti, N.; Bernard, F.X.; Naus, C.C.; Chen, V.C.; Foster, L.J.; Defamie, N.; et al. The gap junction protein Cx43 is involved in the bone-targeted metastatic behaviour of human prostate cancer cells. *Clin. Exp. Metastasis* **2012**, *29*, 111–122. [CrossRef] [PubMed]
133. Chen, Q.; Boire, A.; Jin, X.; Valiente, M.; Er, E.E.; Lopez-Soto, A.; Jacob, L.S.; Patwa, R.; Shah, H.; Xu, K.; et al. Carcinoma–astrocyte gap junctions promote brain metastasis by cGAMP transfer. *Nature* **2016**, *533*, 493–498. [CrossRef] [PubMed]
134. Ramón y Cajal, S.; Capdevila, C.; Hernandez-Losa, J.; De Mattos-Arruda, L.; Ghosh, A.; Lorent, J.; Larsson, O.; Aasen, T.; Postovit, L.M.; Topisirovic, I. Cancer as an ecomolecular disease and a neoplastic consortium. *Biochim. Biophys. Acta (BBA) Rev. Cancer* **2017**, *1868*, 484–499. [CrossRef] [PubMed]
135. Lin, J.H.C.; Takano, T.; Cotrina, M.L.; Arcuino, G.; Kang, J.; Liu, S.; Gao, Q.; Jiang, L.; Li, F.; Lichtenberg-Frate, H.; et al. Connexin 43 Enhances the Adhesivity and Mediates the Invasion of Malignant Glioma Cells. *J. Neurosci.* **2002**, *22*, 4302–4311. [CrossRef] [PubMed]
136. Miekus, K.; Czernik, M.; Sroka, J.; Czyz, J.; Madeja, Z. Contact stimulation of prostate cancer cell migration: The role of gap junctional coupling and migration stimulated by heterotypic cell-to-cell contacts in determination of the metastatic phenotype of Dunning rat prostate cancer cells. *Biol. Cell* **2005**, *97*, 893–903. [CrossRef] [PubMed]
137. Stuhlmann, D.; Ale-Agha, N.; Reinehr, R.; Steinbrenner, H.; Ramos, M.C.; Sies, H.; Brenneisen, P. Modulation of homologous gap junctional intercellular communication of human dermal fibroblasts via a paracrine factor(s) generated by squamous tumor cells. *Carcinogenesis* **2003**, *24*, 1737–1748. [CrossRef] [PubMed]
138. Fujimoto, E.; Sato, H.; Nagashima, Y.; Negishi, E.; Shirai, S.; Fukumoto, K.; Hagiwara, H.; Hagiwara, K.; Ueno, K.; Yano, T. A Src family inhibitor (PP1) potentiates tumor-suppressive effect of connexin 32 gene in renal cancer cells. *Life Sci.* **2005**, *76*, 2711–2720. [CrossRef] [PubMed]
139. Mendoza-Naranjo, A.; Saéz, P.J.; Johansson, C.C.; Ramírez, M.; Mandaković, D.; Pereda, C.; López, M.N.; Kiessling, R.; Sáez, J.C.; Salazar-Onfray, F. Functional Gap Junctions Facilitate Melanoma Antigen Transfer and Cross-Presentation between Human Dendritic Cells. *J. Immunol.* **2007**, *178*, 6949–6957. [CrossRef] [PubMed]
140. Mazzini, E.; Massimiliano, L.; Penna, G.; Rescigno, M. Oral Tolerance Can Be Established via Gap Junction Transfer of Fed Antigens from CX3CR1+ Macrophages to CD103+ Dendritic Cells. *Immunity.* **2014**, *40*, 248–261. [CrossRef] [PubMed]
141. Aucher, A.; Rudnicka, D.; Davis, D.M. MicroRNAs Transfer from Human Macrophages to Hepato-Carcinoma Cells and Inhibit Proliferation. *J. Immunol.* **2013**, *191*, 6250–6260. [CrossRef] [PubMed]
142. Song, B.; Tang, J.-W.; Wang, B.; Cui, X.-N.; Hou, L.; Sun, L.; Mao, L.M.; Zhou, C.H.; Du, Y.; Wang, L.H.; et al. Identify lymphatic metastasis-associated genes in mouse hepatocarcinoma cell lines using gene chip. *World J. Gastroenterol. WJG* **2005**, *11*, 1463–1472. [CrossRef] [PubMed]
143. Furlow, P.W.; Zhang, S.; Soong, T.D.; Halberg, N.; Goodarzi, H.; Mangrum, C.; Wu, Y.G.; Elemento, O.; Tavazoie, S.F. Mechanosensitive pannexin-1 channels mediate microvascular metastatic cell survival. *Nat. Cell Biol.* **2015**, *17*, 943–952. [CrossRef] [PubMed]

144. Jiang, J.X.; Penuela, S. Connexin and pannexin channels in cancer. *BMC Cell Biol.* **2016**, *17*, 12. [CrossRef] [PubMed]
145. Willebrords, J.; Maes, M.; Crespo Yanguas, S.; Vinken, M. Inhibitors of connexin and pannexin channels as potential therapeutics. *Pharmacol. Ther.* **2017**, *180*, 144–160. [CrossRef] [PubMed]
146. Trosko, J.E.; Chang, C.C. Mechanism of up-regulated gap junctional intercellular communication during chemoprevention and chemotherapy of cancer. *Mutat. Res.* **2001**, *480–481*, 219–229. [CrossRef]
147. Fornelli, F.; Leone, A.; Verdesca, I.; Minervini, F.; Zacheo, G. The influence of lycopene on the proliferation of human breast cell line (MCF-7). *Toxicol. In Vitro* **2007**, *21*, 217–223. [CrossRef] [PubMed]
148. Leone, A.; Lecci, R.M.; Durante, M.; Piraino, S. Extract from the zooxanthellate jellyfish Cotylorhiza tuberculata modulates gap junction intercellular communication in human cell cultures. *Mar. Drugs* **2013**, *11*, 1728–1762. [CrossRef] [PubMed]
149. Yamasaki, H.; Katoh, F. Novel method for selective killing of transformed rodent cells through intercellular communication, with possible therapeutic applications. *Cancer Res.* **1988**, *48*, 3203–3207. [PubMed]
150. Safwat, S.; Ishak, R.A.; Hathout, R.M.; Mortada, N.D. Statins anticancer targeted delivery systems: Re-purposing an old molecule. *J. Pharm. Pharmacol.* **2017**, *69*, 613–624. [CrossRef] [PubMed]
151. Cesen-Cummings, K.; Warner, K.A.; Ruch, R.J. Role of protein kinase C in the deficient gap junctional intercellular communication of K-ras-transformed murine lung epithelial cells. *Anticancer Res.* **1998**, *18*, 4343–4346. [PubMed]
152. Touraine, R.L.; Vahanian, N.; Ramsey, W.J.; Blaese, R.M. Enhancement of the herpes simplex virus thymidine kinase/ganciclovir bystander effect and its antitumor efficacy in vivo by pharmacologic manipulation of gap junctions. *Hum. Gene Ther.* **1998**, *9*, 2385–2391. [CrossRef] [PubMed]
153. Wang, L.; Fu, Y.; Peng, J.; Wu, D.; Yu, M.; Xu, C.; Wang, Q.; Tao, L. Simvastatin-induced up-regulation of gap junctions composed of connexin 43 sensitize Leydig tumor cells to etoposide: An involvement of PKC pathway. *Toxicology* **2013**, *312*, 149–157. [CrossRef] [PubMed]
154. Wang, L.; Peng, J.; Huang, H.; Wang, Q.; Yu, M.; Tao, L. Simvastatin protects Sertoli cells against cisplatin cytotoxicity through enhanced gap junction intercellular communication. *Oncol. Rep.* **2015**, *34*, 2133–2141. [CrossRef] [PubMed]
155. Retamal, M.A.; Leon-Paravic, C.G.; Ezquer, M.; Ezquer, F.; Rio, R.D.; Pupo, A.; Martinez, A.D.; Gonzalez, C. Carbon monoxide: A new player in the redox regulation of connexin hemichannels. *IUBMB Life* **2015**, *67*, 428–437. [CrossRef] [PubMed]
156. Leon-Paravic, C.G.; Figueroa, V.A.; Guzman, D.J.; Valderrama, C.F.; Vallejos, A.A.; Fiori, M.C.; Altenberg, G.A.; Reuss, L.; Retamal, M.A. Carbon monoxide (CO) is a novel inhibitor of connexin hemichannels. *J. Biol. Chem.* **2014**, *289*, 36150–36157. [CrossRef] [PubMed]
157. Sato, H.; Iwata, H.; Takano, Y.; Yamada, R.; Okuzawa, H.; Nagashima, Y.; Yamaura, K.; Ueno, K.; Yano, T. Enhanced effect of connexin 43 on cisplatin-induced cytotoxicity in mesothelioma cells. *J. Pharmacol. Sci.* **2009**, *110*, 466–475. [CrossRef] [PubMed]
158. Uzu, M.; Sato, H.; Yamada, R.; Kashiba, T.; Shibata, Y.; Yamaura, K.; Ueno, K. Effect of enhanced expression of connexin 43 on sunitinib-induced cytotoxicity in mesothelioma cells. *J. Pharmacol. Sci.* **2015**, *128*, 17–26. [CrossRef] [PubMed]
159. Uzu, M.; Sato, H.; Shimizu, A.; Shibata, Y.; Ueno, K.; Hisaka, A. Connexin 43 enhances Bax activation via JNK activation in sunitinib-induced apoptosis in mesothelioma cells. *J. Pharmacol. Sci.* **2017**, *134*, 101–107. [CrossRef] [PubMed]
160. Dai, S.; Liu, J.; Sun, X.; Wang, N. Ganoderma lucidum inhibits proliferation of human ovarian cancer cells by suppressing VEGF expression and up-regulating the expression of connexin 43. *BMC Complement. Altern. Med.* **2014**, *14*, 434. [CrossRef] [PubMed]
161. Forster, T.; Rausch, V.; Zhang, Y.; Isayev, O.; Heilmann, K.; Schoensiegel, F.; Liu, L.; Nessling, M.; Richter, K.; Labsch, S.; et al. Sulforaphane counteracts aggressiveness of pancreatic cancer driven by dysregulated Cx43-mediated gap junctional intercellular communication. *Oncotarget* **2014**, *5*, 1621–1634. [CrossRef] [PubMed]
162. Ghatnekar, G.S.; O'Quinn, M.P.; Jourdan, L.J.; Gurjarpadhye, A.A.; Draughn, R.L.; Gourdie, R.G. Connexin43 carboxyl-terminal peptides reduce scar progenitor and promote regenerative healing following skin wounding. *Regen. Med.* **2009**, *4*, 205–223. [CrossRef] [PubMed]

163. Grek, C.L.; Rhett, J.M.; Bruce, J.S.; Abt, M.A.; Ghatnekar, G.S.; Yeh, E.S. Targeting connexin 43 with alpha-connexin carboxyl-terminal (ACT1) peptide enhances the activity of the targeted inhibitors, tamoxifen and lapatinib, in breast cancer: Clinical implication for ACT1. *BMC Cancer* **2015**, *15*, 296. [CrossRef] [PubMed]
164. Murphy, S.F.; Varghese, R.T.; Lamouille, S.; Guo, S.; Pridham, K.J.; Kanabur, P.; Osimani, A.M.; Sharma, S.; Jourdan, J.; Rodgers, C.M.; et al. Connexin 43 Inhibition Sensitizes Chemoresistant Glioblastoma Cells to Temozolomide. *Cancer Res.* **2016**, *76*, 139–149. [CrossRef] [PubMed]
165. Jaraiz-Rodriguez, M.; Tabernero, M.D.; Gonzalez-Tablas, M.; Otero, A.; Orfao, A.; Medina, J.M.; Tabernero, A. A Short Region of Connexin43 Reduces Human Glioma Stem Cell Migration, Invasion, and Survival through Src, PTEN, and FAK. *Stem Cell Rep.* **2017**, *9*, 451–463. [CrossRef] [PubMed]
166. Rhett, J.M.; Calder, B.W.; Fann, S.A.; Bainbridge, H.; Gourdie, R.G.; Yost, M.J. Mechanism of action of the anti-inflammatory connexin43 mimetic peptide JM2. *Am. J. Physiol. Cell Physiol.* **2017**, *313*, C314–C326. [CrossRef] [PubMed]
167. Baklaushev, V.P.; Yusbalieva, G.M.; Tsitrin, E.B.; Gurina, O.I.; Grinenko, N.P.; Victorov, I.V.; Chekhonin, V.P. Visualization of Connexin 43-positive cells of glioma and the periglioma zone by means of intercenously injected monoclonal antibodies. *Drug Deliv.* **2011**, *18*, 331–337. [CrossRef] [PubMed]
168. Chekhonin, V.P.; Baklaushev, V.P.; Yusubalieva, G.M.; Belorusova, A.E.; Gulyaev, M.V.; Tsitrin, E.B.; Grinenko, N.F.; Gurina, O.I.; Pirogov, Y.A. Targeted delivery of liposomal nanocontainers to the peritumoral zone of glioma by means of monoclonal antibodies against GFAP and the extracellular loop of Cx43. *Nanomedicine* **2012**, *8*, 63–70. [CrossRef] [PubMed]
169. Yusubalieva, G.M.; Baklaushev, V.P.; Gurina, O.I.; Gulyaev, M.V.; Pirogov, Y.A.; Chekhonin, V.P. Antitumor effects of monoclonal antibodies to connexin 43 extracellular fragment in induced low-differentiated glioma. *Bull. Exp. Biol. Med.* **2012**, *153*, 163–169. [CrossRef] [PubMed]
170. Nukolova, N.V.; Baklaushev, V.P.; Abakumova, T.O.; Mel'nikov, P.A.; Abakumov, M.A.; Yusubalieva, G.M.; Bychkov, D.A.; Kabanov, A.V.; Chekhonin, V.P. Targeted delivery of cisplatin by small es, Cyrilliconnexin 43 vector nanogels to the focus of experimental glioma C6. *Bull. Exp. Biol. Med.* **2014**, *157*, 524–529. [CrossRef] [PubMed]
171. Baklaushev, V.P.; Nukolova, N.N.; Khalansky, A.S.; Gurina, O.I.; Yusubalieva, G.M.; Grinenko, N.P.; Gubskiy, I.L.; Melnikov, P.A.; Kardashova, K.; Kabanov, A.V.; et al. Treatment of glioma by cisplatin-loaded nanogels conjugated with monoclonal antibodies against Cx43 and BSAT1. *Drug Deliv.* **2015**, *22*, 276–285. [CrossRef] [PubMed]
172. Yusubalieva, G.M.; Baklaushev, V.P.; Gurina, O.I.; Zorkina, Y.A.; Gubskii, I.L.; Kobyakov, G.L.; Golanov, A.V.; Goryainov, S.A.; Gorlachev, G.E.; Konovalov, A.N.; et al. Treatment of poorly differentiated glioma using a combination of monoclonal antibodies to extracellular connexin-43 fragment, temozolomide, and radiotherapy. *Bull. Exp. Biol. Med.* **2014**, *157*, 510–515. [CrossRef] [PubMed]
173. Abakumova, T.; Abakumov, M.; Shein, S.; Chelushkin, P.; Bychkov, D.; Mukhin, V.; Yusubalieva, G.; Grinenko, N.; Kabanov, A.; Nukolova, N.; et al. Connexin 43-targeted T1 contrast agent for MRI diagnosis of glioma. *Contrast Media Mol. Imaging* **2016**, *11*, 15–23. [CrossRef] [PubMed]
174. Jing, Y.; Guo, S.; Zhang, X.; Sun, A.; Tao, F.; Ju, H.; Qian, H. Effects of small interfering RNA interference of connexin 37 on subcutaneous gastric tumours in mice. *Mol. Med. Rep.* **2014**, *10*, 2955–2960. [CrossRef] [PubMed]
175. Hitomi, M.; Deleyrolle, L.P.; Mulkearns-Hubert, E.E.; Jarrar, A.; Li, M.; Sinyuk, M.; Otvos, B.; Brunet, S.; Flavahan, W.A.; Hubert, C.G.; et al. Differential connexin function enhances self-renewal in glioblastoma. *Cell Rep.* **2015**, *11*, 1031–1042. [CrossRef] [PubMed]
176. Munoz, J.L.; Rodriguez-Cruz, V.; Greco, S.J.; Ramkissoon, S.H.; Ligon, K.L.; Rameshwar, P. Temozolomide resistance in glioblastoma cells occurs partly through epidermal growth factor receptor-mediated induction of connexin 43. *Cell Death Dis.* **2014**, *5*, e1145. [CrossRef] [PubMed]
177. Gielen, P.R.; Aftab, Q.; Ma, N.; Chen, V.C.; Hong, X.; Lozinsky, S.; Naus, C.C.; Sin, W.C. Connexin43 confers Temozolomide resistance in human glioma cells by modulating the mitochondrial apoptosis pathway. *Neuropharmacology* **2013**, *75*, 539–548. [CrossRef] [PubMed]
178. Lai, S.W.; Huang, B.R.; Liu, Y.S.; Lin, H.Y.; Chen, C.C.; Tsai, C.F.; Lu, D.Y.; Lin, C. Differential Characterization of Temozolomide-Resistant Human Glioma Cells. *Int. J. Mol. Sci.* **2018**, *19*, E127. [CrossRef] [PubMed]

179. Zhang, J.; O'Carroll, S.J.; Henare, K.; Ching, L.M.; Ormonde, S.; Nicholson, L.F.; Danesh-Meyer, H.V.; Green, C.R. Connexin hemichannel induced vascular leak suggests a new paradigm for cancer therapy. *FEBS Lett.* **2014**, *588*, 1365–1371. [CrossRef] [PubMed]
180. Danesh-Meyer, H.V.; Kerr, N.M.; Zhang, J.; Eady, E.K.; O'Carroll, S.J.; Nicholson, L.F.; Johnson, C.S.; Green, C.R. Connexin43 mimetic peptide reduces vascular leak and retinal ganglion cell death following retinal ischaemia. *Brain* **2012**, *135*, 506–520. [CrossRef] [PubMed]
181. Boyd-Tressler, A.; Penuela, S.; Laird, D.W.; Dubyak, G.R. Chemotherapeutic drugs induce ATP release via caspase-gated pannexin-1 channels and a caspase/pannexin-1- independent mechanism. *J. Biol. Chem.* **2014**, *289*, 27246–27263. [CrossRef] [PubMed]
182. Boyd-Tressler, A.M.; Lane, G.S.; Dubyak, G.R. Up-regulated Ectonucleotidases in Fas-Associated Death Domain Protein- and Receptor-Interacting Protein Kinase 1-Deficient Jurkat Leukemia Cells Counteract Extracellular ATP/AMP Accumulation via Pannexin-1 Channels during Chemotherapeutic Drug-Induced Apoptosis. *Mol. Pharmacol.* **2017**, *92*, 30–47. [PubMed]
183. Saez, P.J.; Vargas, P.; Shoji, K.F.; Harcha, P.A.; Lennon-Dumenil, A.M.; Saez, J.C. ATP promotes the fast migration of dendritic cells through the activity of pannexin 1 channels and P2X7 receptors. *Sci. Signal* **2017**, *10*. [CrossRef] [PubMed]
184. Draganov, D.; Gopalakrishna-Pillai, S.; Chen, Y.R.; Zuckerman, N.; Moeller, S.; Wang, C.; Ann, D.; Lee, P.P. Modulation of P2X4/P2X7/Pannexin-1 sensitivity to extracellular ATP via Ivermectin induces a non-apoptotic and inflammatory form of cancer cell death. *Sci. Rep.* **2015**, *5*, 16222. [CrossRef] [PubMed]
185. Halliwill, K.D.; Quigley, D.A.; Kang, H.C.; Del Rosario, R.; Ginzinger, D.; Balmain, A. Panx3 links body mass index and tumorigenesis in a genetically heterogeneous mouse model of carcinogen-induced cancer. *Genome Med.* **2016**, *8*, 83. [CrossRef] [PubMed]
186. Romano, R.C.; Gardner, J.M.; Shalin, S.C.; Ram, R.; Govindarajan, R.; Montgomery, C.O.; Gilley, J.H.; Nicholas, R.W. High Relative Expression of Pannexin 3 (PANX3) in an Axillary Sweat Gland Carcinoma With Osteosarcomatous Transformation. *Am. J. Dermatopathol.* **2016**, *38*, 846–851. [CrossRef] [PubMed]
187. Di Cesare Mannelli, L.; Marcoli, M.; Micheli, L.; Zanardelli, M.; Maura, G.; Ghelardini, C.; Cervetto, C. Oxaliplatin evokes P2X7-dependent glutamate release in the cerebral cortex: A pain mechanism mediated by Pannexin 1. *Neuropharmacology* **2015**, *97*, 133–141. [CrossRef] [PubMed]
188. Weaver, J.L.; Arandjelovic, S.; Brown Mendu, K.; Schappe, S.; Buckley, M.W.; Chiu, Y.H.; Shu, S.; Kim, J.K.; Chung, J.; Chung, J.; et al. Hematopoietic pannexin 1 function is critical for neuropathic pain. *Sci. Rep.* **2017**, *7*, 42550. [CrossRef] [PubMed]
189. Hanahan, D.; Weinberg, R.A. Hallmarks of cancer: The next generation. *Cell* **2011**, *144*, 646–674. [CrossRef] [PubMed]
190. Mesnil, M.; Aasen, T.; Boucher, J.; Chépied, A.; Cronier, L.; Defamie, N.; Kameritsch, P.; Laird, D.W.; Lampe, P.D.; Lathia, J.D.; et al. An update on minding the gap in cancer. *Biochim. Biophys. Acta* **2018**, *1860*, 237–243. [CrossRef] [PubMed]
191. Sin, W.C.; Crespin, S.; Mesnil, M. Opposing roles of connexin43 in glioma progression. *Biochim. Biophys. Acta* **2012**, *1818*, 2058–2067. [CrossRef] [PubMed]
192. Sin, W.C.; Aftab, Q.; Bechberger, J.F.; Leung, J.H.; Chen, H.; Naus, C.C. Astrocytes promote glioma invasion via the gap junction protein connexin43. *Oncogene* **2016**, *35*, 1504–1516. [CrossRef] [PubMed]
193. Matsuuchi, L.; Naus, C.C. Gap junction proteins on the move: Connexins, the cytoskeleton and migration. *Biochim. Biophys. Acta* **2013**, *1828*, 94–108. [CrossRef] [PubMed]
194. Machtaler, S.; Choi, K.; Dang-Lawson, M.; Falk, L.; Pournia, F.; Naus, C.C.; Matsuuchi, L. The role of the gap junction protein connexin43 in B lymphocyte motility and migration. *FEBS Lett.* **2014**, *588*, 1249–1258. [CrossRef] [PubMed]
195. Elias, L.A.; Wang, D.D.; Kriegstein, A.R. Gap junction adhesion is necessary for radial migration in the neocortex. *Nature* **2007**, *448*, 901–907. [CrossRef] [PubMed]
196. Naus, C.C.; Aftab, Q.; Sin, W.C. Common mechanisms linking connexin43 to neural progenitor cell migration and glioma invasion. *Semin. Cell Dev. Biol.* **2016**, *50*, 59–66. [CrossRef] [PubMed]

9

Novel *TNXB* Variants in Two Italian Patients with Classical-Like Ehlers-Danlos Syndrome

Lucia Micale [1,†,*], Vito Guarnieri [1,†], Bartolomeo Augello [1], Orazio Palumbo [1], Emanuele Agolini [2], Valentina Maria Sofia [2], Tommaso Mazza [3], Antonio Novelli [2], Massimo Carella [1] and Marco Castori [1]

1. Division of Medical Genetics, Fondazione IRCCS-Casa Sollievo della Sofferenza, 71043 San Giovanni Rotondo (Foggia), Italy; v.guarnieri@operapadrepio.it (V.G.); b.augello@operapadrepio.it (B.A.); o.palumbo@operapadrepio.it (O.P.); m.carella@operapadrepio.it (M.C.); m.castori@operapadrepio.it (M.C.)
2. Laboratory of Medical Genetics, IRCCS-Bambino Gesù Children's Hospital, 00146 Rome, Italy; emanuele.agolini@opbg.net (E.A.); vale17l@gmail.com (V.M.S.); antonio.novelli@opbg.net (A.N.)
3. Unit of Bioinformatics, Fondazione IRCCS-Casa Sollievo della Sofferenza, 71043 San Giovanni Rotondo (Foggia), Italy; t.mazza@operapadrepio.it

* Correspondence: l.micale@operapadrepio.it

† These authors equally contributed to the work.

Abstract: *TNXB*-related classical-like Ehlers-Danlos syndrome (*TNXB*-clEDS) is an ultrarare type of Ehlers-Danlos syndrome due to biallelic *null* variants in *TNXB*, encoding tenascin-X. Less than 30 individuals have been reported to date, mostly of Dutch origin and showing a phenotype resembling classical Ehlers-Danlos syndrome without atrophic scarring. *TNXB*-clEDS is likely underdiagnosed due to the complex structure of the *TNXB* locus, a fact that complicates diagnostic molecular testing. Here, we report two unrelated Italian women with *TNXB*-clEDS due to compound heterozygosity for *null* alleles in *TNXB*. Both presented soft and hyperextensible skin, generalized joint hypermobility and related musculoskeletal complications, and chronic constipation. In addition, individual 1 showed progressive finger contractures and shortened metatarsals, while individual 2 manifested recurrent subconjunctival hemorrhages and an event of spontaneous rupture of the brachial vein. Molecular testing found the two previously unreported c.8278C > T p.(Gln2760*) and the c.(2358 + 1_2359 − 1)_(2779 + 1_2780 − 1)del variants in Individual 1, and the novel c.1150dupG p.(Glu384Glyfs*57) and the recurrent c.11435_11524+30del variants in Individual 2. mRNA analysis confirmed that the c.(2358 + 1_2359 − 1)_(2779 + 1_2780 − 1)del variant causes a frameshift leading to a predicted truncated protein [p.(Thr787Glyfs*40)]. This study refines the phenotype recently delineated in association with biallelic *null* alleles in *TNXB*, and adds three novel variants to its mutational repertoire. Unusual digital anomalies seem confirmed as possibly peculiar of *TNXB*-clEDS, while vascular fragility could be more than a chance association also in this Ehlers-Danlos syndrome type.

Keywords: Classical-like; Ehlers-Danlos syndrome; haploinsufficiency; tenascin-X; *TNXB*

---

1. Introduction

Ehlers-Danlos syndromes (EDS) are a clinically variable and genetically heterogeneous group of hereditary connective tissue disorders mainly featured by abnormal skin texture and repair, tissue and vascular fragility, and joint hypermobility. The 2017 international classification identifies 13 EDS types due to deleterious variants in 19 different genes [1]. More recently, a 14th type of EDS with features overlapping classical type and due to recessive variants in the *AEBP1* gene was added to this nosology [2,3]. Among them, classical, vascular, and hypermobile EDS are the most common, while the others are rarer and their frequency in the general population remains mostly unknown.

Classical-like EDS due to biallelic variants in *TNXB*, encoding tenascin-X (*TNXB*-clEDS), is a second EDS type resembling classical EDS but distinguished from the latter by recessive pattern of inheritance and lack of atrophic scarring [1]. Tenascin-X is a large extracellular matrix–forming glycoprotein, whose deficiency was firstly involved in the etiology of EDS in 1997, by the description of a novel contiguous gene syndrome combining congenital adrenal hyperplasia (CAH) and EDS, and due to the deletion of the *CYP21A2* (OMIM 201910) and *TNXB* neighbouring genes [4]. Subsequently, it was clear that this rare type of EDS is a recessive disorder caused by homozygous or compound heterozygous *null* alleles in *TNXB* [5]. Only 24 individuals with *TNXB*-clEDS have been described to date and most of them are of Dutch origin [6]. A recent cross-sectional study on 17 individuals suggests possible phenotypic hallmarks of *TNXB*-clEDS and hypothesizes that it is underdiagnosed with EDS-like symptoms outside The Netherlands due to the complex molecular structure of the *TNXB* locus [7].

TNXB maps on chromosome region 6p23.1 within the human leukocyte antigen histocompatibility complex in a module characterized by highly homologous sequences between functional genes, *CYP21A2* and *TNXB*, and their corresponding pseudogenes *CYP21A1P* and *TNXA*. This genomic structure is prone to non-homologous recombinations. Misalignment events during meiosis result in pathogenic *CYP21A2/CYP21A1P* and *TNXA/TNXB* chimeric genes. To date, three major types of *TNXA/TNXB* chimera have been identified [4,8]. In particular, CAH-X chimera 1 (CH-1) and CAH-X chimera 2 (CH-2) have *TNXB* exons 35–44 and 40–44, respectively, replaced with *TNXA* [4,9,10]. CH-1 is characterized by a 120-bp deletion (c.11435_11524 + 30del) due to the substitution of *TNXB* exon 35 by *TNXA* that is causative of tenascin-X haploinsufficiency in CAH-X CH-1; this region is the only well-documented discrepancy between *TNXB* and *TNXA* homologous portion. CH-2 is characterized by the variant c.12174C > G p.(Cys4058Trp) derived from the substitution of *TNXB* exon 40 by *TNXA* with a likely dominant negative effect [10]. The third chimera, termed CAH-X chimera 3 (CH-3), has *TNXB* exons 41–44 substituted by *TNXA* and is characterized by a cluster of three pseudogene variants: c.12218G > A p.(Arg4073His) in exon 41, and c.12514G > A p.(Asp4172Asn), and c.12524G > A p.(Ser4175Asn) in exon 43. This chimera has been reported in one patient, and its clinical significance is still preliminary [8].

Due to such a complex molecular architecture of the genomic region surrounding *TNXB*, Demirdas et al. [7] proposed a multistep molecular diagnostics workflow including: (i) a mixed approach of next-generation sequencing (NGS) for the non-homologous *TNXB* sequence and Sanger sequencing for the *TNXA/TNXB* homology region to exclude *TNXB* point variants and rare *TNXA/TNXB* chimera, (ii) followed by *TNXB* deletion/duplication analysis aimed to investigate the presence of the recurrent c.11435_11524 + 30del resulting from the common *TNXA/TNXB* chimeric fusion and other rarer rearrangements. Following this approach, this group was able to identify 12 different *TNXB* variants associated with *TNXB*-clEDS [7].

Here, we describe the first two Italian individuals affected by *TNXB*-clEDS. Molecular testing investigated the full range of possible molecular mechanisms leading to *TNXB* null alleles and found three novel variants.

2. Materials and Methods

Patients were enrolled for this study after obtaining written informed consent for publishing pictures (individual 2) and clinical data (both individuals). This study was approved by the local ethical committee, and is in accordance with the 1984 Helsinki declaration and subsequent versions. Part of the results of molecular investigations presented in this work was obtained from the routine clinical diagnostic activities of the involved institutions.

2.1. *Sample Preparation and Next Generation Sequencing Analysis*

Genomic DNA was extracted from patients' and unaffected relatives' peripheral blood leucocytes by using Bio Robot EZ1 (Qiagen, Hilden, Germany) according to the manufacturer's instructions.

The DNA was quantified with Qubit spectrophotometer (Thermo Fisher Scientific, Waltham, MA, USA). Probands' DNA first underwent sequencing with a HaloPlex gene panel (Agilent Technologies, Santa Clara, CA, USA) designed to selectively capture known genes associated with the various forms of EDS (*ADAMTS2, AEBP1, B3GALT6, B4GALT7, CHST14, COL1A1, COL1A2, COL3A1, COL5A1, COL5A2, COL12A1, C1R, C1S, DSE, FKBP14, PLOD1, FLNA, PRDM5, SLC39A13, TNXB* and *ZNF469*) according to the current nosology. For *TNXB*, NGS sequencing is effective for exons 1 to 31 only, which correspond to the non-homologous *TNXB* sequence. Libraries were prepared using the Haloplex target enrichment kit (Agilent Technologies, Santa Clara, CA, USA) following manufacturer's instructions. Targeted fragments were then sequenced on a MiSeq sequencer (Illumina, San Diego, CA, USA) using a MiSeq Reagent kit V3 300 cycles flow cell. Reads were aligned to the GRCh37/hg19 reference genome by BWA (v.0.7.17). BAM files were sorted by SAMtools (v.1.7) and purged from duplicates using Mark Duplicates from the Picard suite (v.2.9.0). Mapped reads were locally realigned using GATK 3.8. Reads with mapping quality scores lower than 20 or with more than one-half nucleotides with quality scores less than 30 were filtered out. The GATK's Haplotype Caller tool was used to identify variants. Variants were annotated by ANNOVAR, with information about allelic frequency (1000 Genomes, dbSNP 151, GO-ESP 6500, ExAC, TOPMED, GnomAD, NCI60, COSMIC), reported or computationally estimated pathogenicity (ClinVar, HGMD, LOVD, or SIFT, Polyphen2, LRT, MutationTaster, MutationAssessor, FATHMM, PROVEAN, VEST3, MetaSVM, MetaLR, M-CAP, CADD, DANN, fathmm-MKL, Eigen, GenoCanyon), and amino acids conservation (fitCons, GERP++, phyloP100way, phyloP20way, phastCons100way vertebrate, phastCons20way mammalian, SiPhy 29way). Selected variants were interpreted according to the American College of Medical Genetics and Genomics/Association for Molecular Pathology (ACMGG/AMP) [11]. Specifically, variants without clinical significance at the time of reporting (i.e., benign and likely benign) were excluded by the presence of one or more criteria for benignity. Variants which passed this preliminary selection were selected for further investigation and classified as pathogenic, likely pathogenic or uncertain significance by using the following criteria: (i) null (nonsense, frameshift) variant in a gene previously described as disease-causing by haploinsufficiency or loss-of-function; (ii) missense variant located in a critical and well-established functional domain; (iii) variant affecting canonical splicing sites (i.e., ±1 or ±2 positions); (iv) variant absent in allele frequency population databases; (v) variant reported in allele frequency population databases but with a minor allele frequency significantly lower than the known disease frequency in the general population; (vi) variant predicted as pathogenic/deleterious in ClinVar and/or LOVD; (vii) missense variant predicted as pathogenic/deleterious in most (≥75%) of the selected *in silico* predictors; (viii) variant co-segregating in two or more affected relatives; ix) the predicted pathogenic effect has been confirmed by an appropriate functional study/studies.

2.2. Sanger Sequencing.

The variants identified by NGS were confirmed by Sanger sequencing. Primer sequences are reported in Table 1. The amplified products were subsequently purified by using ExoSAP-IT PCR Product Cleanup Reagent (Thermo Fisher Scientific, Waltham, MA, USA) and sequenced by using BigDye Terminator v1.1 sequencing kit (Thermo Fisher Scientific, Waltham, MA, USA). The fragments obtained were purified using DyeEx plates (Qiagen, Hilden, Germany) and resolved on ABI Prism 3130 Genetic Analyzer (Thermo Fisher Scientific, Waltham, MA, USA). Sequences were analyzed using the Sequencer software (Gene Codes, Ann Arbor, MI, USA). The identified variant was resequenced in independent experiments.

Table 1. Primers used in this study.

Primers	Sequence	Tm (°C)	Size (bp)
TNXB-LongPCR-F TNXB-LongPCR-R	GTCTCTGCCCTGGGAATGA TGTAAACACAGTGCTGCGA	60	4900
TNXB frag1 For TNXB frag1 Rev	GGCCAAGCCTGGAAGATAAA GATTGGAGACAGAAGCACAC	60	662
TNXB frag2 For TNXB frag2 Rev	CCAGGGAGAGAGGATGGAT GTCCCCAGGAATGGAAGT	60	671
TNXB frag3 For TNXB frag3 Rev	GACCTAGTGCCTCAGCCA GGCTCTCTCTACTCCGTG	60	733
TNXB frag4 For TNXB frag4 Rev	ATGGGTGGGAGTTGAGAG TGGAAGCTGAGCAGGTAG	60	727
TNXB frag5 For TNXB frag5 Rev	TCTCCTCTTCCTGCTTTCCC CCCCATCAGTCTCCATGTC	60	643
TNXB frag6 For TNXB frag6 Rev	CAGGACCAGCACCATCTT TTGAGGTTGGCGTAGTGG	60	741
TNXB frag7 For TNXB frag7 Rev	GCTGTCTCCTACCGAGGG GCAGAGAAGGCTTCCTCC	60	621
TNXB_EX3Fw TNXB_EX3Rv	GGTTGCAGTCAGAGGGGGCG GCCCGCGACCTCTACAGTCG	58	300
TNXB_EX35Fw TNXB_EX35Rv	GGGAGCCTCAGAGTGTGC TCAGCCCCTGGAGTTTCTG	58	480

2.3. *Analysis of the TNXA/TNXB Homology Region*

For the analysis of the *TNXA/TNXB* homology region, the whole genomic sequence of *TNXB*, encompassing exons 32–44 was amplified by employing a Long-PCR reaction using the primers reported in Table 1 and the protocol previously reported [7]. The PCR reaction was performed in a total 50 uL volume reaction containing 5 uL Buffer 1 (10 ×), dNTP (0.625 mM final concentration), primers (10 pmol each), 3U Expand Long Template Enzyme mix (Roche, San Francisco, CA, USA). Cycling conditions were as follows: initial denaturation at 95 °C, 3 min, followed by 30 cycles of 95 °C, 30 s, 62 °C, 30 s, 72 °C, 11 min, final elongation at 72 °C, 7 min. The 4987 bp PCR product was checked on ethidium bromide (EtBr) stained 1% agarose gel and then used as template for seven nested PCR amplifications with the primers listed in Table 1. Reactions were performed in a 25 uL volume reaction containing 2.5 uL Buffer (10 ×), dNTP (0,25 mM final concentration), primers (10 pmol each), 1.25 U AmpliTaq Gold DNA Polymerase (Thermo Fisher Scientific, Waltham, MA, USA). Cycling conditions were the following: initial denaturation at 95 °C, 10 min, followed by 30 cycles of 95 °C, 30 s, 60 °C, 30 s, 72 °C, 30 s, final elongation at 72 °C, 7 min. The overlapping Nested PCR products were then checked on EtBr stained 2% agarose gel, purified with ExoSap-IT kit (Thermo Fisher Scientific, Waltham, MA, USA) and sequenced with a ready reaction kit (BigDye Terminator v1.1 Cycle kit, Thermo Fisher Scientific, Waltham, MA, USA).

2.4. *Multiplex Ligation-Dependent Probe Amplification (MLPA) and Quantitative PCR (qPCR) Analysis*

MLPA was carried out using the commercial kit (SALSA MLPA KIT P155-D2 Ehlers-Danlos syndrome III & IV, MRC Holland, Amsterdam, The Netherlands). The kit includes 17 probes for *TNXB* with amplification products between 130 and 490 nucleotides. This kit also comprises two probes mapping within the region upstream of *TNXB*, located in the *ATF6B* and *BAK1* genes, and two additional probes mapping within *CYP21A2*. Complete probe sequences and the identity of the genes detected by the reference probes is available online. Hybridization, ligation, and PCR amplification were performed according to the manufacturer's instructions. DNAs from three healthy individuals were included as controls. Coffalyser. Net software (MRC Holland, Amsterdam, The Netherlands) was used for data analysis. Detected deletion was confirmed by qPCR. Primers designed for the amplification of DNA fragments by qPCR, including *TNXB* exon 4 to 8 probes, were listed in Table 1.

The qPCR was performed using Power SYBR Green PCR Master Mix (Thermo Fisher Scientific, Waltham, MA, USA) on ABI 7900HT real time PCR system (Thermo Fisher Scientific, Waltham, MA, USA). Control DNA fragments were located on different chromosomes. Samples were run in triplicate using standard conditions.

2.5. *Chromosome Microarrays Analysis (CMA)*

CMA of the individual 1 was performed using the CytoScan™ XON array (Thermo Fisher Scientific, Waltham, MA, USA). This array contains 6.85 million empirically selected probes for whole-genome coverage including 6.5 million copy number probes and 300,000 SNP probes for LOH analysis, duo-trio assessment. The sensitivity of the platform is 95% for the detection of exon-level copy number variations (CNVs). The CytoScan™ XON assay was performed according to the manufacturer's protocol, starting with 100 ng of patient DNA. Data analysis was performed using the Chromosome Analysis Suite software version 4.2 (Thermo Fisher Scientific, Waltham, MA, USA). A CNV was validated if at least 25 contiguous probes showed an abnormal log2 ratio.

2.6. *Conservation of the Variant.*

Evolutionary conservation of p.Gln2760 residue of tenascin-X was investigated with protein sequence alignment generated by Clustal Omega and compared with data provided by UC Santa Cruz Genome Browser

2.7. *Total RNA Analysis.*

Total RNA was extracted using RNeasy Mini Kit (Qiagen, Hilden, Germany), treated with DNase-RNase free (Qiagen, Hilden, Germany), quantified by Nanodrop (Thermo Fisher Scientific, Waltham, MA, USA) and reverse-transcribed using QuantiTect Reverse Transcription Kit (Qiagen, Hilden, Germany) according to the manufacturer's instructions. PCR amplification and Sanger sequencing were carried out with primers listed in Table 1.

2.8. *Variant Designation.*

Nucleotide variant nomenclature follows the format indicated in the Human Genome Variation Society (HGVS) recommendations. DNA variant numbering system refers to cDNA. GenBank Accession Number NM_019105.6 was used as reference sequences for *TNXB*. Nucleotide numbering uses +1 as the A of the ATG translation initiation codon in the reference sequence, with the initiation codon as codon 1.

3. Results

3.1. *Case Report: Individual 1*

This is a 25-year-old woman, first child of healthy and unrelated parents. Her younger brother was described as unaffected. She was born at term, from an uneventful pregnancy and uncomplicated vaginal delivery. Birth parameters were normal. Psychomotor development and education were within normal limits. She recalled congenital contortionism (i.e., positive five-point questionnaire). At 3 years of age, the mother noted trigger fingers of multiple digits in both hands, and this was treated surgically at 16 years of age with complete resolution. She also requested ortodontic therapy for dental crowding and high-arched palate. No visual nor auditory troubles were registered. The patient suffered from constipation since infancy. At 14 years of age, she received the diagnosis of rectal prolapse. She always suffered from easy bruising and tendency to arterial hypotension. More recently, the patient requested rheumatological consultation for proneness to soft-tissue injuries and easy fatigability, although she did never complain of dislocations and fractures. According to the patient's past clinical history, the rheumatologist requested medical genetics consultation for a suspicion of hereditary connective tissue disorder. At examination, she displayed normal upper limb span/height ratio, bilaterally positive wrist sign, bilaterally negative thumb sign, Beighton score (7/9) with genua recurvata, marked hypermobility of the fingers and toes, flatfeet, brachydactyly (due to shortened metatarsals—brachydactyly type E), of the 2nd and 3rd toes bilaterally, brachydactyly type D of the hands (i.e. shortened and broad distal phalanx of the thumbs), soft, doughy and significantly hyperextensible skin, absence of distrophic scars, palmoplantar hyperlinearity, mild palpebral ptosis and bilateral euryblepharon. Of relevance, no other close family members had brachydactyly. Heart ultrasound showed minimal insufficiency of the mitral valve. Bone densitometry showed reduced bone mass at the femoral head (T-score-1.7). Hand X-rays showed "swan neck" deformity of the interphalangeal distal joint of 1st, 2nd and 3rd left fingers.

3.2. Case Report: Individual 2

This is a unique child of unaffected and unrelated parents. Pregnancy and delivery were uneventful, and psychomotor development and education were normal. She came at our medical genetics outpatient service at 26 years of age due to a long history of polyarticular intense pain (visual analogic scale: 7/10) and (sub)luxations of the shoulders, fingers and temporomandibular joints. Additional musculoskeletal and neurological symptoms included moderate pain (visual analogic scale 4-5/10) of the spine, hands and feet, as well as recurrent myalgias, occipital headache, occasional migraine with aura, post-exertional malaise and chronic fatigue. She also reported easy bruising, an episode of spontaneous rupture of the right brachial vein, multiple episodes of ruptures of cystic lesions of the elbows with leakage of a yellowish and filamenotous substance (presumably, molluscoid pseudotumors), eye dryness, recurrent subconjunctival hemorrhages, gastroesophageal reflux with cardia incontinence, esophageal erosions and severe constipation with coprostasis. At examination, at 26 years of age, the patient showed normal anthropometry, Beighton score 7/9, marked hypermobility of the digits, temporomandibular joints and shoulders, bilateral hallux valgus, genua valga, lumbar hyperlordosis, mild thoracic scoliosis, reduced muscle tone, painful movements, soft, doughy and hyperextensible skin (Figure 1a), normal scar formation, residual elbow scars from recurrent ruptures of (likely) mulluscoid pseudotumors (not visible at the time of examination; Figure 1b), a small subcutaneous spheroid of the pretibial region on the left, multiple cutaneous hematomas, piezogenic papules (Figure 1c), palmoplantar hyperlinearity, bluish sclerae, absence of the lingual frenulum and acrocianosis. Heart ultrasound was normal. Bone densitometry showed mildly reduced bone mass at the femural neck. We were also able to carry out physical examination of individual 2's parents and both had positive Beighton score according to age and sex (i.e., generalized joint hypermobility). The father also showed mildly soft and hyperexensible skin, although both did not report any significantly related complaints.

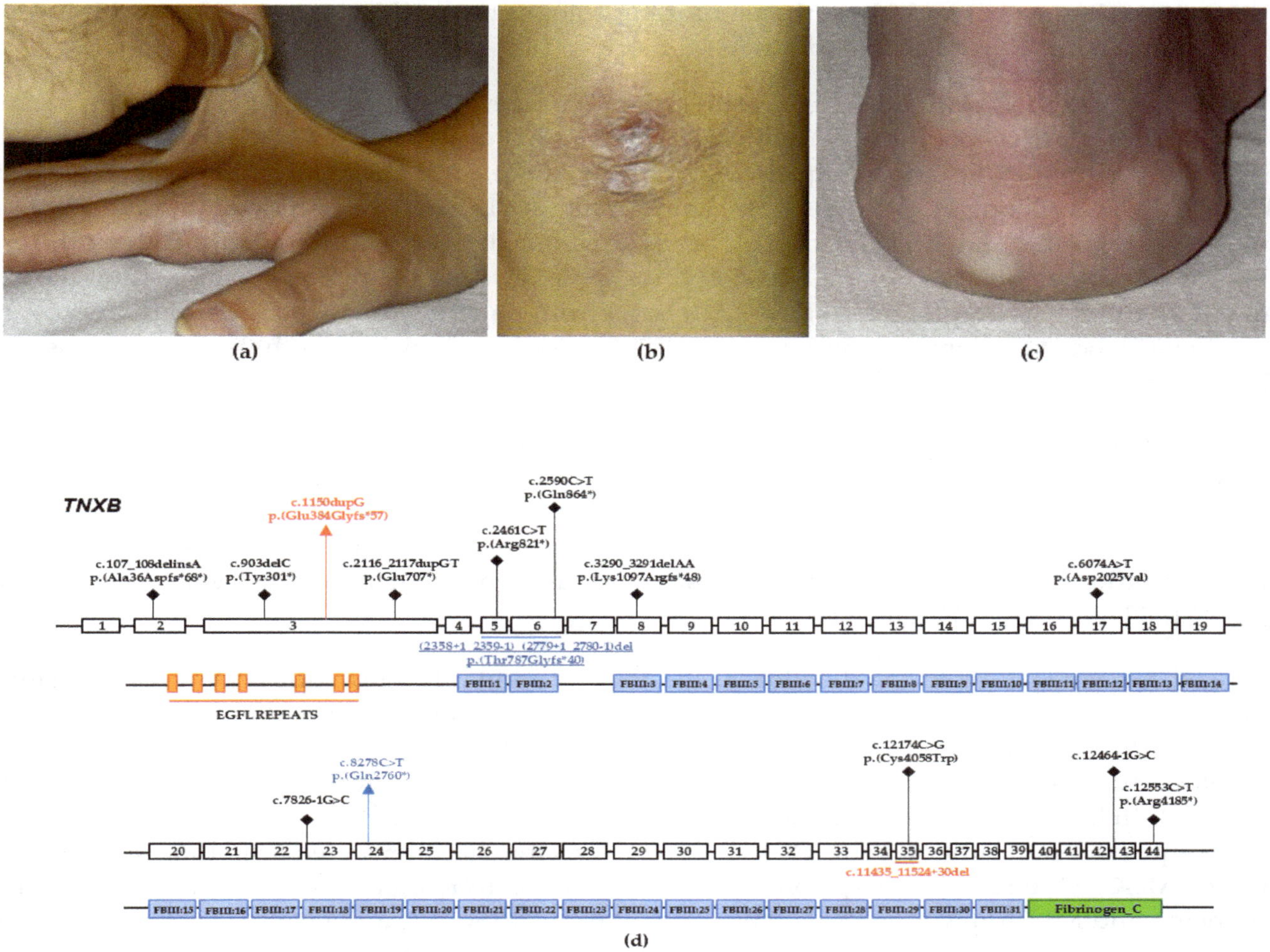

Figure 1. Selected clinical features of individual 2, and schematic diagram showing the genomic structure of *TNXB* and the secondary structure of tenascin-X. (**a**) Markedly hyperextensible skin of the dorsum of the hands. (**b**) Residual scar from recurrent molluscoid pseudotumors of the elbow. (**c**) Piezogenic papules of the heel. (**d**) Coding regions are highlighted with white boxes and introns with black horizontal lines. Tenascin-X is characterized structurally from N-terminus to C-terminus by: (i) an N-terminus with a series of repeats that resemble epidermal growth factor (EGFL repeats); (ii) a stretch of fibronectin type III repeats (FBIII1-31); and (iii) a large C-terminal domain structurally related to fibrinogen (Fibrinogen C). Previously identified variants associated with *TNXB*-clEDS are represented in black. Variants identified in the individuals 1 and 2 are represented in blue and red, respectively.

3.3. Molecular Findings: Individual 1

NGS analysis performed on DNA from individual 1 identified the novel heterozygous c.8278C> T variant located in the exon 24 of *TNXB* (Figure 1d), which is predicted to incorporate a premature stop codon [p.(Gln2760 *)]. No other candidate variants were found in the remaining genes. The c.8278C > T p.(Gln2760 *) variant was not reported in major databases, including dbSNP, ExAC, 1000 Genomes, and GnomAD. This suggests that the variant represents a rare event and was interpreted as likely pathogenic according to the ACMGG/AMP criteria (i.e., a variant absent in population databases and predicted to generate a null allele in a gene previously known as disease-causing with this molecular mechanism). The result was confirmed by direct Sanger sequencing of proband's DNA (Figure 2a). Protein sequences alignment of the homologous regions including the Gln2760 residue of human *TNXB* was generated by using the Clustal Omega tool and showed that the affected residue was evolutionarily conserved (Figure 2b). The Gln2760 residue is located in the 19th fibronectin domain of tenascin-X (Figure 1d) and, thus, the truncated protein presumably loses the last multiple 19–31 fibronectin domains as well as the fibrinogen C motif.

As *TNXB*-clEDS is caused by a complete lack of tenascin-X due to biallelic inactivating variants in *TNXB*, in order to detect the potential presence of a second variant in *TNXB*, we simultaneously performed the long PCR/Sanger sequencing analysis of the *TNXA/TNXB* homologous region and MLPA analysis. The long PCR/Sanger sequencing analysis did not reveal any variant in exons 32–44. On the contrary, MLPA analysis detected a *TNXB* intragenic deletion which includes entirely the exon 5 (Figure 2c). To narrow the proximal deletion breakpoints within the region encompassing the exon 5, qPCR analysis was employed on DNA extracted from patient's, unaffected parents, and control individuals blood. This approach detected a *TNXB* deletion which include both the whole exons 5 and 6 (Figure 2d).

To better molecularly refine the extension of the deletion, we performed a chromosome microarrays analysis using the CytoScan™ XON array. CMA confirmed an interstitial heterozygous microdeletion at chromosome 6p21.33, covered by 62 array probes and spanning 5 Kb, which encompasses the exons 5 and 6 and flanking intronic regions of *TNXB* (Figure 2e). The molecular karyotype of the patient, accordingly with the International System for Human Cytogenomic Nomenclature 2016 was arr [GRCh37] 6p21.33 (32056115_32061375) x1.

Next, we characterized the deletion at the transcriptional level by direct DNA sequencing of in vitro amplified cDNA product generated from total RNA extracted from patients' peripheral blood leucocytes (Figure 2f). We showed that the variant c.(2358 + 1_2359 − 1)_(2779 + 1_2780 − 1)del generates a frameshift with the insertion of a premature stop codon in exon 7 [p.(Thr787Glyfs*40)] (Figure 1d). In light of its absence in population databases, the predicted generation of a null allele and the subsequent demonstration by mRNA study, this variant was interpreted as pathogenic according to the ACMGG/AMP rules. Segregation analysis in both unaffected parents was performed by Sanger sequencing and MLPA/qPCR analysis. We detected the c.8278C > T and (2358 + 1_2359 − 1)_(2779 + 1_2780 − 1)del variants in the proband's father and mother, respectively (Figure 2a,d,f). Both *TNXB* c.8278C > T p.(Gln2760 *) and (2358 + 1_2359 − 1)_(2779 + 1_2780 − 1)del p.(Thr787Glyfs*40) variants have been submitted to the LOVD (Leiden Open Variation Database, https://databases.lovd.nl/shared/variants/0000598484, individual ID # 00266303 https://databases.lovd.nl/shared/variants/0000598485, individual ID # 00266303, respectively).

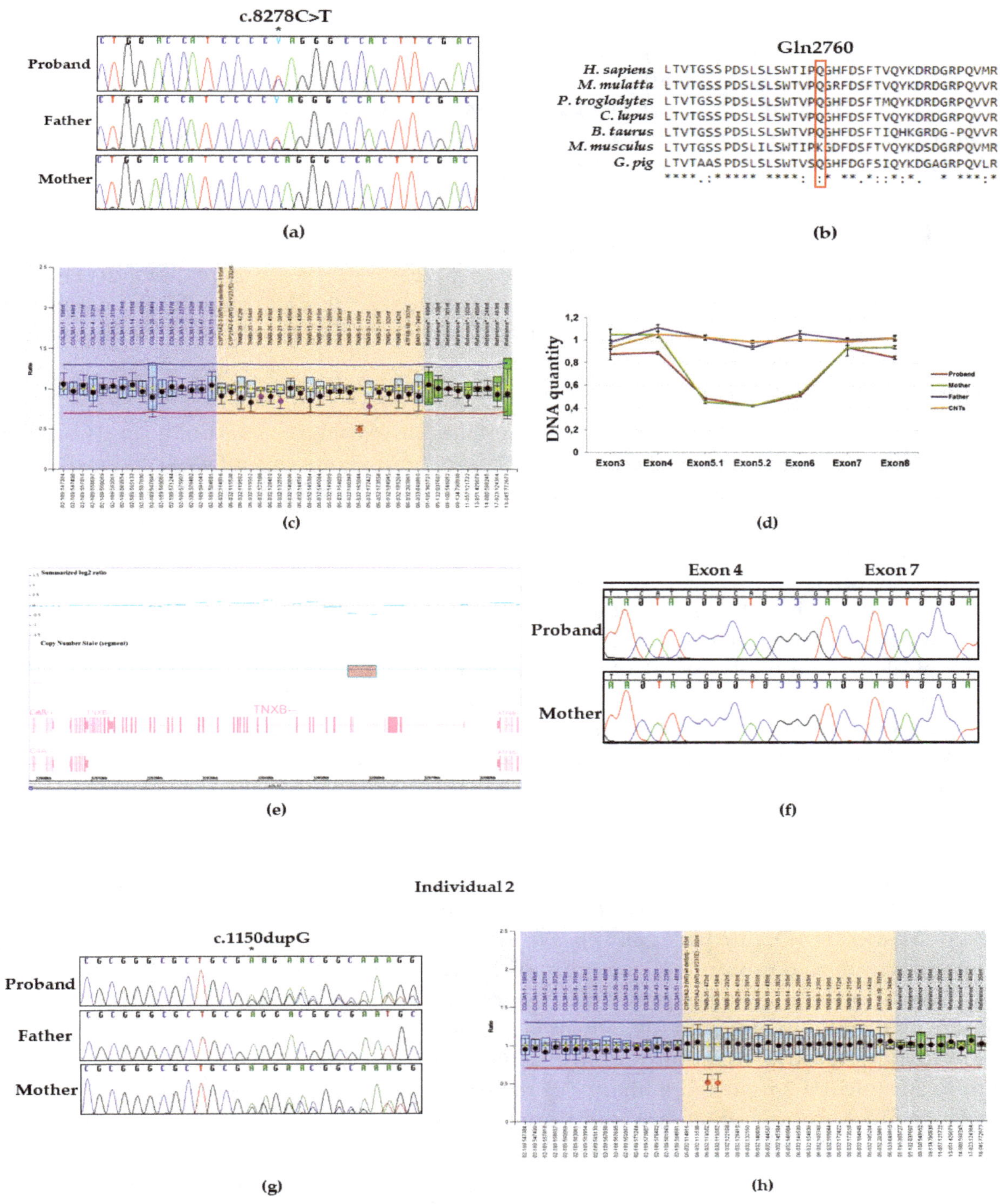

Figure 2. Molecular findings of individuals 1 and 2. (**a**) Electropherograms showing DNA sequencing analysis of PCR product amplified with primers targeting exon 8 of *TNXB*. Nucleotide sequences are provided. The position of the identified variant is indicated with an asterisk. (**b**) Protein sequence alignment of *TNXB* generated by Clustal Omega showed that the affected Gln 2760 residue of tenascin-X is evolutionary conserved. (**c**) Bar chart generated by Coffalyser.net- MLPA analysis software. MLPA was performed on DNA from the individual 1, her unaffected parents and controls (data not showed). A probe ratio of 1 indicates a normal DNA copy number; a probe ratio of 0.5 indicates a heterozygous deletion. MLPA analysis reveals a deletion of exon 5 of *TNXB* in individual 1. (**d**) Profiles of qPCR assay performed to map the deletion breakpoints within the region encompassing the exons 3 to 8 of *TNXB*. Relative DNA quantity of each exon was determined for the patient (red), her asymptomatic

mother and father, (green and purple, respectively), and a pool of DNA controls (CNTs, orange). (**e**) Results of chromosomal microarray analysis in the Individual 1. Intensity data (Summarized log 2 ratio value) of each probe is drawn along chromosome 6 from 32,000 to 32,080 kb (USCS Genome Browser build February 2009, hg19). The red box indicates the interstitial microdeletion (62 probes with decreased signal) identified, encompassing the exons 5 and 6 of the TNXB gene (lower panel). (**f**) Electropherograms showing cDNA Sanger sequencing of a transcript region of *TNXB* amplified with primers targeting exon 3 to 8 of Individual 1 and her mother. (**g**) Sanger sequence of a PCR product amplified with primers targeting exon 3 of *TNXB* of individual 2 and her unaffected parents. The position of the identified variant is indicated with an asterisk. (**h**) Bar chart generated by Coffalyser.ne-MLPA analysis performed on DNA from the individual 2, her unaffected father and controls (data not showed). MLPA analysis reveals the common partial deletion of exon 35 of *TNXB* in individual 2.

3.4. Molecular Findings: Individual 2

NGS platform targeted for EDS genes revealed that individual 2 carries out a single base deletion c.1150dupG located in exon 3 of *TNXB* (Figure 1d). This heterozygous variant was predicted to generate a premature stop codon at residue 441 [p.(Glu384Glyfs*57)]. No other candidate variants were found in the remaining genes. The c.1150dupG variant was not reported in major databases. Therefore, the variant was interpreted as likely pathogenic according to the ACMGG/AMP guidelines. This result was confirmed by direct Sanger sequencing of proband's DNA. The novel variant was also detected in the proband's mother while it was absent in the father (Figure 2g). MLPA analysis (Figure 2h) detected the recurrent pseudogene-derived 120 bps deletion including the exon 35, previously described by Schalkwijk et al. as the likely result of a common *TNXA/TNXB* fusion gene (CAHX-CH1). This variant was inherited from the healthy carrier father.Both TNXB c.1150dupG p.(Glu384Glyfs*57) and c.11435_11524 + 30del variants have been submitted to the LOVD (https://databases.lovd.nl/shared/variants/0000598486, individual ID # 00266304, https://databases.lovd.nl/shared/variants/0000598487, individual ID #00266304, respectively).

4. Discussion

In this work, we described the first two Italian patients with *TNXB*-clEDS, confirming a wider distribution of this rare EDS type in Europe, and the efficacy and reproducibility of the diagnostic approach published by Demirdas et al. [7]. We also identified three novel disease-alleles in *TNXB*, which expand the known mutational spectrum of *TNXB* associated with clEDS (Figure 1d).

These two adults manifest the previously defined phenotypic spectrum of *TNXB*-clEDS. Scarring was apparently normal in our patients, which is in line with the lack of atrophic/dystrophic scarring as a distinguishing feature, together with recessive inheritance, of *TNXB*-clEDS from classical EDS. Intriguingly, individual 2 reported a history of recurrent ruptures of elbow cystic lesions resembling molluscoid pseudotumors, which are additional cutaneous features considered highly suggestive for classical EDS. This expands the cutaneous similarities between *TNXB*-clEDS and classical EDS; a fact that complicates the differential diagnosis of these disorders on clinical groups and reinforces the opportunity to consider *TNXB* molecular testing in all individuals with a clinical diagnosis of classical EDS resulted negative to *COL5A1*, *COL5A2*, and *COL1A1* (recurrent variants) analysis. Individual 2 also testifies for a possible vascular involvement in *TNXB*-clEDS. In fact, this patient reported recurrent subconjunctival hemorrhages, a feature previously annotated in multiples subjects by Demirdas et al. [7], as well as spontaneous rupture of the brachial vein. The latter is an apparently novel feature of *TNXB*-clEDS and could indicate, if confirmed by other observations, a more severe vascular involvement in this condition.

Demirdas et al. [7] pointed out a peculiar appendicular phenotype of *TNXB*-clEDS featured by foot brachydactyly and small joint (apparently acquired) contractures. Our individual 1 supports this hypothesis, as she showed shortened metatarsals and a history of multiple acquired finger contractures with residual swan neck deformities of the left fingers. Furthermore, constipation and evacuation troubles represented major complaints in both individuals. While these features are not rare within the EDS community of syndromes and are highly represented in adults with hypermobile EDS and hypermobility spectrum disorders [12], this observation in *TNXB*-clEDS confirms the opportunity to better investigate the long-range manifestations of these disorders in order to improve quality of life of individuals with EDS.

To date, a total of 15 different *TNXB* deleterious variants, including the three novel reported in this paper were described. These variants are frameshift (7/15), stop codon (4/15), or splicing (2/15) and lead to the insertion of a premature stop codon with a presumed loss of expression of the protein. Two out of these 15 variants (2/15) are missense which have detrimental effects on the proper protein folding and stability [10,13]. Among the 15 variants, 11 are identified in single patients/families. A 2 bp deletion (c.3290_3291del), a 30Kb deletion generating a *TNXB/TNXA* fusion gene, and a pseudogene-derived missense variant (c.12174C > G) were found in more than one patient (Figure 1d). Nevertheless, the current nosology of EDS and related disorders clearly states that only "*null* alleles" in *TNXB* can be considered causative of *TNXB*-clEDS [1,6]. Therefore, missense *TNXB* variants should be considered supportive of the diagnosis in a clinical setting only if they appear convincing for haploinsufficiency.

In this study, individual 1 carries two novel *TNXB* variants, c.8278C>T located in the exon 24 and (2358 + 1_2359 − 1)_(2779 + 1_2780 − 1)del which results in the non in frame deletion of whole exons 5 and 6. Both variants are predicted to generate a premature stop codon. Individual 2 is a compound heterozygote for c.1150dupG and c.11435_11524 + 30del variants. The c.1150dupG is a novel variant located in exon 3 of *TNXB* and is predicted to create a premature stop codon. The c.11435_11524 + 30del variant, which abolishes part of exon 35 and intron 35 of *TNXB*, has been previously described and *TNXA/TNXB* chimeric recombination type 1 [5,7,10]. This deleted region represents the only large *TNXB*-specific sequence in the *TNXA*-homolog region of *TNXB*. The *TNXA*-derived variation is a molecular event which often takes place between a functional gene and a pseudogene. Although this *TNXA/TNXB* fusion gene has been previously characterized, its molecular effect is not yet known. However, tenascin-X serum measurement in affected individuals by previous studies indicate that this variant likely results in a *null* allele [5,9]. In this work, we were not able to carry out a serum dosage of tenascin-X in our patients. Nevertheless, we are confident that the molecular features of the identified variants are convincing for the generation of a not functional allele.

Due to the complex nature of the genomic region spanning around *TNXB*, the underdiagnosis of *TNXB*-clEDS in the routine diagnostic activities of most laboratories is a likely scenario. In fact, molecular testing of *TNXB* is challenging due to the presence of the pseudogene *TNXA*, which is more than 97% identical to *TNXB* at its 3′ end (exons 32–44). With the only exception of exon 35, which partially shows a *TNXB* specific sequence (see above), exon and intron sequences in this region are (nearly) identical in both *TNXB* and *TNXA*. Our experience confirms the need of a multistep and multi-technique approach (comprising NGS for the non-homologous region, Sanger sequencing with a long-PCR and nested-PCR system for the *TNXA/TNXB* homologous segment, and quantitative analysis for intragenic and intergenic rearrangement) for an efficient analysis of the entire *TNXB* coding region, with only slight modifications from the methodology proposed by Demirdas et al. [7] Tenascin-X serum concentration measurement in patients with suspected *TNXB*-clEDS is an alternative in the absence of effective molecular diagnostic facilities.

In summary, we reported two additional individuals with *TNXB*-clEDS. Our findings support the previously defined phenotype, which shows similarities with classical EDS but also include some possible distinguishing features and potentially underreported, clinically relevant manifestations. We also expanded the mutational spectrum of *TNXB* and highlighted the need of a high level of specialty for an efficacious *TNXB* molecular screening in a clinical setting.

Author Contributions: M.C. (Marco Castori), L.M., and V.G. designed the study and wrote the manuscript. L.M., V.G., E.A., and A.N. performed NGS analysis and studies on cDNA. B.A., E.A., V.M.S., and A.N. performed MLPA and qPCR analysis. O.P. and M.C. (Massimo Carella) performed CMA analysis. M.C. (Marco Castori), V.G., and L.M. interpreted molecular data. T.M. carried out the bioinformatics analysis. M.C. (Marco Castori) provided clinical evaluation of the patients. All authors contributed to the writing and reviewing the manuscript and approved its final version.

Acknowledgments: The authors thank the family for their kind availability in sharing the findings within the scientific community.

References

1. Malfait, F.; Francomano, C.; Byers, P.; Belmont, J.; Berglund, B.; Black, J.; Bloom, L.; Bowen, J.M.; Brady, A.F.; Burrows, N.P.; et al. The 2017 international classification of the Ehlers-Danlos syndromes. *Am. J. Med. Genet. C Semin. Med. Genet.* **2017**, *175*, 8–26. [CrossRef] [PubMed]
2. Ritelli, M.; Cinquina, V.; Venturini, M.; Pezzaioli, L.; Formenti, A.M.; Chiarelli, N.; Colombi, M. Expanding the Clinical and Mutational Spectrum of Recessive AEBP1-Related Classical-Like Ehlers-Danlos Syndrome. *Genes (Basel)* **2019**, *10*, 135. [CrossRef] [PubMed]
3. Syx, D.; De Wandele, I.; Symoens, S.; De Rycke, R.; Hougrand, O.; Voermans, N.; De Paepe, A.; Malfait, F. Bi-allelic AEBP1 mutations in two patients with Ehlers-Danlos syndrome. *Hum. Mol. Genet.* **2019**, *28*, 1853–1864. [CrossRef] [PubMed]
4. Burch, G.H.; Gong, Y.; Liu, W.; Dettman, R.W.; Curry, C.J.; Smith, L.; Miller, W.L.; Bristow, J. Tenascin-X deficiency is associated with Ehlers-Danlos syndrome. *Nat. Genet.* **1997**, *17*, 104–108. [CrossRef] [PubMed]
5. Schalkwijk, J.; Zweers, M.C.; Steijlen, P.M.; Dean, W.B.; Taylor, G.; van Vlijmen, I.M.; van Haren, B.; Miller, W.L.; Bristow, J. A recessive form of the Ehlers-Danlos syndrome caused by tenascin-X deficiency. *N. Engl. J. Med.* **2001**, *345*, 1167–1175. [CrossRef] [PubMed]
6. Brady, A.F.; Demirdas, S.; Fournel-Gigleux, S.; Ghali, N.; Giunta, C.; Kapferer-Seebacher, I.; Kosho, T.; Mendoza-Londono, R.; Pope, M.F.; Rohrbach, M.; et al. The Ehlers-Danlos syndromes, rare types. *Am. J. Med. Genet. C Semin. Med. Genet.* **2017**, *175*, 70–115. [CrossRef] [PubMed]
7. Demirdas, S.; Dulfer, E.; Robert, L.; Kempers, M.; van Beek, D.; Micha, D.; van Engelen, B.G.; Hamel, B.; Schalkwijk, J.; Loeys, B.; et al. Recognizing the tenascin-X deficient type of Ehlers-Danlos syndrome: A cross-sectional study in 17 patients. *Clin. Genet.* **2017**, *91*, 411–425. [CrossRef] [PubMed]
8. Chen, W.; Perritt, A.F.; Morissette, R.; Dreiling, J.L.; Bohn, M.F.; Mallappa, A.; Xu, Z.; Quezado, M.; Merke, D.P. Ehlers-Danlos Syndrome Caused by Biallelic TNXB Variants in Patients with Congenital Adrenal Hyperplasia. *Hum. Mutat.* **2016**, *37*, 893–897. [CrossRef] [PubMed]
9. Merke, D.P.; Chen, W.; Morissette, R.; Xu, Z.; Van Ryzin, C.; Sachdev, V.; Hannoush, H.; Shanbhag, S.M.; Acevedo, A.T.; Nishitani, M.; et al. Tenascin-X haploinsufficiency associated with Ehlers-Danlos syndrome in patients with congenital adrenal hyperplasia. *J. Clin. Endocrinol. Metab.* **2013**, *98*, E379–E387. [CrossRef] [PubMed]
10. Morissette, R.; Chen, W.; Perritt, A.F.; Dreiling, J.L.; Arai, A.E.; Sachdev, V.; Hannoush, H.; Mallappa, A.; Xu, Z.; McDonnell, N.B.; et al. Broadening the Spectrum of Ehlers Danlos Syndrome in Patients With Congenital Adrenal Hyperplasia. *J. Clin. Endocrinol. Metab.* **2015**, *100*, E1143–E1152. [CrossRef] [PubMed]
11. Richards, S.; Aziz, N.; Bale, S.; Bick, D.; Das, S.; Gastier-Foster, J.; Grody, W.W.; Hegde, M.; Lyon, E.; Spector, E.; et al. Standards and guidelines for the interpretation of sequence variants: A joint consensus recommendation of the American College of Medical Genetics and Genomics and the Association for Molecular Pathology. *Genet. Med.* **2015**, *17*, 405–424. [CrossRef] [PubMed]
12. Copetti, M.; Morlino, S.; Colombi, M.; Grammatico, P.; Fontana, A.; Castori, M. Severity classes in adults with hypermobile Ehlers-Danlos syndrome/hypermobility spectrum disorders: A pilot study of 105 Italian patients. *Rheumatology (Oxford)* **2019**, *58*, 1722–1730. [CrossRef] [PubMed]
13. Kaufman, C.S.; Butler, M.G. Mutation in TNXB gene causes moderate to severe Ehlers-Danlos syndrome. *World J. Med. Genet.* **2016**, *6*, 17–21. [CrossRef] [PubMed]

10

Impact of Autophagy of Innate Immune Cells on Inflammatory Bowel Disease

Tomoya Iida, Yoshihiro Yokoyama, Kohei Wagatsuma, Daisuke Hirayama and Hiroshi Nakase *

Department of Gastroenterology and Hepatology, Sapporo Medical University School of Medicine, Sapporo 060-8543, Japan; tomoya.iida.0306@gmail.com (T.I.); yoshi_yokoyamaa@yahoo.co.jp (Y.Y.); waga_a05m@yahoo.co.jp (K.W.); hirarin95@yahoo.co.jp (D.H.)

* Correspondence: hiropynakase@gmail.com

Abstract: Autophagy, an intracellular degradation mechanism, has many immunological functions and is a constitutive process necessary for maintaining cellular homeostasis and organ structure. One of the functions of autophagy is to control the innate immune response. Many studies conducted in recent years have revealed the contribution of autophagy to the innate immune response, and relationships between this process and various diseases have been reported. Inflammatory bowel disease is an intractable disorder with unknown etiology; however, immunological abnormalities in the intestines are known to be involved in the pathology of inflammatory bowel disease, as is dysfunction of autophagy. In Crohn's disease, many associations with autophagy-related genes, such as *ATG16L1*, *IRGM*, *NOD2*, and others, have been reported. Abnormalities in the *ATG16L1* gene, in particular, have been reported to cause autophagic dysfunction, resulting in enhanced production of inflammatory cytokines by macrophages as well as abnormal function of Paneth cells, which are important in intestinal innate immunity. In this review, we provide an overview of the autophagy mechanism in innate immune cells in inflammatory bowel disease.

Keywords: autophagy; innate immunity; immune cell; inflammasome; Paneth cell; inflammatory bowel disease; Crohn's disease

---

1. Introduction

The gastrointestinal tract is continuously involved in regulating the gut flora, modulating immune responses to food antigens and other substances, and maintaining homeostasis. Inflammatory bowel disease (IBD) occurs when this homeostasis is disrupted. The innate immune response is indispensable for maintaining homeostasis, and abnormal innate immune activity is deeply involved in the pathogenesis of IBD; research in this field has made substantial advancements in recent years [1–3]. To date, more than 200 IBD disease susceptibility loci have been identified by genome wide association studies (GWASs) [4,5]. Within these 200 loci, based upon single nucleotide polymorphism frequencies in patients with IBD versus controls, are approximately 1500 potential associated genes [6,7]. Numerous molecules involved in producing innate immune responses are also included among these loci.

Cells closely involved in the innate immune response with respect to IBD include blood cells, macrophages, dendritic cells, Paneth cells, and goblet cells, which are also involved in the pathology of IBD [8–10]. These cells have been found to play important roles in the development of abnormalities, including maintaining homeostasis against stress at the cellular level and modulating autophagy.

In this review, we outline the mechanism of autophagy in innate immune cells in IBD.

2. Pathology and Pathogenesis of IBD

IBD is a chronic inflammatory disease involving idiopathic inflammation, primarily in the gastrointestinal tract; when defined more specifically, this condition encompasses ulcerative colitis

(UC) and Crohn's disease (CD). Both are characterized by onset at a young age and the number of affected patients has risen sharply in recent years in Europe, the United States of America, and Japan [11]. Genetic predisposition (innate and acquired immunity, cytokine, and racial difference) and environmental factors (meal, drug, smoking, and infection) are greatly involved in the onset of IBD, and intestinal immune abnormalities are caused by the involvement of the state of dysbiosis, which is believed to cause IBD [11–15] (Figure 1).

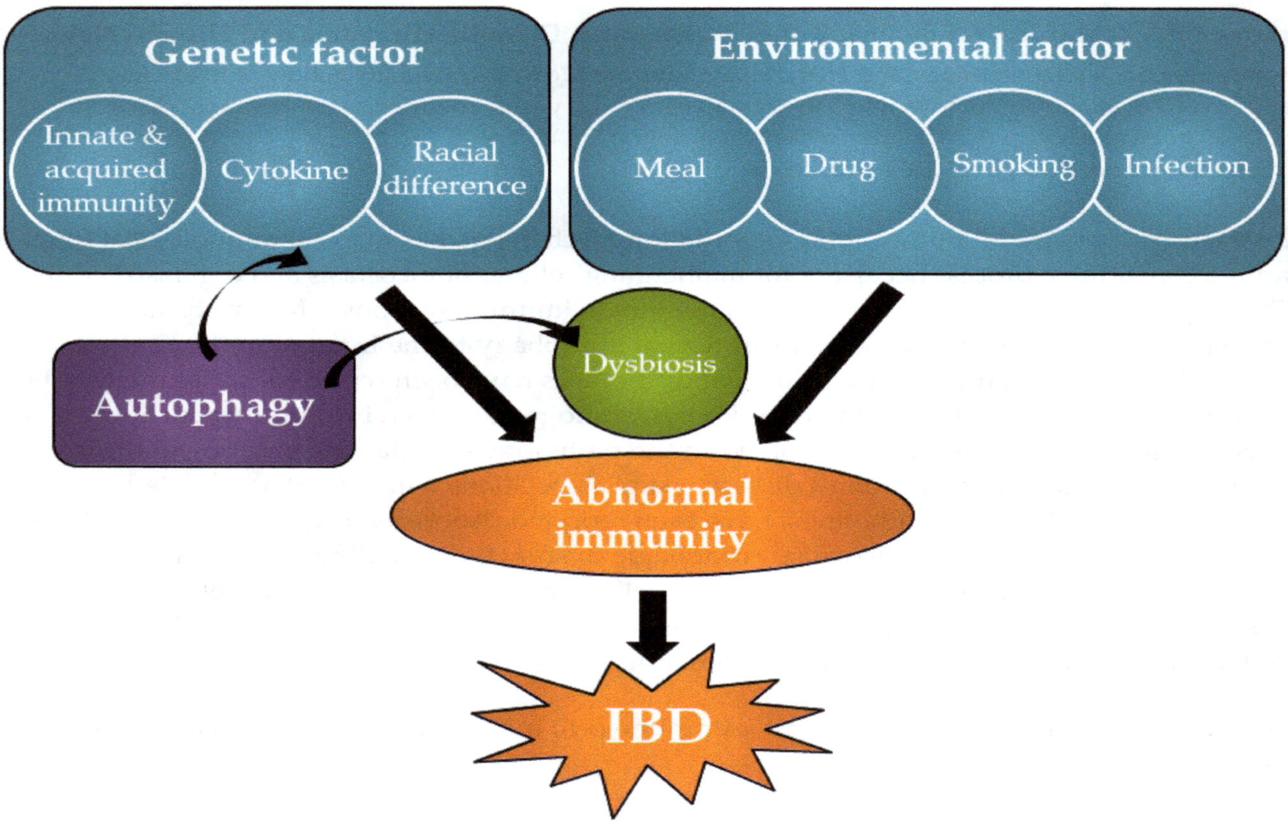

Figure 1. Pathology and pathogenesis of inflammatory bowel disease (IBD). Genetic predisposition and environmental factors are greatly involved in the onset of IBD, and intestinal immune abnormalities are caused by the involvement of the state of dysbiosis, which is believed to cause IBD.

Abnormalities related to genetic predisposition and autophagy are deeply involved in dysbiosis. Representative autophagy-related genes include *nucleotide-binding oligomerization domain containing 2 (NOD2), autophagy-related 16 like 1 (ATG16L1), and immunity-related GTPase family M (IRGM)* [16–18]. Autophagy has been linked to a variety of diseases; however, its link to IBD is currently the subject of much debate.

3. Autophagy

Autophagy is a term derived from a Greek word meaning "self-eating" and is a process that together with the ubiquitin-proteasome system, governs the degradation of intracellular proteins. In addition to immunological functions, such as antigen presentation and protection against infection, autophagy is also involved in the starvation response, carcinogenesis, and quality control of intracellular proteins and is a constitutive process necessary for maintaining proper cell homeostasis and organ health [19–21]. In addition to IBD, autophagy has been shown to be associated with other diseases, such as asthma [22–25], systemic lupus erythematosus [26,27], and Parkinson's disease [28,29].

During the autophagy process, the endoplasmic reticulum or other membranous cellular structures respond to stimuli by generating a double-membrane structure called a phagophore. The

ATG16L1/ATG5/ATG12 complex multimerizes and then lipidates light chain 3 (LC3)-II on this phagophore. Concurrently, the phagophore elongates to envelop the cytoplasm or organelle to be degraded, forming an autophagosome, which is a unique double-membrane organelle. The outer membrane of the autophagosome then integrates with a lysosome and forms an autolysosome. Finally, the inner membrane degrades and absorbs its contents [30] (Figure 2).

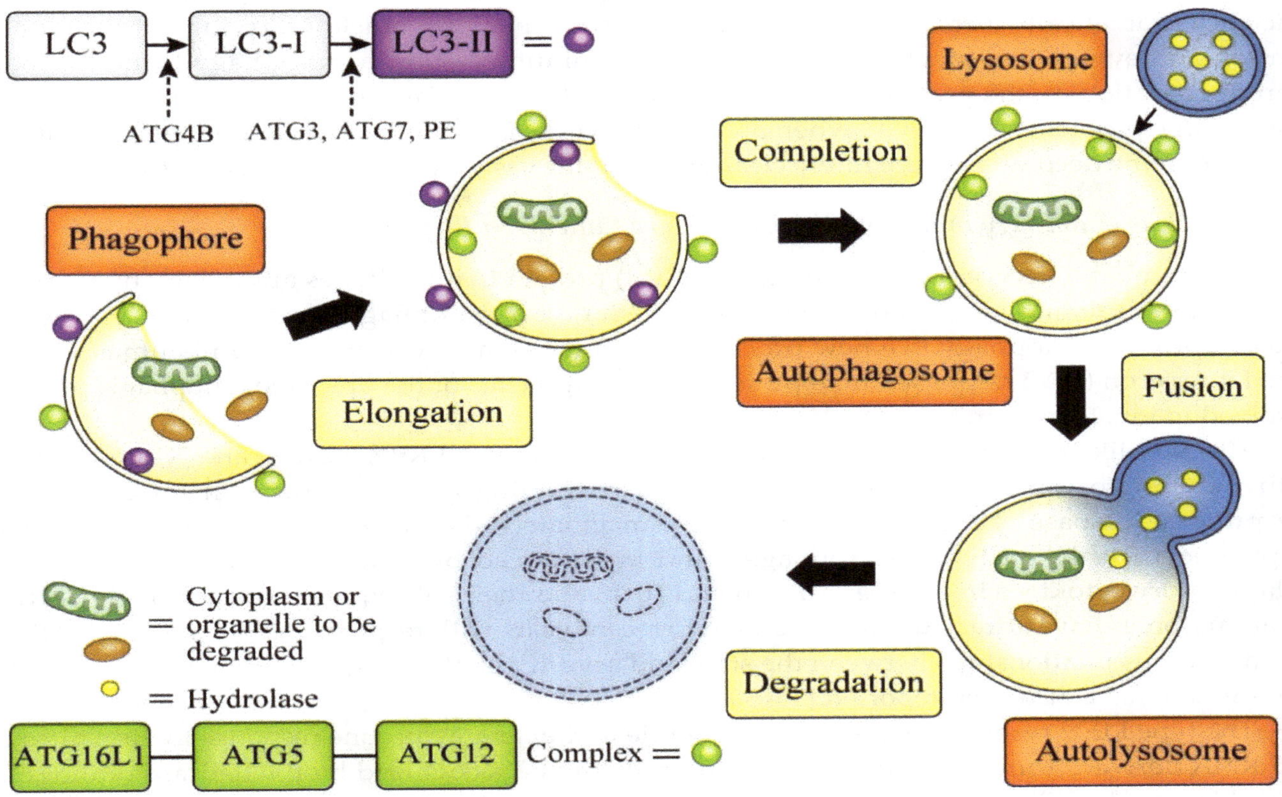

Figure 2. Autophagy mechanism. The endoplasmic reticulum or other membranous cellular structures respond to stimuli by generating a double-membrane structure called a phagophore. ATG16L1-ATG5-ATG12 complex multimerizes and then lipidates light chain 3 (LC3)-II on this phagophore. Concurrently, the phagophore elongates to envelop the cytoplasm or organelle to be degraded, forming an autophagosome. The outer membrane of the autophagosome then integrates with a lysosome and forms an autolysosome. Finally, the inner membrane degrades and absorbs its contents.

4. Role of Autophagy in Innate Immunity

One of the functions of autophagy is control of the innate immune response. Many studies have revealed the involvement of autophagy in innate immune reactions, and extremely precise control mechanisms and pathophysiological roles are becoming more clearly understood and have begun to be elucidated [31,32].

4.1. Xenophagy, Mitophagy

Innate immunity is a mechanism through which almost all multicellular organisms protect themselves from pathogens. This pathway is activated when the constructive patterns of pathogen's components are recognized (i.e., the cell wall components of a bacterial cell or the genome of a virus). Autophagy was initially thought to be a nonspecific mechanism for degrading substances by incorporating them into a membrane structure; however, recent studies have shown that autophagosomes selectively isolate a variety of substrates through sequestosome 1-like receptors, as is observed in autophagy of pathogens (xenophagy) [33–35]. Although the ubiquitin-proteasome system is a well-known selective intracellular degradation system, autophagy can selectively engulf and decompose small substances, such as mitochondria, which are larger than the targets of the ubiquitin-proteasome system, indicating characteristics similar to that of mitophagy [36,37]. The major difference between autophagosomes and other membranous organelles is that autophagosomes have a dynamic structure in which necessary fractions are newly created and disappear with the digestion of contents by fusion with lysosomes; as the necessity increases, as in the starvation state, its production efficiency dramatically increases. These features are convenient for quickly carrying out quantitative control, and even when functioning to control the immune response, autophagy is more suitable than degradation by the proteasome system, and it is believed to be essential for the resolution of quantitative problems. However, when autophagy works in connection with innate immunity, the substrates to be decomposed are rarely clear except in the cases of xenophagy and mitophagy.

4.2. The Role of Autophagy in Inflammasomal and Type I Interferon Response

A controllable receptor tripartite motif (TRIM) protein that facilitates autophagy by recruiting autophagy-regulating factors and recognizing the target of autophagy has recently been reported as a receptor for autophagy in a new process called precision autophagy [38]. Inflammasomal and type I interferon (IFN) responses are representative components of the precision autophagic processes involved in innate immunity.

The Nod-like receptor (NLR) family of proteins, including NLRP1, NLRP3, and NLRC4, together with the apoptosis-associated speck-like protein containing a caspase recruitment domain and the protease caspase-1, functions as downstream innate inflammasomes [39] that are activated in phagocytic cells, such as macrophages, and are induced by caspase-1 via maturation of the inflammatory cytokines interleukin (IL)-1β and IL-18 and their subsequent production [40]. NLRP3 inflammasomes have attracted much attention in recent years with respect to various diseases [41–44], and numerous relationships between the state and severity of *NLRP3* gene polymorphism and IBD presentation have also been reported [45–50].

The type I IFN response plays an essential role in the innate immune response to viral infection, and RNA derived from RNA viruses invading cells can be recognized by the helicase retinoic acid inducible gene 1/melanoma differentiation-associated protein 5 and type I IFN [51]. Because signaling from type I IFN follows the Janus kinase/signal transducer and activator of transcription pathway, this cytokine has also been reported to be associated with IBD [52].

4.2.1. Modulation of NLRP3 Inflammasome Suppression via Autophagy

Gram-negative bacterial lipopolysaccharides (LPSs) stimulate toll-like receptor (TLR) 4 and induce the activation of NLRP3 inflammasomes in a TIR-domain-containing adapter-inducing IFN-β (TRIF)-dependent manner with the information transfer factor. Active oxygen species derived from mitochondria are involved in the activation of NLRP3 inflammasomes. In the TRIF downstream pathway, evolutionarily conserved signaling intermediate in the Toll pathway has been reported as a factor that induces the production of reactive oxygen species (ROS) from mitochondria. This pathway is only slightly activated in wild-type macrophages. In addition, when phagolysosomes are damaged during gram-negative bacterial infection and LPS leaks into cells, NLRP3 inflammasomes are activated via a noncanonical pathway. Activation of the noncanonical pathway is thought to be induced by an unknown LPS sensor present in the cell. In addition, metabolites, such as urate crystals, cholesterol crystals, and free fatty acids, cause damage to phagolysosomes when taken up by macrophages, causing further mitochondrial damage. Adenosine triphosphate, which is known to activate surrounding cells after being released from dead cells, induces mitochondrial damage via the Purinergic 2X7 receptor (P2X7R). Influenza viral infection can cause damage to organelles, such as mitochondria and the Golgi apparatus. When damaged mitochondria produce ROS, NLRP3 inflammasomes become activated. By suppressing this series of pathways, autophagy suppresses the activation of excessive inflammasomes [53–56] (Figure 3).

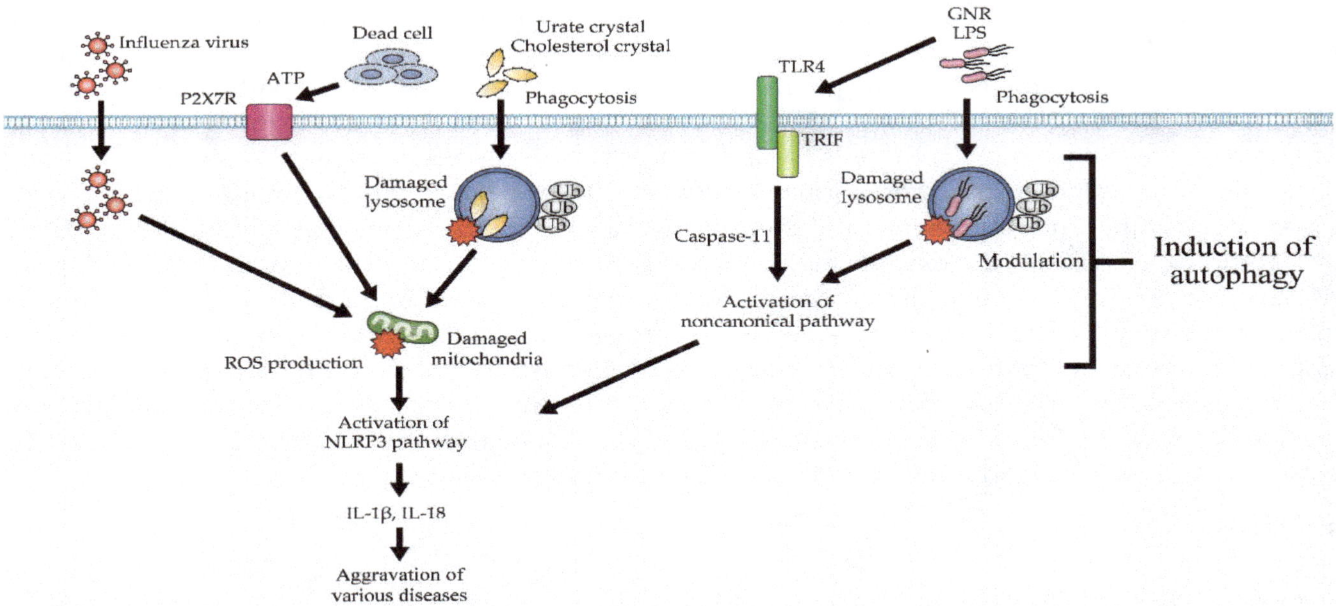

Figure 3. Modulation of NLRP3 inflammasome suppression via autophagy, ATP; adenosine triphosphate, GNR; gram negative rods, IL; interleukin, LPS; lipopolysaccharide, P2X7R; Purinergic 2X7 receptor, ROS; reactive oxygen species, TLR4; Toll-like receptor 4, TRIF; TIR-domain-containing adapter-inducing interferon-β, Ub; ubiquitin.

Autophagy is also believed to cause the decomposition of NLRP3 and AIM2, which are constituent factors of inflammasomes [57,58], and pro-IL-1β has been reported to be degraded by autophagy [59]. Furthermore, as described above, precision autophagy via TRIM protein is also involved in the decomposition of this inflammasome constituent factor by autophagy. TRIM20 binds to NLRP3 and pro-caspase 1, recruits autophagic regulatory factors (e.g., ULK1 and Beclin1), and is degraded by autophagy [38,60,61].

Conversely, autophagy also positively regulates NLRP3 inflammasomes and is involved in both decomposition and secretion. Autophagy is involved in the secretion of cytokines, such as IL-1β, IL-18, and high mobility group box 1 protein, and when inflammasomes become activated [62], folding of IL-1β by heat shock protein 90 is necessary; the IL-1β is then secreted after being transported to the lumen of LC3-II-positive autophagy-related structures [63].

Thus, autophagy plays an important role in the innate immune response by controlling NLRP3 inflammasomes. both positively and negatively.

4.2.2. Modulation of Type I IFN Responses via Autophagy

The TRIM protein regulates type I IFN responses via precision autophagy. TRIM21 binds to the IRF3 dimer, recruits autophagic regulators (e.g., ULK1 and Beclin1), and suppresses type I IFN responses by degrading this dimer via autophagy [61]. Moreover, autophagy also positively controls type I IFN responses. Intracellular viral replication intermediates on endosomes are recognized by TLR7 and cause a type I IFN response, but autophagy promotes type I IFN responses by this TLR7 via viral recognition [64]. As such, autophagy also positively and negatively controls type I IFN responses.

5. Role of Autophagy of Innate Immune Cells in IBD

As discussed above, autophagic abnormalities are deeply involved in the pathology of IBD, particularly CD. Recently, GWASs identified several genetic variants, including variants of *NOD2* [53,65–68], *ATG16L1* [69–77], *IRGM* [78–81], and *XIAP* [82–87] linked to the onset of CD. *NOD2* is the first disease-susceptibility gene discovered for CD [16]. Abnormalities in the *NOD2* gene are found primarily in Westerners and not in Asians. NOD2 is an intracytoplasmic pattern recognition receptor belonging to the NLR family, which recognizes and defends against pathogens and foreign components invading the cytoplasm [88]. NOD2 is strongly expressed by macrophages and dendritic cells (DCs), particularly Paneth cells, and functions through mechanisms involving autophagy, intracellular bacterial sensing, modulation of the antibacterial peptide α-defensin in the Paneth cells of the small intestine, and improvement of immune tolerance by suppressing TLR signals [89]. ATG16L1 is a homolog of ATG16, the existence of which was first reported by Mizushima et al. [69,70]. The *ATG16L1* gene is involved in host immune responses against intracellular parasitic bacteria and viruses via autophagy. In particular, the *ATG16L1* gene is closely associated with Paneth cells and plays an important role in CD pathology. In addition, many genes are associated with various pathologies of IBD in connection with autophagy, and these genes play important roles in immune cells, such as macrophages and DCs, as well as intestinal epithelial cells, including Paneth cells. The relationship between immune cells and autophagy in the IBD state is described below.

5.1. Hematopoietic Cells

5.1.1. Macrophages and DCs

Macrophages and DCs phagocytose foreign substances and bacteria in different tissues, serve as a first line of defense, and act as antigen-presenting cells to exert the functions of the acquired immune system [90,91]. Given the key role of the interactions between host and microbes in the intestine, it is critical to properly regulate pattern recognition receptor (PRR) signals and cytokine secretion. The NLRs in the cytoplasm and TLRs on the cell surface are the two main types of PRRs in innate immune cells [92]. NLRs and TLRs in macrophages are closely associated with autophagy, and macrophage autophagy is highly related to the mediation of innate immune responses in the intestinal wall [16,17]. Additionally, various antigens are degraded by the actions of proteasomes and lysosomes and are then presented by macrophages and DCs via class I and class II MHCs, after which the adaptive immune system is activated. Although it remains unclear as to how intracellular antigens are delivered to lysosomes and decomposed, recent studies have shown that autophagy is deeply involved in this process [93]. In the following section, we describe the relationships among macrophages, DCs, and autophagy in the pathology of IBD with respect to three components: pathogen degradation, suppression of inflammatory cytokine secretion, and antigen presentation.

Pathogen Degradation

NOD2 recruits the autophagy protein ATG16L1 to the plasma membrane at the bacterial entry site; mutant NOD2 fails to recruit ATG16L1 to the plasma membrane, and the wrapping of invading bacteria by the autophagosome is impaired. Thus, patients with CD with *NOD2* variants exhibit autophagy-related disorders [65–68]. Additionally, the capacity for autophagy and the phagocytosis of pathogenic bacteria become impaired in macrophages harboring mutant *NOD2* [94]. Furthermore, autophagy has been reported to be impaired in macrophages transfected with siRNA targeted to ATG16L1 or IRGM, and intracellular adherent-invasive *Escherichia coli* (AIEC) populations increase in the presence of intraperitoneal macrophages in *NOD2*-deficient mice [95]. Moreover, death-receptor activation or starvation-induced metabolic stress in human and murine macrophages increases the degradation of T300A or T316A variants of *ATG16L1*, respectively, resulting in diminished autophagy. In addition, knock-in mice harboring the *ATG16L1* T316A variant show defective clearance of the ileal pathogen *Yersinia enterocolitica* [74]. In an experiment using a cell line originating from macrophages, infection with CD-associated AIEC or administration of LPS or muramyl dipeptide induces IRGM expression [81]. Macrophages and epithelial cells lacking *GPR65* exhibit impaired autophagy for clearance of intracellular bacteria [96].

Suppressing Inflammatory Cytokine Secretion

ATG16L1-deficient macrophages are known to overproduce the inflammatory cytokine IL-1β in response to LPS stimulation, and the importance of ATG16L1 in inflammation has been described based on the finding that intestinal inflammation, induced by dextran sodium sulfate (DSS) intake in bone marrow chimeric mice, results in IL-1β overproduction by hematopoietic cells, leading to increased inflammation and cell fragility [53]. Moreover, in macrophages and DCs, autophagy controls IL-1β secretion by mediating the degradation of pro-IL-1β [59]. Furthermore, macrophages lacking ATG7, another autophagy-related factor, and macrophages that inhibit the activity of Vps34, which is essential for the induction of autophagy, also produce excessive quantities of IL-1β in response to LPS. Macrophages lacking ATG5 have also been reported to produce IL-1β in excess in response to the presence of gram-negative bacteria [97]. These phenomena are caused by the activation of NLRP3 inflammasomes due to autophagic disorders, and in recent years, activation of NLRP3 inflammasomes in response to various stimuli has been found to be controlled by autophagy [54–56] (Figure 3). In another recent report, impairing autophagy using ATG5 siRNA or an autophagy inhibitor (3-MA) was found to induce more robust initiation and activation of the NLRP3 inflammasome combined with increased caspase-1 activation and IL-1β production in peritoneal macrophages treated with LPS/DSS. 3-MA has also been shown to aggravate symptoms of DSS-induced colitis [98].

Loss of the autophagy-related gene *ATG16L1* has been shown to promote accumulation of the adaptor TRIF and enhance production of IFN-β and IL-1β as downstream signaling molecules in macrophages [99]. Macrophages from IBD risk carriers show increased myotubularin-related protein 3 expression and, in turn, decreased autophagy and increased cytokine secretion [100]. DSS and *Saccharomyces cerevisiae* were also inoculated into mice deficient in *ATG16L1*, an autophagy-related gene specific to CD11c+ DCs. Colitis has been reported to be exacerbated by elevated levels of IL-1β and tumor necrosis factor (TNF)-α when exposed to *Salmonella typhimurium* [101].

Antigen Presentation

In DCs, autophagy controls how antigens are processed and presented for antigen presentation [93]. Both *NOD2* 1007fs and *ATG16L1* T300A block muramyl dipeptide induction of autophagy, and this process is associated with defective bacterial handling in DCs and impaired antigen presentation in association with MHC class II at the cell surface [65]. Deletion of *ATG16L1* in a mouse model resulted in increased T-cell stimulation by DCs [102]. Additionally, *ATG7*-deficient mouse DCs are unable to stimulate CD4+ T-cell activation when exposed to *Toxoplasma gondii* antigens [103].

5.1.2. Neutrophils

Neutrophils have strong phagocytic and bacterial killing ability against foreign materials and bacteria, similar to macrophages, and play a central role in innate immunity [104]. Neutrophils react sensitively to stimuli and exhibit various functions. The initial response of neutrophils is quick, and neutrophils are subjected to sophisticated control mechanisms because they are involved in tissue restoration and minimization of injury to surrounding tissues. When this balance is impaired, neutrophils exhibit abnormal activation and are involved in various diseases [105]. Neutrophils are also involved in IBD pathophysiology and have been reported to be associated with cytokines, chemokines, ROS, and elastase [106]. Several reports have described the relationship between neutrophils and autophagy in IBD. For example, impaired *Salmonella typhimurium* clearance and increased ROS production were observed in *ATG16L1*-deficient murine neutrophils [107]. Thus, autophagy-related *ATG16L1* is essential for bacterial clearance and suppression of ROS production by neutrophils. In addition, autophagy receptor optineurin-deficient mice have been shown to be more susceptible to *Citrobacter* colitis and *E. coli* peritonitis and showed reduced levels of TNF-α in serum and diminished neutrophil recruitment to sites of acute inflammation compared with that in wild-type mice [108]. Thus, the autophagy receptor optineurin plays a role in acute inflammation and neutrophil recruitment.

5.1.3. Innate Lymphoid Cells (ILCs)

ILCs are innate immunocompetent cells belonging to the lymphocyte system; some are similar to helper T cells, although cytotoxic natural killer cells (NKs) are also considered ILCs. ILCs are classified into groups 1–3 based on cytokine production. Group I ILCs include ILC1s and NK cells, ILC2s are assigned to group 2 ILCs, and group 3 ILCs include ILC3s. These groups of cells have attracted much attention from researchers interested in IBD pathology and are important for the maintenance of homeostasis and inflammatory immune responses [109]. In addition, autophagy has been shown to be required for ILC development and function. Atg5, an essential component of the autophagy machinery, is required for the development of mature NKs and group 1–3 ILCs [110]. Phosphorylated Forkhead box O (FoxO) 1 is localized in the cytoplasm of immature NKs and interacts with ATG7. FoxO1-mediated autophagy has been shown to be required for NK development and NK-induced innate immunity [111,112].

5.1.4. NKT Cells (NKTs)

NKTs are immunocompetent cells that recognize antigens presented mainly on CDld molecules of antigen-presenting cells and produce cytokines. Because CD1d-restricted NKTs have an invariant T-cell receptor α chain, these cells are expressed as intramucosal NKTs (iNKTs). Mice with oxazolone-induced enteritis are considered a Th2-dominant ulcerative colitis model, and IL-13 produced from iNKTs is an associated cytokine [113]. It has been reported that the number of NKTs is increased in the intestinal mucosa of patients with ulcerative colitis, and IL-13 production is enhanced [114]. Thus, NKTs are thought to be involved in the pathogenesis of IBD, and autophagy is important for the development and differentiation of iNKTs [115,116]. Recent reports have demonstrated that IL-15 induces autophagy of NKTs via TBK-binding protein 1 [117].

5.2. Intestinal Epithelial Cells

5.2.1. Paneth Cells

Paneth cells are found at the base of small intestinal crypts and were first reported in 1888 as epithelial cells with dense coarse granules. Subsequently, α-defensin, an antimicrobial peptide and an innate immune effector, was discovered within Paneth cell granules [118]. Paneth cells play an important role as intestinal epithelial cells responsible for innate immunity [119–121]. In Caucasians, abnormalities in the *NOD2* gene, which was first identified as a CD susceptibility gene, inhibit α-defensin secretion by Paneth cells [122,123]. In addition, in mice with low ATG16L1 expression, significant abnormalities were observed in the secretory pathway of Paneth cell granules, and in patients with CD harboring homozygous *ATG16L1* T300A mutations, abnormal Paneth cells, similar to low ATG16L1 expression mice, were reported to have been found in noninflammatory sites in the ileum [72]. In addition, as described above, autophagic abnormalities are involved in the pathology of CD, and abnormal control of endoplasmic reticulum stress (ERS), ROS, and gut flora by Paneth cells each play important roles.

ER Stress (ERS)

Various intracellular proteins are synthesized in the ER, and these proteins undergo proper folding and are transported to the Golgi apparatus. Unfolded or misfolded proteins accumulate in the ER. The accumulation of proteins with these conformational abnormalities is called ERS, and excessive ERS ultimately induces cell apoptosis. The homeostatic mechanism mediating excessive ERS is known as the unfolded protein response (UPR). The UPR plays an important role in the survival and function of intestinal epithelial cells. In recent studies, the UPR has been shown to control abnormalities involved in the pathogenesis of IBD, and several genes associated with ERS have been reported as disease susceptibility genes by GWASs [12,13,21,89].

As intestinal epithelial cells, Paneth cells are closely related to ERS [12]. ERS results in the induction of autophagy in Paneth cells through three signaling pathways: insulin response element (IRE) 1/c-Jun N-terminal kinase/nuclear factor-κB/X-box binding protein 1 (XBP-1), pancreatic ER kinase/eukaryotic initiation factor (eIF) 2α-activated transcription factor 4, and GRP78-activated transcription factor 6/CCAAT-enhancer-binding protein homologous protein signaling pathways [124–126]. In terms of genetic abnormalities, reports describing the relationships between ERS and autophagy in Paneth cells have focused on the roles of the *NOD2* and *ATG16L1* genes [12,122,127–129]. Secretory autophagy, which is triggered in Paneth cells by bacteria-induced ERS and limited bacterial dissemination, is disrupted in Paneth cells expressing *ATG16L1* T300A [122]. In mice lacking *ATG16L1* specifically in the epithelium, CD-like ileitis occurs spontaneously in an age-dependent manner in Paneth cells, which are ERS sensors and causes changes in IRE1α, which is important for Paneth cell homeostasis [129]. ER stress is induced via deletion of the UPR transcription factor XBP-1 in the intestinal epithelium, resulting in autophagosome formation in Paneth cells via a mechanism involving the eukaryotic translation initiation factor eIF2α [8]. Thus, the involvement of autophagy in ERS may be a new therapeutic target for IBD in the future.

ROS

ROS have been shown to be involved in the pathogenesis of IBD, and many reports have suggested that IBD is associated with an imbalance between ROS and antioxidant activity, causing oxidative stress as a result of either ROS overproduction or decreased antioxidant activity [130–132]. Although many of the details of the relationship between ROS and autophagy have not been elucidated, accumulation of ROS has been reported to be related to induction of autophagy [133]. Notably, mitochondrial dysfunction is known to trigger the accumulation of ROS in Paneth cells, resulting in induction of autophagy through the p53/TP53 induced glycolysis regulatory phosphatase/damage-regulated autophagy modulator, p62-NF-E2-related factor 2, and BCL2/adenovirus E1B 19 kDa protein-interacting protein 3 pathways, thus protecting against cellular damage caused by various stresses [134,135]. Additionally, mutations in Atg promote the production of ROS via mitochondrial insufficiency in Paneth cells [136]. Further studies are needed to fully elucidate the relationship between ROS and autophagy in IBD.

Gut Microbiota

There are in the order of 100 trillion intestinal bacteria present in the human intestinal tract, and these cells play important roles in maintaining host metabolism and immunological homeostasis. Although findings suggesting the involvement of intestinal bacteria in the pathology of IBD are accumulating, it is unclear whether changes in the composition of the gut flora are the cause of IBD. Paneth cells are important factors influencing the gut flora [137], and autophagy abnormalities in Paneth cells are known to be related to alterations in the gut flora [137–139]. Autophagy dysfunction in Paneth cell disrupts the normal intestinal flora and promotes intracellular survival of AIEC and *Salmonella typhimurium* [138]. Vitamin D receptors in the intestinal tract contribute to Paneth cell function, autophagy function, and maintenance of normal intestinal microflora via ATG16L1 [139]. In addition, the microbiota induces basal Paneth cell autophagy by IFN-γ, facilitating the maintenance of intestinal homeostasis [140]. Dysfunction of autophagy by Paneth cells has also been reported to cause not only changes in the gut microbiome, but also improper responses to the altered flora [141]. As described above, the gut flora is closely related to autophagic abnormalities in Paneth cells, and many IBD treatments, particularly those utilizing probiotics, aim to correct intestinal bacterial flora populations [142,143].

5.2.2. Goblet Cells

Goblet cells are intestinal epithelial cells with cytoplasmic granules containing large quantities of mucin, a glycoprotein [144,145]. In the gastrointestinal tract, Goblet cells can be found in both the small intestine and the large intestine, and mucin secreted into the intestinal lumen is thought to contribute to mucosal protection and repair of the intestinal epithelium [146]. Dysfunction in mucin secretion and defects in the mucus layer allow large quantities of bacteria to reach the epithelium and trigger excess host immune responses, which have been shown to be associated with IBD [147].

In recent studies, autophagy has been reported to affect the functions of Goblet cells. Mice or cells lacking autophagy by depletion of autophagy-related proteins, such as ATG5, ATG7, ATG16L1, and LC3, show altered goblet cell morphology and decreased mucin secretion [73,148,149]. In addition, inflammasomes have been shown to be involved in mucin secretion by Goblet cells, and NLRP6 inflammasomes have been reported to promote excocytosis of mucin by Goblet cells through promotion of autophagy [150]. Sonic hedgehog intestinal epithelial conditional knockout mice showed decreased numbers of ileal mucin-secreting Goblet cells accompanied by a significant reduction in autophagy [151]. Apple polysaccharide has been shown to inhibit dysbiosis-associated gut permeability and chronic inflammation due to the induction of autophagy in Goblet cells [152]. As described above, Goblet cells play important roles in the secretion of mucin via autophagy, act to maintain intestinal microflora, and are attracting attention as new therapeutic targets for IBD [149,153,154].

An overview of the autophagy mechanism of innate immunity cells in IBD is shown in Figure 4.

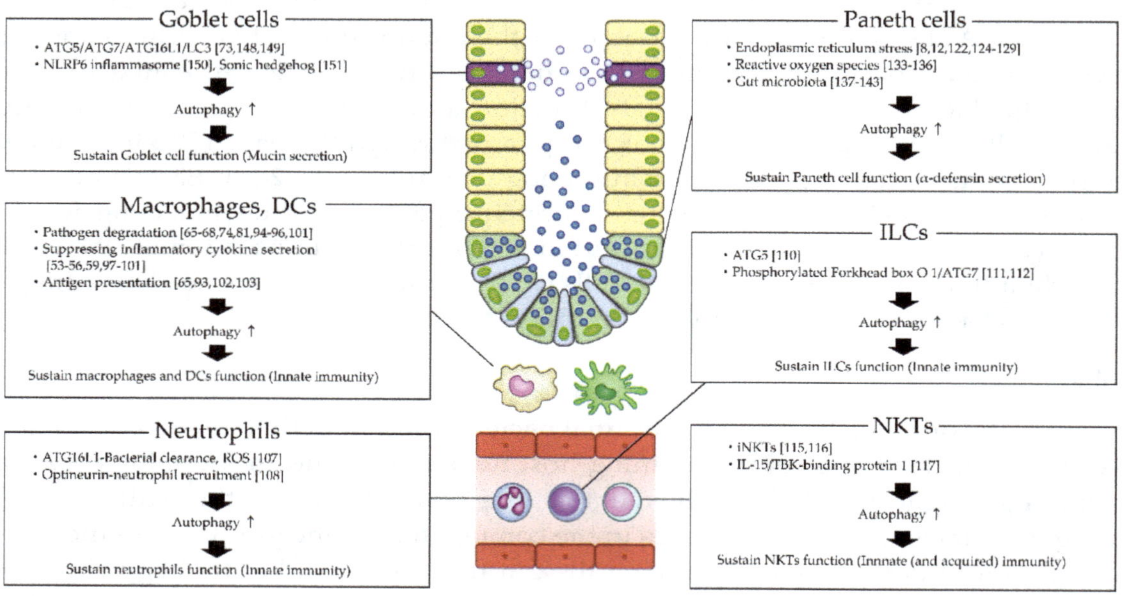

Figure 4. Role of autophagy of innate immune cells on IBD. DCs; dendritic cells, IL; interleukin, ILCs; innate lymphoid cells, NKTs; natural killer T cells, ROS; reactive oxygen species.

6. Conclusions

In this review, we have provided an overview of the autophagy mechanism of innate immune cells in IBD. Numerous studies have revealed that autophagy is an essential key player in controlling inflammatory responses mediated by innate immune cells. We anticipate that in the future, and based on further research, a therapy based on autophagic control will be established for IBD, a condition that does not yet have a curative therapy.

Author Contributions: Conceptualization, T.I. and H.N.; Investigation, T.I., Y.Y., K.W. and D.H.; Writing-Original Draft Preparation, T.I., Y.Y., K.W. and D.H.; Writing-Review & Editing, H.N.; Supervision, H.N.; Funding Acquisition, T.I. and H.N.

References

1. Ebbo, M.; Crinier, A.; Vély, F.; Vivier, E. Innate lymphoid cells: Major players in inflammatory diseases. *Nat. Rev. Immunol.* **2017**, *17*, 665–678. [CrossRef] [PubMed]
2. Choy, M.C.; Visvanathan, K.; De Cruz, P. An overview of the innate and adaptive immune system in inflammatory bowel disease. *Inflamm. Bowel Dis.* **2017**, *23*, 2–13. [CrossRef] [PubMed]
3. Lee, S.H.; Kwon, J.E.; Cho, M.L. Immunological pathogenesis of inflammatory bowel disease. *Intest. Res.* **2018**, *16*, 26–42. [CrossRef] [PubMed]
4. Jostins, L.M.; Ripke, S.; Weersma, R.K.; Duerr, R.H.; McGovern, D.P.; Hui, K.Y.; Lee, J.C.; Schumm, L.P.; Sharma, Y.; Anderson, C.A.; et al. Host-microbe interactions have shaped the genetic architecture of inflammatory bowel disease. *Nature* **2012**, *491*, 119–124. [CrossRef] [PubMed]
5. Liu, J.Z.; van Sommeren, S.; Huang, H.; Ng, S.C.; Alberts, R.; Takahashi, A.; Ripke, S.; Lee, J.C.; Jostins, L.; Shah, T.; et al. Association analyses identify 38 susceptibility loci for IBD and highlight shared genetic risk across populations. *Nat. Genet.* **2015**, *47*, 979–986. [CrossRef] [PubMed]
6. Cho, J.H.; Brant, S.R. Recent insights into the genetics of inflammatory bowel disease. *Gastroenterology* **2011**, *140*, 1704–1712. [CrossRef] [PubMed]
7. Ek, W.E.; D'Amato, M.; Halfvarson, J. The history of genetics in inflammatory bowel disease. *Ann. Gastroenterol.* **2014**, *27*, 294–303. [PubMed]
8. Adolph, T.E.; Tomczak, M.F.; Niederreiter, L.; Ko, H.J.; Böck, J.; Martinez-Naves, E.; Glickman, J.N.; Tschurtschenthaler, M.; Hartwig, J.; Hosomi, S.; et al. Paneth cells as a site of origin for intestinal inflammation. *Nature* **2013**, *503*, 272–276. [CrossRef] [PubMed]
9. Patman, G. Crohn's disease. TCF1 regulates Paneth cell α-defensins. *Nat. Rev. Gastroenterol. Hepatol.* **2014**, *11*, 517. [CrossRef]
10. Eriguchi, Y.; Nakamura, K.; Yokoi, Y.; Sugimoto, R.; Takahashi, S.; Hashimoto, D.; Teshima, T.; Ayabe, T.; Selsted, M.E.; Ouellette, A.J. Essential role of IFN-γ in T cell-associated intestinal inflammation. *JCI. Insight.* **2018**, *20*, pii:121886. [CrossRef]
11. Molodecky, N.A.; Soon, I.S.; Rabi, D.M.; Ghali, W.A.; Ferris, M.; Chernoff, G.; Benchimol, E.I.; Panaccione, R.; Ghosh, S.; Barkema, H.W.; et al. Increasing incidence and prevalence of the inflammatory bowel diseases with time, based on systematic review. *Gastroenterology* **2012**, *142*, 46–54. [CrossRef] [PubMed]
12. Kaser, A.; Blumberg, R.S. Autophagy, microbial sensing, endoplasmic reticulum stress, and epithelial function in inflammatory bowel disease. *Gastroenterology* **2011**, *140*, 1738–1747. [CrossRef] [PubMed]
13. Kaser, A.; Zeissig, S.; Blumberg, R.S. Inflammatory bowel disease. *Annu. Rev. Immunol.* **2010**, *28*, 573–621. [CrossRef] [PubMed]
14. Khor, B.; Gardet, A.; Xavier, R.J. Genetics and pathogenesis of inflammatory bowel disease. *Nature* **2011**, *474*, 307–317. [CrossRef]
15. Weterman, I.T.; Peña, A.S. Familial incidence of Crohn's disease in the Netherlands and a review of the literature. *Gastroenterology* **1984**, *86*, 449–452.
16. Hugot, J.P.; Chamaillard, M.; Zouali, H.; Lesage, S.; Cézard, J.P.; Belaiche, J.; Almer, S.; Tysk, C.; O'Morain, C.A.; Gassull, M.; et al. Association of NOD2 leucine-rich repeat variants with susceptibility to Crohn's disease. *Nature* **2001**, *411*, 599–603. [CrossRef]
17. Ogura, Y.; Bonen, D.K.; Inohara, N.; Nicolae, D.L.; Chen, F.F.; Ramos, R.; Britton, H.; Moran, T.; Karaliuskas, R.; Duerr, R.H.; et al. A frameshift mutation in NOD2 associated with susceptibility to Crohn's disease. *Nature* **2001**, *411*, 603–606. [CrossRef]
18. Goldstein, D.B. Common genetic variation and human traits. *N. Engl. J. Med.* **2009**, *360*, 1696–1698. [CrossRef]
19. Levine, B.; Mizushima, N.; Virgin, H.W. Autophagy in immunity and inflammation. *Nature* **2011**, *469*, 323–325. [CrossRef]
20. Hooper, K.M.; Barlow, P.G.; Stevens, C.; Henderson, P. Inflammatory bowel disease drugs: A focus on autophagy. *J. Crohn's Colitis* **2017**, *11*, 118–127. [CrossRef]
21. Lassen, K.G.; Xavier, R.J. Mechanisms and function of autophagy in intestinal disease. *Autophagy* **2018**, *14*, 216–220. [CrossRef] [PubMed]
22. Zeki, A.A.; Yeganeh, B.; Kenyon, N.J.; Post, M.; Ghavami, S. Autophagy in airway diseases: A new frontier in human asthma? *Allergy* **2016**, *71*, 5–14. [CrossRef] [PubMed]

23. Poon, A.H.; Choy, D.F.; Chouiali, F.; Ramakrishnan, R.K.; Mahboub, B.; Audusseau, S.; Mogas, A.; Harris, J.M.; Arron, J.R.; Laprise, C.; et al. Increased autophagy-related 5 gene expression is associated with collagen expression in the airways of refractory asthmatics. *Front. Immunol.* **2017**, *8*, 355. [CrossRef] [PubMed]
24. Mabalirajan, U. A possible differential role of autophagy in asthma? *J. Allergy Clin. Immunol.* **2017**, *139*, 712. [CrossRef] [PubMed]
25. Racanelli, A.C.; Kikkers, S.A.; Choi, A.M.K.; Cloonan, S.M. Autophagy and inflammation in chronic respiratory disease. *Autophagy* **2018**, *14*, 221–232. [CrossRef] [PubMed]
26. Allison, S.J. Systemic lupus erythematosus: Defective noncanonical autophagy in SLE-like disease. *Nat. Rev. Rheumatol.* **2016**, *12*, 311. [CrossRef] [PubMed]
27. Mistry, P.; Kaplan, M.J. Cell death in the pathogenesis of systemic lupus erythematosus and lupus nephritis. *Clin. Immunol.* **2017**, *185*, 59–73. [CrossRef]
28. Fujikake, N.; Shin, M.; Shimizu, S. Association between autophagy and neurodegenerative diseases. *Front. Neurosci.* **2018**, *12*, 255. [CrossRef]
29. Harper, J.W.; Ordureau, A.; Heo, J.M. Building and decoding ubiquitin chains for mitophagy. *Nat. Rev. Mol. Cell Biol.* **2018**, *19*, 93–108. [CrossRef]
30. Iida, T.; Onodera, K.; Nakase, H. Role of autophagy in the pathogenesis of inflammatory bowel disease. *World J. Gastroenterol.* **2017**, *23*, 1944–1953. [CrossRef]
31. Rogov, V.; Dötsch, V.; Johansen, T.; Kirkin, V. Interactions between autophagy receptors and ubiquitin-like proteins form the molecular basis for selective autophagy. *Mol. Cell* **2014**, *53*, 167–178. [CrossRef] [PubMed]
32. Kawai, T.; Akira, S. The role of pattern-recognition receptors in innate immunity: Update on Toll-like receptors. *Nat. Immunol.* **2010**, *11*, 373–384. [CrossRef] [PubMed]
33. Mizushima, N.; Yoshimori, T.; Ohsumi, Y. The role of Atg proteins in autophagosome formation. *Annu. Rev. Cell Dev. Biol.* **2011**, *27*, 107–132. [CrossRef] [PubMed]
34. Levine, B. Eating oneself and uninvited guests: Autophagy-related pathways in cellular defense. *Cell* **2005**, *120*, 159–162. [CrossRef] [PubMed]
35. Nozawa, T.; Minowa-Nozawa, A.; Aikawa, C.; Nakagawa, I. The STX6-VTI1B-VAMP3 complex facilitates xenophagy by regulating the fusion between recycling endosomes and autophagosomes. *Autophagy* **2017**, *13*, 57–69. [CrossRef]
36. Hailey, D.W.; Rambold, A.S.; Satpute-Krishnan, P.; Mitra, K.; Sougrat, R.; Kim, P.K.; Lippincott-Schwartz, J. Mitochondria supply membranes for autophagosome biogenesis during starvation. *Cell* **2010**, *141*, 656–667. [CrossRef]
37. Yao, Z.; Klionsky, D.J. An unconventional pathway for mitochondrial protein degradation. *Autophagy* **2016**, *12*, 1971–1972. [CrossRef]
38. Kimura, T.; Mandell, M.; Deretic, V. Precision autophagy directed by receptor regulators-emerging examples within the TRIM family. *J. Cell Sci.* **2016**, *129*, 881–891. [CrossRef]
39. Martinon, F.; Burns, K.; Tschopp, J. The inflammasome: A molecular platform triggering activation of inflammatory caspases and processing of proIL-beta. *Mol. Cell* **2002**, *10*, 417–426. [CrossRef]
40. Rathinam, V.A.; Vanaja, S.K.; Fitzgerald, K.A. Regulation of inflammasome signaling. *Nat. Immunol.* **2012**, *13*, 333–342. [CrossRef]
41. Strowig, T.; Henao-Mejia, J.; Elinav, E.; Flavell, R. Inflammasomes in health and disease. *Nature* **2012**, *481*, 278–286. [CrossRef] [PubMed]
42. Guo, H.; Callaway, J.B.; Ting, J.P. Inflammasomes: Mechanism of action, role in disease, and therapeutics. *Nat. Med.* **2015**, *21*, 677–687. [CrossRef] [PubMed]
43. Mangan, M.S.J.; Olhava, E.J.; Roush, W.R.; Seidel, H.M.; Glick, G.D.; Latz, E. Targeting the NLRP3 inflammasome in inflammatory diseases. *Nat. Rev. Drug Discov.* **2018**, *17*, 588–606. [CrossRef] [PubMed]
44. Rathinam, V.A.K.; Chan, F.K. Inflammasome, Inflammation, and Tissue Homeostasis. *Trends Mol. Med.* **2018**, *24*, 304–318. [CrossRef] [PubMed]
45. Becker, C.; Watson, A.J.; Neurath, M.F. Complex roles of caspases in the pathogenesis of inflammatory bowel disease. *Gastroenterology* **2013**, *144*, 283–293. [CrossRef] [PubMed]
46. Opipari, A.; Franchi, L. Role of inflammasomes in intestinal inflammation and Crohn's disease. *Inflamm. Bowel Dis.* **2015**, *21*, 173–181. [CrossRef]
47. de Souza, H.S.; Fiocchi, C. Immunopathogenesis of IBD: Current state of the art. *Nat. Rev. Gastroenterol. Hepatol.* **2016**, *13*, 13–27. [CrossRef]

48. de Souza, H.S.P. Etiopathogenesis of inflammatory bowel disease: Today and tomorrow. *Curr. Opin. Gastroenterol.* **2017**, *33*, 222–229. [CrossRef]
49. Lazaridis, L.D.; Pistiki, A.; Giamarellos-Bourboulis, E.J.; Georgitsi, M.; Damoraki, G.; Polymeros, D.; Dimitriadis, G.D.; Triantafyllou, K. Activation of NLRP3 inflammasome in inflammatory bowel disease: Differences between Crohn's disease and ulcerative colitis. *Dig. Dis. Sci.* **2017**, *62*, 2348–2356. [CrossRef]
50. Mao, L.; Kitani, A.; Similuk, M.; Oler, A.J.; Albenberg, L.; Kelsen, J.; Aktay, A.; Quezado, M.; Yao, M.; Montgomery-Recht, K.; et al. Loss-of-function CARD8 mutation causes NLRP3 inflammasome activation and Crohn's disease. *J. Clin. Investig.* **2018**, *128*, 1793–1806. [CrossRef]
51. Kawai, T.; Akira, S. The roles of TLRs, RLRs and NLRs in pathogen recognition. *Int. Immunol.* **2009**, *21*, 317–337. [CrossRef] [PubMed]
52. Giles, E.M.; Sanders, T.J.; McCarthy, N.E.; Lung, J.; Pathak, M.; MacDonald, T.T.; Lindsay, J.O.; Stagg, A.J. Regulation of human intestinal T-cell responses by type 1 interferon-STAT1 signaling is disrupted in inflammatory bowel disease. *Mucosal Immunol.* **2017**, *10*, 184–193. [CrossRef] [PubMed]
53. Saitoh, T.; Fujita, N.; Jang, M.H.; Uematsu, S.l.; Yang, B.G.; Satoh, T.; Omori, H.; Noda, T.; Yamamoto, N.; Komatsu, M.; et al. Loss of the autophagy protein Atg16L1 enhances endotoxin-induced IL-1beta production. *Nature* **2008**, *456*, 264–268. [CrossRef] [PubMed]
54. Zhou, R.; Yazdi, A.S.; Menu, P.; Tschopp, J. A role for mitochondria in NLRP3 inflammasome activation. *Nature* **2011**, *469*, 221–225. [CrossRef] [PubMed]
55. Wen, H.; Gris, D.; Lei, Y.; Jha, S.; Zhang, L.; Huang, M.T.; Brickey, W.J.; Ting, J.P. Fatty acid-induced NLRP3-ASC inflammasome activation interferes with insulin signaling. *Nat. Immunol.* **2011**, *12*, 408–415. [CrossRef] [PubMed]
56. Lupfer, C.; Thomas, P.G.; Anand, P.K.; Vogel, P.; Milasta, S.; Martinez, J.; Huang, G.; Green, M.; Kundu, M.; Chi, H.; et al. Receptor interacting protein kinase 2-mediated mitophagy regulates inflammasome activation during virus infection. *Nat. Immunol.* **2013**, *14*, 480–488. [CrossRef] [PubMed]
57. Chuang, S.Y.; Yang, C.H.; Chou, C.C.; Chiang, Y.P.; Chuang, T.H.; Hsu, L.C. TLR-induced PAI-2 expression suppresses IL-1β processing via increasing autophagy and NLRP3 degradation. *Proc. Natl. Acad. Sci. USA* **2013**, *110*, 16079–16084. [CrossRef]
58. Shi, C.S.; Shenderov, K.; Huang, N.N.; Kabat, J.; Abu-Asab, M.; Fitzgerald, K.A.; Sher, A.; Kehrl, J.H. Activation of autophagy by inflammatory signals limits IL-1β production by targeting ubiquitinated inflammasomes for destruction. *Nat. Immunol.* **2012**, *13*, 255–263. [CrossRef]
59. Harris, J.; Hartman, M.; Roche, C.; Zeng, S.G.; O'Shea, A.; Sharp, F.A.; Lambe, E.M.; Creagh, E.M.; Golenbock, D.T.; Tschopp, J.; et al. Autophagy controls IL-1beta secretion by targeting pro-IL-1beta for degradation. *J. Biol. Chem.* **2011**, *286*, 9587–9597. [CrossRef]
60. Deretic, V.; Kimura, T.; Timmins, G.; Moseley, P.; Chauhan, S.; Mandell, M. Immunologic manifestations of autophagy. *J. Clin. Investig.* **2015**, *125*, 75–84. [CrossRef]
61. Kimura, T.; Jain, A.; Choi, S.W.; Mandell, M.A.; Schroder, K.; Johansen, T.; Deretic, V. TRIM-mediated precision autophagy targets cytoplasmic regulators of innate immunity. *J. Cell Biol.* **2015**, *210*, 973–989. [CrossRef] [PubMed]
62. Dupont, N.; Jiang, S.; Pilli, M.; Ornatowski, W.; Bhattacharya, D.; Deretic, V. Autophagy-based unconventional secretory pathway for extracellular delivery of IL-1β. *EMBO J.* **2011**, *30*, 4701–4711. [CrossRef] [PubMed]
63. Zhang, M.; Kenny, S.J.; Ge, L.; Xu, K.; Schekman, R. Translocation of interleukin-1β into a vesicle intermediate in autophagy-mediated secretion. *Elife* **2015**, *4*. [CrossRef]
64. Lee, H.K.; Lund, J.M.; Ramanathan, B.; Mizushima, N.; Iwasaki, A. Autophagy-dependent viral recognition by plasmacytoid dendritic cells. *Science* **2007**, *315*, 1398–1401. [CrossRef] [PubMed]
65. Cooney, R.; Baker, J.; Brain, O.; Danis, B.; Pichulik, T.; Allan, P.; Ferguson, D.J.; Campbell, B.J.; Jewell, D.; Simmons, A. NOD2 stimulation induces autophagy in dendritic cells influencing bacterial handling and antigen presentation. *Nat. Med.* **2010**, *16*, 90–97. [CrossRef] [PubMed]
66. Homer, C.R.; Richmond, A.L.; Rebert, N.A.; Achkar, J.P.; McDonald, C. ATG16L1 and NOD2 interact in an autophagy-dependent antibacterial pathway implicated in Crohn's disease pathogenesis. *Gastroenterology* **2010**, *139*, 1630–1641. [CrossRef] [PubMed]
67. Travassos, L.H.; Carneiro, L.A.; Ramjeet, M.; Hussey, S.; Kim, Y.G.; Magalhães, J.G.; Yuan, L.; Soares, F.; Chea, E.; Le Bourhis, L.; et al. Nod1 and Nod2 direct autophagy by recruiting ATG16L1 to the plasma membrane at the site of bacterial entry. *Nat. Immunol.* **2010**, *11*, 55–62. [CrossRef]

68. Negroni, A.; Colantoni, E.; Vitali, R.; Palone, F.; Pierdomenico, M.; Costanzo, M.; Cesi, V.; Cucchiara, S.; Stronati, L. NOD2 induces autophagy to control AIEC bacteria infectiveness in intestinal epithelial cells. *Inflamm. Res.* **2016**, *65*, 803–813. [CrossRef]
69. Mizushima, N.; Noda, T.; Ohsumi, Y. Apg16p is required for the function of the Apg12p-Apg5p conjugate in the yeast autophagy pathway. *EMBO J.* **1999**, *18*, 3888–3896. [CrossRef] [PubMed]
70. Mizushima, N.; Kuma, A.; Kobayashi, Y.; Yamamoto, A.; Matsubae, M.; Takao, T.; Natsume, T.; Ohsumi, Y.; Yoshimori, T. Mouse Apg16L, a novel WD-repeat protein, targets to the autophagic isolation membrane with the Apg12-Apg5 conjugate. *J. Cell Sci.* **2003**, *116*, 1679–1688. [CrossRef]
71. Prescott, N.J.; Fisher, S.A.; Franke, A.; Hampe, J.; Onnie, C.M.; Soars, D.; Bagnall, R.; Mirza, M.M.; Sanderson, J.; Forbes, A.; et al. A nonsynonymous SNP in ATG16L1 predisposes to ileal Crohn's disease and is independent of CARD15 and IBD5. *Gastroenterology* **2007**, *132*, 1665–1671. [CrossRef] [PubMed]
72. Cadwell, K.; Liu, J.Y.; Brown, S.L.; Miyoshi, H.; Loh, J.; Lennerz, J.K.; Kishi, C.; Kc, W.; Carrero, J.A.; Hunt, S.; et al. A key role for autophagy and the autophagy gene Atg16l1 in mouse and human intestinal Paneth cells. *Nature* **2008**, *456*, 259–263. [CrossRef] [PubMed]
73. Lassen, K.G.; Kuballa, P.; Conway, K.L.; Patel, K.K.; Becker, C.E.; Peloquin, J.M.; Villablanca, E.J.; Norman, J.M.; Liu, T.C.; Heath, R.J.; et al. Atg16L1 T300A variant decreases selective autophagy resulting in altered cytokine signaling and decreased antibacterial defense. *Proc. Natl. Acad. Sci. USA* **2014**, *111*, 7741–7746. [CrossRef] [PubMed]
74. Murthy, A.; Li, Y.; Peng, I.; Reichelt, M.; Katakam, A.K.; Noubade, R.; Roose-Girma, M.; DeVoss, J.; Diehl, L.; Graham, R.R.; et al. A Crohn's disease variant in Atg16l1 enhances its degradation by caspase 3. *Nature* **2014**, *506*, 456–462. [CrossRef] [PubMed]
75. Chu, H.; Khosravi, A.; Kusumawardhani, I.P.; Kwon, A.H.; Vasconcelos, A.C.; Cunha, L.D.; Mayer, A.E.; Shen, Y.; Wu, W.L.; Kambal, A.; et al. Gene-microbiota interactions contribute to the pathogenesis of inflammatory bowel disease. *Science* **2016**, *352*, 1116–1120. [CrossRef] [PubMed]
76. Yue, C.; Yang, X.; Li, J.; Chen, X.; Zhao, X.; Chen, Y.; Wen, Y. Trimethylamine N-oxide prime NLRP3 inflammasome via inhibiting ATG16L1-induced autophagy in colonic epithelial cells. *Biochem. Biophys. Res. Commun.* **2017**, *490*, 541–551. [CrossRef] [PubMed]
77. Pott, J.; Kabat, A.M.; Maloy, K.J. Intestinal epithelial cell autophagy is required to protect against TNF-induced apoptosis during chronic colitis in mice. *Cell Host Microbe* **2018**, *23*, 191–202. [CrossRef] [PubMed]
78. Singh, S.B.; Davis, A.S.; Taylor, G.A.; Deretic, V. Human IRGM induces autophagy to eliminate intracellular mycobacteria. *Science* **2006**, *313*, 1438–1441. [CrossRef] [PubMed]
79. McCarroll, S.A.; Huett, A.; Kuballa, P.; Chilewski, S.D.; Landry, A.; Goyette, P.; Zody, M.C.; Hall, J.L.; Brant, S.R.; Cho, J.H.; et al. Deletion polymorphism upstream of IRGM associated with altered IRGM expression and Crohn's disease. *Nat. Genet.* **2008**, *40*, 1107–1112. [CrossRef]
80. Rufini, S.; Ciccacci, C.; Di Fusco, D.; Ruffa, A.; Pallone, F.; Novelli, G.; Biancone, L.; Borgiani, P. Autophagy and inflammatory bowel disease: Association between variants of the autophagy related IRGM gene and susceptibility to Crohn's disease. *Dig. Liver Dis.* **2015**, *47*, 744–750. [CrossRef]
81. Chauhan, S.; Mandell, M.A.; Deretic, V. IRGM governs the core autophagy machinery to conduct antimicrobial defense. *Mol. Cell* **2015**, *58*, 507–521. [CrossRef] [PubMed]
82. Crook, N.E.; Clem, R.J.; Miller, L.K. An apoptosis-inhibiting baculovirus gene with a zinc finger-like motif. *J. Virol.* **1993**, *67*, 2168–2174. [PubMed]
83. Eckelman, B.P.; Salvesen, G.S.; Scott, F.L. Human inhibitor of apoptosis proteins: Why XIAP is the black sheep of the family. *EMBO Rep.* **2006**, *7*, 988–994. [CrossRef] [PubMed]
84. Mizushima, N.; Levine, B.; Cuervo, A.M.; Klionsky, D.J. Autophagy fights disease through cellular self-digestion. *Nature* **2008**, *451*, 1069–1075. [CrossRef] [PubMed]
85. Huang, X.; Wu, Z.; Mei, Y.; Wu, M. XIAP inhibits autophagy via XIAP-Mdm2-p53 signalling. *EMBO J.* **2013**, *32*, 2204–2216. [CrossRef] [PubMed]
86. Zeissig, Y.; Petersen, B.S.; Milutinovic, S.; Bosse, E.; Mayr, G.; Peuker, K.; Hartwig, J.; Keller, A.; Kohl, M.; Laass, M.W.; et al. XIAP variants in male Crohn's disease. *Gut* **2015**, *64*, 66–76. [CrossRef]
87. Schwerd, T.; Pandey, S.; Yang, H.T.; Bagola, K.; Jameson, E.; Jung, J.; Lachmann, R.H.; Shah, N.; Patel, S.Y.; Booth, C.; et al. Impaired antibacterial autophagy links granulomatous intestinal inflammation in Niemann-Pick disease type C1 and XIAP deficiency with NOD2 variants in Crohn's disease. *Gut* **2017**, *66*, 1060–1073. [CrossRef]

88. Elinav, E.; Strowig, T.; Henao-Mejia, J.; Flavell, R.A. Regulation of the antimicrobial response by NLR proteins. *Immunity* **2011**, *34*, 665–679. [CrossRef]
89. Yano, T.; Kurata, S. Intracellular recognition of pathogens and autophagy as an innate immune host defence. *J. Biochem.* **2011**, *150*, 143–149. [CrossRef]
90. Mazzini, E.; Massimiliano, L.; Penna, G.; Rescigno, M. Oral tolerance can be established via gap junction transfer of fed antigens from CX3CR1$^+$ macrophages to CD103$^+$ dendritic cells. *Immunity* **2014**, *40*, 248–261. [CrossRef]
91. Martin, B.; Hirota, K.; Cua, D.J.; Stockinger, B.; Veldhoen, M. Interleukin-17-producing gamma delta T cells selectively expand in response topathogen products and environmental signals. *Immunity* **2009**, *31*, 321–330. [CrossRef] [PubMed]
92. Talero, E.; Garcia-Maurino, S.; Motilva, V. Melatonin, autophagy and intestinal bowel disease. *Curr. Pharm. Des.* **2014**, *20*, 4816–4827. [CrossRef] [PubMed]
93. Münz, C. Autophagy beyond intracellular MHC class II antigen presentation. *Trends. Immunol.* **2016**, *37*, 755–763. [CrossRef] [PubMed]
94. Strisciuglio, C.; Duijvestein, M.; Verhaar, A.P.; Vos, A.C.; van den Brink, G.R.; Hommes, D.W.; Wildenberg, M.E. Impaired autophagy leads to abnormal dendritic cell-epithelial cell interactions. *J. Crohns. Colitis.* **2013**, *7*, 534–541. [CrossRef]
95. Lapaquette, P.; Bringer, M.A.; Darfeuille-Michaud, A. Defects in autophagy favour adherent-invasive Escherichia coli persistence within macrophages leading to increased pro-inflammatory response. *Cell. Microbiol.* **2012**, *14*, 791–807. [CrossRef] [PubMed]
96. Lassen, K.G.; McKenzie, C.I.; Mari, M.; Murano, T.; Begun, J.; Baxt, L.A.; Goel, G.; Villablanca, E.J.; Kuo, S.Y.; Huang, H.; et al. Genetic coding variant in GPR65 alters lysosomal pH and links lysosomal dysfunction with colitis risk. *Immunity* **2016**, *44*, 1392–1405. [CrossRef] [PubMed]
97. Meunier, E.; Dick, M.S.; Dreier, R.F.; Schürmann, N.; Kenzelmann Broz, D.; Warming, S.; Roose-Girma, M.; Bumann, D.; Kayagaki, N.; Takeda, K.; et al. Caspase-11 activation requires lysis of pathogen-containing vacuoles by IFN-induced GTPases. *Nature* **2014**, *509*, 366–370. [CrossRef]
98. Ke, P.; Shao, B.Z.; Xu, Z.Q.; Wei, W.; Han, B.Z.; Chen, X.W.; Su, D.F.; Liu, C. Activation of cannabinoid receptor 2 ameliorates DSS-induced colitis through inhibiting NLRP3 inflammasome in macrophages. *PLoS ONE* **2016**, *11*, e0155076. [CrossRef]
99. Samie, M.; Lim, J.; Verschueren, E.; Baughman, J.M.; Peng, I.; Wong, A.; Kwon, Y.; Senbabaoglu, Y.; Hackney, J.A.; Keir, M.; et al. Selective autophagy of the adaptor TRIF regulates innate inflammatory signaling. *Nat. Immunol.* **2018**, *19*, 246–254. [CrossRef]
100. Fan, K.; Lin, L.; Ai, Q.; Wan, J.; Dai, J.; Liu, G.; Tang, L.; Yang, Y.; Ge, P.; Jiang, R.; et al. Lipopolysaccharide-induced dephosphorylation of AMPK-activated protein kinase potentiates inflammatory injury via repression of ULK1-dependent autophagy. *Front. Immunol.* **2018**, *9*, 1464. [CrossRef]
101. Zhang, H.; Zheng, L.; Chen, J.; Fukata, M.; Ichikawa, R.; Shih, D.Q.; Zhang, X. The protection role of Atg16l1 in CD11c+dendritic cells in murine colitis. *Immunobiology* **2017**, *222*, 831–841. [CrossRef] [PubMed]
102. Baxt, L.A.; Xavier, R.J. Role of autophagy in the maintenance of intestinal homeostasis. *Gastroenterology* **2015**, *149*, 553–562. [CrossRef] [PubMed]
103. Liu, E.; Van Grol, J.; Subauste, C.S. Atg5 but not Atg7 in dendritic cells enhances IL-2 and IFN-γ production by Toxoplasma gondii-reactive CD4+ T cells. *Microbes Infect.* **2015**, *17*, 275–284. [CrossRef] [PubMed]
104. Kolaczkowska, E.; Kubes, P. Neutrophil recruitment and function in health and inflammation. *Nat. Rev. Immunol.* **2013**, *13*, 159–175. [CrossRef] [PubMed]
105. Mantovani, A.; Cassatella, M.A.; Costantini, C.; Jaillon, S. Neutrophils in the activation and regulation of innate and adaptive immunity. *Nat. Rev. Immunol.* **2011**, *11*, 519–531. [CrossRef]
106. Wéra, O.; Lancellotti, P.; Oury, C. The dual role of neutrophils in inflammatory bowel diseases. *Clin. Med.* **2016**, *5*. [CrossRef]
107. Zhang, H.; Zheng, L.; McGovern, D.P.; Hamill, A.M.; Ichikawa, R.; Kanazawa, Y.; Luu, J.; Kumagai, K.; Cilluffo, M.; Fukata, M.; et al. Myeloid ATG16L1 facilitates host-bacteria interactions in maintaining intestinal homeostasis. *J. Immunol.* **2017**, *198*, 2133–2146. [CrossRef] [PubMed]
108. Chew, T.S.; O'Shea, N.R.; Sewell, G.W.; Oehlers, S.H.; Mulvey, C.M.; Crosier, P.S.; Godovac-Zimmermann, J.; Bloom, S.L.; Smith, A.M.; Segal, A.W. Optineurin deficiency in mice contributes to impaired cytokine secretion and neutrophil recruitment in bacteria-driven colitis. *Dis. Model. Mech.* **2015**, *8*, 817–829. [CrossRef] [PubMed]

109. Goldberg, R.; Prescott, N.; Lord, G.M.; MacDonald, T.T.; Powell, N. The unusual suspects–innate lymphoid cells as novel therapeutic targets in IBD. *Nat. Rev. Gastroenterol. Hepatol.* **2015**, *12*, 271–283. [CrossRef] [PubMed]
110. O'Sullivan, T.E.; Geary, C.D.; Weizman, O.E.; Geiger, T.L.; Rapp, M.; Dorn, G.W., 2nd; Overholtzer, M.; Sun, J.C. Atg5 is essential for the development and survival of innate lymphocytes. *Cell Rep.* **2016**, *15*, 1910–1919. [CrossRef]
111. Wang, S.; Xia, P.; Huang, G.; Zhu, P.; Liu, J.; Ye, B.; Du, Y.; Fan, Z. FoxO1-mediated autophagy is required for NK cell development and innate immunity. *Nat. Commun.* **2016**, *7*, 11023. [CrossRef] [PubMed]
112. López-Soto, A.; Bravo-San Pedro, J.M.; Kroemer, G.; Galluzzi, L.; Gonzalez, S. Involvement of autophagy in NK cell development and function. *Autophagy* **2017**, *13*, 633–636. [CrossRef] [PubMed]
113. Heller, F.; Fuss, I.J.; Nieuwenhuis, E.E.; Blumberg, R.S.; Strober, W. Oxazolone colitis, a Th2 colitis model resembling ulcerative colitis, is mediated by IL-13-producing NK-T cells. *Immunity* **2002**, *17*, 629–638. [CrossRef]
114. Fuss, I.J.; Heller, F.; Boirivant, M.; Leon, F.; Yoshida, M.; Fichtner-Feigl, S.; Yang, Z.; Exley, M.; Kitani, A.; Blumberg, R.S.; et al. Nonclassical CD1d-restricted NK T cells that produce IL-13 characterize an atypical Th2 response in ulcerative colitis. *J. Clin. Investig.* **2004**, *113*, 1490–1497. [CrossRef] [PubMed]
115. Salio, M.; Puleston, D.J.; Mathan, T.S.; Shepherd, D.; Stranks, A.J.; Adamopoulou, E.; Veerapen, N.; Besra, G.S.; Hollander, G.A.; Simon, A.K. Essential role for autophagy during invariant NKT cell development. *Proc. Natl. Acad. Sci. USA* **2014**, *111*, E5678–E5687. [CrossRef] [PubMed]
116. Pei, B.; Zhao, M.; Miller, B.C.; Véla, J.L.; Bruinsma, M.W.; Virgin, H.W.; Kronenberg, M. Invariant NKT cells require autophagy to coordinate proliferation and survival signals during differentiation. *J. Immunol.* **2015**, *194*, 5872–5884. [CrossRef]
117. Zhu, L.; Xie, X.; Zhang, L.; Wang, H.; Jie, Z.; Zhou, X.; Shi, J.; Zhao, S.; Zhang, B.; Cheng, X. TBK-binding protein 1 regulates IL-15-induced autophagy and NKT cell survival. *Nat. Commun.* **2018**, *9*, 2812. [CrossRef]
118. Ouellette, A.J.; Hsieh, M.M.; Nosek, M.T.; Cano-Gauci, D.F.; Huttner, K.M.; Buick, R.N.; Selsted, M.E. Mouse Paneth cell defensins: Primary structures and antibacterial activities of numerous cryptdin isoforms. *Infect. Immun.* **1994**, *62*, 5040–5047.
119. Ayabe, T.; Satchell, D.P.; Wilson, C.L.; Parks, W.C.; Selsted, M.E.; Ouellette, A.J. Secretion of microbicidal alpha-defensins by intestinal Paneth cells in response to bacteria. *Nat. Immunol.* **2000**, *1*, 113–118. [CrossRef]
120. Bar Shira, E.; Friedman, A. Innate immune functions of avian intestinal epithelial cells: Response to bacterial stimuli and localization of responding cells in the developing avian digestive tract. *PLoS ONE* **2018**, *13*, e0200393. [CrossRef]
121. Cobo, E.R.; Holani, R.; Moreau, F.; Nakamura, K.; Ayabe, T.; Mastroianni, J.R.; Ouellette, A.; Chadee, K. Entamoeba histolytica alters ileal Paneth cell functions in intact and Muc2 mucin deficiency. *Infect. Immun.* **2018**. [CrossRef] [PubMed]
122. Bel, S.; Pendse, M.; Wang, Y.; Li, Y.; Ruhn, K.A.; Hassell, B.; Leal, T.; Winter, S.E.; Xavier, R.J.; Hooper, L.V. Paneth cells secrete lysozyme via secretory autophagy during bacterial infection of the intestine. *Science* **2017**, *357*, 1047–1052. [CrossRef]
123. Stappenbeck, T.S.; McGovern, D.P.B. Paneth cell alterations in the development and phenotype of Crohn's disease. *Gastroenterology* **2017**, *152*, 322–326. [CrossRef] [PubMed]
124. Urano, F.; Wang, X.; Bertolotti, A.; Zhang, Y.; Chung, P.; Harding, H.P.; Ron, D. Coupling of stress in the ER to activation of JNK protein kinases by transmembrane protein kinase IRE1. *Science* **2000**, *287*, 664–666. [CrossRef] [PubMed]
125. Oyadomari, S.; Mori, M. Roles of CHOP/GADD153 in endoplasmic reticulum stress. *Cell Death Differ.* **2004**, *11*, 381–389. [CrossRef] [PubMed]
126. Kaneko, M.; Niinuma, Y.; Nomura, Y. Activation signal of nuclear factor-kappa B in response to endoplasmic reticulum stress is transduced via IRE1 and tumor necrosis factor receptor-associated factor 2. *Biol. Pharm. Bull.* **2003**, *26*, 931–935. [CrossRef] [PubMed]
127. Fritz, T.; Niederreiter, L.; Adolph, T.; Blumberg, R.S.; Kaser, A. Crohn's disease: NOD2, autophagy and ER stress converge. *Gut* **2011**, *60*, 1580–1588. [CrossRef]
128. Kaser, A.; Blumberg, R.S. ATG16L1 Crohn's disease risk stresses the endoplasmic reticulum of Paneth cells. *Gut* **2014**, *63*, 1038–1039. [CrossRef] [PubMed]

129. Matsuzawa-Ishimoto, Y.; Shono, Y.; Gomez, L.E.; Hubbard-Lucey, V.M.; Cammer, M.; Neil, J.; Dewan, M.Z.; Lieberman, S.R.; Lazrak, A.; Marinis, J.M.; et al. Autophagy protein ATG16L1 prevents necroptosis in the intestinal epithelium. *J. Exp. Med.* **2017**, *214*, 3687–3705. [CrossRef]
130. Balmus, I.M.; Ciobica, A.; Trifan, A.; Stanciu, C. The implications of oxidative stress and antioxidant therapies in Inflammatory Bowel Disease: Clinical aspects and animal models. *Saudi J. Gastroenterol.* **2016**, *22*, 3–17. [CrossRef]
131. Chen, L.; You, Q.; Hu, L.; Gao, J.; Meng, Q.; Liu, W.; Wu, X.; Xu, Q. The antioxidant procyanidin reduces reactive oxygen species signaling in macrophages and ameliorates experimental colitis in mice. *Front. Immunol.* **2018**, *8*, 1910. [CrossRef] [PubMed]
132. Denson, L.A.; Jurickova, I.; Karns, R.; Shaw, K.A.; Cutler, D.J.; Okou, D.T.; Dodd, A.; Quinn, K.; Mondal, K.; Aronow, B.J.; et al. Clinical and genomic correlates of neutrophil reactive oxygen species production in pediatric patients with Crohn's disease. *Gastroenterology* **2018**, *154*, 2097–2110. [CrossRef] [PubMed]
133. Zhang, C.; Li, P.; Zhang, S.; Lei, R.; Li, B.; Wu, X.; Jiang, C.; Zhang, X.; Ma, R.; Yang, L.; et al. Oxidative stress-elicited autophagosome accumulation contributes to human neuroblastoma SH-SY5Y cell death induced by PBDE-47. *Environ. Toxicol. Pharmacol.* **2017**, *56*, 322–328. [CrossRef] [PubMed]
134. Cheung, E.C.; Ludwig, R.L.; Vousden, K.H. Mitochondrial localization of TIGAR under hypoxia stimulates HK2 and lowers ROS and cell death. *Proc. Natl. Acad. Sci. USA* **2012**, *109*, 20491–20496. [CrossRef] [PubMed]
135. Mahalingaiah, P.K.; Singh, K.P. Chronic oxidative stress increases growth and tumorigenic potential of MCF-7 breast cancer cells. *PLoS ONE* **2014**, *9*, e87371. [CrossRef] [PubMed]
136. Tal, M.C.; Sasai, M.; Lee, H.K.; Yordy, B.; Shadel, G.S.; Iwasaki, A. Absence of autophagy results in reactive oxygen species-dependent amplification of RLR signaling. *Proc. Natl. Acad. Sci. USA* **2009**, *106*, 770–775. [CrossRef]
137. Adolph, T.E.; Mayr, L.; Grabherr, F.; Tilg, H. Paneth cells and their antimicrobials in intestinal immunity. *Curr. Pharm. Des.* **2018**, *24*, 1121–1129. [CrossRef]
138. Kostic, A.D.; Xavier, R.J.; Gevers, D. The microbiome in inflammatory bowel disease: Current status and the future ahead. *Gastroenterology* **2014**, *146*, 1489–1499. [CrossRef]
139. Sun, J. VDR/vitamin D receptor regulates autophagic activity through ATG16L1. *Autophagy* **2016**, *12*, 1057–1058. [CrossRef]
140. Burger, E.; Araujo, A.; López-Yglesias, A.; Rajala, M.W.; Geng, L.; Levine, B.; Hooper, L.V.; Burstein, E.; Yarovinsky, F.; et al. Loss of Paneth cell autophagy causes acute susceptibility to Toxoplasma gondii-mediated Inflammation. *Cell Host Microbe* **2018**, *23*, 177–190. [CrossRef]
141. Garrett, W.S.; Gordon, J.I.; Glimcher, L.H. Homeostasis and inflammation in the intestine. *Cell* **2010**, *140*, 859–870. [CrossRef] [PubMed]
142. Kim, D.H.; Kim, S.; Lee, J.H.; Kim, J.H.; Che, X.; Ma, H.W.; Seo, D.H.; Kim, T.I.; Kim, W.H.; Kim, S.W.; et al. Lactobacillus acidophilus suppresses intestinal inflammation by inhibiting endoplasmic reticulum stress. *J. Gastroenterol. Hepatol.* **2018**. [CrossRef] [PubMed]
143. Ganji-Arjenaki, M.; Rafieian-Kopaei, M. Probiotics are a good choice in remission of inflammatory bowel diseases: A meta analysis and systematic review. *J. Cell. Physiol.* **2018**, *233*, 2091–2103. [CrossRef] [PubMed]
144. Verdugo, P. Goblet cells secretion and mucogenesis. *Annu. Rev. Physiol.* **1990**, *52*, 157–176. [CrossRef] [PubMed]
145. Specian, R.D.; Oliver, M.G. Functional biology of intestinal goblet cells. *Am. J. Physiol.* **1991**, *260*, C183–C193. [CrossRef] [PubMed]
146. Itoh, H.; Beck, P.L.; Inoue, N.; Xavier, R.; Podolsky, D.K. A paradoxical reduction in susceptibility to colonic injury upon targeted transgenic ablation of goblet cells. *J. Clin. Investig.* **1999**, *104*, 1539–1547. [CrossRef] [PubMed]
147. Swidsinski, A.; Loening-Baucke, V.; Herber, A. Mucosal flora in Crohn's disease and ulcerative colitis–An overview. *J. Physiol. Pharmacol.* **2009**, *60*, 61–71. [PubMed]
148. Patel, K.K.; Miyoshi, H.; Beatty, W.L.; Head, R.D.; Malvin, N.P.; Cadwell, K.; Guan, J.L.; Saitoh, T.; Akira, S.; Seglen, P.O.; et al. Autophagy proteins control goblet cell function by potentiating reactive oxygen species production. *EMBO J.* **2013**, *32*, 3130–3144. [CrossRef]
149. Johansson, M.E.; Hansson, G.C. Is the intestinal goblet cell a major immune cell? *Cell Host Microbe* **2014**, *15*, 251–252. [CrossRef] [PubMed]

150. Wlodarska, M.; Thaiss, C.A.; Nowarski, R.; Henao-Mejia, J.; Zhang, J.P.; Brown, E.M.; Frankel, G.; Levy, M.; Katz, M.N.; Philbrick, W.M.; et al. NLRP6 inflammasome orchestrates the colonic host-microbial interface by regulating goblet cell mucus secretion. *Cell* **2014**, *156*, 1045–1059. [CrossRef] [PubMed]
151. Gagné-Sansfaçon, J.; Allaire, J.M.; Jones, C.; Boudreau, F.; Perreault, N. Loss of Sonic hedgehog leads to alterations in intestinal secretory cell maturation and autophagy. *PLoS ONE* **2014**, *9*, e98751. [CrossRef] [PubMed]
152. Wang, S.; Li, Q.; Zang, Y.; Zhao, Y.; Liu, N.; Wang, Y.; Xu, X.; Liu, L.; Mei, Q. Apple Polysaccharide inhibits microbial dysbiosis and chronic inflammation and modulates gut permeability in HFD-fed rats. *Int. J. Biol. Macromol.* **2017**, *99*, 282–292. [CrossRef] [PubMed]
153. El-Khider, F.; McDonald, C. Links of Autophagy Dysfunction to Inflammatory Bowel Disease Onset. *Dig. Dis.* **2016**, *34*, 27–34. [CrossRef] [PubMed]
154. Ke, P.; Shao, B.Z.; Xu, Z.Q.; Chen, X.W.; Liu, C. Intestinal Autophagy and Its Pharmacological Control in Inflammatory Bowel Disease. *Front. Immunol.* **2017**, *7*, 695. [CrossRef] [PubMed]

11

The Connexin Mimetic Peptide Gap27 and Cx43-Knockdown Reveal Differential Roles for Connexin43 in Wound Closure Events in Skin Model Systems

Chrysovalantou Faniku [1], Erin O'Shaughnessy [1], Claire Lorraine [1], Scott R. Johnstone [1,2,3], Annette Graham [1], Sebastian Greenhough [1,†] and Patricia E. M. Martin [1,*]

1 Department of Life Sciences, School of Health and Life Sciences, Glasgow Caledonian University, Glasgow G4 0BA, UK; Chrysovalantou.Faniku@gcu.ac.uk (C.F.); Erin.OShaughnessy@gcu.ac.uk (E.O.); clairelorraine@hotmail.co.uk (C.L.); srj6n@eservices.virginia.edu (S.R.J.); ann.graham@gcu.ac.uk (A.G.); S.Greenhough@beatson.gla.ac.uk (S.G.)

2 Robert M. Berne Cardiovascular Research Center, University of Virginia School of Medicine, P.O. Box 801394, Charlottesville, VA 22908, USA

3 Institute of Cardiovascular and Medical Sciences, College of Medical, Veterinary and Life Sciences, University of Glasgow, Glasgow G12 8TT, UK

* Correspondence: patricia.martin@gcu.ac.uk

† Current Address: Cancer Research UK Beatson Institute, Garscube Estate, Switchback Road, Bearsden, Glasgow G61 1BD, UK

Abstract: In the epidermis, remodelling of Connexin43 is a key event in wound closure. However, controversy between the role of connexin channel and non-channel functions exist. We compared the impact of SiRNA targeted to Connexin43 and the connexin mimetic peptide Gap27 on scrape wound closure rates and hemichannel signalling in adult keratinocytes (AK) and fibroblasts sourced from juvenile foreskin (JFF), human neonatal fibroblasts (HNDF) and adult dermal tissue (ADF). The impact of these agents, following 24 h exposure, on *GJA1* (encoding Connexin43), *Ki67* and *TGF-β1* gene expression, and Connexin43 and pSmad3 protein expression levels, were examined by qPCR and Western Blot respectively. In all cell types Gap27 (100 nM–100 μM) attenuated hemichannel activity. In AK and JFF cells, Gap27 (100 nM–100 μM) enhanced scrape wound closure rates by ~50% but did not influence movement in HNDF or ADF cells. In both JF and AK cells, exposure to Gap27 for 24 h reduced the level of Cx43 protein expression but did not affect the level in ADF and HNDF cells. Connexin43-SiRNA enhanced scrape wound closure in all the cell types under investigation. In HDNF and ADF, Connexin43-SiRNA enhanced cell proliferation rates, with enhanced proliferation also observed following exposure of HDNF to Gap27. By contrast, in JFF and AK cells no changes in proliferation occurred. In JFF cells, Connexin43-SiRNA enhanced *TGF-β1* levels and in JFF and ADF cells both Connexin43-SiRNA and Gap27 enhanced pSmad3 protein expression levels. We conclude that Connexin43 signalling plays an important role in cell migration in keratinocytes and foreskin derived fibroblasts, however, different pathways are evoked and in dermal derived adult and neonatal fibroblasts, inhibition of Connexin43 signalling plays a more significant role in regulating cell proliferation than cell migration.

Keywords: wound healing; connexin mimetic peptide; connexin hemichannel; cell migration; SiRNA

---

1. Introduction

Connexin43 (Cx43) is expressed in nearly every tissue in the body where it forms hemichannels and intercellular gap junctions and plays diverse roles in coordinating cellular activities [1].

The connexin mimetic peptide (CMP) Gap27, targeted to the SRPTEKTIFFI sequence (amino acids 204–214) on the second extracellular loop of Cx43 is a versatile inhibitor of connexin-mediated communication (CMC) in tissue networks [2–4]. Early investigations with these peptides by Evans, Griffiths and colleagues [5–8] led to advancement of understanding of the role of connexins in the vasculature and identification of heterocellular communication at the myoendothelial gap junction [9,10]. Other studies employing Gap27 in excitable tissue networks have identified the role of connexins in the coordination of cardiomyocyte activities and calcium wave propagation [11,12], at neuronal synapses and more recently in pathological processes such as epilepsy [13]. In non-excitable tissues, Gap27 blocks the passive exchange of small gap junction permeable dyes such as calcein AM and determined a role for intercellular communication during transendothelial migration [14,15].

Many of the "acute" studies using CMPs have provided evidence for connexin channel signalling in coordinating cellular activities [2]. However, connexins also have reported "non-channel" functions and controversy exists in longer term studies as to whether channel or non-channel activities play key roles in events such as cell adhesion and migration [16]. This is no less evident in the skin where dynamic changes in connexin expression occur during wound healing [17–19]. Antisense oligonucleotides targeted to Cx43 provided the first evidence that connexin based therapies could improve wound healing and resolve inflammation [18,20,21]. Gap27 and other connexin mimetic peptides targeted to the carboxyl terminal domain of Cx43 (such as αCT-1) also improved cell migration rates in 2D and 3D organotypic skin wound model systems [22–25]. In previous studies [22,23], we determined that while Gap27 enhanced migration rates in keratinocytes and fibroblasts isolated from juvenile foreskin discards it was less effective in fibroblasts isolated from adult dermal explants.

In the present work we compared the effect of Gap27 and SiRNA targeted to Cx43, on cell migration in adult keratinocytes (AK) and adult dermal (ADF), juvenile foreskin (JFF) and neonatal foreskin (HDNF) derived fibroblasts. Our findings provide new insights into the effects of Cx43 channel inhibition versus Cx43 gene expression on cell migration, and our results also show that the response of such behaviour varies between cell types (keratinocyte versus fibroblast) and between cells of the same type (skin fibroblasts) but of different tissue origins.

2. Results

2.1. The Impact of Gap27 on Cell Migration Rates in Juvenile Foreskin Fibroblasts

Previously we determined that Gap27 inhibits CMC and enhanced scrape wound closure in fibroblasts and keratinocytes derived from juvenile foreskin explants [22,24]. To further explore the effect of 100 μM Gap27 on cell motility, JFF cells were subject to time-lapse microscopy and images captured every 15 min over a 48 h migration period. The speed of cell movement in non-treated and Gap27 (100 μM) treated cells was analysed: Gap27 treated cells reached 50% scrape closure in approximately half the time taken by non-treated cells (Figure 1A).

Image trajectory analysis was performed to elucidate if the differences observed in JFF scrape closure ± Gap27 were due to variation in cell directionality or speed of movement. Graphical representation of the XY co-ordinate data obtained from tracking the movement of 18 individual cells for each set of JFF images (±100 μM Gap27) illustrated differences in cell migration between the control and peptide treated cells, most noticeably an increase in distance travelled by the Gap27 treated cells, compared to controls, into the scraped area. The data also suggest that the majority of peptide treated cells migrate in straighter lines towards the scraped area compared to controls which had a more lateral movement. Cell tracking data determined that Gap27 treatment in JFF cells significantly increased the average cell velocity over 48 h by 2.5 μm/h compared to controls; the average velocity was 0.23 ± 0.003 μm/min (13.8 μm/h) in control cells and 0.27 ± 0.004 μm/min (16.3 μm/h) in peptide treated cells (Figure 1B). To further explore these differences, data sets of the rate of cell movement at the leading edge (Figure 1C), 0–50 μm (Figure 1D) and 50–100 μm (Figure 1E) behind the wound edge were analysed. At the leading wound edge, the migration of control and peptide treated cells were comparable (Figure 1C). However, in cells located 0–50 μm behind the wound edge cell migration rates in Gap27 was faster, with the greatest difference in velocity occurring 50–100 μm behind the wound edge, where the Gap27 treated cells migrated at a rate of 0.273 ± 0.006 μm/min compared to the non-treated cells that migrated at rates of 0.214 ± 0.004 μm/min (Figure 1D,E). These data indicate that during scrape wound closure in JFF cell monolayers, cell velocity is greater in wound edge cells compared to cells behind the wound edge. However, Gap27 treatment enhances the scrape wound closure in JFF cell monolayers in vitro by increasing cell velocity in cells behind the wound edge.

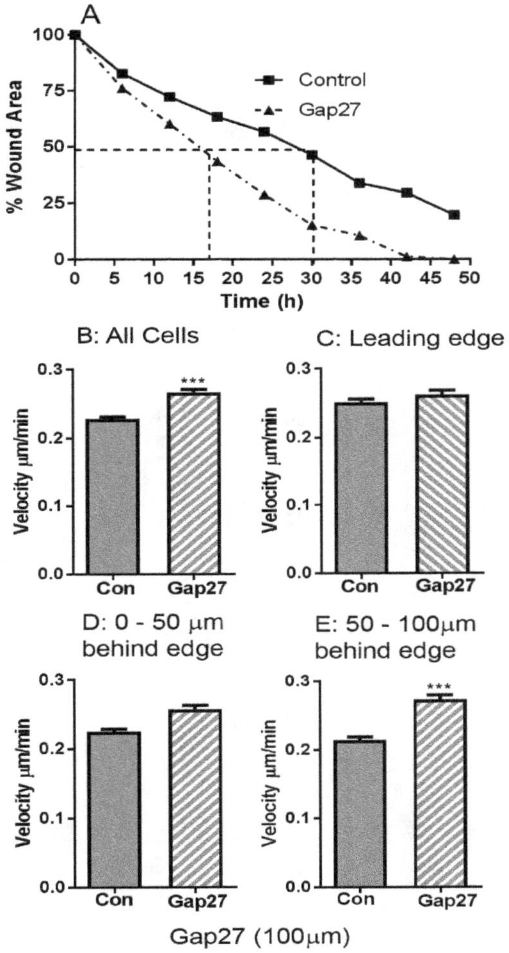

Figure 1. Gap27 (100 μM) influences the speed of Juvenile Foreskin Fibroblasts (JFF) cell migration. (**A**) time-lapse migration data of JFF cells; (**B**) Average cell velocity of JFF cells; (**C**) Cell velocity of JFF cells at the leading edge of the scrape wound; (**D**) Cell velocity of JFF cells 0–50 μm behind the wound edge; (**E**) Cell velocity of JFF cells 50–100 μm behind the wound edge. $n = 18$ cells were tracked in total with 6 cells from each specific area. *** $p < 0.005$.

2.2. *Impact of Gap27 and SiRNA Targeted to Cx43 on Cell Migration in Skin Model Systems*

While both CMPs and antisense Cx43 knockdown strategies are widely accepted to enhance wound closure rates [20,22,26], a direct comparison of their effects on cell migration events has not been reported. We thus explored the impact of Gap27 and SiRNA targeted to Cx43 on scrape wound closure rates in keratinocytes and fibroblasts isolated from adult skin biopsies and compared this to cells derived from juvenile foreskin and neonatal human fibroblasts. Initially a dose response of Gap27 determined that the peptide effectively enhanced scrape wound closure rates in primary adult keratinocytes at 100 nM–100 μM, but was without effect at lower doses (Figure 2A). In these AK cells, SiRNA targeted to Cx43 significantly enhanced the rate of scrape wound closure (Figure 2B). In JFF cells, 100 nM Gap27 and SiRNA targeted to Cx43 significantly enhanced the rate of scrape wound closure with 50% closure rates more than two times faster than non-treated samples (Figure 2C). Multiple studies performed in adult fibroblasts demonstrated that 100 nM–100 μM Gap27 had limited impact on cell migration responses (Figure 2D); by contrast, significant increase in 50% closure rates occurred in adult fibroblasts transfected with SiRNA targeted to Cx43, compared with the SiRNA control (Figure 2D).

To further compare the efficacy of Gap27 on fibroblast cell migration events, scrape wound assays were also performed using commercially sourced human neonatal dermal fibroblasts. Treatment with Gap27 was ineffective in enhancing migration responses at concentrations of 100 nM or 100 μM (Figure 2E,F). By contrast, inhibition of Cx43 expression by transfecting the cells with SiRNA targeted to Cx43 significantly improved cell migration rates suggesting a "non-channel" role for Cx43 in migration of these neonatal fibroblasts (Figure 2E). We also explored the migration responses of HNDF cells on various extracellular matrix components in the presence and absence of 100 μM Gap27. Although the cells migrated slightly faster on both fibronectin and collagen matrices, Gap27 still did not enhance cell migration rates [27].

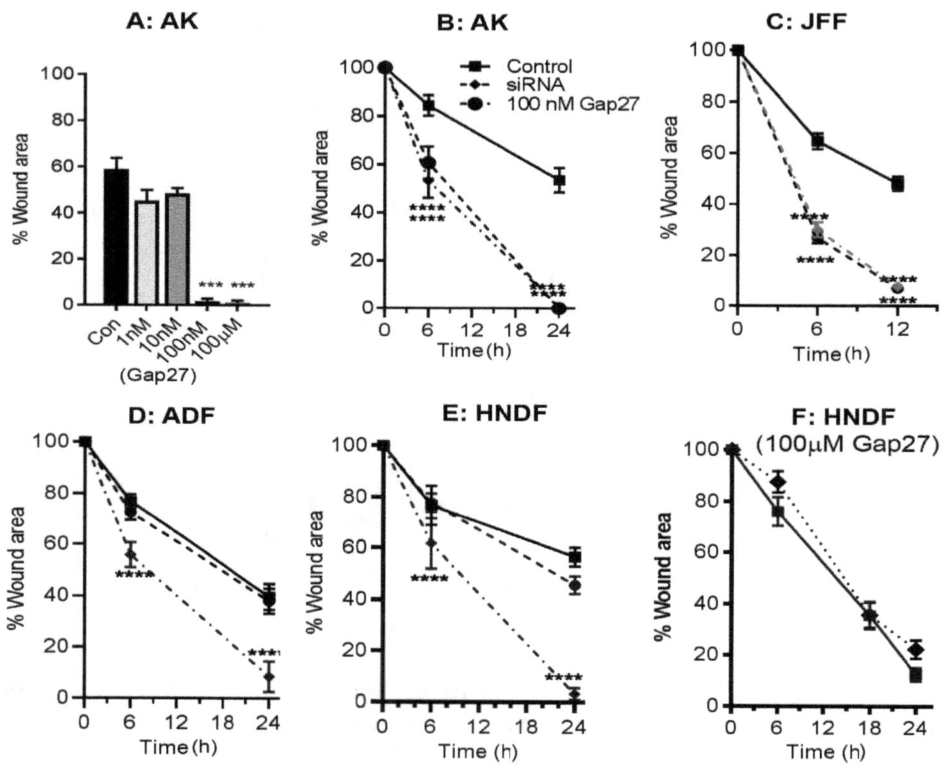

Figure 2. Gap27 and SiRNA targeted to Cx43 have differential effects on scrape wound closure rates in skin cells. Dose response of Gap27 in AK cells (**A**); SiRNA targeted to Cx43 and 100 nM Gap27 enhance scrape wound closure in AK (**B**) and JFF cells (**C**); Gap27 does not enhance cell migration rates in ADF or HNDF cells (**D**–**F**). $n = 3$, ** $p < 0.01$; *** $p < 0.005$.

2.3. Gap27 Attenuates Hemichannel Signalling at Lower Doses than Gap Junction Coupling

In previous studies, microinjection analysis with Alexa 488 determined that Gap27 effectively inhibits gap junction coupling at concentrations of 50 μM in keratinocytes and HeLa43 cells [23,24]. We also previously reported that Gap27 inhibits ATP release in both keratinocytes and fibroblasts isolated from juvenile foreskin tissue discards at concentrations of 100 μM [22,23,28]. In view of the stark contrast in the impact of Gap27 on cell migration rates between the different cell types, we further explored the ability of Gap27 to attenuate hemichannel activity. In all the cell types, Gap27 effectively inhibited ATP release in a dose responsive manner, effective at 10–100 μM concentrations (Figure 3A–D). This data further suggests that in the ADF and HNDF, hemichannel signalling events are unlikely to be involved in controlling cell migration.

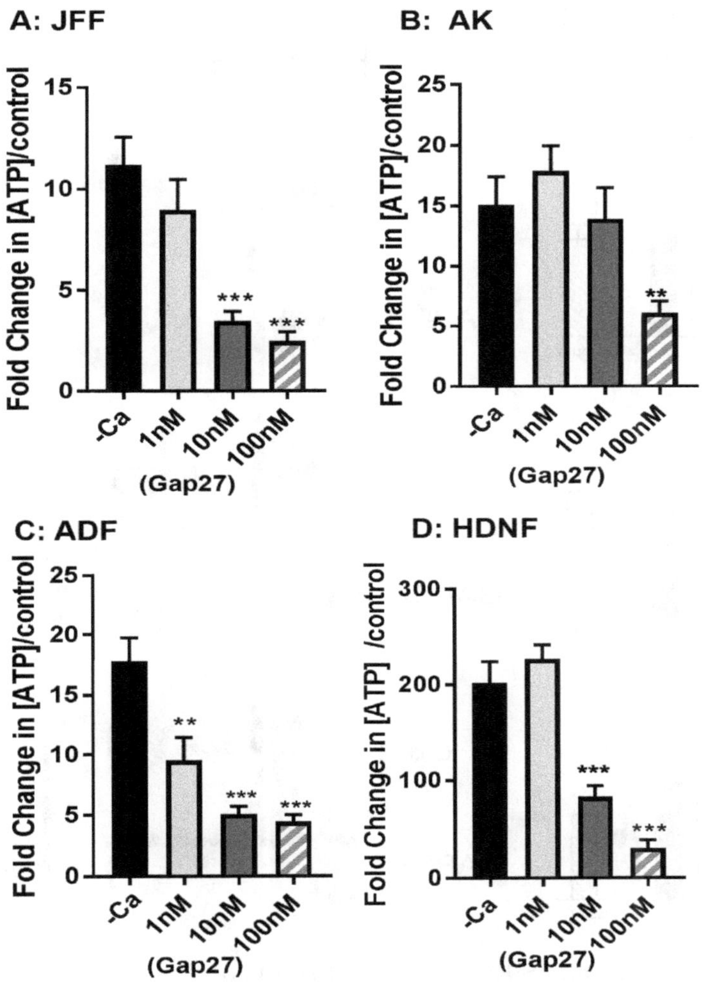

Figure 3. Gap27 inhibits hemichannel signalling. JFF cells (**A**); Keratinocytes (**B**); ADF (**C**) and HNDF (**D**) cells were exposed to a dose response of Gap27 and ATP release assays performed following calcium deprivation. Data are presented at the Fold change in ATP release over control cells that were not subject to calcium challenge. $n = 3$, *** $p < 0.005$, ** $p < 0.01$.

2.4. The Impact of Gap27 and SiRNA Targeted to Cx43 on Gene and Protein Expression Profiles in Skin Model Systems

At the end point of the cell migration assays, RNA and protein were extracted and subject to qPCR and Western blot analysis to determine any significant changes in gene and or protein expression profiles.

SiRNA targeted to Cx43 reduced the level of *Cx43* gene and protein expression by >50% in JFF, AK, ADF and HNDF cells (Figure 4A–D). Exposure to 100 nM Gap27 for up to 24 h reduced *Cx43* gene expression levels in JFF cells but had limited impact on *Cx43* gene expression levels in the other cell types (Figure 4A–D (panel 1)). In ADF and HNDF cells, 100 nM Gap27 did not influence the level of Cx43 protein expression (Figure 4C,D (panels 2 and 3)). However, in JFF cells exposure to 100 nM Gap27 for 24 h caused a >2-fold reduction in the level of Cx43 protein expression and a similar trend, although not as pronounced, was observed in AK cells (Figure 4A,B (panels 2 and 3)).

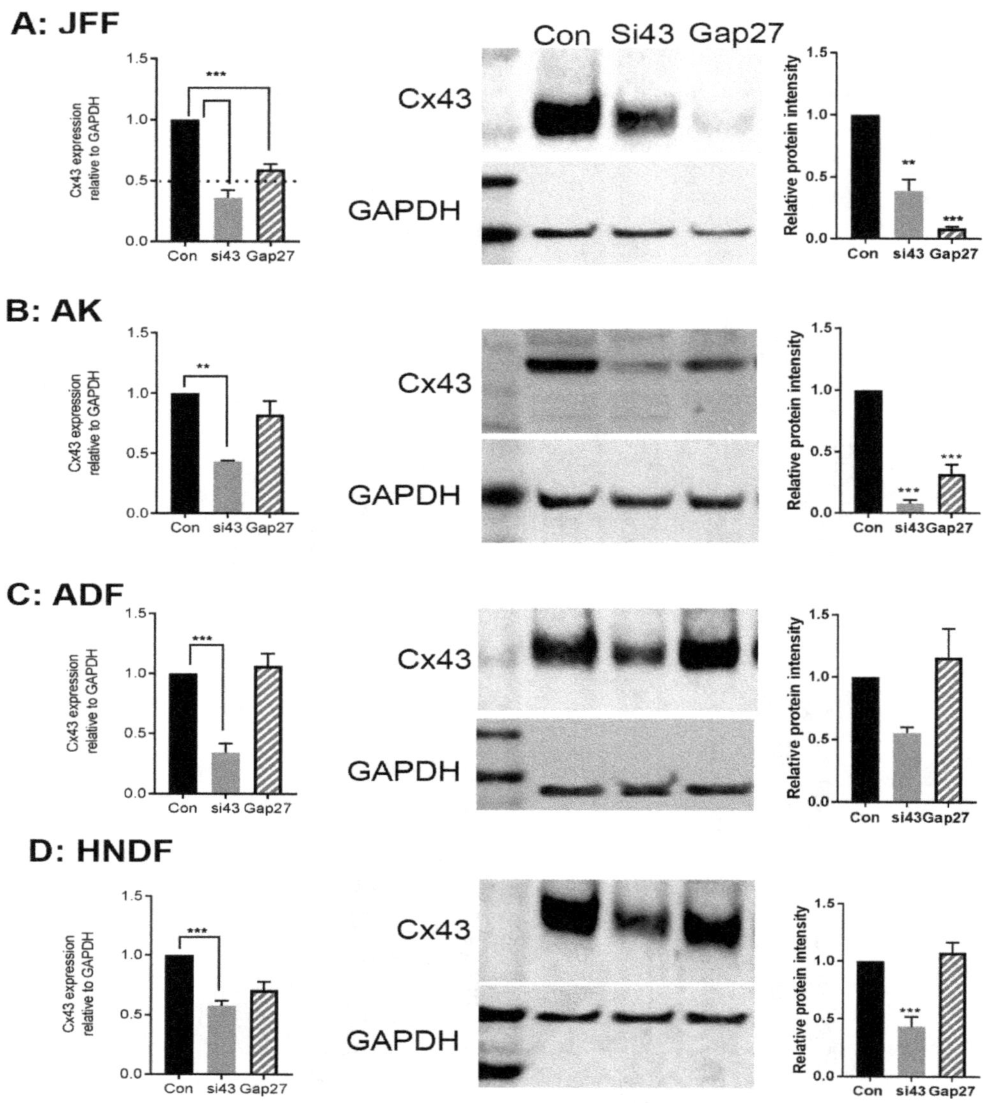

Figure 4. The impact of Gap27 and SiRNA targeted to Cx43 on gene expression. At the end of scrape wound closure assays, RNA and protein was harvested from cells and subject to real time PCR or Western blot analysis to determine levels of Cx43 expression. JFF (**A**); AK (**B**); AF (**C**) and HNDF (**D**). Panel 1 represents changes in gene expression, Panel 2 represents a typical Western blot, Panel 3 represents densitometric analysis of three Western blots. $n = 3$, *** $p < 0.005$, ** $p < 0.01$ a threshold of two fold increase or decrease in expression was considered significant.

2.5. The Impact of Gap27 and SiRNA Targeted to Cx43 on Cell Proliferation, TGF-β1 and SMAD3 Signalling Pathways

To determine if the differences observed in cell migration responses between the various cell groups were related to changes in cell proliferation, the level of *Ki67* gene expression in each of the cell types and treatment groups was determined. In JFF and AK cells, none of the treatments evoked a greater than two-fold increase in the level of *Ki67* gene expression (Figure 5A, AK and JFF panels). By contrast, in ADF cells a 10-fold increase in *Ki67* gene expression was observed in cells exposed to SiRNA targeted to Cx43 but not in those exposed to Gap27 (Figure 5A, ADF panel). In HNDF cells, proliferation was dramatically enhanced in all treatment groups (5-10 fold) compared to non-treated cells (Figure 5A, HNDF panel).

Transforming growth factor β1 (TGF-β1) is a major transcription factor regulating cell signalling events involved in migration. The level of *TGF-β1* gene expression was enhanced ~3–4 fold in JFF cells following knockdown of *Cx43* gene expression and following treatment with 100 nM Gap27 for 24 h (Figure 5B, JFF panel). By contrast, in AK, AF and HNDF cells, Gap27 and SiRNA targeted to Cx43 had limited impact on the level of *TGF-β1* gene expression levels (Figure 5B) at the 24 h time point.

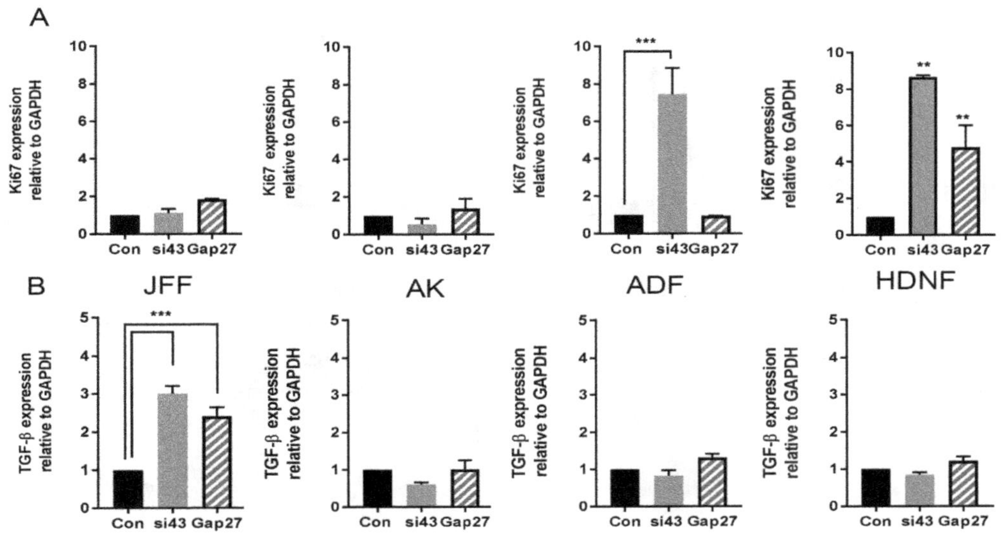

Figure 5. The impact of Gap27 and SiRNA targeted to Cx43 on *Ki67* and *TGF-β1* gene expression. At the end of scrape wound closure assays RNA was harvested from cells and subject to real time PCR analysis to determine changes in gene expression of (**A**) *Ki67* and (**B**) *TGF-β1* $n = 3$, *** $p < 0.005$, ** $p < 0.01$ a threshold of two fold increase or decrease in gene expression was considered significant.

Finally, previous reports identified that phosphorylation of Smad3 is associated with exposure of mucosal derived fibroblasts to Gap27 [29]. Probing the Western blots with an antibody targeting pSmad3 identified that in JFF and ADF cells exposure to SiRNA targeted to Cx43 and 100 nM Gap27 for 24 h enhanced the level of pSmad3 expression (Figure 6A,C). By contrast, in HNDF and AK cells the level remained constant (Figure 6B,D), further suggesting differential signalling pathways are triggered in different compartments of the skin following remodelling of Cx43.

A summary of the combined data is presented in Table 1.

Table 1. Summary of the effect of 100 nM Gap27 (Gap27) and Cx43-SiRNA (SiRNA) on cellular events related to wound closure in JFF, AK, ADF and HDNF cells. Hemichannel activity was monitored following 90 min exposure to peptide and 15 min challenge with Calcium free media. All other assays were recorded 24 h post scrape wounding in the presence or absence of 100 nM Gap27 or Cx43-SiRNA. $n = 3$ in all cases. ND: not determined; NE: no effect; ↑ enhanced effect; ↓ inhibitory effect. For details of experimental design and statistics see text and figures.

Cell Type	Treatment	HC	Migration	Cx43 Protein	Proliferation	TGF-β1	pSmad3
JFF	SiRNA	ND	↑	↓	NE	↑	↑
	Gap27	↓	↑	↓	NE	↑	↑
AK	SiRNA	ND	↑	↓	NE	NE	NE
	Gap27	↓	↑	↓	NE	NE	NE
ADF	SiRNA	ND	↑	↓	↑	↑	↑
	Gap27	↓	NE	NE	NE	NE	↑
HDNF	SiRNA	ND	↑	↓	↑	NE	NE
	Gap27	↓	NE	NE	↑	NE	NE

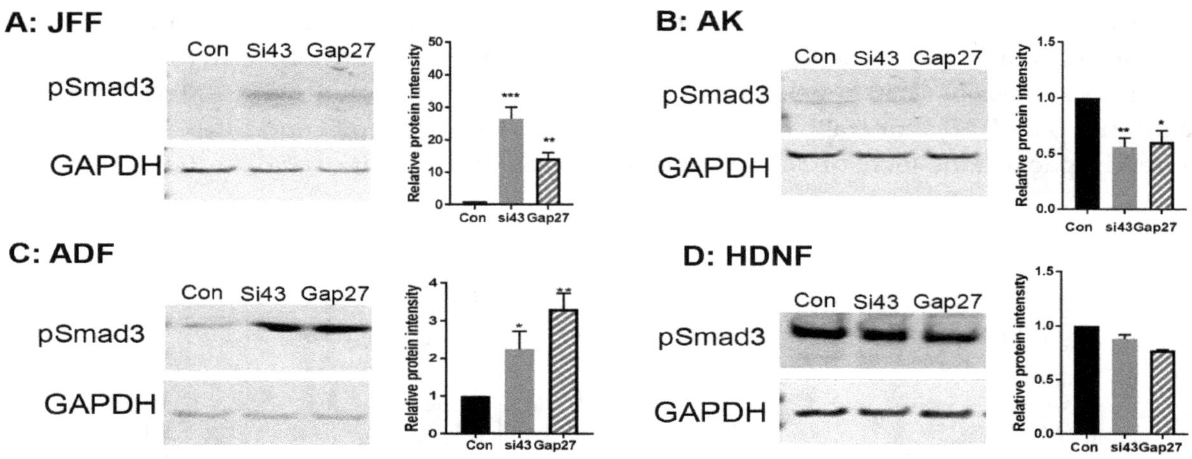

Figure 6. The impact of Gap27 and SiRNA targeted to Cx43 on pSmad3 expression. At the end of scrape, wound closure assays protein was harvested from cells and subject to Western blot analysis. Blots were probed with an antibody targeted to pSmad3 and GAPDH. Representative blots are presented for each cell type JFF (**A**); AK (**B**); AF (**C**) and HNDF (**D**) (panel 1). Panel 2 represents densitometric analysis of triplicate blots and relative pSmad3 protein levels compared to GAPDH. $n = 3$, *** $p < 0.005$, ** $p < 0.01$; * $p < 0.5$.

3. Discussion

In the present study we compared the effect of Gap27 and SiRNA targeted to Cx43 on scrape wound closure rates in fibroblasts derived from neonatal, juvenile foreskin and adult dermal explants and matched adult keratinocytes. Both of these reagents enhanced scrape wound closure in the JFF cells and adult keratinocytes with Gap27 enhancing cell migration rates at concentrations of 100 nM, reflecting the dose of peptide that inhibited hemichannel signalling and supporting the concept that ATP release via hemichannels is required for keratinocyte galvanotaxis [30]. By contrast, in the AF and HNDF cells, SiRNA targeted to Cx43 enhanced scrape wound closure, but treatment with Gap27 was without effect, extending studies where we reported limited effects of Gap27 on adult fibroblast migration rates [22,23]. Profound differences in cell migration, proliferation and the TGF-β1/pSmad3 signalling axis occurred between the cells isolated from different skin compartments. The data provides new insights into the controversy surrounding Cx43 channel versus non-channel functions in cell migration and wound repair responses [16] and suggests that inhibition of hemichannel signalling alone is insufficient to modify cell migration events in adult dermal fibroblasts.

Within epithelial tissues, including the skin and cornea, it is widely accepted that downregulation of Cx43 is favourable to wound closure, as reported in the skin of connexin-deficient mice [19] and by the development of Cx43 anti-sense oligonucleotides, that have proven effective in rat models and in human clinical trials [18,26,31,32]. Other studies by Gourdie and colleagues used a peptide targeting the carboxyl tail of Cx43 and its binding site with the PDZ domain to improve wound healing, resolve inflammation and reduce scarring in rat models and recently in human clinical trials [33–35]. Studies using Pep5, based on the Gap27 sequence, have shown remarkable effects on tissue repair and inflammation in the retina, cornea and spinal cord [36–38]. Recent studies using Gap27 have also shown that this peptide is effective in improving rabbit corneal wound healing [39] and in primary human gingival fibroblasts, isolated from donors aged 26–48 years of age [29]. A further peptide TAT-Gap19, has also recently been reported to enhance scrape wound closure of human gingival fibroblasts [40]. TAT-Gap19, targeted to the intracellular loop of Cx43, was designed as a cell permeant peptide and has been extensively used to characterise interactions between the intracellular loop of Cx43 and the carboxy terminal tail [41,42]. This peptide effectively blocks hemichannel activity but has no effect on gap junction coupling, in contrast to Gap27 which blocks all forms of connexin mediated communication. Thus, inhibiting *Cx43* gene expression and blocking channel function both have a positive influence on wound closure events; however, comparisons of the mechanisms underlying the modes of action of these different means of remodelling Cx43 remains unresolved.

In the present study we have identified profound differences in wound healing events in skin cells isolated from different sources, and between adult epidermal and stromal derived fibroblasts, which relate to whether Cx43 channel function or gene expression is regulated.

In the case of JFF cells, derived from juvenile foreskin discards (a thin layer of tissue) and in adult keratinocytes, both Gap27 and SiRNA targeted to Cx43 enhanced scrape wound closure. Further, in both of these cell types at the end point of the migration time course, neither knockdown of Cx43 expression or inhibition of channel function by Gap27 had any effect on cell proliferation as monitored by *Ki67* gene expression. This re-enforces our previous findings where irradiated juvenile fibroblasts were used and Gap27 effectively enhanced wound closure [22]. Hence in JFF cells and keratinocytes proliferation factors are not involved in the enhanced cell migration response, suggesting hemichannel signalling plays an important role in co-ordinating cellular responses [30,40].

By contrast, in ADF and HNDF while SiRNA targeted to Cx43 accelerated the rates of scrape wound closure, exposure to Gap27 had a limited effect on cell migration rates. In AF cells, Gap27 did not influence the gene expression of *Ki67* but decreasing *Cx43* gene expression enhanced cell proliferation. In the HNDF cells, exposure to Gap27 and to SiRNA targeted to Cx43 enhanced cell proliferation, but only SiRNA targeted to Cx43 enhanced cell migration rates. It is also noteworthy that at the end point of the migration assays, while SiRNA targeted to Cx43 reduced Cx43 gene and protein expression in all cell types by >50% exposure to Gap27 had no effect on Cx43 protein levels in AF cells. By contrast, in the JFF and AK cells Gap27 reduced the level of Cx43 protein expression by ~50%, however it had a limited effect on *Cx43* gene expression, suggesting Cx43 changes were post-transcriptional. A similar effect was also observed in adult human gingival fibroblasts where Gap27 also enhanced wound closure rates [29]. Studies using mouse NIH3T3 fibroblasts also determined that Gap27 reduced Cx43 protein expression in line with our observations in JFF cells [43]. Studies in our lab also determined that Gap27 improved cell migration rates in primary neonatal mouse fibroblasts [27] and keratinocytes [44]. Taken together, this data suggests that in human adult dermal fibroblasts and neonatal fibroblasts, non-channel functions of Cx43 may be more important than acute hemichannel signalling in regulating cell migratory behaviour.

Previously, we identified changes in expression of a panel of genes associated with extracellular matrix (ECM) deposition in JFF cells following exposure to Gap27, including metalloproteinase 9 (MMP-9) and connective tissue growth factor (CTGF) [23]. Several other reports have indicated a link between altered Cx43 expression and ECM regulation, including in fibroblasts isolated from a patient harbouring a non-functional Cx43 mutation associated with the Cx-channelopathy oculodentodigital dysplasia [45]. Modifying Cx43 expression or function by antisense oligonucleotides and peptide αCTI have also been associated with alterations in ECM deposition [20,33]. Further studies by Tarzemany et al. systematically reviewed the impact of Gap27 and more recently TAT-Gap19 on gene expression and cell signalling pathways involved in wound closure events in human adult gingival fibroblasts [29,40]. Both peptides effectively enhanced wound closure rates and gene array analysis after 24 h indicated changes in expression of a panel of genes related to ECM deposition including a number of MMP proteins and CTGF, in agreement with our previous studies on JFF cells [23].

The TGF-β signalling pathway is important in controlling cell migration events, and a number of studies have suggested links between TGF-β1 and Cx43 expression in wound healing scenarios [20,46]. Treatment with either Gap27 or SiRNA targeted to Cx43 enhanced the gene expression of *TGF-β1* in JFF cells, but had little impact following 24 h exposure to these reagents in the adult keratinocytes and fibroblasts. However, it remains possible that expression of *TGF-β1* is transiently induced at earlier time points, since TGF-β1 has been reported to stimulate chemotactic migration of human fibroblasts [47].

The TGF-β/Smad3 signalling axis plays an important role in cell migration events, and has been linked with Cx43 expression. In line with this in both JFF and ADF cells, levels of pSmad3 were increased following 24 h exposure to Gap27 and SiRNA targeted to Cx43. A profound increase in pSmad3 was also reported in gingival fibroblasts exposed to Gap27 for 24 h [29]. Smad3 and the carboxyl terminal tail of Cx43 both compete for a similar 'microtubule binding domain' [48]. Thus, alteration in Cx43 expression levels or function may modify the interaction. Upon translocation to the nucleus, Smad3 is phosphorylated to pSmad3 and exerts transcriptional control on a range of genes involved in regulation of inflammation, cell proliferation and re-epithelisation in both positive and negative tissue-specific ways. Given the diverse pathways that pSmad3 can regulate, it is highly likely that in the ADF cells, where Gap27 did not influence cell migration, other key cellular events may be affected. Although no evidence of induction of pSmad3 expression was observed in the keratinocytes, a host of other signalling pathways including the ERK1/2 and JNK pathways may be influenced [49] and this is subject to further investigation. In the present studies, the influence of modulation of Cx43 was assessed in monocultures. In the future it will be important to exploit our 3D organotypic models as it is well established that keratinocytes and fibroblasts can influence responses of adjacent cells as part of a coordinated tissue event [50].

4. Materials and Methods

4.1. Cell Culture

Primary juvenile human dermal fibroblasts (JFF cells) were derived from paediatric foreskins discarded at surgery following informed consent with ethical approval by Yorkhill Hospital Trust Research Ethics Committee, Glasgow, or were kindly gifted by Prof J Brandner, University Hamburg, with their use approved by the ethics committee of the Aerztekammer Hamburg (060900) as previously described [22]. Human neonatal dermal fibroblasts (HNDF) were sourced from Invitrogen (Cat No.: C0045C, Paisley, UK) and human adult dermal fibroblasts (AF) and keratinocytes (AK) were obtained from the GCU Skin Research Tissue Bank, which has NHS and GCU research ethical approval (NHS REC Ref 16/ES/0069). Fibroblasts and keratinocytes were isolated from tissue explants and cultured as previously described [22,24]. All cells were maintained at 37 °C, 5% CO_2. Monolayers of all fibroblasts were maintained in DMEM (Lonza, Wokingham, UK) supplemented with 10% (v/v) foetal calf serum, 2 mM glutamine, 50 Units/mL penicillin/streptomycin (Lonza, Wokingham, UK), hereafter termed "complete" DMEM (cDMEM). Keratinocytes were maintained in EPILIFE medium as previously described [51] (Thermo Fisher, Paisley, UK). Cells were seeded at appropriate densities on 24-well plates for ATP assays (~0.5×10^5 per well) or 6-well plates (~1×10^6 cells per well) for all other assays.

4.2. Inhibition of Connexin Mediated Communication

For the purpose of this study, Gap27 (MW 1305) (Zealand Pharma, Glostrop, Denmark) was used in aqueous solution at doses ranging from 1–100 μM for 15 min–48 h depending on experimental requirements. The peptide and media were replaced at 8 h intervals.

4.3. Knockdown of Cx43 Expression by siRNA

SiRNA duplex sequences targeted to Cx43 (TriFECTa®RNAi Kit from Integrated DNA Technologies (Tyne & Wear, UK)) along with a fluorescently-labelled scrambled transfection control duplex: TYE 563™ was used to knockdown Cx43 expression. SiRNA transfection was carried out using Lipofectamine 3000 transfection reagent (Invitrogen, Paisley, UK). Transfection reagents and siRNAs were combined and incubated for 20 min at room temperature for complex formation. Cells were transfected with a final concentration of 5 nM siRNA diluted in 1.5 mL of EPILIFE medium for primary keratinocytes and serum free DMEM (SFM) for fibroblasts. Twenty hours post transfection scrape wound assays were performed and cells subsequently harvested for endpoint analysis as described below. Transfection efficiency of control SiRNA, determined by fluorescent microscopy analysis of the scrambled SiRNA control was ~90% for all cell types.

4.4. Hemichannel Functionality Assays

Hemichannel activity was assessed by ATP release assays with minor modifications to that previously described [51]. Briefly, cells were seeded on 24-well plates and grown to ~80% confluency overnight. Cells were then washed three times in SFM and incubated in SFM for 1 h prior to exposure to Gap27 for 90 min. Following this, one half of the plate was challenged with Ca^{2+} and Mg^{2+} free PBS in the presence or absence of Gap27 for 15 min. Supernatants were collected and microcentrifuged at 10,000 rpm for 5 min prior to addition of 25 μL of supernatant to a well of an opaque-walled Nunc 96 well plate containing 25 μL ATP assay mix diluted 1:10 with ATP dilution buffer (Sigma-Aldrich, Gillingham, UK). ATP standards (25 μL) 0–10 nM diluted in SFM, and in PBS, were also added in duplicate. Luminescence was measured in relative luminescence units (RLU) using the Fluostar Optima plate reader (BMG Labtech, Aylesbury, UK). Experiments were performed in triplicate per treatment group, and each experiment was carried out a minimum of three times (n = 3). Data is represented as the fold change in ATP released between control and peptide treated wells.

4.5. Scrape Wound Assays and Time-Lapse Microscopic Analysis of Cell Migration

Cells were pre-exposed to peptide or SFM for 90 min, or were transfected with SiRNA targeting Cx43 for 20 h, prior to introducing a scrape wound to confluent cell monolayers using a sterile 100 μL pipette tip. Cell migration was monitored by taking triplicate images of wound area 0, 6, 12 and 24 h post scraping on a CMEX-3200 camera [51]. The scrape wound area was measured at each time point using Image J software. Values were normalised by comparing with the corresponding initial wound size. For time-lapse microscopy analysis, images were recorded on a Zeiss Axiovert 100 microscope (Cambridge, UK) linked up to a CCD camera (Nikon Eclipse TS10, Kingston Upon Thames, UK). Image capture was controlled by AQMsoftware (Kinetic Imaging Ltd., Nottingham, UK). Images were captured every 15 min for up to 48 h [52]. The movement of 18 individual cells for each set of JFF time-lapse images in the presence or absence of 100 μM Gap27, were tracked using Image J software tracking plug-in. The size of each image was 512 × 512 pixels with a diameter of ~500 μm, therefore, at ×100 magnification each pixel represented approximately 1 μm. This value was used as the x/y calibration value with a time interval value of 15 min. Cells were tracked by clicking on the leading edge of a cell on sequential images representing every 15 min over the 48 h period. Six cells were randomly chosen from each of (1) wound edge; (2) 0–50 μm from the wound edge and (3) 50–100 μm from the wound edge. The data output produced by Image J software included the XY co-ordinates together with distance and velocity values. The XY co-ordinates were plotted on a graph using Excel software, providing an individual track for each cell, enabling visualisation of cell movement over 48 h.

4.6. RNA Extraction and Real Time PCR

The Bioline ISOLATE RNA Kit (Bioline, London, UK) was used according to manufacturer's instructions to extract RNA from cell monolayers (usually 2 wells for a 6 well plate). RNA concentrations were determined using a Nanodrop ND-100 at 260/280 nm. cDNA was prepared from the RNA samples using cDNA synthesis kit from Primerdesign and real-time PCR was performed using Primerdesign Master Mix kit (Primer Design, Chandlers Ford, UK). Primers amplifying human *Cx43*, human *Ki67*, human *TGF-β1* and the house keeping gene *GAPDH* were purchased from IDT (Tyne & Wear, UK) (Table S1). All reactions were performed in an ABI 7500 FA Real-Time PCR system (Applied Biosystems, Warrington, UK). The mRNA expression level for each gene was determined using the ΔC_t method and each sample was run in triplicate.

The CT value obtained for the target gene in all samples was first normalised with the CT value obtained for the housekeeping gene. The resulting change in CT (ΔC_t) calculated for test samples was then normalised with the ΔC_t calculated for the control sample, giving a $\Delta\Delta C_t$ value. The gene expression ratio was calculated using $2^{-\Delta\Delta Ct}$, providing a fold increase or decrease in gene expression compared to the control sample. Gene fold changes $\geq\pm2$ were considered significant.

4.7. Western Blot Analysis

Protein was harvested from cells in 100 µL lysis buffer (1% (*v*/*v*) SDS, 30 mM Na_3VO_4, 1 µM DTT, protease inhibitor cocktail (Sigma-Aldrich) and phenylmethanosulfonylfluoride (PMSF)) prepared in 1xPBS as previously described [52].

Equivalent amounts of protein (30–80 µg) were mixed with 5 µL loading buffer (NuPAGE® LDS Sample Buffer (4X)) and the volume adjusted to 20 µL with lysis buffer. Samples were mixed for 15 min at 20 rpm followed by brief centrifugation and separated by 4–12% sodium dodecyl sulphate polyacrylamide gel electrophoresis (SDS-PAGE) (NuPAGE® Novex® Bis-Tris Mini Gels; Thermo Fisher) followed by electrophoretic transfer to a nitrocellulose membrane using an I-Blot transfer system (Invitrogen) following manufacturer's instructions. Transfer efficiency was determined by staining the blots with Ponceau S (0.1% (*w*/*v*) in 5% acetic acid) (Sigma-Aldrich) for 15 s, prior to rinsing in distilled water and probing for relevant protein expression using appropriate primary antibodies as previously described [52]. Membranes were probed with primary antibodies to detect Cx43 (Rivedal polylclonal antibody 1:2000 dilution, kindly gifted by Edward Leithe [53]), GAPDH (mouse monoclonal antibody, Santa Cruz (LOCATION) (1:5000 dilution)) and pSmad3 (rabbit polyclonal antibody Abcam (Cambridge, UK) (1:2000 dilution)) expression as appropriate. Secondary antibodies were IRDye® 800CW goat anti-rabbit IgG or IRDye® 680CW goat anti-mouse IgG (Licor 1:15,000 dilution) as appropriate. Blots were developed by exposing the image for a period of 15 s to 5 min according to the intensity of the signal using an Odyssey FC Dual Mode Licor imaging system (LI-COR Biosceinces UK Ltd, Lincoln, UK). Densitometric values were quantified using the Odyssey software. To enable normalisation of the blots and comparison of the effect of different treatments on protein expression, the intensity of the protein bands were compared to the house keeping protein.

4.8. Statistical Analysis

Experiments were performed in triplicate per setting and on three separate occasions with at least 2 different patient samples. Results were compiled in GraphPad Prism software (La Jolla, San Diego, CA, USA) and all data is expressed as mean ± SEM unless otherwise stated. Statistical tests were performed on the data using Student's unpaired *t*-test or one-way ANOVA and Dunnett's post-test as appropriate, with statistical significance inferred at $p < 0.05$.

5. Conclusions

In conclusion, we provide an in-depth study on the comparative effects of Gap27 with a Cx43-SiRNA knockdown approach to improve wound healing and identify significant differences in the cell signalling pathways that are controlled by Cx43 in fibroblasts and keratinocytes. Further work is now warranted to define the molecular pathways by which Cx43 exerts its effects in the skin which will aide in identifying new therapeutic strategies and applications for specific types of wounds.

Acknowledgments: We thank Professor Joanna Brandner, University of Hamburg for the supply of the Juvenile Foreskin Fibroblasts used in the latter part of this project. Chrysovalantou Faniku and Claire Lorraine were funded by GCU studentships and Erin O'Shaughnessy by a Ph.D. studentship from the Psoriasis Association (Grant No.: ST3 15). We thank, Professor Rachel Errington (University of Cardiff) for access to time lapse microscopy, Dr. Bjarne Due Larsen (Zealand Pharma) for supply of Gap27 and a grant from Animal Free Research (AG) for support of the GCU Skin Research Tissue Bank. We are also indebted to Professor Malcolm Hodgins for helpful discussions and inputs. No funds for covering the costs to publish in open access were awarded.

Author Contributions: Patricia E.M. Martin, Claire Lorraine, Chrysovalantou Faniku conceived and designed the experiments; Claire Lorraine, Chrysovalantou Faniku and Erin O'Shaughnessy performed the experiments and Scott R. Johnstone performed the initial timelapse experiments; Claire Lorraine, Chrysovalantou Faniku, Erin O'Shaughnessy and Patricia E.M. Martin analysed the data; Sebastian Greenhough, Annette Graham and Scott R. Johnstone contributed reagents/materials/analysis tools and Sebastian Greenhough, funded by Animal Free Research, did not participate in any experiments involving animals or animal tissue; Claire Lorraine and Chrysovalantou Faniku contributed initial drafts and Patricia E.M. Martin wrote the final manuscript that was critically proof read by Annette Graham.

Abbreviations

Cx	connexin
CMP	connexin mimetic peptide
CMC	connexin mediated communication
JFF	human juvenile foreskin derived fibroblasts
HNDF	human neonatal dermal fibroblasts
AF	adult dermal derived fibroblasts
AK	adult keratinocytes
SFM	serum free media

References

1. Evans, W.H.; Martin, P.E. Gap junctions: Structure and function (Review). *Mol. Membr. Biol.* **2002**, *19*, 121–136. [CrossRef] [PubMed]
2. Evans, W.H.; Bultynck, G.; Leybaert, L. Manipulating connexin communication channels: Use of peptidomimetics and the translational outputs. *J. Mem. Biol.* **2012**, *245*, 437–449. [CrossRef] [PubMed]
3. Evans, W.H.; Leybaert, L. Mimetic peptides as blockers of connexin channel-facilitated intercellular communication. *Cell. Commun. Adhes.* **2007**, *14*, 265–273. [CrossRef] [PubMed]
4. Willebrords, J.; Maes, M.; Crespo Yanguas, S.; Vinken, M. Inhibitors of connexin and pannexin channels as potential therapeutics. *Pharmacol. Ther.* **2017**, *180*, 144–160. [CrossRef] [PubMed]
5. Chaytor, A.T.; Evans, W.H.; Griffith, T.M. Peptides homologous to extracellular loop motifs of connexin 43 reversibly abolish rhythmic contractile activity in rabbit arteries. *J. Physiol.* **1997**, *503 Pt 1*, 99–110. [CrossRef] [PubMed]
6. Chaytor, A.T.; Martin, P.E.; Evans, W.H.; Randall, M.D.; Griffith, T.M. The endothelial component of cannabinoid-induced relaxation in rabbit mesenteric artery depends on gap junctional communication. *J. Physiol.* **1999**, *520*, 539–550. [CrossRef] [PubMed]
7. Dora, K.A.; Martin, P.E.; Chaytor, A.T.; Evans, W.H.; Garland, C.J.; Griffith, T.M. Role of heterocellular Gap junctional communication in endothelium-dependent smooth muscle hyperpolarization: inhibition by a connexin-mimetic peptide. *Biochem. Biophys. Res. Commun.* **1999**, *254*, 27–31. [CrossRef] [PubMed]
8. Hutcheson, I.R.; Chaytor, A.T.; Evans, W.H.; Griffith, T.M. Nitric oxide-independent relaxations to acetylcholine and A23187 involve different routes of heterocellular communication. Role of Gap junctions and phospholipase A2. *Circ. Res.* **1999**, *84*, 53–63. [CrossRef] [PubMed]
9. Griffith, T.M.; Chaytor, A.T.; Edwards, D.H. The obligatory link: Role of gap junctional communication in endothelium-dependent smooth muscle hyperpolarization. *Pharmacol. Res.* **2004**, *49*, 551–564. [CrossRef] [PubMed]
10. Straub, A.C.; Zeigler, A.C.; Isakson, B.E. The myoendothelial junction: connections that deliver the message. *Physiology* **2014**, *29*, 242–249. [CrossRef] [PubMed]
11. Verma, V.; Hallett, M.B.; Leybaert, L.; Martin, P.E.; Evans, W.H. Perturbing plasma membrane hemichannels attenuates calcium signalling in cardiac cells and HeLa cells expressing connexins. *Eur. J. Cell. Biol.* **2009**, *88*, 79–90. [CrossRef] [PubMed]
12. Boitano, S.; Evans, W.H. Connexin mimetic peptides reversibly inhibit Ca^{2+} signaling through gap junctions in airway cells. *Am. J. Physiol. Lung Cell. Mol. Physiol.* **2000**, *279*, L623–L630. [CrossRef] [PubMed]
13. Yoon, J.J.; Nicholson, L.F.; Feng, S.X.; Vis, J.C.; Green, C.R. A novel method of organotypic brain slice culture using connexin-specific antisense oligodeoxynucleotides to improve neuronal survival. *Brain Res.* **2010**, *1353*, 194–203. [CrossRef] [PubMed]
14. Oviedo-Orta, E.; Errington, R.J.; Evans, W.H. Gap junction intercellular communication during lymphocyte transendothelial migration. *Cell. Biol. Int.* **2002**, *26*, 253–263. [CrossRef] [PubMed]
15. Oviedo-Orta, E.; Evans, W.H. Gap junctions and connexins: potential contributors to the immunological synapse. *J. Leukoc. Biol.* **2002**, *72*, 636–642. [PubMed]
16. Kameritsch, P.; Pogoda, K.; Pohl, U. Channel-independent influence of connexin 43 on cell migration. *BBA-Bioenergetics* **2012**, *1818*, 1993–2001. [CrossRef] [PubMed]

17. Brandner, J.M.; Houdek, P.; Husing, B.; Kaiser, C.; Moll, I. Connexins 26, 30, and 43: Differences among spontaneous, chronic, and accelerated human wound healing. *J. Investig. Dermatol.* **2004**, *122*, 1310–1320. [CrossRef] [PubMed]
18. Becker, D.L.; Thrasivoulou, C.; Phillips, A.R. Connexins in wound healing; perspectives in diabetic patients. *BBA-Bioenergetics* **2012**, *1818*, 2068–2075. [CrossRef] [PubMed]
19. Kretz, M.; Euwens, C.; Hombach, S.; Eckardt, D.; Teubner, B.; Traub, O.; Willecke, K.; Ott, T. Altered connexin expression and wound healing in the epidermis of connexin-deficient mice. *J. Cell. Sci.* **2003**, *116 Pt 16*, 3443–3452. [CrossRef] [PubMed]
20. Mori, R.; Power, K.T.; Wang, C.M.; Martin, P.; Becker, D.L. Acute downregulation of connexin43 at wound sites leads to a reduced inflammatory response, enhanced keratinocyte proliferation and wound fibroblast migration. *J. Cell. Sci.* **2006**, *119 Pt 24*, 5193–5203. [CrossRef] [PubMed]
21. Mendoza-Naranjo, A.; Cormie, P.; Serrano, A.E.; Hu, R.; O'Neill, S.; Wang, C.M.; Thrasivoulou, C.; Power, K.T.; White, A.; Serena, T.; et al. Targeting Cx43 and N-cadherin, which are abnormally upregulated in venous leg ulcers, influences migration, adhesion and activation of Rho GTPases. *PLoS ONE* **2012**, *7*, e37374. [CrossRef] [PubMed]
22. Pollok, S.; Pfeiffer, A.C.; Lobmann, R.; Wright, C.S.; Moll, I.; Martin, P.E.; Brandner, J.M. Connexin 43 mimetic peptide Gap27 reveals potential differences in the role of Cx43 in wound repair between diabetic and non-diabetic cells. *J. Cell. Mol. Med.* **2011**, *15*, 861–873. [CrossRef] [PubMed]
23. Wright, C.S.; Pollok, S.; Flint, D.J.; Brandner, J.M.; Martin, P.E. The connexin mimetic peptide Gap27 increases human dermal fibroblast migration in hyperglycemic and hyperinsulinemic conditions in vitro. *J. Cell. Physiol.* **2012**, *227*, 77–87. [CrossRef] [PubMed]
24. Wright, C.S.; van Steensel, M.A.; Hodgins, M.B.; Martin, P.E. Connexin mimetic peptides improve cell migration rates of human epidermal keratinocytes and dermal fibroblasts in vitro. *Wound Repair Regen.* **2009**, *17*, 240–249. [CrossRef] [PubMed]
25. Ghatnekar, G.S.; Grek, C.L.; Armstrong, D.G.; Desai, S.C.; Gourdie, R.G. The effect of a connexin43-based Peptide on the healing of chronic venous leg ulcers: a multicenter, randomized trial. *J. Investig. Dermatol.* **2015**, *135*, 289–298. [CrossRef] [PubMed]
26. Qiu, C.; Coutinho, P.; Frank, S.; Franke, S.; Law, L.Y.; Martin, P.; Green, C.R.; Becker, D.L. Targeting connexin43 expression accelerates the rate of wound repair. *Curr. Biol.* **2003**, *13*, 1697–1703. [CrossRef] [PubMed]
27. Lorraine, C. The role of connexins in skin wound healing events. Ph.D. Thesis, Glasgow Caledonian University, Glasgow, UK, available through British Library Electronic Theses Online System. 2015.
28. Wright, J.A.; Richards, T.; Becker, D.L. Connexins and diabetes. *Cardiol. Res. Pract.* **2012**, *2012*, 496904. [CrossRef] [PubMed]
29. Tarzemany, R.; Jiang, G.; Larjava, H.; Hakkinen, L. Expression and function of connexin 43 in human gingival wound healing and fibroblasts. *PLoS ONE* **2015**, *10*, e0115524. [CrossRef] [PubMed]
30. Riding, A.; Pullar, C.E. ATP Release and P2 Y Receptor Signaling are Essential for Keratinocyte Galvanotaxis. *J. Cell. Physiol.* **2016**, *231*, 181–191. [CrossRef] [PubMed]
31. Grupcheva, C.N.; Laux, W.T.; Rupenthal, I.D.; McGhee, J.; McGhee, C.N.; Green, C.R. Improved corneal wound healing through modulation of gap junction communication using connexin43-specific antisense oligodeoxynucleotides. *Investig. Ophthalmol. Vis. Sci.* **2012**, *53*, 1130–1138. [CrossRef] [PubMed]
32. Ormonde, S.; Chou, C.Y.; Goold, L.; Petsoglou, C.; Al-Taie, R.; Sherwin, T.; McGhee, C.N.; Green, C.R. Regulation of connexin43 gap junction protein triggers vascular recovery and healing in human ocular persistent epithelial defect wounds. *J. Memb. Biol.* **2012**, *245*, 381–388. [CrossRef] [PubMed]
33. Ghatnekar, G.S.; O'Quinn, M.P.; Jourdan, L.J.; Gurjarpadhye, A.A.; Draughn, R.L.; Gourdie, R.G. Connexin43 carboxyl-terminal peptides reduce scar progenitor and promote regenerative healing following skin wounding. *Regen. Med.* **2009**, *4*, 205–223. [CrossRef] [PubMed]
34. Moore, K.; Bryant, Z.J.; Ghatnekar, G.; Singh, U.P.; Gourdie, R.G.; Potts, J.D. A synthetic connexin 43 mimetic peptide augments corneal wound healing. *Exp. Eye Res.* **2013**, *115*, 178–188. [CrossRef] [PubMed]
35. Soder, B.L.; Propst, J.T.; Brooks, T.M.; Goodwin, R.L.; Friedman, H.I.; Yost, M.J.; Gourdie, R.G. The connexin43 carboxyl-terminal peptide ACT1 modulates the biological response to silicone implants. *Plast. Reconstr. Surg.* **2009**, *123*, 1440–1451. [CrossRef] [PubMed]

36. Danesh-Meyer, H.V.; Kerr, N.M.; Zhang, J.; Eady, E.K.; O'Carroll, S.J.; Nicholson, L.F.; Johnson, C.S.; Green, C.R. Connexin43 mimetic peptide reduces vascular leak and retinal ganglion cell death following retinal ischaemia. *Brain* **2012**, *135 Pt 2*, 506–520. [CrossRef] [PubMed]
37. Guo, C.X.; Mat Nor, M.N.; Danesh-Meyer, H.V.; Vessey, K.A.; Fletcher, E.L.; O'Carroll, S.J.; Acosta, M.L.; Green, C.R. Connexin43 Mimetic Peptide Improves Retinal Function and Reduces Inflammation in a Light-Damaged Albino Rat Model. *Investig. Ophthalmol. Vis.Sci.* **2016**, *57*, 3961–3973. [CrossRef] [PubMed]
38. Mao, Y.; Nguyen, T.; Tonkin, R.S.; Lees, J.G.; Warren, C.; O'Carroll, S.J.; Nicholson, L.F.B.; Green, C.R.; Moalem-Taylor, G.; Gorrie, C.A. Characterisation of Peptide5 systemic administration for treating traumatic spinal cord injured rats. *Exp. Brain Res.* **2017**, *235*, 3033–3048. [CrossRef] [PubMed]
39. Elbadawy, H.M.; Mirabelli, P.; Xeroudaki, M.; Parekh, M.; Bertolin, M.; Breda, C.; Cagini, C.; Ponzin, D.; Lagali, N.; Ferrari, S. Effect of connexin43 inhibition by the mimetic peptide Gap27 on corneal wound healing, inflammation and neovascularization. *Br. J. Pharmacol.* **2016**, *173*, 2880–2893. [CrossRef] [PubMed]
40. Tarzemany, R.; Jiang, G.; Jiang, J.X.; Larjava, H.; Hakkinen, L. Connexin43 Hemichannels Regulate the Expression of Wound Healing-Associated Genes in Human Gingival Fibroblasts. *Sci. Rep.* **2017**, *7*, 14157. [CrossRef] [PubMed]
41. Abudara, V.; Bechberger, J.; Freitas-Andrade, M.; De Bock, M.; Wang, N.; Bultynck, G.; Naus, C.C.; Leybaert, L.; Giaume, C. The connexin43 mimetic peptide Gap19 inhibits hemichannels without altering gap junctional communication in astrocytes. *Front. Cell. Neurosci.* **2014**, *8*, 306. [CrossRef] [PubMed]
42. Iyyathurai, J.; Wang, N.; D'Hondt, C.; Jiang, J.X.; Leybaert, L.; Bultynck, G. The SH3—Binding domain of Cx43 participates in loop/tail interactions critical for Cx43—hemichannel activity. *CMLS* **2017**. [CrossRef] [PubMed]
43. Glass, B.J.; Hu, R.G.; Phillips, A.R.; Becker, D.L. The action of mimetic peptides on connexins protects fibroblasts from the negative effects of ischemia reperfusion. *Biol. Open* **2015**, *4*, 1473–1480. [CrossRef] [PubMed]
44. Kandyba, E.E.; Hodgins, M.B.; Martin, P.E. A murine living skin equivalent amenable to live-cell imaging: Analysis of the roles of connexins in the epidermis. *J. Investig. Dermatol.* **2008**, *128*, 1039–1049. [CrossRef] [PubMed]
45. Kelly, J.J.; Esseltine, J.L.; Shao, Q.; Jabs, E.W.; Sampson, J.; Auranen, M.; Bai, D.; Laird, D.W. Specific functional pathologies of Cx43 mutations associated with oculodentodigital dysplasia. *Mol. Biol. Cell.* **2016**, *27*, 2172–2185. [CrossRef] [PubMed]
46. Hills, C.E.; Siamantouras, E.; Smith, S.W.; Cockwell, P.; Liu, K.K.; Squires, P.E. TGFbeta modulates cell-to-cell communication in early epithelial-to-mesenchymal transition. *Diabetologia* **2012**, *55*, 812–824. [CrossRef] [PubMed]
47. Postlethwaite, A.E.; Keski-Oja, J.; Moses, H.L.; Kang, A.H. Stimulation of the chemotactic migration of human fibroblasts by transforming growth factor beta. *J. Exp. Med.* **1987**, *165*, 251–256. [CrossRef] [PubMed]
48. Dai, P.; Nakagami, T.; Tanaka, H.; Hitomi, T.; Takamatsu, T. Cx43 mediates TGF-beta signaling through competitive Smads binding to microtubules. *Mol. Biol. Cell.* **2007**, *18*, 2264–2273. [CrossRef] [PubMed]
49. Leivonen, S.K.; Lazaridis, K.; Decock, J.; Chantry, A.; Edwards, D.R.; Kahari, V.M. TGF-β-elicited induction of tissue inhibitor of metalloproteinases (TIMP)-3 expression in fibroblasts involves complex interplay between Smad3, p38α, and ERK1/2. *PLoS ONE* **2013**, *8*, e57474. [CrossRef] [PubMed]
50. Huang, P.; Bi, J.; Owen, G.R.; Chen, W.; Rokka, A.; Koivisto, L.; Heino, J.; Hakkinen, L.; Larjava, H. Keratinocyte Microvesicles Regulate the Expression of Multiple Genes in Dermal Fibroblasts. *J. Investig. Dermatol.* **2015**, *135*, 3051–3059. [CrossRef] [PubMed]
51. Wright, C.S.; Berends, R.F.; Flint, D.J.; Martin, P.E. Cell motility in models of wounded human skin is improved by Gap27 despite raised glucose, insulin and IGFBP-5. *Exp. Cell. Res.* **2013**, *319*, 390–401. [CrossRef] [PubMed]
52. Johnstone, S.R.; Best, A.K.; Wright, C.S.; Isakson, B.E.; Errington, R.J.; Martin, P.E. Enhanced connexin 43 expression delays intra-mitotic duration and cell cycle traverse independently of gap junction channel function. *J. Cell. Biochem.* **2010**, *110*, 772–782. [CrossRef] [PubMed]
53. Leithe, E.; Rivedal, E. Ubiquitination and down-regulation of gap junction protein connexin-43 in response to 12-*O*-tetradecanoylphorbol 13-acetate treatment. *J. Biol. Chem.* **2004**, *279*, 50089–50096. [CrossRef] [PubMed]

12

Autophagy in Neurotrauma: Good, Bad or Dysregulated

Junfang Wu [1,2,3,*] and Marta M. Lipinski [1,2]

1 Department of Anesthesiology and Center for Shock, Trauma and Anesthesiology Research (STAR), University of Maryland School of Medicine, Baltimore, MD 21201, USA
2 Department of Anatomy and Neurobiology, University of Maryland School of Medicine, Baltimore, MD 21201, USA
3 Center to Advance Chronic Pain Research, University of Maryland, Baltimore, MD 21201, USA
* Correspondence: junfang.wu@som.umaryland.edu

Abstract: Autophagy is a physiological process that helps maintain a balance between the manufacture of cellular components and breakdown of damaged organelles and other toxic cellular constituents. Changes in autophagic markers are readily detectable in the spinal cord and brain following neurotrauma, including traumatic spinal cord and brain injury (SCI/TBI). However, the role of autophagy in neurotrauma remains less clear. Whether autophagy is good or bad is under debate, with strong support for both a beneficial and detrimental role for autophagy in experimental models of neurotrauma. Emerging data suggest that autophagic flux, a measure of autophagic degradation activity, is impaired in injured central nervous systems (CNS), and interventions that stimulate autophagic flux may provide neuroprotection in SCI/TBI models. Recent data demonstrating that neurotrauma can cause lysosomal membrane damage resulting in pathological autophagosome accumulation in the spinal cord and brain further supports the idea that the impairment of the autophagy–lysosome pathway may be a part of secondary injury processes of SCI/TBI. Here, we review experimental work on the complex and varied responses of autophagy in terms of both the beneficial and detrimental effects in SCI and TBI models. We also discuss the existing and developing therapeutic options aimed at reducing the disruption of autophagy to protect the CNS after injuries.

Keywords: spinal cord injury; traumatic brain injury; autophagy; autophagic flux; neuronal cell death; lysosomal damage

1. Introduction

The role of autophagy after the central nervous system (CNS) insults is under perusal, as investigation has begun to determine how autophagy and related pathways contribute to secondary injury and functional recovery following neurotrauma [1–5], including spinal cord injury (SCI) and traumatic brain injury (TBI). Whether detected autophagic responses to injury are protective or detrimental remains controversial, with experimental reports revealing protective effects of both enhancing and hindering autophagy [1,6].

Autophagy is a vital intracellular degradation pathway that delivers cytoplasmic constituents to the lysosomes for degradation [7]. There are three different types of autophagy that have been descripted so far, including macroautophagy, microautophagy, and chaperone-mediated autophagy [8–10]. In addition, several types of targeted autophagy have been described, including mitophagy, which is a selective form of macroautophagy that specifically targets and degrades damaged mitochondria. Macroautophagy involves the formation of a cytoplasmic membrane that engulfs cargo and eventually elongates to form double-membrane vesicles termed autophagosomes. It culminates in the fusion of cargo-containing autophagosomes to the lysosomes and the degradation of the cargo by lysosomal hydrolases [11]. As macroautophagy is the best characterized form of autophagy, hereafter, the term autophagy refers to macroautophagy unless otherwise specified. Under normal conditions, autophagy is an essential physiological process that maintains a balance between the manufacture of cellular components and breakdown of damaged organelles and other toxic cellular constituents. Its processing is strictly regulated under physiological conditions [12]. Recent considerable progress has demonstrated that autophagy is dysregulated in injured CNS following trauma, and may play either beneficial or detrimental functions after injury, depending on the context and the mechanisms leading to its perturbation [1,6,13,14]. Emerging data also suggest that the restoration and/or augmentation of proper autophagy function, for example by inducing lysosomal biogenesis, may be a potential therapeutic target for TBI and SCI.

This review explores the current research on the function and mechanisms of autophagy in two models of CNS injury: SCI and TBI. Cell-type specific responses of autophagy are discussed according to different locations, severity, and time windows of traumatic injury. We discuss recent findings suggesting that impairment of the autophagy–lysosomal pathway may be part of the secondary injury processes of SCI/TBI. We also review recent studies and novel mechanistic discoveries on cytosolic phospholipase A2 (cPLA2) participation in lysosomal damage, and provide therapeutic options, with an emphasis on the pharmacological modulation of autophagy and lysosomal biogenesis for neuroprotection and the prevention of neuroinflammation after CNS trauma.

2. Traumatic Spinal Cord and Brain Injury and Their Injury Mechanisms

According to the National Spinal Cord Injury Statistical Center [NSCISC, 2018], in the United States (U.S.), there are approximately 288,000 people living with SCI, and 17,000 new SCI cases occur each year. The impact of these injuries is devastating for individuals, and the health care costs associated with the injury are some of the highest in the U.S. [15,16]. Experimental and clinical studies [17–21] have indicated that acute SCI is a two-step process involving primary and secondary mechanisms. Primary injury of the spinal cord refers to the initial mechanical tissue damage. It also includes ruptured microvessels in the spinal cord, and subsequent hemorrhage and edema that are associated with secondary injury. SCI-mediated secondary injury processes include a cascade of biochemical and cellular events [22], such as free-radical formation, excitatory amino acid release, axonal damage, neuronal and oligodendroglial cell death, the infiltration of macrophages and peripheral immune cells, microglia, and astrocyte activation/glial scar formation. These delayed secondary injury processes can occur over hours, days, and months after initial impact [23,24], contributing to progressive neuronal degeneration and neurological dysfunction. Despite considerable research over the past 30 years, there is still no established effective treatment to improve recovery following SCI. In part, this reflects an incomplete understanding of the complex secondary pathobiological mechanisms involved.

TBI represents a major public health problem, with more than 1.7 million new cases annually in the United States [25] and accounting for 60% of all trauma deaths in the U.S. [26]. Similar to SCI, TBI causes cell loss and neurological functional deficits through both the direct physical damage of tissue (primary injury), and through subsequent biochemical changes (secondary injury). The latter reflects delayed and potentially reversible molecular and cellular pathophysiological mechanisms [27,28], which begin within seconds to minutes after the primary insult, and may continue for months to years [29,30]. Such secondary injury processes, similar in SCI, lead to cellular changes that include neuronal and oligodendroglial cell death, as well as microglia and astrocyte activation and glial scar formation. Although most of the research to date has been directed at early cellular and molecular events, both experimental and clinical evidence suggests that CNS trauma-mediated pathophysiological changes may continue for years [30–33], leading to chronic post-mitotic cell loss and microglial/astrocytes activation, and contributing to chronic functional deficits.

Cell death after neurotrauma is a major cause of neurological deficits and mortality. Although CNS injury induces changes in multiple cell types such as neurons and oligodendrocytes, the mechanisms of neuronal cell death have been the predominant focus. There are multiple cell death mechanisms in injured CNS following trauma [34,35]. Three main morphological types of cell death include apoptosis, autophagic cell death, and necrosis. Molecular and biochemical pathways that are involved in cell death after both TBI and SCI include, among others, caspases-dependent apoptosis (the Bcl-2 family), cell cycle activation-dependent pathways, the autophagy-related (ATG) protein family-mediated cell death (autophagy), caspase-independent programmed cell death [including extracellular-signal-regulated kinase 2 (ERK2), poly[Adenosine diphosphate (ADP)-ribose] polymerase (PARP)-1, apoptosis-inducing factor (AIF)], calpains and cathepsis-mediated calcium-dependent cell death, and the c-Jun N-terminal kinase-mediated non-apoptotic cell death (oncosis) [34,36,37]. Interestingly, apoptosis and autophagy share many regulatory factors, including the Bcl-2 family proteins [38]. The pro-apoptotic B-cell lymphoma 2 (Bcl-2) proteins Bim, Bid, and Bax, are known mediators of lysosomal membrane permeabilization (LMP) [39–42], while the anti-apoptotic Bcl-1 and Mcl-1 negatively regulate autophagy through interaction with Beclin 1. Additionally, necroptosis, the regulated receptor interacting protein kinase (RIPK)-dependent necrosis pathway, may also contribute to secondary neuronal cell death after CNS insults [3,43,44]. Obstacles to successful therapy against neurotrauma-induced neuronal cell death include the diversity of cell death pathways, which have both overlapping and distinct molecular mechanisms, and the narrow therapeutic windows for some types of neuronal cell death [34,45]. Thus, we emphasize that the effective neuroprotective strategies will need to concurrently modulate multiple signaling pathways to reflect the spatial and temporal changes underlying the diversity of neuronal cell death.

Stimulation by pro-inflammatory cytokines, chemokines, or alterations in the CNS environment induces microglial activation and the attraction of macrophages to the injury site [46,47]. Activated microglia undergo a transition from a resting, ramified phenotype to a phagocytosis-capable, 'macrophage-like' phenotype that is virtually indistinguishable from blood-borne macrophages [48–50]. Microglia and macrophages are found in the injured CNS within 12 to 24 h post-injury, with maximal concentration at four to eight days post-injury [49,51]. These cells produce free radicals, nitric oxide, and arachidonic acid derivatives, as well as a number of cytokines and chemokines in an effort to remove debris and dysfunctional cells. However, excessive inflammation may also result in the death of neighboring undamaged cells [52–56]. It is reported [57] that the activation of microglia-associated inflammatory factors may continue indefinitely after CNS trauma: certainly, it lasts for many months in rodents.

3. Autophagy, Autophagy Flux, and the Lysosomal Functions in Neurotrauma

3.1. Autophagy and Autophagy Flux

The process of autophagy includes several essential steps, including the induction, sequestration of cargo within the autophagosomal membrane, maturation of the autophagosomes, and degradation [12,58]. While baseline autophagy proceeds at all times, in adverse conditions such as environmental stress, nutrient starvation, or acute cellular injury, it is further activated. Cytoplasmic components including damaged organelles and toxic protein aggregates are sequestered by a unique membrane called the phagophore or isolation membrane. Complete sequestration by the elongating phagophore results in the formation of the autophagosome, which is typically a double-membraned vesicle. Then, autophagosomes are transported within the cell and fuse with lysosomes. Then, the inner membrane of the autophagosome and the cytoplasm-derived materials contained in the autophagosome are degraded by lysosomal hydrolases. The whole process of autophagy is referred to autophagic flux [7], which represents the dynamic process of autophagy from cargo sequestration to its degradation.

Completion of the autophagic flux requires the coordinated activity of various members of the autophagy-related (ATG) protein family [59,60]. For example, ATG13, ATG101, and FIP200 (homolog of yeast ATG17) are part of the ULK1 kinase complex that initiates autophagy. ATG9 also mediates an essential function in early autophagosome formation. Expansion of the autophagosomal membrane depends on two ubiquitin-like conjugating systems: the ATG12–ATG5–ATG16L system and the phosphatidylethanolamine (PE)–LC3 system. LC3 is the commonly used name for microtubule-associated protein 1 light chain 3β (MAP1LC3B). Upon activation of the autophagic pathway, the cytosolic, proteolytically processed form of LC3 (termed LC3-I) is lipidated to form LC3–PE (termed LC3-II), which is specifically recruited to the phagophore membrane. LC3-II accumulates on autophagosomal membranes and—through interaction with adaptor proteins—helps recruit substrates that are tagged for autophagic degradation. Thus, LC-II levels correlate well with autophagosome numbers. In addition, rapamycin complex 1 (MTORC1) operates as a central suppressor of autophagy. Conversely, beclin 1 (BECN1), a regulatory subunit of the type III phosphatidylinositol (PI) 3 kinase, promotes autophagy by promoting the formation of phosphatidylinositol 3 phosphate, which is necessary for autophagosome formation [60]. Moreover, ubiquitylated structures, including protein aggregated and in some cases mitochondria, are bound by the autophagic adaptor sequestosome 1 (SQSTM1; also known as p62), which enables their uptake by autophagosomes through LC3-II [61]. p62/SQSTM1 is one of several factors that target specific cargoes for autophagy, also including NBR1 [neighbor of breast cancer type 1 (BRCA1) gene], NDP52 (nuclear domain 10 protein 52), and OPTN (optineurin).

A number of methods are currently utilized to assess autophagic flux [62]. Transmission electron microscopy can be used for the partial analysis of the autophagosome pool size in vitro and in vivo without a time dimension. One of the most common ways to monitor autophagy is by measuring LC3-II protein turnover, which is incorporated into autophagosomes and then degraded in the lysosome. There are many different ways to measure LC3-II protein levels, including Western blot and immunofluorescent microscopy. However, these methods are complicated by the LC3-II levels increasing with autophagy induction due to increased autophagosomal formation, but also decreasing as these autophagosomes are turned over. Thus, a more reliable way to accurately monitor LC3-II levels is with a flux assay that uncouples autophagosome formation from its degradation by using lysosomal inhibitors such as bafilomycin-A1 (V-ATPase inhibitor) or chloroquine (a lysosomotropic compound that neutralizes lysosomal pH). As the flux is a rate, an analysis of both LC3-II and p62 levels over time in the presence and absence of lysosomal inhibitor is required. Another possibility in vitro is monitoring the half-life of labeled long-lived proteins that are known to be degraded via autophagy [63]. Fluorescence microscopy is an extremely valuable tool for the assessment of autophagic flux and the autophagosome pool size per cell. Use of the green fluorescent protein (GFP)–LC3 reporter allowing direct visualization of autophagosomes has been especially valuable. It is widely used for the evaluation of autophagy flux in vitro via image-based flux assay and live cell microscopy, and of the autophagosome pool in vivo using transgenic *GFP-LC3* reporter mice. Recent developments of the dual RFP-GFP-LC3 reporter further improved the evaluation of autophagy flux. It takes advantage of differential pH sensitivity of GFP (acid labile) and RFP (acid stable) to directly assess the fusion of autophagosomes (red and green) with lysosomes to form autolysosomes (red only) [62]. However, it remains challenging to employ these techniques in vivo in a manner that uniformly expresses autophagic flux quantitatively and assesses the magnitude of change in flux.

3.2. *Impairment of Autophagy Flux in SCI and TBI*

Increased markers of autophagy have been observed in different experimental SCI models [64–68]. Several reports indicate that the accumulation of autophagosomes is initiated very early during secondary injury, in some cases within hours after the initial impact. In SCI, depending on the injury models and severities as well as different species and sex, some reported significant increases in expression levels of the autophagosome marker LC3-II during the first 24 h after SCI [3,4,67,69,70], whereas others have only detected a delayed increase of this marker three to seven days after injury [64,65,68,71–73]. In some cases, the expression of Beclin 1, a key protein in the initiation of autophagy [74], has been reported to increase after SCI, supporting the hypothesis that SCI may lead to an increase of autophagy initiation [64,65,73,75,76]. However, other works have reported unaltered levels of Beclin 1 and other upstream mediators and regulators of autophagy [4,68], suggesting that increased autophagy initiation is unlikely to account for an increase in the number of autophagosomes. The p62/SQSTM1 protein, similar to all autophagy cargo adaptors, is degraded by autophagy along with its cargo. Therefore, provided no changes in transcription/synthesis are observed, p62 levels can be often used to approximate the autophagy-dependent degradation rate, with low levels of p62 protein associated with high autophagy flux (high degradation) and high p62 levels associated with low autophagy flux (inhibited degradation). Most reports describe the accumulation of both LC3 and p62 in the damaged spinal cord tissues [3,4,68]. Since p62/*Sqstm1* mRNA expression is not changed after SCI, this suggests that an accumulation of autophagosomes after SCI is likely a result of inhibited autophagy flux rather than its increased initiation [1]. This includes diverse injury models such as acute contusion SCI in male rat [4] and male mouse [3] and chronic spinal cord compression in both sexes [66,77]. The inhibition of autophagy flux was also recently reported following moderate contusion SCI in *GFP–LC3* male mice [3], and demonstrated the accumulation of both GFP–LC3 positive autophagosomes and p62 in the same cells near the injury site. Although autophagic changes in response to SCI show some discrepancies observed among studies, species, injury models, and injury severities, the vast majority of data support the inhibition of autophagic flux in the damaged spinal cord.

Increased markers of autophagy, including LC3-II, beclin1, p62, and autophagosomes, have been reported in human TBI autopsy samples [78,79], as well as in cerebrospinal fluid (CSF) [80]. TBI-mediated accumulation of p62 in both brain autopsy samples [78] and CSF [80] is associated with injury severity and worse recovery [80], and likely reflects an impairment of autophagic flux. Similarly, in experimental models of TBI, LC3-II expression levels as well as the accumulation of autophagosomes observed by electron microscope [81] has been demonstrated in the injured brain [79,82–84]. However, autophagy flux has not been directly assessed until more recently [62]. Interestingly, these data indicate that unlike in the spinal cord, in the brain, the autophagic flux capacity may be dependent on injury severity [14]. Supporting this possibility, the accumulation of p62 appears most pronounced at or near the lesion area after moderate to severe injury in both rodent TBI models [5,85] and human TBI brain samples [78]. The initiation of autophagy is not changed after moderate/severe injury in a controlled cortical impact (CCI) model [85]. Recently, an inhibition of autophagy flux was also reported in *GFP–LC3* mice after moderate CCI [5], and further confirmed by ex vivo flux assay in organotypic brain slices in the presence or absence of a lysosomal inhibitor (chloroquine). Conversely, in a mild CCI model [85], p62 was reduced in the ipsilateral cortex accompanied by increased beclin 1, ATG5, and ATG12, suggesting the enhancement of autophagy initiation. Increased autophagy has also been reported in rat models of TBI following a fluid percussion injury [83] and CCI [86,87]. Bayir et al. [88] reported that increased LC3-II after moderate CCI injury on postnatal day 17 rats is more prominent in male versus female rats, suggesting that trauma-induced autophagy is not limited to the mature mammalian brain, and that similar to nutrient deprivation studies in vitro [89], there are sex-dependent differences in the autophagic response. The divergent findings in autophagy flux following TBI may be explained by the different lesion paradigms and tissue sampling or time windows after injury. Nonetheless, autophagy flux is impaired in most models of moderate to severe brain injury.

3.3. Lysosomal Functions In Neurotrauma

Lysosomes are membrane-enclosed organelles that contain an array of enzymes that are capable of breaking down all types of biological polymers: proteins, nucleic acids, carbohydrates, and lipids [90–93]. Lysosomes function as the digestive system of the cell, serving both to degrade material taken up from outside the cell and the obsolete or superfluous components of the cell itself. Autophagic degradation is dependent on lysosomal proteases. Defects in the lysosomal function have been demonstrated in various neurodegenerative diseases and aging. In many of these disease paradigms, lysosomal dysfunction can be caused by the increase in lysosomal membrane permeability (LMP) [94–99]. We and others [3–5,100] demonstrated that decreased protein levels and activity of lysosomal enzymes accompanied the inhibition of autophagy flux in both TBI and SCI. The altered intracellular localization of soluble lysosomal enzymes including cathepsin D (CTSD) diffuse rather than discrete punctate, which further suggests the possibility that LMP allows the leakage of CTSD into cytosol, resulting in decreased lysosomal activity and the inhibition of autophagy flux after neurotrauma. In addition to its detrimental effect on autophagy, the leakage of the highly degradative lysosomal enzymes into the cytosol could lead to significant damage to other cellular components.

Similar to most cellular organelles, lysosomes are surrounded by a single-layer phospholipid membrane. Therefore, they are vulnerable to the activation of phospholipases. There are three major phospholipases present in the CNS: namely, calcium-dependent secretory phospholipase A2 (sPLA2), calcium-dependent cytosolic phospholipase A2 (cPLA2), and calcium-independent phospholipase A2 (iPLA2) [101,102]. Among these, cPLA2 is considered to be the most important PLA2 isoform, because it exhibits a strong preference for the deacylation of arachidonic acid (AA) over other fatty acids, and has been implicated as an effector in the receptor-mediated release of AA [103,104]. Both the expression levels and activity of cPLA2 are increased in several neurodegenerative diseases [101,105–108] as well as following SCI [109,110] and TBI [111]. cPLA2 cleaves the fatty acyl linkage of glycerophospholipids at the sn-2 position, releasing AA and leaving lysophospholipids remaining in the membrane [101,102,112–115]. Then, AA is oxygenated and further transformed into a variety of products such as prostaglandins, leukotrienes, and thromboxanes, which mediate or modulate inflammatory reactions. The accumulation of lysophospholids can affect the membrane properties, including its fluidity and permeability [112,113,115]. Although the signaling function of cPLA2 metabolites has been widely studied, the consequences of its action on the properties of the affected membranes and organelles are less well understood.

We recently used mass spectrometry (MS)-based in vivo lysosomal lipidomics to demonstrate an increase in several classes of lysosophospholipids, which are the products of phospholipases A (PLAs), as well as the accumulation of PLA activators and ceramides in lysosomes purified from the injured brain [111] and spinal cord [110]. Further in vitro and in vivo data indicated that cPLA2-mediated LMP leads to release of lysosomal enzymes into the cytosol, the inhibition of autophagy flux, and neuronal cell death. Taken together, our data implicate cPLA2 in the mediation of the lysosomal defects observed in the pathophysiology of neurotrauma. cPLA2-mediated lysosomal damage in turn causes the inhibition of autophagy flux and autophagosome accumulation, which are associated with neuronal cell death (Figure 1). Interestingly, our in vitro results indicate that the inhibition of cPLA2 can also limit amyloid-β-induced LMP and the inhibition of autophagy [111], suggesting that similar mechanisms may also contribute to Alzheimer's and potentially other neurodegenerative diseases.

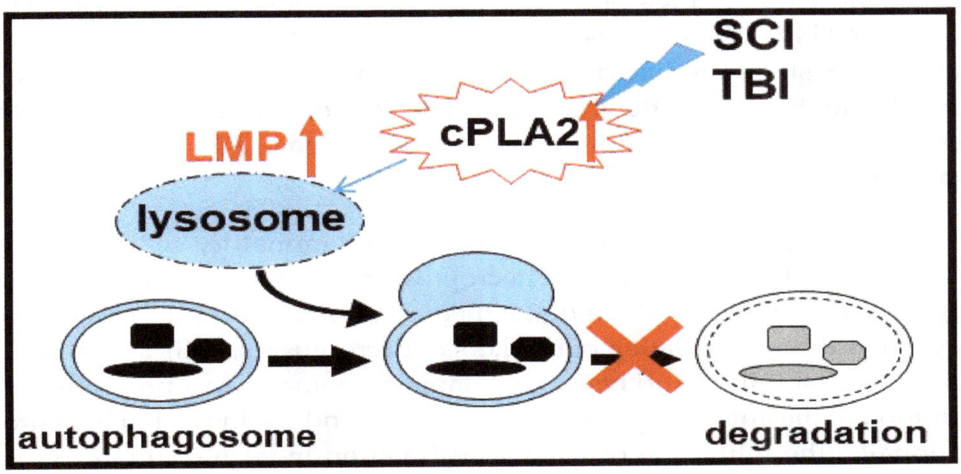

Figure 1. Spinal cord injury (SCI) and traumatic brain injury (TBI) activate cytosolic phospholipase A2 (cPLA2), mediating increased lysosomal membrane permeability (LMP), and leading to lysosomal damage and the inhibition of autophagy after SCI and TBI.

4. Beneficial or Detrimental Effects of Autophagy in CNS Cells After Trauma

4.1. Function of Autophagy in Neurons after Neurotrauma

Neurons, the fundamental units of the CNS, are post-mitotic cells, and most neurons have a cell body, an axon, and dendrites. CNS trauma causes progressive secondary injury processes including neuronal cell death and axonal damage, contributing to neurological dysfunction. Neurons are also the cell type that are most commonly associated with dysregulated autophagy after both TBI and SCI [1]. Afterwards, TBI markers of autophagy are predominantly reported in the neurons of the ipsilateral cortex and hippocampus, and appear within 24 h after injury [5,79,83]. In a mouse closed head injury model, Diskin et al. [82] reported that 17–37% of Beclin-1+ neurons were also terminal deoxynucleotidyl transferase dUTP (2′-deoxyuridine 5′-triphosphate) nick end labeling (TUNEL) positive, suggesting that cell death was associated with autophagy. In agreement with this observation, we observed significant numbers of GFP-LC3+ and p62+ neurons expressing cleaved caspase-3 in the injured cortex at day (d) 1 and 3 after injury in a mouse controlled cortical impact CCI model [5]. In addition, neuronal GFP-LC3 and p62 also co-localized with markers of caspase-independent cell death (such as AIF), indicating that impaired autophagy flux may contribute to both apoptotic and non-apoptotic neuronal cell death.

In SCI, changes in neuronal autophagy appear to be dependent on both the injury model and neuronal subtype. In rat and mouse contusion SCI models, the accumulation of both LC3 and p62 was greater in the ventral horn motor neurons as compared to the dorsal horn sensory neurons, despite the latter being located closer to the impact site [3,4,68]. This suggests that motor neurons may be relatively more vulnerable to the disruption of autophagy flux. Moreover, in these models, motor neurons with impaired autophagy also expressed higher levels of caspase12 and cleaved caspase 3 [4], supporting a role for impaired autophagy in mediating neuronal apoptosis. However, the inhibition of autophagy flux in the dorsal horn neurons was observed in spinal nerve ligation, which is a model of neuropathic pain [116,117], suggesting that neuronal subclasses may respond differentially to specific types of injury. That autophagy flux was inhibited even in this mild injury model also suggests that overall, spinal cord neurons may be more prone to the inhibition of autophagy flux as compared to brain neurons.

Endoplasmic reticulum (ER) stress induces a variety of neuronal cell death pathways, and has been implicated in the secondary injury processes after CNS trauma [118,119], but its mechanisms remain unclear. The induction of ER stress and activation of caspase 12 following TBI and SCI have been previously reported [4,5,118]. ER stress is a potent inducer of autophagy [120,121], and autophagy can protect cells from ER stress-mediated cell death [122]. Consistently, several studies indicate that markers of inhibited autophagy flux after injury correlate with the exacerbation of ER stress, suggesting a connection between the inhibition of autophagy and induction of ER stress-mediated neuronal cell death after neurotrauma [4,5] (Figure 2).

Necroptosis is a programmed form of necrosis, or inflammatory cell death, mediated by the RIPK1/RIPK3 complex [123]. The inhibition of necroptosis can improve functional recovery after both SCI and TBI, suggesting that it is involved in the mediation of the secondary injury [43,44]. A recent study [3] demonstrated the accumulation of markers of necroptosis specifically in neurons displaying signs of autophagy flux inhibition and lysosomal damage, pointing to a previously unexplored link between the inhibition of the autophagy-lysosomal pathway and the induction of neuronal necroptosis after SCI. Additionally, the inhibition of lysosomal function in vitro resulted in the accumulation of necroptosis mediators RIPK1 and RIPK3. Therefore, the inhibition of lysosomal function and autophagy in CNS trauma could also contribute to neuronal necroptosis (Figure 2).

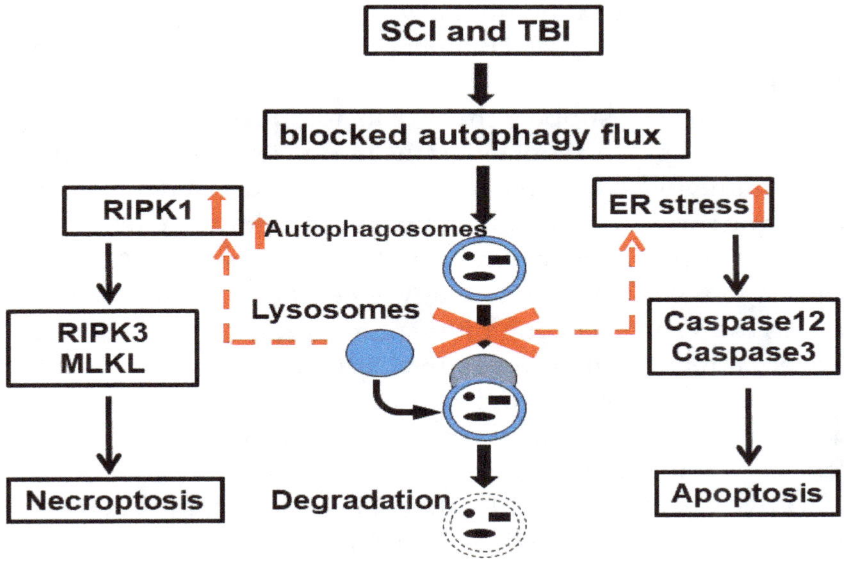

Figure 2. Lysosomal damage after spinal cord injury (SCI) and traumatic brain injury (TBI) cause endoplasmic reticulum (ER) stress and the accumulation of receptor interacting protein kinases (RIPK1/RIPK3), leading to neuronal apoptosis and necroptosis.

Recent findings have identified another type of cell death called 'autosis', which is an autophagy-dependent non-apoptotic form of cell death with unique features. It is characterized by enhanced cell-substrate adhesion, focal ballooning of the perinuclear space, and the dilation and fragmentation of ER. Autosis is mediated by the Na^+, K^+-ATPase pump in the mitochondria, and it is triggered by autophagy-inducing peptides, starvation, and neonatal cerebral hypoxia–ischemia. Whether or not autophagy-dependent autosis participates in neuronal cell death in injured CNS is unknown. While it's known that autophagy can mediate the execution of cell death in the absence of other death pathways, it is difficult to determine in vivo whether cell death is caused by high autophagy or if it is the by-product of other processes that happen alongside autophagy.

In addition to neuronal cell bodies, autophagosome accumulation has been reported to occur in damaged axons after both TBI and SCI [68,79,124]. While autophagy has been proposed to participate in the process of axonal degeneration in vitro, it is currently not known whether it is involved in axonal damage after neurotrauma. Another possibility is that axonal accumulation of autophagosomes could reflect the inhibition of autophagy flux due to lysosomal defects and cytoskeletal collapse, similar to what is observed in neurodegenerative diseases.

4.2. Role of Autophagy in Oligodendrocyte Survival after Neurotrauma

Oligodendrocytes (OLs), also called oligodendroglia, are a type of neuroglia whose main functions are to provide support and insulation to axons, and are the myelinating cells of the CNS [125]. Mature OLs are the end product of oligodendrocyte precursor cells (OPCs), which have to undergo a complex and precisely timed program of proliferation, migration, differentiation, and myelination to finally produce the insulating sheath of axons. Due to this complex differentiation program, and due to their unique metabolism and physiology, OLs count among the most vulnerable cells of the CNS. It is known that OLs undergo apoptosis following CNS trauma, thus the loss and demyelination of OLs contribute as major pathological processes to secondary damages after injury [126]. Increased numbers of autophagosomes have been reported in OLs after both TBI and SCI [4,5,65,66,68,127]. The accumulation of phagophores and autophagosomes in OLs was observed at three to seven days post-injury [4,5,68], which is later than in neurons in most reports. In a mouse contusion SCI model [127], myelin fractions purified from injured spinal cord tissues at eight days post-injury showed enrichment in autophagic proteins, including LC3-II, Atg5, and beclin 1. This study [127] has also demonstrated the increased co-localization of p62 with Olig2 at 3 days post-SCI, indicating impaired autophagic flux in OLs. Additionally, after TBI, increased LC3+ cells have been observed not only in mature OLs, but also in NG2+ OPCs [5].

While the current data strongly support changes in autophagy in OLs during functional recovery after CNS trauma, much less is known about either the mechanisms or the function of autophagy in OL and OPC cells. It has been previously demonstrated in a rat model of demyelination that autophagy is necessary to support oligodendrocyte precursor survival and myelin development [128]. Thus, it is possible that autophagy in OPCs/OLs may play a similar function after CNS trauma. Using transgenic mice with OL-specific loss of the essential autophagy gene *Atg5*, Saraswat et al. reported [127] that the loss of autophagy in OLs exacerbates the inhibition of the autophagic flux in OLs and correlates with worse functional recovery after SCI and greater myelin loss.

ER stress is also a potent inducer of autophagy in OLs [127]. In vitro, a pharmacological blockade of ER stress-induced autophagy in OPCs increases survival. *Atg5* deletion specifically in OLs increased ER stress and reduced cell viability in vitro and in vivo after SCI, indicating a critical regulation of ER stress by autophagy in OLs. This is consistent with the beneficial contribution of *Atg5* and autophagy to OPC/OL health after SCI. Whether or not *Atg5* and ER stress in OLs/OPCs play a similar function following TBI needs to be determined.

4.3. Function of Autophagy in Microglia and Astrocytes after CNS Trauma

Microglia are a type of glial cell that is located throughout the CNS. They account for 10–15% of all cells found within the brain. As the resident macrophage cells, microglia act as the first and main form of active immune defense in the CNS. Microglia are activated in response to injury and are one of the main drivers of inflammatory responses after both TBI and SCI [129]. An increase in markers of autophagy has been reported in microglia after both TBI and SCI [4,5,66]. Interestingly, only the most activated CD68-expressing microglia with amoeboid morphology were reported to accumulate autophagosomes and p62 after TBI in a mouse CCI model [5]. This is consistent with the recently discovered function for autophagy in the regulation of inflammatory responses in macrophages and other immune cells [130,131], including microglia [132]. In general, high levels of autophagy flux are associated with anti-inflammatory properties and the inhibition of flux, with pro-inflammatory phenotypes [133]. Several autophagy genes are also linked to inflammatory and autoimmune diseases [133,134]. On the mechanistic level, autophagy is thought to control the activity of the inflammasomes, both directly by degrading components of activated NLRP3 (nucleotide-binding oligomerization domain, leucine rich repeat and pyrin domain containing 3) and AIM2 (absent in melanoma 2) inflammasomes, and indirectly by limiting mitochondrial damage and reactive oxygen species (ROS) production [135–137]. Additionally, autophagy can modulate inflammatory polarization through its influence on NFκB (nuclear factor kappa B subunit) activity by directly targeting the RELA/p65 protein and by affecting the availability of the p62 protein, which is needed for NFκB activation [138–140]. Conversely, a pro-inflammatory environment may also regulate levels of autophagy, as in primary cultured mouse microglia, where interleukin 1 Beta (IL-1β) induced the accumulation of many acidic vesicles loaded with autophagic markers (p62 and LC3) [141]. It is possible that autophagy may similarly be regulated by and contribute to the regulation of inflammatory responses in microglia and/or infiltrating macrophages after CNS injury.

Astrocytes are the largest and most numerous types of glial cells in the CNS, and are known to have a wide variety of physiological functions, including the maintenance of neurons, formation of the blood–brain barrier, and regulation of synaptic function. Similarly, to microglia, in response to injury, astrocytes are activated and become hypertrophic. Several groups reported that glial fibrillary acid protein (GFAP)-positive astrocytes accumulate autophagosomes after neurotrauma [65,66,82,84]. In mouse contusion SCI, reactive astrocytes accumulated phagophores and autophagosomes at seven d post-injury. Unlike other cell types, this was associated with increased autophagy initiation rather than its inhibition [68]. Much less is known about either the mechanisms or the function of autophagy in astrocytes. Autophagy has been implicated in protective cellular responses in astrocytes [142–144]; however, further work will be necessary to determine how it may affect astrocyte survival and function after CNS trauma.

4.4. Beneficial or Detrimental Effects of Autophagy Activation in Neurotrauma

Defects in autophagy are thought to contribute to Parkinson's disease [145], Alzheimer's disease [146], and other age-related dementias. The accumulated evidence suggests that autophagy deficiency contributes to neurodegenerative diseases by perturbing protein homeostasis, as well as by directly contributing to neuronal cell death, axonal degeneration, and synaptic dysfunction. Conversely, the upregulation of autophagy has been proposed as a potential therapeutic strategy and shows considerable promise in both pre-clinical and clinical studies. However, the function of autophagy in neurodegeneration after traumatic CNS injury has been more controversial [1], with both beneficial and detrimental roles proposed. This may reflect that, as discussed above, either the induction or inhibition of autophagy flux may occur after acute CNS injury, especially in the brain. Since the function of autophagy is dependent on its flux, in cases where flux is inhibited, such as moderate to severe TBI or most cases of SCI, it would be expected to contribute to neuronal cell death and exacerbate other pathological phenotypes. Conversely, in cases where autophagy flux is increased, such as mild TBI, it would be expected to promote cell survival and improve outcomes. Thus, in each neurotrauma model, it is pertinent to ascertain whether observed changes in autophagy are the result of its induction or the inhibition of flux.

5. Therapeutic Potential of Autophagy–Lysosomal Pathway Modulation in Neurotrauma

5.1. Neuroprotection

The most common drugs used to manipulate autophagy in vivo are the mTOR (mechanistic target of Rapamycin kinase) inhibitor rapamycin, which is used to stimulate autophagy, and the type III PI3 kinase inhibitor 3-methyladenine (3-MA), which inhibits autophagosome formation. In general, pharmacological modulations that promote autophagy flux have been shown to provide neuroprotection in both TBI and SCI. However, in addition to autophagy, rapamycin is known to affect other cellular functions such protein synthesis, cell proliferation, and immune responses. Therefore, it is important to confirm that the neuroprotective effects of rapamycin are mediated via the restoration of the autophagy–lysosomal pathway. In a neonatal hypoxia–ischemia injury model, the protective effects of rapamycin were attenuated in animals treated with 3-MA [147]. Rapamycin-induced neuroprotection was also attenuated by AKT1 inhibition, suggesting that both autophagy and AKT1 signaling may be involved downstream of mTOR. Involvement of this pathway in TBI and SCI remains to be confirmed. However, as an improvement in functional recovery was reported after both pharmacologically enhancing [64,148] or blocking autophagy [149,150] after a thoracic SCI, further studies are warranted.

Another complicated factor is that activity of the target of rapamycin, mTOR, plays a vital role in oligodendrocyte differentiation [151] and myelination, and is also involved in axonal sprouting [152], which are both necessary for functional recovery after CNS injury, especially in the spinal cord. Therefore, the inhibition of mTOR may not be optimal as a treatment for CNS injury in general, and SCI in particular. In agreement with this, some [127,149] reported no effects of rapamycin on functional recovery after SCI. This suggests that drugs that are able to promote autophagy flux without inhibiting mTOR function may offer the best therapeutic benefits after neurotrauma. Trehalose is a naturally occurring sugar containing two glucose molecules, and has been reported as a novel mTOR-independent autophagy enhancer [153,154]. Trehalose has been shown to improve outcomes in rodent models of neurodegenerative diseases [155,156] and in a rabbit model of spinal cord ischemia [157]. However, trehalose is known to also act as a chemical chaperone [153], which could attenuate injury and improve recovery independently of autophagy. A specific mTOR inhibitor, Torin 1 [158,159], has been reported to increase autophagy flux. Both trehalose and Torin 1 induce lysosomal biogenesis via activation of the transcriptional factor E-box (TFEB) [160] and increase autophagy flux but are known to act through different molecular pathways (mTOR-independent and mTOR-dependent, respectively). However, whether or not a combination of trehalose and Torin 1 is able to overcome the block of autophagy flux after neurotrauma and lead to improved functional outcomes needs to be investigated.

As lysosomal function is necessary to support autophagy flux, increasing lysosomal biogenesis has been shown to augment autophagy flux and improve outcomes in animal models of neurodegenerative diseases [161]. Enhancing lysosomal function by reducing lysosomal damage or promoting lysosomal biogenesis may also provide an attractive approach for therapy after neurotrauma. In both contusion TBI and SCI mice models, we recently demonstrated that the early administration of cPLA2 inhibitor arachidonyl trifluoromethyl ketone (AACOCF3) reduced lysosomal damage, improved autophagy flux, limited neuronal cell death, and improved functional outcomes [110,111]. Another possibility is the enhancing activity of the transcription factor EB (TFEB). TFEB is the master regulator of lysosomal biogenesis and is negatively regulated by mTOR [162]. The enhancement of autophagic flux by activating TFEB is protective in experimental brain injuries produced by cadmium [163]. This supports the notion that enhancing autophagy flux by stimulating lysosomal biogenesis may represent a potential treatment strategy after neurotrauma.

There are also other autophagy inducers reported in the context of neurotruama. Baicalin (7-D-glucuronic acid-5,6-dihydroxyflavone) is a major flavonoid in traditional Chinese medicinal herb isolated from the radix of Scutellaria baicalensis that was found to increase expression levels of LC3, Beclin 1, and p62 at 24 h following the weight-drop TBI model in mice [164]. Salubrinal is the selective phosphatase inhibitor of p-eIF2α. Wang et al. reported [165] that salubrinal reduced the expression of the ER stress marker as well as the number of CHOP+/TUNEL+ and CHOP+/LC3+ cells at 48 h after mouse TBI, which was associated with neuroprotection and improved recovery. Omega-3 polyunsaturated fatty acids (ω-3 PUFA) are known to have anti-oxidative and anti-inflammatory effects. ω-3 PUFA supplementation increased Beclin-1 deacetylation and its nuclear export, and induced direct interactions between cytoplasmic Beclin-1 and Bcl-2 by increasing the sirtuin family of proteins (SIRT1) activity following a weight-drop TBI model in rat [166]. Valproic acid (VPA), a class I/II histone deacetylase inhibitor, is able to significantly increase expression levels of the autophagic markers (LC3-II, Beclin, ATG-3, and ATG-7) at one day after TBI in rat [167]. These data are consistent with the notion that enhancing autophagy may be beneficial after neurotrauma. However, while the treatments affected the expression of autophagy markers after neurotrauma, their influence on autophagy flux remains to be assessed. Additionally, none of the compounds used are specific for autophagy, and have many additional cellular and organismal effects. Therefore, it remains to be determined if their beneficial effects are in fact dependent on autophagy.

5.2. *Neuroinflammation*

The crosstalk between autophagy and inflammation has been reported [168] in diseases associated with inflammation, such as inflammatory bowel diseases [169], type 2 diabetes [170], cardiac disorders [171], and cystic fibrosis [172]. Autophagy is known to be involved in the development, homeostasis, and survival of all inflammatory cells, including macrophages, neutrophils, and lymphocytes, thus playing critical roles in the development and pathogenesis of inflammation. In a mouse Alzheimer's disease model, a recent study [173] demonstrated positive correlation between Beclin-1, IL-1β, and TNF-α (tumor necrosis factor alpha) in the cortex and/or hippocampus, suggesting a relationship between inflammatory responses and autophagy. It remains to be determined whether a similar relationship exists after neurotrauma, and whether enhancing autophagy can be used to manipulate neuroinflammatory responses in this context. Conversely, as inflammation can affect cellular autophagy [1], the anti-inflammatory treatments could also improve autophagy flux.

Neurotrauma-induced neuroinflammation can cause the excessive generation of reactive oxygen species (ROS), which non-selectively damages neurons and glia, and thus participates in pathophysiology [174]. ROS can also regulate autophagy in both a positive and negative manner, depending on the levels and context [175,176]. Excessive ROS as well as reactive nitrogen species (RNS) can inhibit autophagy through the S-nitrosylation of proteins in the JNK (c-Jun N-terminal kinase) and mTOR pathways, which are important for the regulation of autophagy [177]. Lysosomal membranes can also be directly subjected to oxidative damage, leading to LMP. This suggests that ROS could be an important factor contributing to alterations in autophagy levels after neurotrauma. Conversely, autophagy can also be stimulated by ROS through its influence on ATG4 activity. Therefore, depending on the injury severity and mechanism, CNS injury-mediated ROS and RNS could either stimulate or inhibit autophagy flux.

6. Conclusions and Perspectives

When the CNS is injured, many cellular processes are activated that attempt to heal the damage. The activation of other cellular responses can increase damage over time. In case of autophagy, both protective and pathological functions are possible. Although we need to more thoroughly understand the complex and heterogeneous autophagic response triggered by the CNS trauma, in general, the enhancement of autophagy is considered protective in many injury paradigms, and helps restore homeostasis. Autophagy-enhancing drugs could positively affect multiple cell types, promoting neuron and oligodendrocyte survival, oligodendrocyte differentiation, and decreasing neuroinflammation. So, while we need to understand the mechanisms in more detail, the enhancement of autophagy after TBI and SCI carries a promise of a potential pleiotropic treatment that could target multiple cell types and pathways.

Author Contributions: Writing—original draft preparation, J.W.; figure drawing, J.W.; writing—review and editing, M.M.L. and J.W.

References

1. Lipinski, M.M.; Wu, J.; Faden, A.I.; Sarkar, C. Function and Mechanisms of Autophagy in Brain and Spinal Cord Trauma. *Antioxid. Redox Signal.* **2015**, *23*, 565–577. [CrossRef] [PubMed]
2. Lipinski, M.M.; Wu, J. Modification of autophagy-lysosomal pathway as a neuroprotective treatment for spinal cord injury. *Neural Regen. Res.* **2015**, *10*, 892–893. [CrossRef] [PubMed]
3. Liu, S.; Li, Y.; Choi, H.M.C.; Sarkar, C.; Koh, E.Y.; Wu, J.; Lipinski, M.M. Lysosomal damage after spinal cord injury causes accumulation of RIPK1 and RIPK3 proteins and potentiation of necroptosis. *Cell Death Dis.* **2018**, *9*, 476. [CrossRef] [PubMed]
4. Liu, S.; Sarkar, C.; Dinizo, M.; Faden, A.I.; Koh, E.Y.; Lipinski, M.M.; Wu, J. Disrupted autophagy after spinal cord injury is associated with ER stress and neuronal cell death. *Cell Death Dis.* **2015**, *6*, e1582. [CrossRef] [PubMed]
5. Sarkar, C.; Zhao, Z.; Aungst, S.; Sabirzhanov, B.; Faden, A.I.; Lipinski, M.M. Impaired autophagy flux is associated with neuronal cell death after traumatic brain injury. *Autophagy* **2014**, *10*, 2208–2222. [CrossRef]
6. Galluzzi, L.; Bravo-San Pedro, J.M.; Blomgren, K.; Kroemer, G. Autophagy in acute brain injury. *Nat. Rev. Neurosci.* **2016**, *17*, 467–484. [CrossRef] [PubMed]
7. Mizushima, N.; Levine, B.; Cuervo, A.M.; Klionsky, D.J. Autophagy fights disease through cellular self-digestion. *Nature* **2008**, *451*, 1069–1075. [CrossRef]
8. Cuervo, A.M.; Wong, E. Chaperone-mediated autophagy: Roles in disease and aging. *Cell Res.* **2014**, *24*, 92–104. [CrossRef]
9. Li, W.W.; Li, J.; Bao, J.K. Microautophagy: Lesser-known self-eating. *Cell. Mol. Life Sci.* **2012**, *69*, 1125–1136. [CrossRef]
10. Levine, B.; Klionsky, D.J. Development by self-digestion: Molecular mechanisms and biological functions of autophagy. *Dev. Cell* **2004**, *6*, 463–477. [CrossRef]
11. Lamb, C.A.; Yoshimori, T.; Tooze, S.A. The autophagosome: Origins unknown, biogenesis complex. *Nat. Rev. Mol. Cell Biol.* **2013**, *14*, 759–774. [CrossRef] [PubMed]
12. Mizushima, N. Autophagy: Process and function. *Genes Dev.* **2007**, *21*, 2861–2873. [CrossRef]
13. Smith, C.M.; Chen, Y.; Sullivan, M.L.; Kochanek, P.M.; Clark, R.S. Autophagy in acute brain injury: Feast, famine, or folly? *Neurobiol. Dis.* **2011**, *43*, 52–59. [CrossRef] [PubMed]

14. Wolf, M.S.; Bayir, H.; Kochanek, P.M.; Clark, R.S.B. The role of autophagy in acute brain injury: A state of flux? *Neurobiol. Dis.* **2019**, *122*, 9–15. [CrossRef] [PubMed]
15. Ackery, A.; Tator, C.; Krassioukov, A. A global perspective on spinal cord injury epidemiology. *J. Neurotrauma* **2004**, *21*, 1355–1370. [CrossRef] [PubMed]
16. Wood-Dauphinee, S.; Exner, G.; Bostanci, B.; Exner, G.; Glass, C.; Jochheim, K.A.; Kluger, P.; Koller, M.; Krishnan, K.R.; Post, M.W.; et al. Quality of life in patients with spinal cord injury–basic issues, assessment, and recommendations. *Restor. Neurol. Neurosci.* **2002**, *20*, 135–149. [PubMed]
17. Tator, C.H. Experimental and clinical studies of the pathophysiology and management of acute spinal cord injury. *J. Spinal Cord Med.* **1996**, *19*, 206–214. [CrossRef]
18. Tator, C.H.; Fehlings, M.G. Review of the secondary injury theory of acute spinal cord trauma with emphasis on vascular mechanisms. *J. Neurosurg.* **1991**, *75*, 15–26. [CrossRef]
19. Beattie, M.S.; Farooqui, A.A.; Bresnahan, J.C. Review of current evidence for apoptosis after spinal cord injury. *J. Neurotrauma* **2000**, *17*, 915–925. [CrossRef]
20. Osterholm, J.L. The pathophysiological response to spinal cord injury. The current status of related research. *J. Neurosurg.* **1974**, *40*, 5–33. [CrossRef]
21. Mautes, A.E.; Weinzierl, M.R.; Donovan, F.; Noble, L.J. Vascular events after spinal cord injury: Contribution to secondary pathogenesis. *Phys. Ther.* **2000**, *80*, 673–687. [PubMed]
22. Zhang, B.; Gensel, J.C. Is neuroinflammation in the injured spinal cord different than in the brain? Examining intrinsic differences between the brain and spinal cord. *Exp. Neurol.* **2014**, *258*, 112–120. [CrossRef] [PubMed]
23. Beck, K.D.; Nguyen, H.X.; Galvan, M.D.; Salazar, D.L.; Woodruff, T.M.; Anderson, A.J. Quantitative analysis of cellular inflammation after traumatic spinal cord injury: Evidence for a multiphasic inflammatory response in the acute to chronic environment. *Brain* **2010**, *133*, 433–447. [CrossRef] [PubMed]
24. Wu, J.; Pajoohesh-Ganji, A.; Stoica, B.A.; Dinizo, M.; Guanciale, K.; Faden, A.I. Delayed expression of cell cycle proteins contributes to astroglial scar formation and chronic inflammation after rat spinal cord contusion. *J. Neuroinflammation* **2012**, *9*, 169. [CrossRef] [PubMed]
25. Faul, M.X.L.; Wald, M.M.; Coronado, V.G. *Traumatic Brain Injury in the United States: Emergency Department Visits, Hospitalizations, and Deaths*; Centers for Disease Control and Prevention NcfIPaC: Atlanta, GA, USA, 2010.
26. Dutton, R.P.; Stansbury, L.G.; Leone, S.; Kramer, E.; Hess, J.R.; Scalea, T.M. Trauma mortality in mature trauma systems: Are we doing better? An analysis of trauma mortality patterns, 1997-2008. *J. Trauma* **2010**, *69*, 620–626. [CrossRef] [PubMed]
27. Panter, S.S.; Faden, A.I. Biochemical changes and secondary injury from stroke and trauma, Chapter 4. In *Principles and Practice of Restorative Neurology*; Butterworth's: New York, NY, USA, 1992; pp. 32–52.
28. Keane, R.W.; Davis, A.R.; Dietrich, W.D. Inflammatory and apoptotic signaling after spinal cord injury. *J. Neurotrauma* **2006**, *23*, 335–344. [CrossRef] [PubMed]
29. Hall, E.D.; Springer, J.E. Neuroprotection and acute spinal cord injury: A reappraisal. *NeuroRx* **2004**, *1*, 80–100. [CrossRef]
30. Bramlett, H.M.; Dietrich, W.D. Progressive damage after brain and spinal cord injury: Pathomechanisms and treatment strategies. *Prog. Brain Res.* **2007**, *161*, 125–141.
31. Sidaros, A.; Engberg, A.W.; Sidaros, K.; Liptrot, M.G.; Herning, M.; Petersen, P.; Paulson, O.B.; Jernigan, T.L.; Rostrup, E. Diffusion tensor imaging during recovery from severe traumatic brain injury and relation to clinical outcome: A longitudinal study. *Brain* **2008**, *131*, 559–572. [CrossRef]
32. Ramlackhansingh, A.F.; Brooks, D.J.; Greenwood, R.J.; Bose, S.K.; Turkheimer, F.E.; Kinnunen, K.M.; Gentleman, S.; Heckemann, R.A.; Gunanayagam, K.; Gelosa, G.; et al. Inflammation after trauma: Microglial activation and traumatic brain injury. *Ann. Neurol.* **2011**, *70*, 374–383. [CrossRef]
33. Faden, A.I. Microglial activation and traumatic brain injury. *Ann. Neurol.* **2011**, *70*, 345–346. [CrossRef] [PubMed]
34. Stoica, B.A.; Faden, A.I. Cell death mechanisms and modulation in traumatic brain injury. *Neurotherapeutics* **2010**, *7*, 3–12. [CrossRef] [PubMed]
35. Schoch, K.M.; Madathil, S.K.; Saatman, K.E. Genetic manipulation of cell death and neuroplasticity pathways in traumatic brain injury. *Neurotherapeutics* **2012**, *9*, 323–337. [CrossRef] [PubMed]
36. Bredesen, D.E. Key note lecture: Toward a mechanistic taxonomy for cell death programs. *Stroke* **2007**, *38*, 652–660. [CrossRef] [PubMed]

37. Bredesen, D.E. Programmed cell death mechanisms in neurological disease. *Curr. Mol. Med.* **2008**, *8*, 173–186. [CrossRef] [PubMed]
38. Pattingre, S.; Tassa, A.; Qu, X.; Garuti, R.; Liang, X.H.; Mizushima, N.; Packer, M.; Schneider, M.D.; Levine, B. Bcl-2 antiapoptotic proteins inhibit Beclin 1-dependent autophagy. *Cell* **2005**, *122*, 927–939. [CrossRef]
39. Frankel, L.B.; Lund, A.H. MicroRNA regulation of autophagy. *Carcinogenesis* **2012**, *33*, 2018–2025. [CrossRef]
40. Xu, J.; Wang, Y.; Tan, X.; Jing, H. MicroRNAs in autophagy and their emerging roles in crosstalk with apoptosis. *Autophagy* **2012**, *8*, 873–882. [CrossRef]
41. Alqurashi, N.; Hashimi, S.M.; Wei, M.Q. Chemical Inhibitors and microRNAs (miRNA) Targeting the Mammalian Target of Rapamycin (mTOR) Pathway: Potential for Novel Anticancer Therapeutics. *Int. J. Mol. Sci.* **2013**, *14*, 3874–3900. [CrossRef]
42. Johansson, A.C.; Appelqvist, H.; Nilsson, C.; Kagedal, K.; Roberg, K.; Ollinger, K. Regulation of apoptosis-associated lysosomal membrane permeabilization. *Apoptosis* **2010**, *15*, 527–540. [CrossRef]
43. You, Z.; Savitz, S.I.; Yang, J.; Degterev, A.; Yuan, J.; Cuny, G.D.; Moskowitz, M.A.; Whalen, M.J. Necrostatin-1 reduces histopathology and improves functional outcome after controlled cortical impact in mice. *J. Cereb. Blood Flow Metab.* **2008**, *28*, 1564–1573. [CrossRef] [PubMed]
44. Wang, Y.; Wang, H.; Tao, Y.; Zhang, S.; Wang, J.; Feng, X. Necroptosis inhibitor necrostatin-1 promotes cell protection and physiological function in traumatic spinal cord injury. *Neuroscience* **2014**, *266*, 91–101. [CrossRef] [PubMed]
45. Faden, A.I. Neuroprotection and traumatic brain injury: Theoretical option or realistic proposition. *Curr. Opin. Neurol.* **2002**, *15*, 707–712. [CrossRef] [PubMed]
46. Gomes-Leal, W.; Corkill, D.J.; Freire, M.A.; Picanco-Diniz, C.W.; Perry, V.H. Astrocytosis, microglia activation, oligodendrocyte degeneration, and pyknosis following acute spinal cord injury. *Exp. Neurol.* **2004**, *190*, 456–467. [CrossRef] [PubMed]
47. Smith, M.E.; van der Maesen, K.; Somera, F.P. Macrophage and microglial responses to cytokines in vitro: Phagocytic activity, proteolytic enzyme release, and free radical production. *J. Neurosci. Res.* **1998**, *54*, 68–78. [CrossRef]
48. Suh, H.S.; Kim, M.O.; Lee, S.C. Inhibition of Granulocyte-Macrophage Colony-Stimulating Factor Signaling and Microglial Proliferation by Anti-CD45RO: Role of Hck Tyrosine Kinase and Phosphatidylinositol 3-Kinase/Akt. *J. Immunol.* **2005**, *174*, 2712–2719. [CrossRef] [PubMed]
49. Popovich, P.G.; Wei, P.; Stokes, B.T. Cellular inflammatory response after spinal cord injury in Sprague-Dawley and Lewis rats. *J. Comp. Neurol.* **1997**, *377*, 443–464. [CrossRef]
50. Watanabe, T.; Yamamoto, T.; Abe, Y.; Saito, N.; Kumagai, T.; Kayama, H. Differential activation of microglia after experimental spinal cord injury. *J. Neurotrauma* **1999**, *16*, 255–265. [CrossRef] [PubMed]
51. Carlson, S.L.; Parrish, M.E.; Springer, J.E.; Doty, K.; Dossett, L. Acute inflammatory response in spinal cord following impact injury. *Exp. Neurol.* **1998**, *151*, 77–88. [CrossRef] [PubMed]
52. Dehghani, F.; Conrad, A.; Kohl, A.; Korf, H.W.; Hailer, N.P. Clodronate inhibits the secretion of proinflammatory cytokines and NO by isolated microglial cells and reduces the number of proliferating glial cells in excitotoxically injured organotypic hippocampal slice cultures. *Exp. Neurol.* **2004**, *189*, 241–251. [CrossRef]
53. Delves, P.J.; Roitt, I.M. The immune system. First of two parts. *N. Engl. J. Med.* **2000**, *343*, 37–49. [CrossRef] [PubMed]
54. McTigue, D.M.; Tani, M.; Krivacic, K.; Chernosky, A.; Kelner, G.S.; Maciejewski, D.; Maki, R.; Ransohoff, R.M.; Stokes, B.T. Selective chemokine mRNA accumulation in the rat spinal cord after contusion injury. *J. Neurosci. Res.* **1998**, *53*, 368–376. [CrossRef]
55. Pan, J.Z.; Ni, L.; Sodhi, A.; Aguanno, A.; Young, W.; Hart, R.P. Cytokine activity contributes to induction of inflammatory cytokine mRNAs in spinal cord following contusion. *J. Neurosci. Res.* **2002**, *68*, 315–322. [CrossRef] [PubMed]
56. Wang, C.X.; Olschowka, J.A.; Wrathall, J.R. Increase of interleukin-1beta mRNA and protein in the spinal cord following experimental traumatic injury in the rat. *Brain Res.* **1997**, *759*, 190–196. [CrossRef]
57. Byrnes, K.R.; Garay, J.; Di Giovanni, S.; De Biase, A.; Knoblach, S.M.; Hoffman, E.P.; Movsesyan, V.; Faden, A.I. Expression of two temporally distinct microglia-related gene clusters after spinal cord injury. *Glia* **2006**, *53*, 420–433. [CrossRef] [PubMed]

58. Nikoletopoulou, V.; Papandreou, M.E.; Tavernarakis, N. Autophagy in the physiology and pathology of the central nervous system. *Cell Death Differ.* **2015**, *22*, 398–407. [CrossRef] [PubMed]
59. Lee, J.A. Neuronal autophagy: A housekeeper or a fighter in neuronal cell survival? *Exp. Neurobiol.* **2012**, *21*, 1–8. [CrossRef]
60. Noda, N.N.; Inagaki, F. Mechanisms of Autophagy. *Annu. Rev. Biophys.* **2015**, *44*, 101–122. [CrossRef]
61. Narendra, D.; Kane, L.A.; Hauser, D.N.; Fearnley, I.M.; Youle, R.J. P62/SQSTM1 is required for Parkin-induced mitochondrial clustering but not mitophagy; VDAC1 is dispensable for both. *Autophagy* **2010**, *6*, 1090–1106. [CrossRef]
62. Klionsky, D.J.; Abdelmohsen, K.; Abe, A.; Abedin, M.J.; Abeliovich, H.; Acevedo Arozena, A.; Adachi, H.; Adams, C.M.; Adams, P.D.; Adeli, K.; et al. Guidelines for the use and interpretation of assays for monitoring autophagy (3rd edition). *Autophagy* **2016**, *12*, 1–222. [CrossRef]
63. Zhao, J.; Brault, J.J.; Schild, A.; Cao, P.; Sandri, M.; Schiaffino, S.; Lecker, S.H.; Goldberg, A.L. FoxO3 coordinately activates protein degradation by the autophagic/lysosomal and proteasomal pathways in atrophying muscle cells. *Cell Metab.* **2007**, *6*, 472–483. [CrossRef] [PubMed]
64. Sekiguchi, A.; Kanno, H.; Ozawa, H.; Yamaya, S.; Itoi, E. Rapamycin promotes autophagy and reduces neural tissue damage and locomotor impairment after spinal cord injury in mice. *J. Neurotrauma* **2012**, *29*, 946–956. [CrossRef] [PubMed]
65. Kanno, H.; Ozawa, H.; Sekiguchi, A.; Yamaya, S.; Itoi, E. Induction of autophagy and autophagic cell death in damaged neural tissue after acute spinal cord injury in mice. *Spine* **2011**, *36*, E1427–E1434. [CrossRef] [PubMed]
66. Tanabe, F.; Yone, K.; Kawabata, N.; Sakakima, H.; Matsuda, F.; Ishidou, Y.; Maeda, S.; Abematsu, M.; Komiya, S.; Setoguchi, T. Accumulation of p62 in degenerated spinal cord under chronic mechanical compression: Functional analysis of p62 and autophagy in hypoxic neuronal cells. *Autophagy* **2011**, *7*, 1462–1471. [CrossRef] [PubMed]
67. Hao, H.H.; Wang, L.; Guo, Z.J.; Bai, L.; Zhang, R.P.; Shuang, W.B.; Jia, Y.J.; Wang, J.; Li, X.Y.; Liu, Q. Valproic acid reduces autophagy and promotes functional recovery after spinal cord injury in rats. *Neurosci. Bull.* **2013**, *29*, 484–492. [CrossRef]
68. Munoz-Galdeano, T.; Reigada, D.; Del Aguila, A.; Velez, I.; Caballero-Lopez, M.J.; Maza, R.M.; Nieto-Diaz, M. Cell Specific Changes of Autophagy in a Mouse Model of Contusive Spinal Cord Injury. *Front. Cell. Neurosci.* **2018**, *12*, 164. [CrossRef]
69. Chen, H.C.; Fong, T.H.; Lee, A.W.; Chiu, W.T. Autophagy is activated in injured neurons and inhibited by methylprednisolone after experimental spinal cord injury. *Spine* **2012**, *37*, 470–475. [CrossRef]
70. Hou, H.; Zhang, L.; Zhang, L.; Tang, P. Acute spinal cord injury in rats should target activated autophagy. *J. Neurosurg. Spine* **2014**, *20*, 568–577. [CrossRef] [PubMed]
71. Zhang, H.Y.; Wang, Z.G.; Wu, F.Z.; Kong, X.X.; Yang, J.; Lin, B.B.; Zhu, S.P.; Lin, L.; Gan, C.S.; Fu, X.B. Regulation of autophagy and ubiquitinated protein accumulation by bFGF promotes functional recovery and neural protection in a rat model of spinal cord injury. *Mol. Neurobiol.* **2013**, *48*, 452–464. [CrossRef]
72. Zhang, Q.; Huang, C.; Meng, B.; Tang, T.S.; Yang, H.L. Changes in autophagy proteins in a rat model of spinal cord injury. *Chin. J. Traumatol.* **2014**, *17*, 193–197.
73. Berliocchi, L.; Maiaru, M.; Varano, G.P.; Russo, R.; Corasaniti, M.T.; Bagetta, G.; Tassorelli, C. Spinal autophagy is differently modulated in distinct mouse models of neuropathic pain. *Mol. Pain* **2015**, *11*, 3. [CrossRef] [PubMed]
74. He, C.; Levine, B. The Beclin 1 interactome. *Curr. Opin. Cell Biol.* **2010**, *22*, 140–149. [CrossRef] [PubMed]
75. Wang, Z.Y.; Lin, J.H.; Muharram, A.; Liu, W.G. Beclin-1-mediated autophagy protects spinal cord neurons against mechanical injury-induced apoptosis. *Apoptosis* **2014**, *19*, 933–945. [CrossRef] [PubMed]
76. Kanno, H.; Ozawa, H.; Sekiguchi, A.; Itoi, E. Spinal cord injury induces upregulation of Beclin 1 and promotes autophagic cell death. *Neurobiol. Dis.* **2009**, *33*, 143–148. [CrossRef] [PubMed]
77. Chen, Z.; Fu, Q.; Shen, B.; Huang, X.; Wang, K.; He, P.; Li, F.; Zhang, F.; Shen, H. Enhanced p62 expression triggers concomitant autophagy and apoptosis in a rat chronic spinal cord compression model. *Mol. Med. Rep.* **2014**, *9*, 2091–2096. [CrossRef] [PubMed]
78. Sakai, K.; Fukuda, T.; Iwadate, K. Immunohistochemical analysis of the ubiquitin proteasome system and autophagy lysosome system induced after traumatic intracranial injury: Association with time between the injury and death. *Am. J. Forensic. Med. Pathol.* **2014**, *35*, 38–44. [CrossRef]

79. Clark, R.S.; Bayir, H.; Chu, C.T.; Alber, S.M.; Kochanek, P.M.; Watkins, S.C. Autophagy is increased in mice after traumatic brain injury and is detectable in human brain after trauma and critical illness. *Autophagy* **2008**, *4*, 88–90. [CrossRef]
80. Au, A.K.; Aneja, R.K.; Bayir, H.; Bell, M.J.; Janesko-Feldman, K.; Kochanek, P.M.; Clark, R.S.B. Autophagy Biomarkers Beclin 1 and p62 are Increased in Cerebrospinal Fluid after Traumatic Brain Injury. *Neurocrit. Care* **2017**, *26*, 348–355. [CrossRef]
81. Lai, Y.; Hickey, R.W.; Chen, Y.; Bayir, H.; Sullivan, M.L.; Chu, C.T.; Kochanek, P.M.; Dixon, C.E.; Jenkins, L.W.; Graham, S.H.; et al. Autophagy is increased after traumatic brain injury in mice and is partially inhibited by the antioxidant gamma-glutamylcysteinyl ethyl ester. *J. Cereb. Blood Flow Metab.* **2008**, *28*, 540–550. [CrossRef]
82. Diskin, T.; Tal-Or, P.; Erlich, S.; Mizrachy, L.; Alexandrovich, A.; Shohami, E.; Pinkas-Kramarski, R. Closed head injury induces upregulation of Beclin 1 at the cortical site of injury. *J. Neurotrauma* **2005**, *22*, 750–762. [CrossRef]
83. Liu, C.L.; Chen, S.; Dietrich, D.; Hu, B.R. Changes in autophagy after traumatic brain injury. *J. Cereb. Blood Flow Metab.* **2008**, *28*, 674–683. [CrossRef] [PubMed]
84. Erlich, S.; Alexandrovich, A.; Shohami, E.; Pinkas-Kramarski, R. Rapamycin is a neuroprotective treatment for traumatic brain injury. *Neurobiol. Dis.* **2007**, *26*, 86–93. [CrossRef] [PubMed]
85. Zeng, X.J.; Li, P.; Ning, Y.L.; Zhao, Y.; Peng, Y.; Yang, N.; Zhao, Z.A.; Chen, J.F.; Zhou, Y.G. Impaired autophagic flux is associated with the severity of trauma and the role of A2AR in brain cells after traumatic brain injury. *Cell Death Dis.* **2018**, *9*, 252. [CrossRef] [PubMed]
86. Zhang, Y.B.; Li, S.X.; Chen, X.P.; Yang, L.; Zhang, Y.G.; Liu, R.; Tao, L.Y. Autophagy is activated and might protect neurons from degeneration after traumatic brain injury. *Neurosci. Bull.* **2008**, *24*, 143–149. [CrossRef] [PubMed]
87. Sadasivan, S.; Dunn, W.A.; Jr Hayes, R.L.; Wang, K.K. Changes in autophagy proteins in a rat model of controlled cortical impact induced brain injury. *Biochem. Biophys. Res. Commun.* **2008**, *373*, 478–481. [CrossRef] [PubMed]
88. Bayir, H.; Tyurin, V.A.; Tyurina, Y.Y.; Viner, R.; Ritov, V.; Amoscato, A.A.; Zhao, Q.; Zhang, X.J.; Janesko-Feldman, K.L.; Alexander, H.; et al. Selective early cardiolipin peroxidation after traumatic brain injury: An oxidative lipidomics analysis. *Ann. Neurol.* **2007**, *62*, 154–169. [CrossRef] [PubMed]
89. Du, L.; Hickey, R.W.; Bayir, H.; Watkins, S.C.; Tyurin, V.A.; Guo, F.; Kochanek, P.M.; Jenkins, L.W.; Ren, J.; Gibson, G.; et al. Starving neurons show sex difference in autophagy. *J. Biol. Chem.* **2009**, *284*, 2383–2396. [CrossRef] [PubMed]
90. Xu, H.; Ren, D. Lysosomal physiology. *Annu. Rev. Physiol.* **2015**, *77*, 57–80. [CrossRef]
91. Kilpatrick, B.S.; Eden, E.R.; Hockey, L.N.; Futter, C.E.; Patel, S. Methods for monitoring lysosomal morphology. *Methods. Cell Biol.* **2015**, *126*, 1–19.
92. de Duve, D. The peroxisome: A new cytoplasmic organelle. *Proc. R. Soc. Lond.Ser. B Biol. Sci.* **1969**, *173*, 71–83.
93. Luzio, J.P.; Pryor, P.R.; Bright, N.A. Lysosomes: Fusion and function. *Nat. Rev. Mol. Cell Biol.* **2007**, *8*, 622–632. [CrossRef]
94. Gomez-Sintes, R.; Ledesma, M.D.; Boya, P. Lysosomal cell death mechanisms in aging. *Ageing Res. Rev.* **2016**, *32*, 150–168. [CrossRef] [PubMed]
95. Rodriguez-Muela, N.; Hernandez-Pinto, A.M.; Serrano-Puebla, A.; Garcia-Ledo, L.; Latorre, S.H.; de la Rosa, E.J.; Boya, P. Lysosomal membrane permeabilization and autophagy blockade contribute to photoreceptor cell death in a mouse model of retinitis pigmentosa. *Cell Death Differ.* **2015**, *22*, 476–487. [CrossRef] [PubMed]
96. Aits, S.; Jaattela, M. Lysosomal cell death at a glance. *J. Cell Sci.* **2013**, *126*, 1905–1912. [CrossRef] [PubMed]
97. Boya, P.; Kroemer, G. Lysosomal membrane permeabilization in cell death. *Oncogene* **2008**, *27*, 6434–6451. [CrossRef] [PubMed]
98. Yamashima, T.; Oikawa, S. The role of lysosomal rupture in neuronal death. *Prog. Neurobiol.* **2009**, *89*, 343–358. [CrossRef] [PubMed]
99. Cuervo, A.M.; Dice, J.F. When lysosomes get old. *Exp. Gerontol.* **2000**, *35*, 119–131. [CrossRef]

100. Yin, Y.; Li, E.; Sun, G.; Yan, H.Q.; Foley, L.M.; Andrzejczuk, L.A.; Attarwala, I.Y.; Hitchens, T.K.; Kiselyov, K.; Dixon, C.E.; et al. Effects of DHA on Hippocampal Autophagy and Lysosome Function After Traumatic Brain Injury. *Mol. Neurobiol.* **2018**, *55*, 2454–2470. [CrossRef] [PubMed]
101. Lee, J.C.; Simonyi, A.; Sun, A.Y.; Sun, G.Y. Phospholipases A2 and neural membrane dynamics: Implications for Alzheimer's disease. *J. Neurochem.* **2011**, *116*, 813–819. [CrossRef]
102. Burke, J.E.; Dennis, E.A. Phospholipase A2 structure/function, mechanism, and signaling. *J. Lipid Res.* **2009**, *50*, S237–S242. [CrossRef]
103. Farooqui, A.A.; Yang, H.C.; Rosenberger, T.A.; Horrocks, L.A. Phospholipase A2 and its role in brain tissue. *J. Neurochem.* **1997**, *69*, 889–901. [CrossRef] [PubMed]
104. Clark, J.D.; Schievella, A.R.; Nalefski, E.A.; Lin, L.L. Cytosolic phospholipase A2. *J. Lipid Mediat. Cell Signal.* **1995**, *12*, 83–117. [CrossRef]
105. Sanchez-Mejia, R.O.; Newman, J.W.; Toh, S.; Yu, G.Q.; Zhou, Y.; Halabisky, B.; Cisse, M.; Scearce-Levie, K.; Cheng, I.H.; Gan, L.; et al. Phospholipase A2 reduction ameliorates cognitive deficits in a mouse model of Alzheimer's disease. *Nat. Neurosci.* **2008**, *11*, 1311–1318. [CrossRef] [PubMed]
106. Leslie, C.C. Cytosolic phospholipase A(2): Physiological function and role in disease. *J. Lipid Res.* **2015**, *56*, 1386–1402. [CrossRef] [PubMed]
107. Phillis, J.W.; O'Regan, M.H. A potentially critical role of phospholipases in central nervous system ischemic, traumatic, and neurodegenerative disorders. *Brain Res. Rev.* **2004**, *44*, 13–47. [CrossRef] [PubMed]
108. Zhang, Z.; Lee, Y.C.; Kim, S.J.; Choi, M.S.; Tsai, P.C.; Saha, A.; Wei, H.; Xu, Y.; Xiao, Y.J.; Zhang, P.; et al. Production of lysophosphatidylcholine by cPLA2 in the brain of mice lacking PPT1 is a signal for phagocyte infiltration. *Hum. Mol. Genet.* **2007**, *16*, 837–847. [CrossRef] [PubMed]
109. Liu, N.K.; Deng, L.X.; Zhang, Y.P.; Lu, Q.B.; Wang, X.F.; Hu, J.G.; Oakes, E.; Bonventre, J.V.; Shields, C.B.; Xu, X.M. Cytosolic phospholipase A2 protein as a novel therapeutic target for spinal cord injury. *Ann. Neurol.* **2014**, *75*, 644–658. [CrossRef]
110. Li, Y.; Jones, J.W.; Choi, H.M.C.; Sarkar, C.; Kane, M.A.; Koh, E.Y.; Lipinski, M.M.; Wu, J. cPLA2 activation contributes to lysosomal defects leading to impairment of autophagy after spinal cord injury. *Cell Death Dis.* **2019**, in press.
111. Sarkar, C.; Jones, J.W.; Hegdekar, N.; Thayer, J.A.; Kumar, A.; Faden, A.I.; Kane, M.A.; Lipinski, M.M. PLA2G4A/cPLA2-mediated lysosomal membrane damage leads to inhibition of autophagy and neurodegeneration after brain trauma. *Autophagy* **2019**, 1–20. [CrossRef]
112. Farooqui, A.A.; Horrocks, L.A. Brain phospholipases A2: A perspective on the history. *Prostaglandin. Leukot. Essent. Fatty Acids* **2004**, *71*, 161–169. [CrossRef]
113. Gijon, M.A.; Leslie, C.C. Regulation of arachidonic acid release and cytosolic phospholipase A2 activation. *J. Leukoc. Biol.* **1999**, *65*, 330–336. [CrossRef] [PubMed]
114. Murakami, M.; Taketomi, Y.; Miki, Y.; Sato, H.; Hirabayashi, T.; Yamamoto, K. Recent progress in phospholipase A(2) research: From cells to animals to humans. *Prog. Lipid Res.* **2011**, *50*, 152–192. [CrossRef]
115. Farooqui, A.A.; Ong, W.Y.; Horrocks, L.A. Inhibitors of brain phospholipase A2 activity: Their neuropharmacological effects and therapeutic importance for the treatment of neurologic disorders. *Pharmacol. Rev.* **2006**, *58*, 591–620. [CrossRef]
116. Berliocchi, L.; Russo, R.; Maiaru, M.; Levato, A.; Bagetta, G.; Corasaniti, M.T. Autophagy impairment in a mouse model of neuropathic pain. *Mol. Pain* **2011**, *7*, 83. [CrossRef]
117. Zhang, E.; Yi, M.H.; Ko, Y.; Kim, H.W.; Seo, J.H.; Lee, Y.H.; Lee, W.; Kim, D.W. Expression of LC3 and Beclin 1 in the spinal dorsal horn following spinal nerve ligation-induced neuropathic pain. *Brain Res.* **2013**, *1519*, 31–39. [CrossRef] [PubMed]
118. Larner, S.F.; Hayes, R.L.; McKinsey, D.M.; Pike, B.R.; Wang, K.K. Increased expression and processing of caspase-12 after traumatic brain injury in rats. *J. Neurochem.* **2004**, *88*, 78–90. [CrossRef] [PubMed]
119. Ohri, S.S.; Hetman, M.; Whittemore, S.R. Restoring endoplasmic reticulum homeostasis improves functional recovery after spinal cord injury. *Neurobiol. Dis.* **2013**, *58*, 29–37. [CrossRef]
120. Yorimitsu, T.; Nair, U.; Yang, Z.; Klionsky, D.J. Endoplasmic reticulum stress triggers autophagy. *J. Biol. Chem.* **2006**, *281*, 30299–30304. [CrossRef] [PubMed]

121. Kouroku, Y.; Fujita, E.; Tanida, I.; Ueno, T.; Isoai, A.; Kumagai, H.; Ogawa, S.; Kaufman, R.J.; Kominami, E.; Momoi, T. ER stress (PERK/eIF2alpha phosphorylation) mediates the polyglutamine-induced LC3 conversion, an essential step for autophagy formation. *Cell Death Differ.* **2007**, *14*, 230–239. [CrossRef] [PubMed]
122. Boyce, M.; Lipinski, M.M.; Py, B.F.; Yuan, J. Endoplasmic reticulum stress response in cell death and cell survival. In *Apoptosis: Physiology and Pathology*, 1st ed.; Reed, J.C., Green, D.R., Eds.; Cambridge University Press: Cambridge, UK, 2011; pp. 51–62.
123. Vandenabeele, P.; Galluzzi, L.; Vanden Berghe, T.; Kroemer, G. Molecular mechanisms of necroptosis: An ordered cellular explosion. *Nat. Rev. Mol. Cell Biol.* **2010**, *11*, 700–714. [CrossRef]
124. Ribas, V.T.; Schnepf, B.; Challagundla, M.; Koch, J.C.; Bahr, M.; Lingor, P. Early and sustained activation of autophagy in degenerating axons after spinal cord injury. *Brain Pathol.* **2015**, *25*, 157–170. [CrossRef] [PubMed]
125. Bradl, M.; Lassmann, H. Oligodendrocytes: Biology and pathology. *Acta Neuropathol.* **2010**, *119*, 37–53. [CrossRef]
126. Beattie, M.S.; Hermann, G.E.; Rogers, R.C.; Bresnahan, J.C. Cell death in models of spinal cord injury. *Prog. Brain Res.* **2002**, *137*, 37–47. [PubMed]
127. Saraswat Ohri, S.; Bankston, A.N.; Mullins, S.A.; Liu, Y.; Andres, K.R.; Beare, J.E.; Howard, R.M.; Burke, D.A.; Riegler, A.S.; Smith, A.E.; et al. Blocking Autophagy in Oligodendrocytes Limits Functional Recovery after Spinal Cord Injury. *J. Neurosci.* **2018**, *38*, 5900–5912. [CrossRef]
128. Smith, C.M.; Mayer, J.A.; Duncan, I.D. Autophagy promotes oligodendrocyte survival and function following dysmyelination in a long-lived myelin mutant. *J. Neurosci.* **2013**, *33*, 8088–8100. [CrossRef] [PubMed]
129. Loane, D.J.; Byrnes, K.R. Role of microglia in neurotrauma. *Neurotherapeutics* **2010**, *7*, 366–377. [CrossRef] [PubMed]
130. Messer, J.S. The cellular autophagy/apoptosis checkpoint during inflammation. *Cell. Mol. Life Sci.* **2017**, *74*, 1281–1296. [CrossRef]
131. Zhong, Z.; Sanchez-Lopez, E.; Karin, M. Autophagy, Inflammation, and Immunity: A Troika Governing Cancer and Its Treatment. *Cell* **2016**, *166*, 288–298. [CrossRef]
132. Su, P.; Zhang, J.; Wang, D.; Zhao, F.; Cao, Z.; Aschner, M.; Luo, W. The role of autophagy in modulation of neuroinflammation in microglia. *Neuroscience* **2016**, *319*, 155–167. [CrossRef]
133. Sil, P.; Muse, G.; Martinez, J. A ravenous defense: Canonical and non-canonical autophagy in immunity. *Curr. Opin. Immunol.* **2018**, *50*, 21–31. [CrossRef]
134. Cadwell, K.; Liu, J.Y.; Brown, S.L.; Miyoshi, H.; Loh, J.; Lennerz, J.K.; Kishi, C.; Kc, W.; Carrero, J.A.; Hunt, S.; et al. A key role for autophagy and the autophagy gene Atg16l1 in mouse and human intestinal Paneth cells. *Nature* **2008**, *456*, 259–263. [CrossRef] [PubMed]
135. Cho, M.H.; Cho, K.; Kang, H.J.; Jeon, E.Y.; Kim, H.S.; Kwon, H.J.; Kim, H.M.; Kim, D.H.; Yoon, S.Y. Autophagy in microglia degrades extracellular beta-amyloid fibrils and regulates the NLRP3 inflammasome. *Autophagy* **2014**, *10*, 1761–1775. [CrossRef] [PubMed]
136. Nakahira, K.; Haspel, J.A.; Rathinam, V.A.; Lee, S.J.; Dolinay, T.; Lam, H.C.; Englert, J.A.; Rabinovitch, M.; Cernadas, M.; Kim, H.P.; et al. Autophagy proteins regulate innate immune responses by inhibiting the release of mitochondrial DNA mediated by the NALP3 inflammasome. *Nat. Immunol.* **2011**, *12*, 222–230. [CrossRef] [PubMed]
137. Shi, C.S.; Shenderov, K.; Huang, N.N.; Kabat, J.; Abu-Asab, M.; Fitzgerald, K.A.; Sher, A.; Kehrl, J.H. Activation of autophagy by inflammatory signals limits IL-1beta production by targeting ubiquitinated inflammasomes for destruction. *Nat. Immunol.* **2012**, *13*, 255–263. [CrossRef] [PubMed]
138. Duran, A.; Linares, J.F.; Galvez, A.S.; Wikenheiser, K.; Flores, J.M.; Diaz-Meco, M.T.; Moscat, J. The signaling adaptor p62 is an important NF-kappaB mediator in tumorigenesis. *Cancer Cell* **2008**, *13*, 343–354. [CrossRef] [PubMed]
139. Lee, H.M.; Shin, D.M.; Yuk, J.M.; Shi, G.; Choi, D.K.; Lee, S.H.; Huang, S.M.; Kim, J.M.; Kim, C.D.; Lee, J.H.; et al. Autophagy negatively regulates keratinocyte inflammatory responses via scaffolding protein p62/SQSTM1. *J. Immunol.* **2011**, *186*, 1248–1258. [CrossRef] [PubMed]
140. Chang, C.P.; Su, Y.C.; Hu, C.W.; Lei, H.Y. TLR2-dependent selective autophagy regulates NF-kappaB lysosomal degradation in hepatoma-derived M2 macrophage differentiation. *Cell Death Differ.* **2013**, *20*, 515–523. [CrossRef] [PubMed]

141. Francois, A.; Terro, F.; Janet, T.; Rioux Bilan, A.; Paccalin, M.; Page, G. Involvement of interleukin-1beta in the autophagic process of microglia: Relevance to Alzheimer's disease. *J. Neuroinflammation* **2013**, *10*, 151. [CrossRef] [PubMed]
142. Shen, C.; Xian, W.; Zhou, H.; Chen, L.; Pei, Z. Potential protective effects of autophagy activated in MPP+ treated astrocytes. *Exp. Ther. Med.* **2016**, *12*, 2803–2810. [CrossRef] [PubMed]
143. Pla, A.; Pascual, M.; Guerri, C. Autophagy Constitutes a Protective Mechanism against Ethanol Toxicity in Mouse Astrocytes and Neurons. *PLoS ONE* **2016**, *11*, e0153097. [CrossRef]
144. Cao, L.; Fu, M.; Kumar, S.; Kumar, A. Methamphetamine potentiates HIV-1 gp120-mediated autophagy via Beclin-1 and Atg5/7 as a pro-survival response in astrocytes. *Cell Death Dis.* **2016**, *7*, e2425. [CrossRef] [PubMed]
145. Lynch-Day, M.A.; Mao, K.; Wang, K.; Zhao, M.; Klionsky, D.J. The role of autophagy in Parkinson's disease. *Cold Spring Harb. Perspect. Med.* **2012**, *2*, a009357.
146. Bordi, M.; Berg, M.J.; Mohan, P.S.; Peterhoff, C.M.; Alldred, M.J.; Che, S.; Ginsberg, S.D.; Nixon, R.A. Autophagy flux in CA1 neurons of Alzheimer hippocampus: Increased induction overburdens failing lysosomes to propel neuritic dystrophy. *Autophagy* **2016**, *12*, 2467–2483. [CrossRef] [PubMed]
147. Carloni, S.; Girelli, S.; Scopa, C.; Buonocore, G.; Longini, M.; Balduini, W. Activation of autophagy and Akt/CREB signaling play an equivalent role in the neuroprotective effect of rapamycin in neonatal hypoxia-ischemia. *Autophagy* **2010**, *6*, 366–377. [CrossRef] [PubMed]
148. Chen, H.C.; Fong, T.H.; Hsu, P.W.; Chiu, W.T. Multifaceted effects of rapamycin on functional recovery after spinal cord injury in rats through autophagy promotion, anti-inflammation, and neuroprotection. *J. Surg. Res.* **2013**, *179*, e203–e210. [CrossRef]
149. Hu, L.Y.; Sun, Z.G.; Wen, Y.M.; Cheng, G.Z.; Wang, S.L.; Zhao, H.B.; Zhang, X.R. ATP-mediated protein kinase B Akt/mammalian target of rapamycin mTOR/p70 ribosomal S6 protein p70S6 kinase signaling pathway activation promotes improvement of locomotor function after spinal cord injury in rats. *Neuroscience* **2010**, *169*, 1046–1062. [CrossRef]
150. Walker, C.L.; Walker, M.J.; Liu, N.K.; Risberg, E.C.; Gao, X.; Chen, J.; Xu, X.M. Systemic bisperoxovanadium activates Akt/mTOR, reduces autophagy, and enhances recovery following cervical spinal cord injury. *PLoS ONE* **2012**, *7*, e30012. [CrossRef]
151. Wahl, S.E.; McLane, L.E.; Bercury, K.K.; Macklin, W.B.; Wood, T.L. Mammalian target of rapamycin promotes oligodendrocyte differentiation, initiation and extent of CNS myelination. *J.Neurosci.* **2014**, *34*, 4453–4465. [CrossRef]
152. Lee, D.H.; Luo, X.; Yungher, B.J.; Bray, E.; Lee, J.K.; Park, K.K. Mammalian target of rapamycin's distinct roles and effectiveness in promoting compensatory axonal sprouting in the injured CNS. *J. Neurosci.* **2014**, *34*, 15347–15355. [CrossRef]
153. Sarkar, S.; Davies, J.E.; Huang, Z.; Tunnacliffe, A.; Rubinsztein, D.C. Trehalose, a novel mTOR-independent autophagy enhancer, accelerates the clearance of mutant huntingtin and alpha-synuclein. *J. Biol. Chem.* **2007**, *282*, 5641–5652. [CrossRef]
154. Dehay, B.; Bove, J.; Rodriguez-Muela, N.; Perier, C.; Recasens, A.; Boya, P.; Vila, M. Pathogenic lysosomal depletion in Parkinson's disease. *J Neurosci.* **2010**, *30*, 12535–12544. [CrossRef] [PubMed]
155. Schaeffer, V.; Lavenir, I.; Ozcelik, S.; Tolnay, M.; Winkler, D.T.; Goedert, M. Stimulation of autophagy reduces neurodegeneration in a mouse model of human tauopathy. *Brain* **2012**, *135*, 2169–2177. [CrossRef] [PubMed]
156. Zhang, X.; Chen, S.; Song, L.; Tang, Y.; Shen, Y.; Jia, L.; Le, W. MTOR-independent, autophagic enhancer trehalose prolongs motor neuron survival and ameliorates the autophagic flux defect in a mouse model of amyotrophic lateral sclerosis. *Autophagy* **2014**, *10*, 588–602. [CrossRef] [PubMed]
157. Takahashi, S.; Isaka, M.; Hamaishi, M.; Imai, K.; Orihashi, K.; Sueda, T. Trehalose protects against spinal cord ischemia in rabbits. *J. Vasc. Surg.* **2014**, *60*, 490–496. [CrossRef] [PubMed]
158. Thoreen, C.C.; Kang, S.A.; Chang, J.W.; Liu, Q.; Zhang, J.; Gao, Y.; Reichling, L.J.; Sim, T.; Sabatini, D.M.; Gray, N.S. An ATP-competitive mammalian target of rapamycin inhibitor reveals rapamycin-resistant functions of mTORC1. *J. Biol. Chem.* **2009**, *284*, 8023–8032. [CrossRef]
159. Liu, Q.; Chang, J.W.; Wang, J.; Kang, S.A.; Thoreen, C.C.; Markhard, A.; Hur, W.; Zhang, J.; Sim, T.; Sabatini, D.M.; et al. Discovery of 1-(4-(4-propionylpiperazin-1-yl)-3-(trifluoromethyl)phenyl)-9-(quinolin-3-yl)benzo[h][1,6]naphthyridin-2(1H)-one as a highly potent, selective mammalian target of rapamycin (mTOR) inhibitor for the treatment of cancer. *J. Med. Chem.* **2010**, *53*, 7146–7155. [CrossRef]

160. Sardiello, M.; Palmieri, M.; di Ronza, A.; Medina, D.L.; Valenza, M.; Gennarino, V.A.; Di Malta, C.; Donaudy, F.; Embrione, V.; Polishchuk, R.S.; et al. A gene network regulating lysosomal biogenesis and function. *Science* **2009**, *325*, 473–477. [CrossRef]
161. Bove, J.; Martinez-Vicente, M.; Vila, M. Fighting neurodegeneration with rapamycin: Mechanistic insights. *Nat. Rev. Neurosci.* **2011**, *12*, 437–452. [CrossRef]
162. Pena-Llopis, S.; Vega-Rubin-de-Celis, S.; Schwartz, J.C.; Wolff, N.C.; Tran, T.A.; Zou, L.; Xie, X.J.; Corey, D.R.; Brugarolas, J. Regulation of TFEB and V-ATPases by mTORC1. *EMBO J.* **2011**, *30*, 3242–3258. [CrossRef]
163. Pi, H.; Li, M.; Tian, L.; Yang, Z.; Yu, Z.; Zhou, Z. Enhancing lysosomal biogenesis and autophagic flux by activating the transcription factor EB protects against cadmium-induced neurotoxicity. *Sci. Rep.* **2017**, *7*, 43466. [CrossRef]
164. Fang, J.; Zhu, Y.; Wang, H.; Cao, B.; Fei, M.; Niu, W.; Zhou, Y.; Wang, X.; Li, X.; Zhou, M. Baicalin Protects Mice Brain From Apoptosis in Traumatic Brain Injury Model Through Activation of Autophagy. *Front. Neurosci.* **2018**, *12*, 1006. [CrossRef]
165. Wang, Z.F.; Gao, C.; Chen, W.; Gao, Y.; Wang, H.C.; Meng, Y.; Luo, C.L.; Zhang, M.Y.; Chen, G.; Chen, X.P.; et al. Salubrinal offers neuroprotection through suppressing endoplasmic reticulum stress, autophagy and apoptosis in a mouse traumatic brain injury model. *Neurobiol. Learn. Mem.* **2019**, *161*, 12–25. [CrossRef] [PubMed]
166. Chen, X.; Pan, Z.; Fang, Z.; Lin, W.; Wu, S.; Yang, F.; Li, Y.; Fu, H.; Gao, H.; Li, S. Omega-3 polyunsaturated fatty acid attenuates traumatic brain injury-induced neuronal apoptosis by inducing autophagy through the upregulation of SIRT1-mediated deacetylation of Beclin-1. *J. Neuroinflammation* **2018**, *15*, 310. [CrossRef]
167. Chen, X.; Wang, H.; Zhou, M.; Li, X.; Fang, Z.; Gao, H.; Li, Y.; Hu, W. Valproic Acid Attenuates Traumatic Brain Injury-Induced Inflammation in Vivo: Involvement of Autophagy and the Nrf2/ARE Signaling Pathway. *Front. Mol. Neurosci.* **2018**, *11*, 117. [CrossRef]
168. Qian, M.; Fang, X.; Wang, X. Autophagy and inflammation. *Clin. Transl. Med.* **2017**, *6*, 24. [CrossRef]
169. Randall-Demllo, S.; Chieppa, M.; Eri, R. Intestinal epithelium and autophagy: Partners in gut homeostasis. *Front. Immunol.* **2013**, *4*, 301. [CrossRef] [PubMed]
170. Marselli, L.; Bugliani, M.; Suleiman, M.; Olimpico, F.; Masini, M.; Petrini, M.; Boggi, U.; Filipponi, F.; Syed, F.; Marchetti, P. Beta-Cell inflammation in human type 2 diabetes and the role of autophagy. *Diabetes Obes. Metab.* **2013**, *15* (Suppl. 3), 130–136. [CrossRef]
171. Pan, L.; Li, Y.; Jia, L.; Qin, Y.; Qi, G.; Cheng, J.; Qi, Y.; Li, H.; Du, J. Cathepsin S deficiency results in abnormal accumulation of autophagosomes in macrophages and enhances Ang II-induced cardiac inflammation. *PLoS ONE* **2012**, *7*, e35315. [CrossRef] [PubMed]
172. Junkins, R.D.; McCormick, C.; Lin, T.J. The emerging potential of autophagy-based therapies in the treatment of cystic fibrosis lung infections. *Autophagy* **2014**, *10*, 538–547. [CrossRef]
173. Francois, A.; Rioux Bilan, A.; Quellard, N.; Fernandez, B.; Janet, T.; Chassaing, D.; Paccalin, M.; Terro, F.; Page, G. Longitudinal follow-up of autophagy and inflammation in brain of APPswePS1dE9 transgenic mice. *J. Neuroinflammation* **2014**, *11*, 139. [CrossRef]
174. von Leden, R.E.; Yauger, Y.J.; Khayrullina, G.; Byrnes, K.R. Central Nervous System Injury and Nicotinamide Adenine Dinucleotide Phosphate Oxidase: Oxidative Stress and Therapeutic Targets. *J. Neurotrauma* **2016**, *34*, 755–764. [CrossRef] [PubMed]
175. Filomeni, G.; De Zio, D.; Cecconi, F. Oxidative stress and autophagy: The clash between damage and metabolic needs. *Cell Death Differ.* **2014**, *22*, 377. [CrossRef] [PubMed]
176. Lipinski, M.M.; Zheng, B.; Lu, T.; Yan, Z.; Py, B.F.; Ng, A.; Xavier, R.J.; Li, C.; Yankner, B.A.; Scherzer, C.R.; et al. A genome-wide analysis reveals differential regulation of autophagy in normal brain aging and in Alzheimer's disease. *Proc. Natl. Acad. Sci. USA* **2010**, *107*, 14164–14169. [CrossRef] [PubMed]
177. Sarkar, S.; Korolchuk, V.I.; Renna, M.; Imarisio, S.; Fleming, A.; Williams, A.; Garcia-Arencibia, M.; Rose, C.; Luo, S.; Underwood, B.R.; et al. Complex inhibitory effects of nitric oxide on autophagy. *Mol. Cell* **2011**, *43*, 19–32. [CrossRef] [PubMed]

13

Differential Association of Cx37 and Cx40 Genetic Variants in Atrial Fibrillation with and without Underlying Structural Heart Disease

Sebastian Carballo [1,*], Anna Pfenniger [2], David Carballo [3], Nicolas Garin [1], Richard W James [4], François Mach [3], Dipen Shah [3,†] and Brenda R Kwak [2,†]

1 Service of General Internal medicine, University Hospitals of Geneva, 1211 Geneva, Switzerland; nicolas.garin@hcuge.ch
2 Department of Pathology and Immunology, University of Geneva, 1211 Geneva, Switzerland; anna.pfenniger@gmail.com (A.P.); Brenda.KwakChanson@unige.ch (B.R.K.)
3 Service of Cardiology, University Hospitals of Geneva, 1211 Geneva, Switzerland; david.carballo@hcuge.ch (D.C.); francois.mach@hcuge.ch (F.M.); dipen.shah@hcuge.ch (D.S.)
4 Service of Endocrinology and Diabetes, University Hospitals of Geneva, 1211 Geneva, Switzerland; richard.james@hcuge.ch
* Correspondence: sebastian.carballo@hcuge.ch
† These authors contributed equally to this work.

Abstract: Atrial fibrillation (AF) appears in the presence or absence of structural heart disease. The majority of foci causing AF are located near the ostia of pulmonary veins (PVs), where cardiomyocytes and vascular smooth muscle cells interdigitate. Connexins (Cx) form gap junction channels and participate in action potential propagation. Genetic variants in genes encoding Cx40 and Cx37 affect their expression or function and may contribute to PV arrhythmogenicity. DNA was obtained from 196 patients with drug-resistant, symptomatic AF with and without structural heart disease, who were referred for percutaneous catheter ablation. Eighty-nine controls were matched for age, gender, hypertension, and BMI. Genotyping of the Cx40 $-44G > A$, Cx40 $+71A > G$, Cx40 $-26A > G$, and Cx37 $1019C > T$ polymorphisms was performed. The promoter A Cx40 polymorphisms ($-44G > A$ and $+71A > G$) showed no association with non-structural or structural AF. Distribution of the Cx40 promoter B polymorphism ($-26A > G$) was different in structural AF when compared to controls ($p = 0.03$). There was no significant difference with non-structural AF ($p = 0.50$). The distribution of the Cx37 $1019C > T$ polymorphism was different in non-structural AF ($p = 0.03$) but not in structural AF ($p = 0.08$) when compared to controls. Our study describes for the first time an association of drug-resistant non-structural heart disease AF with the Cx37 $1019C > T$ gene polymorphism. We also confirmed the association of the Cx40 $-26G > A$ polymorphism in patients with AF and structural disease.

Keywords: atrial fibrillation; connexin; polymorphism; genetic variant

---

1. Introduction

Atrial fibrillation (AF) is the most common sustained cardiac arrhythmia, its incidence increasing with age to reach up to 35 new cases per 1000 population in the elderly [1,2]. In the general population, its prevalence is estimated at 1.5–2%. AF is associated with increased risk of stroke, incidence of heart failure, and an overall higher mortality [3,4]. Diagnosis of AF is based on electrocardiographic characteristics such as rapid, irregular, fibrillatory waves, varying in size, shape, and timing [1]. Five clinical types of AF are recognized, mainly based on duration [2–5]: paroxysmal AF, persistent AF, long-standing persistent AF, and permanent AF. Whilst controversial, the term idiopathic or lone AF is used in reference to AF appearing in the absence of structural disease such as atrial left enlargement or valvular heart disease [6]. This historical concept and term should probably and progressively be avoided as understanding of the multiple complex etiologies of AF is improved [7].

When underlying structural heart disease is present, such as in patients with hypertensive heart disease, valvulopathy, or ischemic heart disease, this may trigger progressive remodeling of both the ventricles and atria [3,4]. Structural abnormalities will induce remodeling of the myocardium by affecting the extracellular matrix and cardiomyocytes through inflammatory processes and increased fibrosis [3,4]. Electrophysiological alterations and remodeling are instrumental in maintaining AF after its onset [8]. Initiation of AF is thought to depend on a combination of abnormal impulse formation, conduction and a propensity for reentry at the ostia of pulmonary veins (PVs), where sheets of cardiomyocytes and vascular smooth muscle cells (VSMCs) interdigitate [9,10]. However, the molecular mechanism underlying this regional specificity remains to be discovered.

Variants in genes encoding for membrane channels have been associated with both familial and other forms of AF, including genes encoding potassium channels such as *KCNQ1* and *KCNA5* [11–13]. Interestingly, atrial vulnerability to AF has been associated with polymorphisms in the Connexin40 (Cx40) gene, *GJA5* [14–17]. In addition, specific somatic mutations in the same gene have been discovered in idiopathic AF [18]. Other clinical AF presentations have been described with mosaicism in another connexin gene, *GJA1* encoding for Cx43 [19].

Connexins are gap junction proteins playing an essential role in direct cell–cell communication in the vast majority of tissues in the body, including in electrical propagation in the heart [20]. There are 20 different connexins in humans, each forming channels with distinct properties and with specific expression patterns [21]. Cx40, encoded by *GJA5*, is expressed by endothelial cells (ECs), by coronary VSMCs, by atrial cardiomyocytes, and in the cardiac conduction system. Cx37, encoded by *GJA4*, is found in ECs, pulmonary vein VSMCs, monocyte/macrophages, and platelets. Cx43, encoded by *GJA1*, is expressed by ventricular and atrial cardiomyocytes, VSMCs, ECs, and monocyte/macrophages [22]. Several polymorphisms have been described in *GJA4* and *GJA5*, which affect either their connexin expression level or gap junction channel function, some of which may contribute to the arrhythmogenicity of the PVs [15]. In animal studies, downregulation of either Cx40 or Cx43 expression increases susceptibility to AF [23,24].

Variants in the Cx37 (*GJA4*) gene have been associated with atherosclerosis and coronary heart disease, most likely through their influence on monocyte adhesion, thereby regulating the extent of local inflammation [25]. Both systemic and local inflammation appear to influence the development of AF in various situations, in patients having undergone cardiac surgery as well as non-post-operative patients [26].

Here, we investigated the relation between polymorphisms in *GJA5* and *GJA4* in defined AF populations. Within the AF population, a distinction was made between patients with no underlying structural cardiomyopathy, for the purpose of clarity referred to as non-structural AF, and those with clearly documented structural disease, referred to as structural AF. All AF patients that were included had undergone a trial of anti-arrhythmic drugs and were referred for catheter ablation because of poor response.

2. Results

A total of 285 individuals were included in this study; 92 patients in the non-structural AF group, 104 patients with structural AF, and 89 controls. Characteristics of the study population are summarized in Table 1.

Table 1. Characteristics and cardiovascular risk factors in the three cohorts.

Characteristics	Controls $n = 89$	Non-Structural AF $n = 92$	Structural AF $n = 104$
Age, years (SD)	61.79 (7.81)	64.09 (8.87)	60.04 (9.96)
Males (%)	74.2	84.8	76.9
Smokers (%)	66.3	56.5	32.7 *
Diabetes (%)	10.1	3.3	13.4
Dyslipidemia (%)	17.0	26.1	42.3 *
Hypertension (%)	42.5	30.4	42.3
BMI (Kg/m^2) (SD)	27.54 (4.48)	27.15 (5.70)	27.65 (5.77)

Controls were matched against the atrial fibrillation groups for age, gender, hypertension, and BMI. SD: standard deviation; BMI: body mass index. Qualitative values compared with Fisher's exact test. Quantitative values compared with the Student's t-test. * $p < 0.05$.

The type of cardiomyopathy present in the structural AF group is detailed in Table 2. Valvular disease and dilated atria were the main structural abnormalities.

Table 2. Characteristics of heart disease in the structural AF group. (More than one type of cardiomyopathy was possible in each patient).

Characteristics	Numbers
Type of Heart Disease	**Total n (%) ($n = 104$)**
Valvular heart disease	
- Mitral regurgitation	71 (68.3)
- Mitral stenosis	2 (1.9)
- Aortic regurgitation	29 (27.9)
- Aortic stenosis	4 (3.8)
Ischemic heart disease	9 (8.6)
Other (HCM, interatrial communication, etc.)	34 (32.7)
Dilated left atrium (>20 cm^2)	61 (58.7)
Echocardiography values	
Average LVEF (%)	56
Average left atrial surface, cm^2 (SD)	23 (6.9)
Average left ventricular ejection fraction, % (SD)	56.2 (10.1)

HCM: hypertrophic cardiomyopathy, LVEF: Left Ventricular Ejection Fraction, SD: standard deviation.

2.1. *Cx40 − 44G > A/+71A > G Polymorphisms*

Analysis of the two promoter A Cx40 polymorphisms ($-44G > A$ and $+71A > G$) showed an almost complete linkage disequilibrium of the $-44G/+71A$ and $-44A/+71G$ alleles. The overall genotype distribution in the control group was $-44GG/+71AA$ = 67.4%, $-44AG/+71AG$ = 28.1% and $-44AA/+71GG$ = 4.5%. This genotype distribution was not significantly different in either of the AF groups (non-structural AF: $p = 0.846$; structural AF: $p = 0.132$) (Table 3). There was also no significant difference in between the two AF groups ($p = 0.275$).

2.2. *Cx40 − 26G > A Polymorphism*

The specific genotype distribution of the Cx40 $- 26G > A$ polymorphism in the control group was $-26GG$ = 25.8%, $-26AG$ = 47.2%, and $-26AA$ = 27.0%. This distribution was significantly different in the structural AF group: $-26GG$ = 26.0%, $-26AG$ = 61.5%, and $-26AA$ = 12.5% ($p = 0.029$). There was no significant difference between the control and the non-structural AF group ($p = 0.511$) (Table 3) or between the two AF groups ($p = 0.3$).

2.3. Cx37 1019C > T Polymorphism

The specific genotype distribution of the Cx37 *1019C > T* polymorphism in the control group was *1019CC* = 42.7%, *1019CT* = 34.8%, and *1019TT* = 22.5%. This distribution was significantly different in the non-structural AF group: *1019CC* = 46.7%, *1019CT* = 44.6%, and 1019TT = 8.7% (p = 0.034). There was no significant difference between the control and the structural AF group (p = 0.080) (Table 3) or between the two AF groups (p = 0.85).

Table 3. Allele distributions of the Cx40 (*GJA5*) and Cx37 (*GJA4*) polymorphisms in the control, non-structural AF, and structural AF groups. Proportions were compared with Fisher's exact test.

Genotype		*Gene*			*p Value vs. Control Group*
Cx40 −44G > A	***GG (n, %)***	***AG (n, %)***	***AA (n, %)***	***Total***	
Control	*60 (67.4)*	*25 (28.1)*	*4 (4.5)*	*89*	
Non-Structural AF	*59 (64.1)*	*27 (29.3)*	*6 (6.5)*	*92*	*p = 0.846*
Structural AF	*55 (52.9)*	*41 (39.5)*	*8 (7.7)*	*104*	*p = 0.132*
Cx40 +71A > G	***AA (n, %)***	***AG (n, %)***	***GG (n, %)***	***Total***	
Control	*60 (67.4)*	*25 (28.1)*	*4 (4.5)*	*89*	
Non-Structural AF	*61 (66.3)*	*26 (28.3)*	*5 (5.4)*	*92*	*p = 1.000*
Structural AF	*55 (52.9)*	*41 (39.4)*	*8 (7.7)*	*104*	*p = 0.133*
Cx40 − 26G > A	***GG (n, %)***	***AG (n, %)***	***AA (n, %)***	***Total***	
Control	*23 (25.8)*	*42 (47.2)*	*24 (27.0)*	*89*	
Non-Structural AF	*26 (28.3)*	*48 (52.2)*	*18 (19.6)*	*92*	*p = 0.511*
Structural AF	*27 (26.0)*	*64 (61.5)*	*13 (12.5)*	*104*	***p = 0.029***
Cx37 1019C > T	***CC (n, %)***	***CT (n, %)***	***TT (n, %)***	***Total***	
Control	*38 (42.7)*	*31 (34.8)*	*20 (22.5)*	*89*	
Non-Structural AF	*43 (46.7)*	*41 (44.6)*	*8 (8.7)*	*92*	***p = 0.034***
Structural AF	*50 (48.1)*	*43 (41.3)*	*11 (10.6)*	*104*	*p = 0.080*

In bold the genes and genotypes.

3. Discussion

Our study describes for the first time an association of the Cx37 *1019C > T* gene polymorphism with drug-resistant non-structural AF, but not with structural AF. The potential differences in gene susceptibility between non-structural and structural AF were further underlined by the fact that we found an association of the Cx40 − *26G > A* polymorphism with structural AF and not with non-structural AF.

These results suggest that there are potential differences in the genetic susceptibility to AF in given populations. Patients who develop AF in whom there is no underlying structural cardiac disease appear to have an increased frequency of Cx37 *1019C* alleles than patients who do not develop AF. This genetic polymorphism has previously been described in populations with coronary heart disease and myocardial infarction [27,28]. The *GJA4* genotype may predict survival after an acute coronary syndrome [29]. Cx37 is principally expressed in endothelial cells, VSMCs, monocyte/macrophages, and platelets. The *1019C > T* polymorphism in *GJA4* causes a Proline-to-Serine substitution at amino acid 319 (P319S) in the cytoplasmic tail of Cx37, which in turn alters channel conductance and permeability [25,30]. The Cx37 polymorphism has been shown to affect monocyte adhesion as well as platelet aggregation [25,31]. Both mechanisms are thought to underlie the development of CAD [25]. Inflammation and its associated immune response are increasingly recognized to be involved in the initiation and maintenance of atrial fibrillation [32]. Thus, the Cx37 *1019C > T* polymorphism might affect the susceptibility to non-structural AF by virtue of its effect on monocyte adhesion. Alternatively, initiation of non-structural AF is thought to depend on a combination of abnormal impulse formation and conduction [9]. As Cx37 is also expressed in VSMCs at the ostia of pulmonary veins (PVs), where sheets of cardiomyocytes and VSMCs interdigitate, the differences in gap junction channel electrophysiological properties associated with the Cx37 *1019C > T* polymorphism may accentuate the latter mechanism [33].

Our results also show an association of the Cx40 − *26G > A* polymorphism in patients with AF with underlying cardiomyopathy, with the −26G allele being more frequent than in control patients. This single nucleotide polymorphism (SNP) in the promoter B region of *GJA5*, the *Cx40* gene, which alters the TATA box sequence and modulates mRNA expression levels of Cx40, has previously been associated with AF [34]. Of note, our study did not show any association of AF (either structural or non-structural) with the promoter A polymorphisms, Cx40 − *44/+71*; these polymorphisms were also shown to reduce *GJA5* expression in vitro by about 50%; however, Wirka et al. showed no effect on *GJA5* expression in atrial tissue, suggesting that promoter A is not necessary to Cx40 expression in atrial myocytes [34]. In patients with structural AF, atrial remodeling is often present at a structural, electrophysiological, and molecular level with changes in the refractory period and cardiomyocyte contractility [8,10]. Some of these atrial cardiomyocyte characteristics can be explained by changes in potassium channel properties and important changes to calcium handling [8]. Inconsistent observations have been made with respect to Cx40 expression levels in patients with AF, with both higher and lower levels being reported [35–37]. However, only few patients were included in these studies—10 and 12, respectively—and almost exclusively with mitral valve disease. Complete deletion of Cx40 in murine models leads to decreased atrial conduction velocity and increased atrial stability [8,38]. Somatic mutations in *GJA5* have been shown to predispose patients to idiopathic AF by either impairing the assembly of Cx40 into gap junctions or by affecting the electrical coupling itself [14,18]. Importantly, a recent study revealed that one of the reported Cx40 mutations (A96S) caused decreased atrial conduction velocities and sustained episodes of induced atrial fibrillation in mice and rat [39,40].

The strength of our study is the distinction between patients with or without underlying cardiomyopathy. This enables a more precise association study and a dissection of possible different pathophysiological mechanism leading to AF. We chose to include patients in whom anti-arrhythmic treatment was not successful in order to have long-standing or permanent AF. It may be interesting in the future to include all AF. The main limitation of our study is nevertheless the relatively small sample size, which increases the risk of falsely positive results. Furthermore, we acknowledge that non-structural AF is a misnomer and an exhaustive search of underlying etiology reduces the number of instances when there is truly no explanation for AF [7]. We also acknowledge that the link between the severity of valvular disease, in particular mitral valve disease, and AF may be complex. This may be an important aspect to further investigate. Associations between smoking or serum lipid levels and Cx40 have never been reported; it is, however, quite unlikely that one of these confounding factors would induce a significant association of the Cx40 − *26G > A* polymorphism with structural AF.

4. Materials and Methods

4.1. Patients

Three patient cohorts were studied, namely patients with AF and no underlying structural cardiac disease (non-structural AF), patients with AF and documented structural cardiac disease (structural AF), and a control population with no AF or underlying cardiac disease. This study protocol conforms to the ethical guidelines of the 1975 Declaration of Helsinki, as reflected in prior approval by the institution's human research committee, namely the Internal Medicine Departmental Ethics Committee, Geneva University Hospital (Protocol 03-167, 3 April 2010). Informed consent was obtained from all patients.

The non-structural AF group consisted of patients undergoing catheter ablation of AF by radiofrequency ablation through pulmonary vein isolation (RFAPVI). Inclusion criteria were an age > 18 years, documented paroxysmal or persistent AF (for <2 years) with or without typical flutter (ECG or Holter) after failure of at least one anti-arrhythmic treatment of Class I or III, with planned and clinically indicated RFAPVI. Exclusion criteria were reversible AF, clinical heart failure, increased left atrial size (>20 cm^2 four chamber view), decreased left ventricular ejection fraction, any valvulopathy, or a history of prior AF or flutter ablation. The structural AF group consisted of patients undergoing RFAPVI but in whom there was underlying cardiomyopathy, be it structural or valvular disease, or documented ischemic heart disease (history of acute or chronic coronary disease, angiographically proven disease). Inclusion criteria were an age > 18 years, documented paroxysmal or persistent AF (for <2 years) with or without typical flutter (ECG or Holter) and with planned and clinically indicated RFAPVI. Inclusion and exclusion criteria for these groups are detailed in Table 4. Demographics and characteristics of each group are detailed in Table 1. The type of cardiomyopathy present in the structural AF group is detailed in Table 1. The control group was considered as a whole and variables were matched to the AF groups with priority given to age, gender, hypertension, and BMI, these being major risk factors associated with AF development. These individuals were from the same population basin as AF patients, seen in the same clinic, and were undergoing elective coronary angiography at the Geneva University Hospital due to symptoms of suspected CAD or unrelated conditions requiring angiographic evaluation [41]. Participants gave written informed consent for a blood draw at the time of angiography for use in confidential studies approved by the hospital's institutional review board. Exclusion criteria for this control group were AF or a history of AF, or arrhythmia on 12 lead ECG, a history of coronary heart disease, any significant angiographic lesions on coronary angiography, or any known heart disease including valvulopathy.

Table 4. Inclusion and exclusion criteria for the non-structural and structural atrial fibrillation and control groups.

Criteria	Non-Structural AF	Structural AF	Control Group
Inclusion criteria	Age > 18 years Paroxysmal or persistent AF Failure of at least 1 anti-arrhythmic drug of class I or III	Age > 18 years Any valvulopathy Left ventricular or atrial dilatation Documented ischemic heart disease Hypertrophic cardiomyopathy Any structural disease	Age > 18 years
Exclusion criteria	Reversible AF Clinical heart failure Decrease left ejection fraction Any valvulopathy		History or documented AF Any heart disease including coronary heart disease or significant coronary lesion on angiography Any valvulopathy

AF: atrial fibrillation; NYHA: New York Heart Association heart failure classification.

4.2. Echocardiography

Echocardiography was performed on a HP/Philips 5500, Philips Electronics North American Corporation, Andover, MA, USA, with digitalization of images and analyzed according to a standardized protocol in a core lab.

4.3. DNA Extraction and Genotyping

DNA was extracted from the peripheral blood and genotyping of the Cx40 − *44G > A*, Cx40 + *71A > G*, Cx40 − *26A > G*, and Cx37 *1019C > T* polymorphisms was performed by polymerase chain reaction (PCR) and restriction fragment length polymorphism (RFLP) assays using previously established methods [34,42,43].

4.4. Statistical Analysis

Clinical, biological, and echocardiographic characteristics are presented using descriptive statistics and a number of cases with a percentage in parentheses for categorical variables. In view of skewed allele distribution and small numbers of certain genotypes, we used non-parametric tests. Proportions/categorical data were compared with the Fisher's exact test.

5. Conclusions

Our study suggests that there may be a different genetic predisposition to non-structural AF as compared to AF appearing in the context of underlying heart disease. We report here for the first time that the Cx37 *1019C > T* variant is associated with non-structural AF. Mechanistically, this might involve effects of altered Cx37 channel function on the inflammatory response (monocyte adhesion) or on abnormal impulse conduction (communication between VSMCs and atrial cardiomyocytes). In addition, we confirmed that the Cx40 $-$ *26G > A* polymorphism affecting the expression level of this protein in atrial cardiomyocytes is associated with structural AF.

Acknowledgments: The authors thank Katia Galan and Bernard Foglia for technical assistance with DNA extraction and genotyping. This work was partly supported by the Research Fund of the Department of Internal Medicine of the University Hospital and the Faculty of Medicine of Geneva; this Fund receives an unrestricted grant from AstraZeneca Switzerland. Anna Pfenniger was supported by a joint grant from the Swiss National Science Foundation, the Swiss Academy of Medical Sciences, and the Velux Foundation (323630-123735), and Brenda R Kwak by a grant of the Swiss National Science Foundation (310030_162579).

Author Contributions: Sebastian Carballo, David Carballo, and Brenda R Kwak conceived and designed the experiments; Anna Pfenniger performed the experiments; Anna Pfenniger and Sebastian Carballo analyzed the data; Dipen Shah and Richard W James contributed to the recruitment of the patients and controls; Sebastian Carballo, Brenda R Kwak, David Carballo, Nicolas Garin, and François Mach wrote the manuscript.

References

1. Chugh, S.S.; Havmoeller, R.; Narayanan, K.; Singh, D.; Rienstra, M.; Benjamin, E.J.; Gillum, R.F.; Kim, Y.H.; McAnulty, J.H., Jr.; Zheng, Z.J.; et al. Worldwide epidemiology of atrial fibrillation: A Global Burden of Disease 2010 Study. *Circulation* **2014**, *129*, 837–847. [CrossRef] [PubMed]
2. January, C.T.; Wann, L.S.; Alpert, J.S.; Calkins, H.; Cigarroa, J.E.; Cleveland, J.C., Jr.; Conti, J.B.; Ellinor, P.T.; Ezekowitz, M.D.; Field, M.E.; et al. 2014 AHA/ACC/HRS guideline for the management of patients with atrial fibrillation: A report of the American College of Cardiology/American Heart Association Task Force on Practice Guidelines and the Heart Rhythm Society. *J. Am. Coll. Cardiol.* **2014**, *64*, e1–e76. [PubMed]
3. Camm, A.J.; Kirchhof, P.; Lip, G.Y.; Schotten, U.; Savelieva, I.; Ernst, S.; Van Gelder, I.C.; Al-Attar, N.; Hindricks, G.; Prendergast, B.; et al. Guidelines for the management of atrial fibrillation: The Task Force for the Management of Atrial Fibrillation of the European Society of Cardiology (ESC). *Eur. Heart J.* **2010**, *31*, 2369–2429. [PubMed]
4. Kirchhof, P.; Benussi, S.; Kotecha, D.; Ahlsson, A.; Atar, D.; Casadei, B.; Castella, M.; Diener, H.C.; Heidbuchel, H.; Hendriks, J.; et al. 2016 ESC Guidelines for the management of atrial fibrillation developed in collaboration with EACTS. *Eur. Heart J.* **2016**, *37*, 2893–2962. [CrossRef] [PubMed]
5. Camm, A.J.; Lip, G.Y.; De Caterina, R.; Savelieva, I.; Atar, D.; Hohnloser, S.H.; Hindricks, G.; Kirchhof, P. 2012 focused update of the ESC Guidelines for the management of atrial fibrillation: An update of the 2010 ESC Guidelines for the management of atrial fibrillation. Developed with the special contribution of the European Heart Rhythm Association. *Eur. Heart J.* **2012**, *33*, 2719–2747. [CrossRef] [PubMed]
6. Weijs, B.; Pisters, R.; Nieuwlaat, R.; Breithardt, G.; Le Heuzey, J.Y.; Vardas, P.E.; Limantoro, I.; Schotten, U.; Lip, G.Y.; Crijns, H.J. Idiopathic atrial fibrillation revisited in a large longitudinal clinical cohort. *Europace* **2012**, *14*, 184–190. [CrossRef] [PubMed]
7. Wyse, D.G.; Van Gelder, I.C.; Ellinor, P.T.; Go, A.S.; Kalman, J.M.; Narayan, S.M.; Nattel, S.; Schotten, U.; Rienstra, M. Lone atrial fibrillation: Does it exist? *J. Am. Coll. Cardiol.* **2014**, *63*, 1715–1723. [CrossRef] [PubMed]
8. Schotten, U.; Verheule, S.; Kirchhof, P.; Goette, A. Pathophysiological mechanisms of atrial fibrillation: A translational appraisal. *Physiol. Rev.* **2011**, *91*, 265–325. [CrossRef] [PubMed]
9. Haissaguerre, M.; Jais, P.; Shah, D.C.; Takahashi, A.; Hocini, M.; Quiniou, G.; Garrigue, S.; Le Mouroux, A.; Le Metayer, P.; Clementy, J. Spontaneous initiation of atrial fibrillation by ectopic beats originating in the pulmonary veins. *N. Engl. J. Med.* **1998**, *339*, 659–666. [CrossRef] [PubMed]
10. Wijffels, M.C.; Kirchhof, C.J.; Dorland, R.; Allessie, M.A. Atrial fibrillation begets atrial fibrillation. A study in awake chronically instrumented goats. *Circulation* **1995**, *92*, 1954–1968. [CrossRef] [PubMed]

11. Chen, Y.H.; Xu, S.J.; Bendahhou, S.; Wang, X.L.; Wang, Y.; Xu, W.Y.; Jin, H.W.; Sun, H.; Su, X.Y.; Zhuang, Q.N.; et al. KCNQ1 gain-of-function mutation in familial atrial fibrillation. *Science* **2003**, *299*, 251–254. [CrossRef] [PubMed]
12. Fatkin, D.; Otway, R.; Vandenberg, J.I. Genes and atrial fibrillation: A new look at an old problem. *Circulation* **2007**, *116*, 782–792. [CrossRef] [PubMed]
13. Olson, T.M.; Alekseev, A.E.; Liu, X.K.; Park, S.; Zingman, L.V.; Bienengraeber, M.; Sattiraju, S.; Ballew, J.D.; Jahangir, A.; Terzic, A. Kv1.5 channelopathy due to KCNA5 loss-of-function mutation causes human atrial fibrillation. *Hum. Mol. Genet.* **2006**, *15*, 2185–2191. [CrossRef] [PubMed]
14. Christophersen, I.E.; Holmegard, H.N.; Jabbari, J.; Sajadieh, A.; Haunso, S.; Tveit, A.; Svendsen, J.H.; Olesen, M.S. Rare variants in GJA5 are associated with early-onset lone atrial fibrillation. *Can. J. Cardiol.* **2013**, *29*, 111–116. [CrossRef] [PubMed]
15. Firouzi, M.; Ramanna, H.; Kok, B.; Jongsma, H.J.; Koeleman, B.P.; Doevendans, P.A.; Groenewegen, W.A.; Hauer, R.N. Association of human connexin40 gene polymorphisms with atrial vulnerability as a risk factor for idiopathic atrial fibrillation. *Circ. Res.* **2004**, *95*, e29–e33. [CrossRef] [PubMed]
16. Juang, J.M.; Chern, Y.R.; Tsai, C.T.; Chiang, F.T.; Lin, J.L.; Hwang, J.J.; Hsu, K.L.; Tseng, C.D.; Tseng, Y.Z.; Lai, L.P. The association of human connexin 40 genetic polymorphisms with atrial fibrillation. *Int. J. Cardiol.* **2007**, *116*, 107–112. [CrossRef] [PubMed]
17. Hailati, J.; Yang, Y.C.; Zhang, L.; He, P.Y.; Baikeyi, M.; Muhuyati, W.; Liu, Z.Q. Association between −44G/A and +71A/G polymorphisms in the connexin 40 gene and atrial fibrillation in Uyghur and Han populations in Xinjiang, China. *Genet. Mol. Res.* **2016**, *15*. [CrossRef] [PubMed]
18. Gollob, M.H.; Jones, D.L.; Krahn, A.D.; Danis, L.; Gong, X.Q.; Shao, Q.; Liu, X.; Veinot, J.P.; Tang, A.S.; Stewart, A.F.; et al. Somatic mutations in the connexin 40 gene (GJA5) in atrial fibrillation. *N. Engl. J. Med.* **2006**, *354*, 2677–2688. [CrossRef] [PubMed]
19. Thibodeau, I.L.; Xu, J.; Li, Q.; Liu, G.; Lam, K.; Veinot, J.P.; Birnie, D.H.; Jones, D.L.; Krahn, A.D.; Lemery, R.; et al. Paradigm of genetic mosaicism and lone atrial fibrillation: Physiological characterization of a connexin 43-deletion mutant identified from atrial tissue. *Circulation* **2010**, *122*, 236–244. [CrossRef] [PubMed]
20. Jansen, J.A.; van Veen, T.A.; de Bakker, J.M.; van Rijen, H.V. Cardiac connexins and impulse propagation. *J. Mol. Cell. Cardiol.* **2010**, *48*, 76–82. [CrossRef] [PubMed]
21. Pfenniger, A.; Wohlwend, A.; Kwak, B.R. Mutations in connexin genes and disease. *Eur. J. Clin. Investig.* **2011**, *41*, 103–116. [CrossRef] [PubMed]
22. Pfenniger, A.; Chanson, M.; Kwak, B.R. Connexins in atherosclerosis. *Biochim. Biophys. Acta* **2013**, *1828*, 157–166. [CrossRef] [PubMed]
23. Chaldoupi, S.M.; Loh, P.; Hauer, R.N.; de Bakker, J.M.; van Rijen, H.V. The role of connexin40 in atrial fibrillation. *Cardiovasc. Res.* **2009**, *84*, 15–23. [CrossRef] [PubMed]
24. Fontes, M.S.; van Veen, T.A.; de Bakker, J.M.; van Rijen, H.V. Functional consequences of abnormal Cx43 expression in the heart. *Biochim. Biophys. Acta* **2012**, *1818*, 2020–2029. [CrossRef] [PubMed]
25. Wong, C.W.; Christen, T.; Roth, I.; Chadjichristos, C.E.; Derouette, J.P.; Foglia, B.F.; Chanson, M.; Goodenough, D.A.; Kwak, B.R. Connexin37 protects against atherosclerosis by regulating monocyte adhesion. *Nat. Med.* **2006**, *12*, 950–954. [CrossRef] [PubMed]
26. Aranki, S.F.; Shaw, D.P.; Adams, D.H.; Rizzo, R.J.; Couper, G.S.; VanderVliet, M.; Collins, J.J., Jr.; Cohn, L.H.; Burstin, H.R. Predictors of atrial fibrillation after coronary artery surgery. Current trends and impact on hospital resources. *Circulation* **1996**, *94*, 390–397. [CrossRef] [PubMed]
27. Wen, D.; Du, X.; Nie, S.P.; Dong, J.Z.; Ma, C.S. Association of Connexin37 C1019T with myocardial infarction and coronary artery disease: A meta-analysis. *Exp. Gerontol.* **2014**, *58*, 203–207. [CrossRef] [PubMed]
28. Listi, F.; Candore, G.; Lio, D.; Russo, M.; Colonna-Romano, G.; Caruso, M.; Hoffmann, E.; Caruso, C. Association between C1019T polymorphism of connexin37 and acute myocardial infarction: A study in patients from Sicily. *Int. J. Cardiol.* **2005**, *102*, 269–271. [CrossRef] [PubMed]
29. Lanfear, D.E.; Jones, P.G.; Marsh, S.; Cresci, S.; Spertus, J.A.; McLeod, H.L. Connexin37 (GJA4) genotype predicts survival after an acute coronary syndrome. *Am. Heart J.* **2007**, *154*, 561–566. [CrossRef] [PubMed]
30. Derouette, J.P.; Desplantez, T.; Wong, C.W.; Roth, I.; Kwak, B.R.; Weingart, R. Functional differences between human Cx37 polymorphic hemichannels. *J. Mol. Cell. Cardiol.* **2009**, *46*, 499–507. [CrossRef] [PubMed]

31. Angelillo-Scherrer, A.; Fontana, P.; Burnier, L.; Roth, I.; Sugamele, R.; Brisset, A.; Morel, S.; Nolli, S.; Sutter, E.; Chassot, A.; et al. Connexin 37 limits thrombus propensity by downregulating platelet reactivity. *Circulation* **2011**, *124*, 930–939. [CrossRef] [PubMed]
32. Hu, Y.F.; Chen, Y.J.; Lin, Y.J.; Chen, S.A. Inflammation and the pathogenesis of atrial fibrillation. *Nat. Rev. Cardiol.* **2015**, *12*, 230–243. [CrossRef] [PubMed]
33. Verheule, S.; Wilson, E.E.; Arora, R.; Engle, S.K.; Scott, L.R.; Olgin, J.E. Tissue structure and connexin expression of canine pulmonary veins. *Cardiovasc. Res.* **2002**, *55*, 727–738. [CrossRef]
34. Wirka, R.C.; Gore, S.; Van Wagoner, D.R.; Arking, D.E.; Lubitz, S.A.; Lunetta, K.L.; Benjamin, E.J.; Alonso, A.; Ellinor, P.T.; Barnard, J.; et al. A common connexin-40 gene promoter variant affects connexin-40 expression in human atria and is associated with atrial fibrillation. *Circ. Arrhythm. Electrophysiol.* **2011**, *4*, 87–93. [CrossRef] [PubMed]
35. Nao, T.; Ohkusa, T.; Hisamatsu, Y.; Inoue, N.; Matsumoto, T.; Yamada, J.; Shimizu, A.; Yoshiga, Y.; Yamagata, T.; Kobayashi, S.; et al. Comparison of expression of connexin in right atrial myocardium in patients with chronic atrial fibrillation versus those in sinus rhythm. *Am. J. Cardiol.* **2003**, *91*, 678–683. [CrossRef]
36. Polontchouk, L.; Haefliger, J.A.; Ebelt, B.; Schaefer, T.; Stuhlmann, D.; Mehlhorn, U.; Kuhn-Regnier, F.; De Vivie, E.R.; Dhein, S. Effects of chronic atrial fibrillation on gap junction distribution in human and rat atria. *J. Am. Coll. Cardiol.* **2001**, *38*, 883–891. [CrossRef]
37. Gemel, J.; Levy, A.E.; Simon, A.R.; Bennett, K.B.; Ai, X.; Akhter, S.; Beyer, E.C. Connexin40 abnormalities and atrial fibrillation in the human heart. *J. Mol. Cell. Cardiol.* **2014**, *76*, 159–168. [CrossRef] [PubMed]
38. Hagendorff, A.; Schumacher, B.; Kirchhoff, S.; Luderitz, B.; Willecke, K. Conduction disturbances and increased atrial vulnerability in Connexin40-deficient mice analyzed by transesophageal stimulation. *Circulation* **1999**, *99*, 1508–1515. [CrossRef] [PubMed]
39. Lubkemeier, I.; Andrie, R.; Lickfett, L.; Bosen, F.; Stockigt, F.; Dobrowolski, R.; Draffehn, A.M.; Fregeac, J.; Schultze, J.L.; Bukauskas, F.F.; et al. The Connexin40A96S mutation from a patient with atrial fibrillation causes decreased atrial conduction velocities and sustained episodes of induced atrial fibrillation in mice. *J. Mol. Cell. Cardiol.* **2013**, *65*, 19–32. [CrossRef] [PubMed]
40. Kanthan, A.; Fahmy, P.; Rao, R.; Pouliopoulos, J.; Alexander, I.E.; Thomas, S.P.; Kizana, E. Human Connexin40 Mutations Slow Conduction and Increase Propensity for Atrial Fibrillation. *Heart Lung Circ.* **2018**, *27*, 114–121. [CrossRef] [PubMed]
41. James, R.W.; Leviev, I.; Righetti, A. Smoking is associated with reduced serum paraoxonase activity and concentration in patients with coronary artery disease. *Circulation* **2000**, *101*, 2252–2257. [CrossRef] [PubMed]
42. Wong, C.W.; Christen, T.; Pfenniger, A.; James, R.W.; Kwak, B.R. Do allelic variants of the connexin37 1019 gene polymorphism differentially predict for coronary artery disease and myocardial infarction? *Atherosclerosis* **2007**, *191*, 355–361. [CrossRef] [PubMed]
43. Pfenniger, A.; van der Laan, S.W.; Foglia, B.; Dunoyer-Geindre, S.; Haefliger, J.A.; Winnik, S.; Mach, F.; Pasterkamp, G.; James, R.W.; Kwak, B.R. Lack of association between connexin40 polymorphisms and coronary artery disease. *Atherosclerosis* **2012**, *222*, 148–153. [CrossRef] [PubMed]

Permissions

All chapters in this book were first published by MDPI; hereby published with permission under the Creative Commons Attribution License or equivalent. Every chapter published in this book has been scrutinized by our experts. Their significance has been extensively debated. The topics covered herein carry significant findings which will fuel the growth of the discipline. They may even be implemented as practical applications or may be referred to as a beginning point for another development.

The contributors of this book come from diverse backgrounds, making this book a truly international effort. This book will bring forth new frontiers with its revolutionizing research information and detailed analysis of the nascent developments around the world.

We would like to thank all the contributing authors for lending their expertise to make the book truly unique. They have played a crucial role in the development of this book. Without their invaluable contributions this book wouldn't have been possible. They have made vital efforts to compile up to date information on the varied aspects of this subject to make this book a valuable addition to the collection of many professionals and students.

This book was conceptualized with the vision of imparting up-to-date information and advanced data in this field. To ensure the same, a matchless editorial board was set up. Every individual on the board went through rigorous rounds of assessment to prove their worth. After which they invested a large part of their time researching and compiling the most relevant data for our readers.

The editorial board has been involved in producing this book since its inception. They have spent rigorous hours researching and exploring the diverse topics which have resulted in the successful publishing of this book. They have passed on their knowledge of decades through this book. To expedite this challenging task, the publisher supported the team at every step. A small team of assistant editors was also appointed to further simplify the editing procedure and attain best results for the readers.

Apart from the editorial board, the designing team has also invested a significant amount of their time in understanding the subject and creating the most relevant covers. They scrutinized every image to scout for the most suitable representation of the subject and create an appropriate cover for the book.

The publishing team has been an ardent support to the editorial, designing and production team. Their endless efforts to recruit the best for this project, has resulted in the accomplishment of this book. They are a veteran in the field of academics and their pool of knowledge is as vast as their experience in printing. Their expertise and guidance has proved useful at every step. Their uncompromising quality standards have made this book an exceptional effort. Their encouragement from time to time has been an inspiration for everyone.

The publisher and the editorial board hope that this book will prove to be a valuable piece of knowledge for researchers, students, practitioners and scholars across the globe.

List of Contributors

Agnieszka Paradowska-Gorycka, Anna Wajda, Barbara Stypinska and Ewa Walczuk
Department of Molecular Biology, National Institute of Geriatrics, Rheumatology and Rehabilitation, Warsaw 02-637, Poland

Marcela Walczyk, Anna Felis-Giemza, Aleksandra Poluch-Lewandowska and Marzena Olesińska
Department of Connective Tissue Diseases, National Institute of Geriatrics, Rheumatology and Rehabilitation, Warsaw 02-637, Poland

Sup Kim
Department of Microbiology, Chungnam National University School of Medicine, Daejeon 35015, Korea
Department of Medical Science, Chungnam National University School of Medicine, Daejeon 35015, Korea
Infection Control Convergence Research Center, Chungnam National University School of Medicine, Daejeon 35015, Korea
Department of Radiation Oncology, Chungnam National University Hospital, 282, Munwha-ro, Jung-gu, Daejeon 34952, Korea

Hyuk Soo Eun
Department of Internal Medicine, Chungnam National University Hospital, 282, Munwha-ro, Jung-gu, Daejeon 34952, Korea
Department of Internal Medicine, School of Medicine, Chungnam National University, 266, Munwha-ro, Jung-gu, Daejeon 35015, Korea

Eun-Kyeong Jo
Department of Microbiology, Chungnam National University School of Medicine, Daejeon 35015, Korea
Department of Medical Science, Chungnam National University School of Medicine, Daejeon 35015, Korea
Infection Control Convergence Research Center, Chungnam National University School of Medicine, Daejeon 35015, Korea

Jean X. Jiang
Department of Biochemistry and Structural Biology, University of Texas, Health Science Center, 7703 Floyd Curl Drive, San Antonio, TX 78229, USA

Xavier F. Figueroa
Departamento de Fisiología, Faculdad de Ciencias Biológicas, Pontifica Universidad Católica de Chile, Santiago 8330025, Chile

Brant E. Isakson
Robert M. Berne Cardiovascular Research Center, University of Virginia School of Medicine, Charlottesville, VA 22908, USA
Department of Molecular Physiology and Biophysics, University of Virginia School of Medicine, Charlottesville, VA 22908, USA

Jonathan M. Gibbins
Institute for Cardiovascular & Metabolic Research, School of Biological Sciences, Harborne Building, University of Reading, Reading RG6 6AS, UK

Marc Chanson and Alice Zoso
Department of Pediatrics and Cell Physiology & Metabolism, Geneva University Hospitals and University of Geneva, 1211 Geneva, Switzerland

Masakatsu Watanabe
Graduate School of Frontier Biosciences, Osaka University, Osaka 565-0871, Japan

Csilla Viczenczova, Branislav Kura, Tamara Egan Benova, Jan Slezak, Narcis Tribulova and Barbara Szeiffova Bacova
Institute for Heart Research, Center of Experimental Medicine, Slovak Academy of Sciences, Bratislava 841 04, Slovak Republic

Mahmoud Noureldin, Honghong Chen and Donglin Bai
Department of Physiology and Pharmacology, University of Western Ontario, London, ON, N6A 5C1 Canada

Sheila V. Graham
Centre for Virus Research, Institute of Infection Immunity and Inflammation, College of Medical Veterinary and Life Sciences, Room 254 Jarrett Building, Garscube Estate, University of Glasgow, Glasgow G61 1QH, UK

Filippo Molica and Brenda R. Kwak
Department of Pathology and Immunology, University of Geneva, CH-1211 Geneva, Switzerland

Marc Mesnil
STIM Laboratory, ERL 7003CNRS/Building B36, University of Poitiers, 1 rue Georges BonnetTSA 51 106, 86073 Poitiers, CEDEX 09, France

Mélanie Busby and Isabelle Plante
INRS-Institut Armand-Frappier, Laval, QC H7V 1B7, Canada

Michael T. Hallett
Centre for Structural and Functional Genomics, Department of Biology, Concordia University, Montreal, QC H4B 1R6, Canada

Nobuko Iikawa
Department of Molecular and Tumour Pathology, Akita University Graduate School of Medicine, Akita 010-8543, Japan
Department of Otorhinolaryngology and Head-and-Neck Surgery, Akita University Graduate School of Medicine, Akita 010-8543, Japan

Yohei Yamamoto, Aki Nishijima-Matsunobu, Maya Suzuki and Yasufumi Omori
Department of Molecular and Tumour Pathology, Akita University Graduate School of Medicine, Akita 010-8543, Japan

Yohei Kawasaki and Takechiyo Yamada
Department of Otorhinolaryngology and Head-and-Neck Surgery, Akita University Graduate School of Medicine, Akita 010-8543, Japan

Chang Yin and Rakesh C. Kukreja
Division of Cardiology, Medical College of Virginia, Virginia Commonwealth University, Richmond, VA 23298, USA

Jonathan Boucher, Claire Simonneau, Golthlay Denet, Annie-Claire Balandre, Marc Mesnil, Laurent Cronier and Arnaud Monvoisin
CNRS ERL 7003, Laboratoire "Signalisation & Transports Ioniques Membranaires", University of Poitiers, 86073 Poitiers, France

Jonathan Clarhaut
CNRS UMR 7285, Institut de Chimie des Milieux et des Matériaux de Poitiers (IC2MP), University of Poitiers, 86073 Poitiers, France
CHU de Poitiers, 86021 Poitiers, France

Myo Htet, Jane E. Nally, Andrew Shaw, Bradley E. Foote, Patricia E. Martin, Erin M. O'Shaughnessy, Chrysovalantou Faniku, Claire Lorraine, Annette Graham, Erin O'Shaughnessy, Patricia E. M. Martin, Sebastian Greenhough and Yvonne Dempsie
Department of Life Sciences, School of Health and Life Sciences, Glasgow Caledonian University, Glasgow G4 0BA, UK

Scott R. Johnstone
Department of Life Sciences, School of Health and Life Sciences, Glasgow Caledonian University, Glasgow G4 0BA, UK
Robert M. Berne Cardiovascular Research Center, University of Virginia School of Medicine, Charlottesville, VA 22908, USA
Institute of Cardiovascular and Medical Sciences, College of Medical, Veterinary and Life Sciences, University of Glasgow, Glasgow G12 8TT, UK

Sebastian Carballo and Nicolas Garin
Service of General Internal medicine, University Hospitals of Geneva, 1211 Geneva, Switzerland

Anna Pfenniger and Brenda R Kwak
Department of Pathology and Immunology, University of Geneva, 1211 Geneva, Switzerland

David Carballo, François Mach and Dipen Shah
Service of Cardiology, University Hospitals of Geneva, 1211 Geneva, Switzerland

Richard W James
Service of Endocrinology and Diabetes, University Hospitals of Geneva, 1211 Geneva, Switzerland

Index

S

T

U

V

W

Printed in the USA
CPSIA information can be obtained
at www.ICGtesting.com
LVHW081319310823
756829LV00007B/293

9 781646 475940